Handbook of Obesity Prevention

Shiriki Kumanyika

Ross C. Brownson
Editors

Handbook of Obesity Prevention

A Resource for Health Professionals

Foreword by Dr. David Satcher

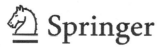 Springer

Editors
Shiriki Kumanyika, PhD, RD, MPH
Center for Clinical Epidemiology
  and Biostatistics
University of Pennsylvania School
  of Medicine
423 Guardian Drive
Philadelphia 19104-6021

Ross Brownson, PhD
St. Louis University School
  of Public Health
3545 Lafayette Ave
St. Louis MO, USA 63104

ISBN-13: 978-0-387-47859-3   e-ISBN-13: 978-0-387-47860-9

Library of Congress Control Number: 2007926434

springer.com

To Christiaan and Chenjerai, who provide strength and inspiration.

S.K.K.

To Carol, for her support, guidance, and good humor.

R.C.B.

Foreword

In the Surgeon General's Report: *A Surgeon General's Call to Action to Prevent and Reduce Overweight and Obesity,* we referred to the "epidemic" of overweight and obesity. This was an unusual designation for a chronic disease or condition but we felt it quite appropriate. In public health, where "epidemic" has generally referred to an unusual outbreak or increase in incidence of an infectious disease, this application of the term to a chronic condition such as obesity was unusual but appropriate. The increase in overweight and obesity in America over the last two to three decades has been both dramatic and unprecedented and certainly unexpected. We reported that in children overweight had increased two-fold from 1980 to 2000 and almost tripled in adolescents. A similar trend was also seen in adults in America. There was no sign of abatement of this increase as we entered the 21st century.

Although this dramatic increase in overweight and obesity affected all groups in the nation it impacted some much more than others. African Americans, Hispanics and American Indians were most severely impacted. These were the groups which had been targeted for improvement in health outcomes with the 2010 goal of eliminating disparities in health. But the epidemic of overweight and obesity not only threatens to derail this goal but it also threatens to undue much of the progress in control of chronic diseases that we made in the last half of the 21st century. The concern about overweight and obesity was not about cosmetics and appearances, as we pointed out in the report, it was about health. There are beautiful people who are overweight and obese and there are beautiful people who are thin but this epidemic is about health. The epidemic of overweight and obesity is a threat to our health now and in the future. It was and is a threat to increase morbidity and mortality from diabetes, cardiovascular disease, cancer and osteoarthritis. It interferes with learning in children by increasing risks for asthma and other causes of absenteeism from school and the ability to concentrate in school. It also dramatically increases costs in the healthcare system. Children who are overweight, and especially into their adolescent years are most likely to be obese as adults. Thus childhood overweight must be particularly targeted.

The cause of this epidemic of overweight and obesity is not altogether clear but it is clear that two major forces in our society have contributed greatly to the epidemic. Those two forces have been the pressures for us to consume more calories and at the same time to be less physically active. With the production and sale of more and more food, the pressure to consume more calories faces us on every corner and with every other commercial. More fast foods have not only meant faster food but also more fat, more sugar and more salt. The other force has been the growing disincentive for us to be physically active. In 1996 the Surgeon General's Report on Physical Activity was released. As director of the CDC I was involved in the development of that report. We pointed to the dramatic decrease in physical activity by American children and adults. We found, for example, that less than 30% of teenagers were taking physical education in school, and this represented a trend for all students. Physical education was seen as competing with classroom activities geared toward preparing children for standardized exams. Of course we know now that physical activity and good nutrition can improve learning and performance by children on math and reading tests, as well as writing. But the trend to eat more and to be less physically active is not easy to reverse in children or adults.

While it is true that treatment is sometimes indicated and possible to deal with obesity, as with other epidemics, it is not the answer to the epidemic. The challenge we face is to prevent overweight and obesity, especially in children but also in adults. In a nation and in a health system where health promotion and disease prevention have never been priorities, except for infectious diseases, we are faced with a daunting challenge to prevent overweight and obesity. Most studies show that we as a nation spend less than two to three percent of our health budget on population based prevention, and population based prevention is what is needed to fight this epidemic. In the language of McKinlay and others this epidemic must be fought, downstream, midstream, and upstream.

Downstream we must educate, motivate and mobilize individuals and families toward healthy lifestyles that militate against overweight and obesity. As surgeon general I took seriously my designation as "The Nation's Doctor" and among other things wrote an actual prescription for the American people. On this prescription I encourage physical activity at least 30 minutes a day, five days a week. I also prescribed good nutrition focusing on the consumption of at least five servings of fruits and vegetables per day. The other recommendations related to the avoidance of toxins and being responsible in one's sexual behavior. Clearly individuals and families must respond to the epidemic by increasing physical activity and consuming a more nutritious, low fat, low calorie diet and becoming significantly more physically active. But this is not enough.

We must also act at *midstream* or in the community where environments can facilitate or militate against healthy lifestyles or eating habits. The school curriculum, the safety of our streets and the general quality of the natural and built environments are critical to allowing and encouraging healthy lifestyles. In the community there must be a commitment especially to creating the kind of environment that encourages children to develop lifetime habits of physical activity and good nutrition. Today children are most susceptible to our "obesogenic" environments, from fast foods to T.V. watching and their related advertisements. Finally, overlooking what individuals can and will be incentivized to do as well as how communities and their institutions respond to this epidemic are the local, state and federal policies. This *upstream* function is critical to our success in stopping and reversing the trend of overweight and obesity.

At the end of the Surgeon General's Call to Action to Prevent and Decrease Overweight in Obesity we listed several settings for action. Among those settings we included the home and community, schools, workplace, healthcare, and media/communication. These settings are all very important for attacking the epidemic of overweight and obesity. In many cases they must work together. The program "Action for Healthy Kids," which we started in the Fall of 2002 and is now nationwide with over 6,000 volunteers, begins by encouraging schools to return to physical education K-12 and to model good nutrition as well as to educate parents, teachers, students and others about the value of physical activity and good nutrition. This strategy is geared toward habituating children to healthy lifestyles in such a way that they will be on the path to good health for life.

But this midstream intervention was given new life and a major boost in 2004 when congress passed the Wellness Act (upstream). This act required local school districts that received federal funds for programs such as free breakfast and lunches to put in place policies and programs to help children develop habits of regular physical activity and good nutrition. Already we have seen major movement on the part of school districts to respond to this federal policy.

In one program, we are attempting to attack the problem of overweight and obesity at all three levels. This is the 100 Black Men's Health Challenge started in Atlanta and recently discussed and described in the January issue of the *Journal of Health Education*. *Downstream* the program focuses on getting black men to change their lifestyle toward more physical activity and better nutrition. There is close monitoring and group challenge and support for these changes. In *midstream* the program takes advantage of the men's power/influence in the community and the fact that they often serve as mentors of children from the housing projects. They are in a very good position to work to make the community more supportive of physical activity and good nutrition. They can help to make the streets safer and the parks more attractive. *Upstream*, these men often occupy positions on the school board and even in the legislature and can help to get policies in place that lead to environments which encourage/support healthy lifestyles. Thus the 100 Black Men Health Challenge is a three-dimensional challenge

It is especially great to attempt to pull together in one handbook virtually all that we know about the nature and distribution of overweight and obesity and about the various strategies for intervening to prevent and reduce overweight and obesity. Those who are on the front line of the battle against overweight and obesity have come together to put forth the status of our knowledge and experience with the efforts to reverse this dangerous public health trend. This sharing of knowledge and experiences and research strategies is critical if we are to be successful in our efforts. As many new minds and bodies join the efforts against this epidemic they do not need to start from scratch or "reinvent the wheel." What is already known and experienced in terms of strategies that work and do not work and methodologies that are being applied to further advance knowledge are available in this ***Handbook of Obesity Prevention.*** The editors of this handbook are well established and respected for their leadership in public health and especially research related to the nature and causes of overweight and obesity and the assessment of strategies for ameliorating this problem. Thus the book reflects their oversight and the tremendous input of several outstanding investigators and program developers.

Dr. David Satcher
Director, Center of Excellence on Health Disparities and
The Satcher Health Leadership Institute Initiative
Poussaint-Satcher-Cosby Chair in Mental Health
Morehouse School of Medicine
Atlanta, Georgia

Preface

The statistics are alarming. Over the past decades we have watched the weight levels of the U.S. population shift steadily upward. Media coverage of obesity conveys a continuing sense of crisis—for the population at large, especially children and youth, and for the health care system. We hear threats of spiraling health and societal costs related to obesity within the United States as well as dour predictions of the millions affected globally by obesity and its adverse health consequences. It is now clear that the society at large, not just the health sector, has a stake in ensuring that obesity is controlled. So we know that obesity must be controlled. The question is how to control it.

Without being overly technical, we frame, organize, and explain information relevant to obesity prevention, providing general background and perspective and reviewing how solutions to the problem might proceed within different settings or with different audiences. This book attempts to get to the "nuts and bolts" of how to halt and eventually reverse the obesity epidemic. In so doing, we are not starting at the beginning. In fact, the high level of action, energy, and discourse devoted to curbing the obesity epidemic has given us both the motivation and mandate for developing this book. Efforts are underway in the population at large, in community organizations, in local, state, and federal government agencies, in voluntary organizations, and within the commercial sector and the media. Some are relatively spontaneous; others have developed more purposely. These efforts encompass a spectrum of initiatives directed both to individual behavior and to aspects of the environments that influence individual behavior. Numerous reports and evidence reviews have been developed. There are national, state, and local action plans that spell out what needs to be done broadly as well as more specific guidelines and tools, while research to build the evidence base is ongoing. Yet, as described in the book, many of the ongoing efforts are not well coordinated and therefore are not obtaining maximum synergy.

This book comes at a time when obesity *prevention* has emerged as a specific topic within the broader fields of public health, health promotion, and preventive medicine—and especially as distinct from the well established clinical and research focus on obesity *treatment*. In part, we attempt to counter the tendency to talk about obesity "prevention and treatment" while allowing the more familiar, treatment perspective to dominate. Stopping the epidemic means preventing the gain of unhealthy excess weight in the population at large, and this can only be done through preventive strategies. Obesity treatment will continue to be important in obesity control efforts, but treatment affects the problem very far "downstream", i.e., after the problem has already taken hold. Treatment may be only partly effective over the long term, and—even when successful—is unlikely to reverse all of the long term effects of having carried the excess weight. Most important, if the forces underlying the epidemic remain unchecked, the numbers who need to be treated will continue to rise far beyond our capacity to provide individualized treatment to all who need it—especially as the potential to gain excess weight is lifelong.

Population-based, public health approaches are needed to address the underlying forces that influence—at a population level—how people eat and how physically active they are. These forces are "upstream" of the individual-level. Individual choices about eating and physical activity ultimately determine their weight levels (within very flexible physiological boundaries). Obesity prevention must alter the relevant physical, economic, and social environments and the policies that structure these environments in ways that make choices conducive to healthy weights easier or more desirable than others. Changing these environments will require collaboration and coordination across diverse sectors such as public health, agriculture, urban planning, and transportation. A significant challenge, yet entirely within our reach when one considers other major challenges that have been faced and met by public health initiatives in the past, including the eradication of smallpox or the reduction in tobacco-related diseases.

We have aimed for comprehensiveness, with a focus on the most recent literature, highlighting aspects of obesity prevention from multiple vantage points that, taken together, will tell the entire story. A key objective is to focus obesity prevention on *both* children and adults rather than in children only—as some might expect. Another is to increase understanding of the environmental and policy influences on obesity prevention, particularly in areas heretofore unfamiliar or insufficiently appreciated as affecting the success of lifestyle change programs (e.g., How might new school policies affect rates of childhood obesity?). A third objective is to facilitate strategic approaches to planning and executing obesity prevention initiatives in a way that draws upon established principles of public health practice and social change to find new approaches.

The three main sections of the book: *Overview*, *Understanding the Landscape*, and *Crafting Solutions*—progress from upstream, societal-level perspectives to downstream, community- and individual-level perspectives. This organization roughly follows the now widespread application of ecological frameworks in addressing public health issues. Considerations underlying interventions for adults and children have been integrated where appropriate, but important differences by life stage are highlighted in separate chapters. Intervention options are addressed separately for settings and population groups—to fit with these two different but related approaches to programming. For example, there are chapters on interventions in school and child care settings and in worksites, but there are also chapters on interventions in children and youth by developmental stage and in adults. Almost all chapters integrate issues related to both food and physical activity. Several chapters highlight special issues for subgroups defined by ethnicity or socioeconomic status, because these are the population groups with the highest current and future potential burden of obesity.

Our goal is to offer guidance and inspiration for the teachers, students, and professionals from the diverse array of disciplines whose efforts are needed in order to solve the obesity problem. We hope the book will be useful for academic institutions, state and local health agencies, non-profit organizations, health care organizations, and national public health agencies—to help these various audiences to use the information about obesity prevention that we have now and that will develop in the coming years to keep pace with continuing cultural and other environmental changes.

While we focus mainly on the U.S. context, the principles and approaches apply in most other countries. The problem is inherently global in nature, and both the problem of obesity and its eventual solutions must extend across the globe. However, the character of the epidemic and the potential feasibility and effectiveness of various solutions varies across countries and, within countries, in different regions, localities, and neighborhoods.

In spite of the rapidly increasing rates of obesity and the future implications of these trends, there is considerable hope for change and improvement. Many sectors of society now recognize the importance of obesity prevention, and we have more information and tools at our fingertips than ever before to meet this challenge. We therefore offer this handbook to all who can be enlisted in crafting solutions to the obesity problem and to foster the societal transformation that this implies.

Shiriki Kumanyika and Ross C. Brownson

Acknowledgments

We are only the editors of this book and, therefore, attribute any value that it will have to the talents of the authors who have generously given their time and energies to produce the chapters. We were extremely fortunate in attracting an outstanding group of contributors—scholars who are leading the science and practice on diverse aspects of obesity prevention and for whom the opportunity to share the insights they have gleaned to date became an irresistible challenge. We are deeply indebted to these very busy people, and to the people who have worked with them behind the scenes, for their willingness to sign on to this project and for their exceptionally collaborative spirit in shaping the individual chapters to fit with our vision and organizational schema. We also acknowledge the key role of Bill Tucker at Springer for his initiative in suggesting this project initially to Shiriki and for his ongoing encouragement and support throughout the writing and editing process.

Contents

Section 3. Crafting Solutions

Part 1: Influencing Systems and Institutions

Part 2. Influencing Individuals and Families

Section 4. Conclusion

About the Editors

Shiriki K. Kumanyika, PhD, RD, MPH, is Professor of Epidemiology in Biostatistics and Epidemiology and Pediatrics (Nutrition), Associate Dean for Health Promotion, and Disease Prevention, and was the Founding Director of the Graduate Program in Public Health Studies at the University of Pennsylvania School of Medicine (Penn). At Penn she is also a Senior Fellow in the Center for Clinical Epidemiology and Biostatistics, the Leonard Davis Institute for Health Economics, and the Institute on Aging and is a Faculty Associate at the Penn Institute for Urban Research. Dr. Kumanyika holds a B.A. in Psychology from Syracuse University, an M.S. in Social Work from Columbia University, PhD in Human Nutrition from Cornell University, and Master of Public Health (MPH) from the Johns Hopkins University School of Public Health. She has authored or co-authored more than 200 scientific articles, book chapters and monographs related to nutritional epidemiology, obesity and minority health.

Dr. Kumanyika directs a National Institutes of Health (NIH)-funded Project EXPORT Center of Excellence whose focus is on research, outreach and training to reduce obesity and related health disparities. She is also engaged in the development of AACORN (African American Collaborative Obesity Research Network) a national initiative which she created to further the quality and quantity of research to foster healthy weights in African American communities. Dr. Kumanyika is an elected member of the Institute of Medicine (IOM) of the National Academy of Sciences and has served on three IOM committees related to obesity prevention and weight control. She currently serves on the NIH Clinical Obesity Research Panel and, since 1996, has chaired the Prevention Group of the International Obesity Task Force of the International Association for the Study of Obesity. Dr. Kumanyika has been actively engaged in public health research and training for more than 30 years and currently serves as Vice Chair of the Executive Board of the American Public Health Association.

Ross C. Brownson, PhD, is Professor of Epidemiology and Director of the Prevention Research Center at Saint Louis University School of Public Health, St. Louis, MO. He also is a Research Member and Co-Director for Prevention and Control at the Siteman Cancer Center at Washington University School of

Medicine. Dr. Brownson directs the Centre for Evidence-Based Chronic Disease Prevention, which is sponsored by the World Health Organization and the Pan American Health Organization. He is a chronic disease epidemiologist whose research has focused on tobacco use prevention, promotion of physical activity, evaluation of community-level interventions, and the influence of environmental and policy factors on chronic disease risk. He received his Ph.D. in environmental health and epidemiology at Colorado State University and was formerly a Division Director with the Missouri Department of Health. In the state health department, Dr. Brownson was responsible for overall administration and direction of research activities for the state programs in chronic disease prevention including representation to the Missouri General Assembly, voluntary health agencies, federal agencies, and health care providers.

Dr. Brownson's research is funded by the Centers for Disease Control and Prevention, the National Institutes of Health, and the Robert Wood Johnson Foundation. He was a member of two Institute of Medicine Committees on Obesity Prevention in Children and Youth. He is an associate editor of the Annual Review of Public Health and serves on four editorial boards. Dr. Brownson also was a founding member of the 15-person CDC Task Force developing the Guide to Community Preventive Services. He is active in numerous professional associations, including the American Public Health Association and the Missouri Public Health Association. He has authored or co-authored more than 200 scientific articles, book chapters and monographs and is the editor or author of the books: *Chronic Disease Epidemiology and Control, Applied Epidemiology, Evidence-Based Public Health, Community-Based Prevention,* and *Communicating Public Health Information Effectively: A Guide for Practitioners.*

Contributors

Alice Ammerman, Dr.P.H., R.D., Center for Health Promotion and Disease Prevention and Department of Nutrition, Schools of Public Health and Medicine University of North Carolina at Chapel Hill, Chapel Hill, North Carolina, U.S.A.

Kelly D. Brownell, Ph.D., Departments of Psychology, Epidemiology and Public Health, Yale Center for Weight and Eating Disorders, Institute for Social Policy Studies, and Rudd Center for Food Policy and Obesity, Yale University, New Haven, Connecticut, U.S.A.

Ross C. Brownson, Ph.D., Prevention Research Center and Department of Community Health, School of Public Health, St. Louis University, St. Louis, Missouri, U.S.A,

Meghan Butryn, M.S., The Miriam Hospital and Brown Medical School, Providence, Rhode Island, U.S.A.

Kelly Clifton, Ph.D., Urban Studies and Planning Program, University of Maryland, College Park, Maryland, U.S.A.

Graham A. Colditz, M.D., Dr.P.H., Department of Surgery and Alvin J. Siteman Cancer Center, Washington University School of Medicine, St. Louis, Missouri, U.S.A.

Brian L. Cole, Dr. P.H., Department of Health Services, University of California at Los Angeles, School of Public Health, Los Angeles, California, U.S.A.

Lisa Craypo, M.P.H., R.D., Samuels & Associates, Oakland, California, U.S.A.

Lori Dorfman, Dr. P.H., Berkeley Media Studies Group, Oakland, California, U.S.A.

Nancy C. Edwards, Ph.D., School of Nursing and Department of Epidemiology and Community Medicine, University of Ottawa, Ontario, Canada

Eva Epstein, M.A., Department of Psychology, Temple University, Philadelphia, Pennsylvania, U.S.A.

Myles S. Faith, Ph.D., Center for Weight and Eating Disorders, Department of Psychiatry, University of Pennsylvania School of Medicine and The Children's Hospital of Philadelphia, Philadelphia, Pennsylvania, U.S.A.

Zubaida Faridi, M.B.B.S., M.P.H., Prevention Research Center, Yale University School of Medicine, Derby, Connecticut, U.S.A.

Alison E. Field, Sc.D., Division of Adolescent/Young Adult Medicine, Children's Hospital Boston and Harvard Medical School and Channing Laboratory, Department of Medicine, Brigham and Women's Hospital and Harvard Medical School, Boston, Massachusetts, U.S.A.

Christopher Fleming, M.P.H., Obesity Prevention Center and Department of Community Health, School of Public Health, St. Louis University, St. Louis, Missouri, U.S.A.

Eileen G. Ford, M.S., R.D., Center for Obesity Research and Education, Temple University, Philadelphia, Pennsylvania, U.S.A.

Gary D. Foster, Ph.D., Center for Obesity Research and Education, Temple University, Philadelphia, Pennsylvania, U.S.A.

John M. Garcia, M.Sc., Division of Preventive Oncology, Cancer Care Ontario and Ontario Tobacco Research Unit, Toronto, Ontario, Canada

Debra Haire-Joshu, Ph.D., Obesity Prevention Center and Department of Community Health, School of Public Health, St. Louis University, St. Louis, Missouri, U.S.A.

Susan Handy, Ph.D., Department of Environmental Science and Policy, University of California Davis, Davis, California, U.S.A.

David L. Katz, M.D., M.P.H., F.A.C.P.M., F.A.C.P., Prevention Research Center, Yale University School of Medicine, Derby, Connecticut, U.S.A.

Robert J. Kuczmarski, Dr. P.H., Obesity Prevention and Treatment Program, Division of Digestive Diseases and Nutrition, National Institute of Diabetes and Digestive and Kidney Diseases, National Institutes of Health, Bethesda, Maryland, U.S.A.

Shiriki Kumanyika, Ph.D., R.D. M.P.H., Center for Clinical Epidemiology and Biostatistics, Departments of Biostatistics and Epidemiology and Pediatrics (Nutrition), University of Pennsylvania School of Medicine, Philadelphia Pennsylvania, U.S.A.

Sally Lawrence, M.P.H., Samuels & Associates, Oakland, California, U.S.A.

May May Leung, M.S., R.D, Department of Nutrition, School of Public Health, University of North Carolina at Chapel Hill, North Carolina, U.S.A.

Elena O. Lingas, Dr. P.H., M.P.H., Berkeley Media Studies Group, Berkeley, California, U.S.A.

Marilyn S. Nanney, Ph.D., M.P.H., R.D., Program in Health Disparities, Department of Family Medicine and Community Health, University of Minnesota, Minneapolis, Minnesota, U.S.A.

Amy E. Paxton, Department of Nutrition, School of Public Health, University of North Carolina at Chapel Hill, Chapel Hill, North Carolina, U.S.A.

John C. Peters, Ph.D., Nutrition Science Institute, Food and Beverage Technology Division, The Procter & Gamble Company, Cincinnati, Ohio, U.S.A.

Suzanne Phelan, Ph.D., The Miriam Hospital and Brown Medical School, Providence, Rhode Island, U.S.A.

Barry M. Popkin, Ph.D., School of Public Health and Carolina Population Center, University of North Carolina at Chapel Hill, Chapel Hill, North Carolina, U.S.A.

Nico P. Pronk, Ph.D., M.A., F.A.C.S.M., F.A.W.H.P., Center for Health Promotion, HealthPartners Research Foundation, HealthPartners, Minneapolis, Minnesota, U.S.A.

Barbara L. Riley, Ph.D., National Cancer Institute of Canada/Canadian Cancer Society, Centre for Behavioural Research and Program Evaluation and Department of Health Studies and Gerontology, University of Waterloo, Waterloo, Ontario, Canada

Carmen D. Samuel-Hodge, Ph.D., M.S., R.D., Department of Nutrition, Schools of Public Health and Medicine, University of North Carolina, Chapel Hill, North Carolina, U.S.A.

Sarah E. Samuels, Dr..P.H., President, Samuels & Associates, Oakland, California, U.S.A.

David Satcher, M.D., Ph.D., Center of Excellence on Health Disparities and the Satcher Health Leadership Institute, Morehouse School of Medicine, Atlanta, Georgia, U.S.A.

Rebecca Schermbeck, M.P.H., M.S., R.D., Obesity Prevention Center and Department of Community Health, School of Public Health, St. Louis University, St. Louis, Missouri, U.S.A.

Janice K. Sommers, M.P.H., Center for Health Promotion and Disease Prevention, University of North Carolina at Chapel Hill, Chapel Hill, North Carolina, U.S.A.

Cynthia Stein, M.D., M.P.H., Harvard Center for Cancer Prevention, Harvard School of Public Health and Channing Laboratory, Department of Medicine, Brigham and Women's Hospital and Harvard Medical School, Boston, Massachusetts, U.S.A.

Nicolas Stettler, M.D., M.S.C.E., The Children's Hospital of Philadelphia and Center for Clinical Epidemiology and Biostatistics, University of Pennsylvania School of Medicine, Philadelphia, Pennsylvania, U.S.A.

Stephanie S. Vander Veur, M.P.H., Center for Obesity Research and Education, Temple University, Philadelphia, Pennsylvania, U.S.A.

Maihan B. Vu, Dr.P.H., M.P.H., Center for Health Promotion and Disease Prevention, University of North Carolina at Chapel Hill, Chapel Hill, North Carolina, U.S.A.

Youfa Wang, M.D., Ph.D., Center for Human Nutrition, Departments of International Health and Epidemiology, Bloomberg School of Public Health, Johns Hopkins University, Baltimore, Maryland, U.S.A.

Brian Wansink, Ph.D., Department of Applied Economics and Management, Johnson Graduate School of Management, Cornell University, Ithaca, New York, U.S.A.

Rena R. Wing, Ph.D., The Miriam Hospital and Brown Medical School, Providence, Rhode Island, U.S.A.

Antronette K. Yancey, M.D., M.P.H., F.A.C.P.M., Department of Health Services and Center to Eliminate Health Disparities. University of California at Los Angeles, School of Public Health, Los Angeles, California, U.S.A.

Chapter 1

Why Obesity Prevention?

Shiriki Kumanyika and Ross C. Brownson

Introduction

Obesity prevention means prevention of excess weight gain, where "excess" means weight gain beyond that considered favorable to short and long term health and where the excess weight is characterized by excess fat. The weight ranges considered harmful to health are termed "overweight" and "obese". Obesity indicates a greater amount of excess weight with a greater likelihood of associated health complications. In adults who have reached full height and are not underweight, obesity prevention can be interpreted to mean prevention of any net increments in weight over time outside of weight gain that occurs in conjunction with pregnancy. In children and adolescents, weight gain is expected as part of normal growth and development. Obesity prevention during these developmental periods relates to weight gain that is judged to be in excess of the normal growth trajectory (see Chapter 2). Positively stated, the goal of obesity prevention is to achieve and maintain healthy weight. This goal relates to *primary prevention*, i.e., prevention of the development of overweight and obesity rather than only preventing further weight gain among those who are already overweight or obese.

This chapter is an introduction to the remainder of this Handbook. Here we clarify what is meant by obesity prevention, why it is important, and what it entails. This sets the stage for the content of the sections and chapters that follow.

Background

Obesity in the general population (as opposed the type of obesity that is caused by certain rare genetic disorders such as Prader-Willi Syndrome (Dietz, 2002)) requires an underlying genetic susceptibility for which there are undoubtedly many different genes involved, as well as environmental circumstances that allow for positive energy balance to occur (Comuzzie, 2002). Given the rapid rise in the prevalence of obesity over the past few decades, changes in genetic make-up alone are unlikely to be major contributors to the epidemic. Humans vary in their innate regulatory capacity and susceptibility to gain weight under 'obesogenic' environmental circumstances (French, Story, & Jeffery, 2001; Hill & Peters, 1998; Hill, Wyatt, Reed, & Peters, 2003), but global patterns and trends in obesity suggest that increasing numbers of people are gaining excess weight (World Health Organization, 2000). There is still variation in the tendency of individuals to gain excess weight but, increasingly, this seems to be a matter of how much rather than any excess weight. We have apparently not yet seen the upper limit in obesity prevalence in the United States and, especially, globally given the continued emergence of social and environmental conditions predisposing to a relative excess of energy intake in many countries.

There is an important evolutionary backdrop to obesity. Obesity has been observed throughout human history (Bray, 2002). The ability to accumulate excess fat, apparently observed as far back as the Stone Ages, has clearly been beneficial for human survival—allowing people to take advantage of times when food was plentiful to store fat as a defense against hunger in times of food shortages (Bray, 2002; Brown & Konner, 1987). Friedman (2003) has suggested that our early existence as hunter-gatherers (in times of frequent famine) may have favored genes for energy storage and survival, making modern humans maladapted in an age of food abundance and sedentary living (the so called "thrifty gene hypothesis").

Concern about obesity has evolved in a variety of disciplines and settings. For example, recognition of the adverse health consequences of obesity has been longstanding in clinical medicine, dating back to the time of Hippocrates and Galen (Bray, 2002; Papavramidou, Papavramidis, & Christopoulou-Aletra, 2004). In the business sector, the life insurance industry is concerned about the contribution of obesity to mortality and the resulting costs (Lew, 1985). From both clinical and business perspectives, the problem has heretofore been viewed as affecting a minority of the population. The obesity epidemic is now forcing a shift in societal attitudes about the nature of the problem and the importance of addressing it on a population-wide level.

In the United States, obesity received serious attention as a public health issue when national nutrition monitoring data from health examination surveys began to show evidence of a gradual, and then more marked increase in adult obesity prevalence between the 1960–62 and 1988–91 surveys (Kuczmarski, 1992; Kuczmarski, Flegal, Campbell, & Johnson, 1994). These data were augmented by data from the Behavioral Risk Factor Surveillance System for 1991–99 showing an increasing number of states with a significant proportion of adults meeting the definition of obesity (Mokdad, Serdula, Dietz, Bowman, Marks, & Koplan, 1999; 2000).

Public health focus on the obesity issue was increased further by changes in the thresholds used to define overweight and obesity, which had the effect of increasing the number of people considered to be at risk (National Heart, Lung, and Blood Institute, 1998; Flegal, Carroll, Kuczmarski, & Johnson, 1998; World Health Organization, 2000). By these new definitions, more than half of U.S. men were classified as overweight or obese beginning in 1971–74 and more than half of U.S. women were classified as overweight or obese beginning in 1988–94 (National Center for Health Statistics, 2006). In 2003–2004, 62 and 71% of U.S. women and men, respectively, were overweight or obese (Ogden et al., 2006).

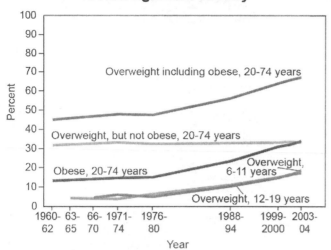

SOURCES Centers for Disease Control and Prevention, National Center for Health Statistics, *Health, United States, 2006*, Figure 13. Data from the National Health and Nutrition Examination Survey.

Figure 1.1 Overweight and obesity in U.S. children and adults, 1960–62 to 2003–2004.

Source: National Center for Health Statistics, 2006.

A striking increase in pediatric obesity approximately paralleled the trends in adults (Gortmaker et al., 1987; Troiano et al., 1995) (see Figure 1.1), suggesting that more and more children and adolescents were being exposed to the adverse health and social consequences of obesity. For example, given current prevalence and trends, a significant subset of obese youth would develop type 2 diabetes—a condition previously considered to be of adult onset (Dietz & Gortmaker, 2001). As of 2003–2004, about 34% of children and adolescents ages 2 to 19 years were either overweight or obese[1], and about 17% were obese (Ogden et al., 2006).

The scenario has also been playing out globally. An expert group convened in 1997 by the World Health Organization (2000) concluded:

"Obesity is a chronic disease, prevalent in both developed and developing countries, and affecting children as well as adults. Indeed, it is now so common that it is replacing the more traditional public health concerns, including undernutrition and infectious diseases, as one of the most significant contributors to ill health. Furthermore, as obesity is a key risk factor in the natural history of other chronic and noncommunicable diseases (NCDs), it is only a mater of time before the same high mortality rates for such diseases will be seen in developing countries as those prevailing 30 years ago in industrialized countries with well established market economies (pp. 1–2)."

The validity of this assessment has been confirmed by many subsequent reports and updates on global prevalence and trends and on the increasing burden of obesity related chronic diseases (Kumanyika et al., 2002; Ebbeling, Pawlak, & Ludwig, 2002; James, 2006; Wang & Lobstein, 2006; World Health Organization, 2003). The global context of the obesity epidemic is discussed in detail in Chapter 11.

---

[1] The Centers for Disease Control uses the terminology "overweight" and "at risk of overweight" when referring, respectively, to obesity and overweight in children (see Chapter 2).

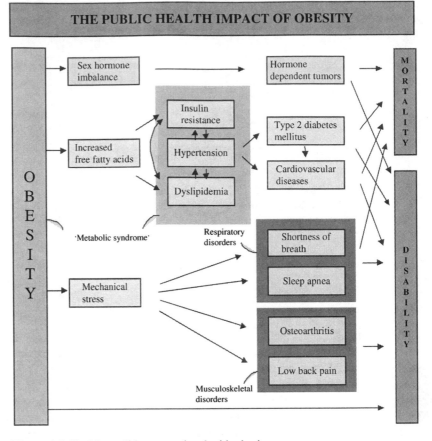

Figure 1.2 Health conditions associated with obesity.

From: Visscher & Seidell, 2001. Reprinted, with permission, from the Annual Review of Public Health, Volume 22(c)2001 by Annual Reviews.

The public health and broader societal concerns about the high levels of obesity relate largely to its health impacts. As shown in Figure 1.2, obesity is associated with metabolic disease and both cardiovascular diseases and cancer—the major causes of disability and death in U.S. adults—as well as respiratory and musculoskeletal problems (Visscher & Seidell, 2001; World Health Organization, 2000). The relative magnitude of these different obesity related risks differs, as shown in Table 1.1. A notable feature of these data involves the number of conditions for which obesity increases the risk by a 3:1 ratio or more. For major chronic diseases, "weak associations" (those with relative risk values less than two or three (Wynder, 1987; Szklo, 2001)) are the most common. These relatively large increased risks for obesity are important illustrations of the magnitude of this issue.

Obesity-related health problems pose a burden to the affected individuals and their families. In addition, as explained in Chapter 4, the treatment of diseases to which obesity has been linked causally can be extremely expensive, and these costs may increase as more adverse health effects of obesity are identified. For example, non-alcoholic fatty liver disease, which can lead to chronic liver disease and even to cirrhosis, is now recognized as a complication of obesity in both adults and children (Sadchev, Riely, & Maden, 2006).

Table 1.1 Relative risk of health problems associated with obesity[a].

Greatly increased (relative risk >3)	Moderately increased (relative risk 2–3)	Slightly increased (relative risk 1–2)
Type 2 diabetes	Coronary heart disease	Cancer[b]
Gallbladder disease	Hypertension	Reproductive hormone abnormalities
Dyslipidemia	Osteoarthritis (Knees)	Polycystic ovary syndrome
		Impaired fertility
Insulin resistance	Hyperuricemia and gout	Low back pain
Breathlessness		Anesthesia complications
Sleep apnea		Fetal defects

[a] All relative risk values are approximate
[b] Breast cancer in postmenopausal women, endometrial cancer, colon cancer
Source: World Health Organization, 2000; Table 4.1, page 43. Reprinted with permission.

The consequences of obesity in children and adolescents impact their physical, emotional, and social health (Table 1.2).

If the obesity epidemic remains unchecked, the demand for the treatment of conditions resulting from obesity will become increasingly difficult to meet within the United States and likely impossible to meet in less developed

Table 1.2 Physical, social, and emotional health consequences of obesity in children and youth.

Physical Health
- Glucose intolerance and insulin resistance
- Type 2 diabetes
- Dyslipidemia
- Fatty liver disease
- Gallstones
- Sleep apnea
- Menstrual abnormalities
- Impaired balance
- Orthopedic problems

Emotional Health
- Low self-esteem
- Negative body image
- Depression

Social Health
- Stigma
- Negative stereotyping
- Discrimination
- Teasing and bullying
- Social marginalization

Source: Institute of Medicine (2005). Preventing Childhood Obesity: Health in the Balance, Table 2–1 (p. 71).

countries with markedly fewer health care resources (World Health Organization, 2000). In addition to the health care costs, there are the costs to society of obesity-related absenteeism and loss of productivity from school or work.

Given this backdrop, why have we chosen to focus on obesity *prevention*? We need obesity prevention not only because it is the right thing to do, i.e., promote healthy weights in the population, but also because there is no other way to curb the rising epidemic of excess weight gain. Obesity impairs physical functioning and quality of life. Short term weight losses are relatively achievable under the right circumstances but permanent weight loss is extremely difficult to achieve. People enrolled in the National Weight Control Registry, who have previously lost an average of 30 pounds and maintained the loss for at least 5 years, report an average of 90 minutes of physical activity per day to maintain this weight loss in addition to following a low-fat, low-calorie diet (Wing & Phelan, 2005). Bariatric surgery as a means to long term weight loss has shown a large increase in use—from an annual average of about 10,000 to more than 100,000 procedures—between 1996–98 and 2002–2004 (National Center for Health Statistics, 2006)—but cannot be viewed as a long-term, cost-effective solution to the obesity epidemic because of acceptability, cost and associated morbidity and mortality. Even when weight loss is achieved, not all of the longstanding consequences of obesity are necessarily reversible. Depending on when in the course of obesity the weight loss occurs, the damage might already have been done (Harris, Savage, Tell, Haan, Kumanyika & Lynch, 1997). Most fundamentally, however, reliance on treatment will never address the root causes that are leading so many people to become obese (see Chapter 5). Addressing root causes is the focus of prevention, which has shown remarkable successes and potential over the past 100 years (Centers for Disease Control, 1999).

Understanding the Task: What are we Trying to Accomplish?

Food Intake, Physical Activity, and Energy Balance

The principle of energy balance is fundamental for an understanding of obesity prevention. The components of energy balance are shown in Figure 1.3 (World Health Organization, 2000). Energy (calories) is consumed in foods and beverages, as fat, protein, carbohydrate, or alcohol. Energy is used for basal metabolism, to digest food, and in physical activity. Calories not needed for these purposes or for growth (during development) are deposited as fat. Obesity develops as a consequence of consuming more calories[2] than the body expends—termed "positive energy balance"—chronically and beyond the ability of the body's regulatory systems to compensate. Preventing obesity requires achieving energy balance through regulation of food intake and physical activity. We have complex physiological mechanisms to regulate body weight, but cannot rely solely on these regulatory systems, i.e., on instinctive or spontaneous compensatory behaviors (World Health Organization, 2000). These systems seem to

---

[2] "Energy intake and expenditure", terms that are used throughout this book, are the more technical terms for caloric intake and expenditure.

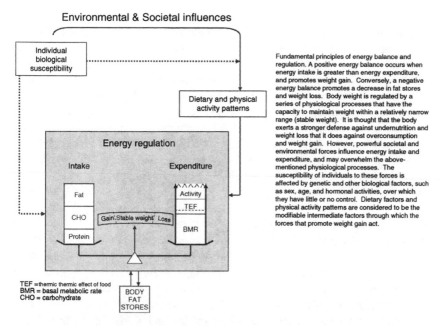

Environmental & Societal influences

Individual biological susceptibility

Dietary and physical activity patterns

Energy regulation

Intake

Expenditure

Fat

Activity

TEF

CHO

Gain\Stable weight/ Loss

Protein

BMR

TEF = thermic thermic effect of food
BMR = basal metabolic rate
CHO = carbohydrate

BODY FAT STORES

Fundamental principles of energy balance and regulation. A positive energy balance occurs when energy intake is greater than energy expenditure, and promotes weight gain. Conversely, a negative energy balance promotes a decrease in fat stores and weight loss. Body weight is regulated by a series of physiological processes that have the capacity to maintain weight within a relatively narrow range (stable weight). It is thought that the body exerts a stronger defense against undernutrition and weight loss that it does against overconsumption and weight gain. However, powerful societal and environmental forces influence energy intake and expenditure, and may overwhelm the above-mentioned physiological processes. The susceptibility of individuals to these forces is affected by genetic and other biological factors, such as sex, age, and hormonal activities, over which they have little or no control. Dietary factors and physical activity patterns are considered to be the modifiable intermediate factors through which the forces that promote weight gain act.

Figure 1.3 Influences on energy balance and weight gain (energy regulation).
From: World Health Organization, 2000, Figure 7.1 p.103. Reprinted with permission.

work much more effectively to prevent weight loss than they do to prevent weight gain. From an evolutionary perspective, our bodies and minds are much more strongly geared to preventing hunger and undernutrition than to compensating for excesses (Friedman, 2003). However, from a societal perspective we have now made conditions conducive to a relative excess of calories—positive energy balance—into a way of life (Kumanyika et al. 2002; Swinburn, Seidell, Caterson, & James, 2004; World Health Organization, 2000). It has become more and more difficult to maintain energy balance, as the opportunities for food and beverage consumption have increased and opportunities to be physically active have decreased.

Although approaches to obesity prevention must impact energy balance via food and beverage intake and physical activity, it is very difficult to quantify the specific size of the relative excess of calories on a per-person-per day basis (World Health Organization, 2000; Wang, Gortmaker, Sobol, & Kuntz, 2006). Whereas the caloric deficit needed to produce weight loss is relatively easy to describe, specifying and assessing the boundaries of energy balance associated with weight maintenance are more difficult and make the task of obesity prevention so challenging. Simplistically, one pound is gained when an excess of 3,500 kilocalories has occurred. However, in "real world" conditions, several factors are important to consider: (1) the difficulty of precisely measuring energy intake and expenditure outside of controlled laboratory settings, (2) individual variability in body weight regulation, and (3) changes in the dynamics of energy balance in different phases of weight gain and weight loss. For these reasons, specification of obesity prevention goals and outcomes tends to rely on weight levels and body mass to infer the energy balance and weight gain effects of changes in food intake and physical activity.

Various attempts have been made to quantify the amount of excess calories driving the current epidemic at the population level and also to identify the relative contributions of excess calorie consumption versus insufficient caloric expenditure. Hill (2003) suggests that relatively small behavior changes (adding a 15 minute walk and eating a few bites less at meals) to influence energy balance by about 100 kilocalories per day could prevent weight gain. Modeling of the "energy gap", as the caloric excess is termed, suggests the need for an adjustment of between 100 and 200 kilocalories for younger children and by as much as 600–1,000 kilocalories for adolescents (Wang, et al., 2006).

Adult respondents in the National Health and Nutrition Examination Survey (NHANES) reported approximately 200 to 300 kilocalories more in 1999–2002 compared to 1971–74 (National Center for Health Statistics, 2006), although some of this difference might be an artifact of improved dietary interview techniques. Less inactivity but similar levels of regular physical activity were reported by adult respondents in national surveys between 1998 and 2004, but these data do not permit quantification of any net change in energy expenditure.

Both food and beverage intake and physical activity levels have effects on health that are independent of their effects on obesity. Dietary recommendations to lower the risks of cardiovascular disease and cancer include avoiding fats that are unhealthy, such as saturated fat and *trans* fat, eating ample quantities of fruits and vegetables and whole grains, minimizing the intake of sodium, and consuming alcohol only in moderation, if at all (U.S. Department of Health and Human Services & U.S. Department of Agriculture, 2005). Consuming limited amounts of free sugar or added sugar is also recommended in order to give priority to consumption of calories from foods that also contain other nutrients. Moderate or vigorous physical activity on a regular basis improves physical fitness and lowers the risk of cardiovascular disease, diabetes, and certain cancers. These behaviors can, therefore, be recommended to the entire population, including those with existing weight problems.

In fact, some data suggest that up to a certain level of overweight, these behaviors will convey more health benefit than modest weight loss (Lee, Blair, & Jackson, 1999; Wei, Kampert, Barlow, Nichaman, Gibbons, & Paffenbarger, 1999). However, while this argument might have validity in some individuals or population groups, it does not preclude the need for attention to obesity prevention, especially in groups at high risk of excess weight gain. Strategies to prevent weight gain over time are needed for the population at large, and in a timely manner for high risk individuals. In addition, "fat yet fit" findings do not hold equally well for all obesity related outcomes (e.g., the relationship is stronger for cardiovascular diseases than for all cause mortality) and population subgroups.

Reducing Incidence and Prevalence

At the level of the population, obesity prevention means achieving and maintaining a distribution of body mass index (BMI) in which a maximum number of people are at a healthy weight, i.e., with a minimum number who are undernourished and a minimum who are obese (World Health Organization, 2000). For both clinical and public health purposes, overweight and obesity are defined by somewhat arbitrary cutoffs on a continuous distribution of BMI (calculated as weight (in kilograms) ÷ height (in meters) squared). The ranges that define overweight and obesity for adults are, respectively, a BMI of 25–29.9 and 30 or greater (National Heart, Lung, and Blood Institute, 1998). As an example, a 5' 9" adult who weighs 203 pounds is considered obese at a BMI of 30. For children and adolescents the ranges are, respectively the 85th–94.9th and 95th age–sex reference percentile of the BMI reference curves (Kuczmarski, Ogden, Grummer-Strawn, et al., 2000). According to the World Health Organization, the mean BMI in such an optimal distribution for adults is probably around 21 kg/m2 (World Health Organization, 2000). As discussed in detail in Chapter 2, weight-related risk occurs along a continuum, and the development of obesity is not an "event" such that risk is present after but not before the threshold is reached.

In the United States, the establishment and tracking of numerical goals is crucial in setting priorities and assessing public health progress. The U.S. Public Health Service has set 15% and 5% as targets for obesity prevalence in adults in 2003–2004 and children, respectively (U.S. Department of Health and Human Services, 2000), but we have actually moved substantially away from those goals since they were set. As shown in Table 1.3, the prevalence of obesity in adults in 2003–2004, based on measured height and weight in a representative sample of the U.S. population, was from 2 to more than 3 times higher than the target of 15%. Not only did obesity prevalence fail to decrease toward the targeted levels, but it actually increased by 5 to 13% points over the levels observed around 1990, depending on the subgroup considered. Table 1.4 shows a similar situation in children. The prevalence of obesity in children in 2001–2004 was 3 to 5 times the target of 5%, with increases of 2 to 9% since around 1990. What makes obesity stand out in this public health scenario is the trajectory of increase, combined with the associated increases in the incidence and prevalence of type 2 diabetes

Table 1.3 Changes in obesity prevalence in U.S. adults compared to Healthy People 2010 goal of 15% prevalence.

	Prevalence		
	1988–94	2001–2004	Change
All adults ages 20 years	23	31	+7%
Below100% poverty level	26	33	+7%
100% to less than 200% of poverty level	24	33	+9%
200% or more above poverty level	21	31	+10%
Non-Hispanic White Males	20	30	+10%
Non-Hispanic White Females	23	31	+8%
Non-Hispanic Black Males	21	31	+10%
Non-Hispanic Black Females	38	51	+13%
Mexican American Males	24	29	+5%
Mexican American Females	35	39	+5%

Data are for ages 20 years and over, age adjusted to the 2000 standard population. Obesity is defined as BMI ≥ 30.0.

Persons of Mexican-American origin may be any race

Poverty level is based on family income and family size

Prevalence estimates are rounded to whole numbers

Change is by subtraction

Source: National Center for Health Statistics, CDC, Health U.S. 2006, Table 73

Table 1.4 Changes in obesity prevalence in U.S. children and youth ages 6–19, compared to Healthy People 2010 goal of 5% prevalence.

	Prevalence		
	1988–94	**2001–2004**	**Change**
All children and youth ages 6–11	11	18	+7%
Below 100% poverty level	11	20	+9%
100% to less than 200% of poverty level	11	18	+7%
200% or more above poverty level	11	15	+4%
Non-Hispanic White Males	12	17	+5%
Non-Hispanic White Females	10*	16	+6%
Non-Hispanic Black Males	18	26	+8%
Non-Hispanic Black Females	17	25	+8%
Mexican American Males	11	16	+5%
Mexican American Females	15	17	+2%
All children and youth ages 12–19	11	17	+7%
Below 100% poverty level	16	18	+2%
100% to less than 200% of poverty level	11	17	+6%
200% or more above poverty level	8	16	+8%
Non-Hispanic White Males	12	18	+6%
Non-Hispanic White Females	9	15	+6%
Non-Hispanic Black Males	11	18	+7%
Non-Hispanic Black Females	16	24	+8%
Mexican American Males	14	20	+6%
Mexican American Females	13*	17	+4%

Overweight is defined for ages 6–19 years as BMI ≥ gender- and age-specific 95th percentile from the 2000 CDC Growth Charts for the United States.
Persons of Mexican-American origin may be any race
Poverty level is based on family income and family size
Prevalence estimates are rounded to whole numbers
Change is by subtraction
* indicates that estimates are considered unreliable (standard error of 20% to 30%)
Source: National Center for Health Statistics, CDC, Health U.S. 2006, Table 74

occurring at increasingly younger ages and in an aging adult population (U.S. Department of Health and Human Services, 2002). The Centers for Disease Control (CDC) notes that "because of the dynamics of an aging population, the societal costs will increase, even if the increase in prevalence is halted" (U.S. Department of Health and Human Services, 2002, page 2).

This situation was anticipated because of obesity prevalence and trends when Healthy People goals were set. The less ambitious Healthy People 2000 weight goal for adults—20% prevalence of overweight[3]—was far out of reach

---

[3] The Healthy People 2000 goal, and the analysis cited here used BMI 27.8 and 27.3 kg/m^2, respectively to define the weight target for adult males and females and the term "overweight" rather than "obesity" was used for people at or above these thresholds.

soon after it was set. Using a 1994 baseline of 24.7% overweight estimated from the National Health and Nutrition Examination Follow up Study, Russell, Williamson, & Byers (1995) estimated that "the 20% prevalence objective could be reached if all overweight persons were to lose 11.2 kg (24.6 lb) of body weight or by combining the prevention of all weight gain by the non-overweight with a weight loss of 6.6 kg (14.5 lb) in all overweight adults". They concluded that "it is highly unlikely that such population-wide weight changes will occur in the U.S. over the next 6 years." The challenge with respect to African American women, identified as a high risk group because their starting prevalence of overweight was substantially higher than for whites or black men, was even greater, although the HP 2000 goal had been set higher in consideration of the higher baseline 30%. "Reaching the 30% prevalence objective would require that all overweight African American women lose and maintain a 12.2 kg (26.8 lb) loss of weight, or that all weight gain be prevented in combination with the loss of 9.3 (20.5 lb) of weight by all over-weight African American women."

The establishment of and progress toward public health goals for obesity raise several issues. They make the point, indirectly, that strategies involving weight loss among those already overweight or obese do not influence the increasing numbers of people crossing the thresholds to become obese. This is a classic scenario in public health that illustrates the inability of treatment to address the underlying causes of a problem. To address the obesity issue on a population-wide level, it is particularly risky to rely primarily on treatment approaches partly because of the still uncertain prospects for reaching affected individuals with treatments that are effective over the long term (U.S. Preventive Services Task Force, 2003; Whitlock,Williams, Gold, Smith, & Shipman, 2005). Efforts to improve the long term effectiveness and reach of weight loss programs will continue to be of high priority to improve the health and quality of life and reduce health care costs among the obese. However, as noted previously, only prevention can address the underlying causes of epidemic—by eliminating them, by diminishing them, by working around them, by rendering people less vulnerable to them, or by all of these routes—so that the number of people who gain weight to overweight and obese levels eventually stabilizes and then decreases (see Chapter 5). It also is highly likely that if we create an environment favorable for obesity prevention, efforts for treatment will be greatly enhanced.

Identifying Modifiable Determinants

The framework in Figure 1.4 was developed specifically to identify and show relationships among determinants of healthy eating and physical activity, thus informing intervention approaches. The development of the framework and conceptualization of each layer are described elsewhere in detail (Booth, Sallis, Ritenbaugh, Hill, Birch, Frank, Glanz, Himmelgreen, Mudd, Popkin, Rickard, St Jeor, & Hays, 2001; Wetter, Goldberg, King, Sigman-Grant, Baer, Crayton, Devine, Drewnowski, Dunn, Johnson, Pronk, Saelens, Snyder, Novelli, Walsh, & Warland, 2001). Although not specifically focused on obesity, the framework is very useful for understanding these two key of influences on obesity in context and as a reference point for which factors to consider when thinking through intervention possibilities. The framework

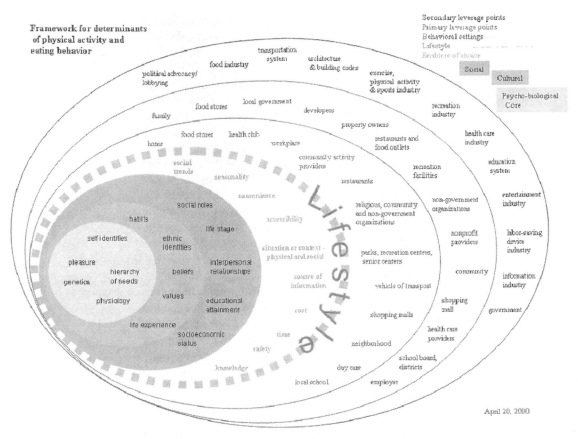

Figure 1.4 Framework for determinants of physical activity and eating behavior, developed by the Partnership to Promote Healthy Eating and Active Living
Source: Booth S.L. et al. (2001). Environmental and Societal Factors Affect Food Choice and Physical Activity: Rationale, Infuences, and Leverage Points. *Nutrition Reviews 59 (3 Part 2),* S21-S29. Reprinted with permission of the International Life Sciences Institue (ILSI)

uses an ecological model (see Chapter 5) to show multiple layers of interacting individual, societal and environmental variables that influence eating and physical activity behaviors in populations.

As noted in the discussion of energy balance, influences in the "psychobiologic core" are geared to avoiding hunger but are under-developed with respect to setting limits at the upper end of caloric intake. Few of the social and cultural variables are directly modifiable through health interventions, but they are critical aspects of the contexts in which such interventions take place and in which any associated behavior changes must be achieved and maintained. Influences identified within the layer of "enablers of choice"—the outer layer of what is labeled as "lifestyle"—may be the targets of interventions that focus on individuals or on their environments. For example, social marketing may be used to shape knowledge or affect trends, and policies may be developed to increase access to recommended options for healthy eating and physical activity.

An emphasis on identifying ways to exert influence through environmental and policy changes has increased generally in the related fields of public health and health promotion (Association of State and Territorial Directors of Health Promotion and Public Health Education, 2001; Institute of Medicine,

2003; Satcher, 2006; Smedley & Syme, 2000; Wallack & Dorfman, 1996) and is central to the current understanding of obesity prevention both within the United States and globally (Institute of Medicine, 2005; Kumanyika et al., 2002; Swinburn et al., 2004; World Health Organization, 2000, 2003). Finding solutions that affect whole populations but are remote from both the control and the personal behaviors of individuals is often termed working "upstream", in contrast to working with "downstream" influences more likely to affect individuals directly (see Chapter 5). Upstream issues and approaches are discussed in many of the chapters in this book, particularly in Section 2, which describes the "landscape" for obesity prevention, and also in Part 1 of Section 3, on influencing settings and organizations.

Overall, the task of obesity prevention is complex and challenging, involving determinants that extend from the innermost psychobiology of the individual to the broadest conceivable, global levels of agriculture, commerce, development, media, and marketing. For several of the levels in this model, there is presently limited knowledge of the causal influence of various factors and even less understanding of the interaction of factors *across* levels. Obesity is part of the larger picture of chronic disease risk, i.e., along with cardiovascular diseases, diabetes, and certain cancers. These conditions are influenced independently by changes in food intake and physical activity levels. Tobacco is also an important part of this equation, affecting cancers and cardiovascular diseases directly, and partly related to obesity in that concern about weight gain after smoking cessation may be a deterrent to smoking cessation.

Identifying Populations of Interest

Whole Population Approaches
The population of interest for obesity prevention is everyone. The concept of obesity prevention applies to the entire population throughout the life course. That is, it is never too early or too late to consider the elements needed to support healthy weight gain patterns or the achievement and maintenance of healthy weight. Within the United States, underweight now occurs only in conjunction with certain clinical or psychosocial disorders that are of relatively low frequency and is not a general public health concern. Hence, the focus is on prevention of excess weight gain and the factors that lead to it. During gestation and infancy this means setting a course for healthy early growth and development through appropriate maternal weight gain and infant feeding (see Chapter 18). During childhood and adolescence this means maintaining or adjusting growth and development trajectories to avoid excess weight gain, through the promotion of healthful eating and physical activity, thus maintaining energy balance (see Chapters 19 and 20). During adulthood this means maintaining eating and physical activity behaviors to avoid the 0.5 to 1 kg lifestyle-related annual weight gain (Lewis, Jacobs, McCreath, Kiefe, Schreiner, Smith, & Williams, 2000) or the larger weight gains that may occur during certain life transitions (e.g., early college years) or, in women, as a result of weight retained after pregnancy (see Chapter 21).

An enduring and elegant argument for a whole population focus was made by the British epidemiologist, Geoffrey Rose, in his classic book *The Strategy of Preventive Medicine* (1992) and is discussed in more detail in Chapter 5. Rose explains that for risk factors or conditions with a continuous distribution and graded risk, the objective of prevention is to reduce the prevalence by fostering a downward shift in the average levels in the population. As more people gain excess weight, the average BMI increases, the distribution widens, and the proportion of people above the cut off point of BMI 30 increases. The lower the population mean BMI, the smaller the proportion of people whose BMI levels will fall in the obese range. Rose also pointed out that population wide approaches are the most applicable and cost-effective when prevalence is high, as is the case for overweight and obesity in the United States. Even when such approaches are implemented on a large scale, the cost effectiveness relates to the savings on time- and cost-intensive screening and counseling programs, which are not needed when the entire population or community is to be reached (World Health Organization, 2000).

Many people, including health care professionals—who are attuned to a focus on interpersonal interventions and individual benefit—may be skeptical about or at least unfamiliar with the ability to mount effective population wide approaches or about their ultimate impact on individual behavior (Antipatis, Kumanyika, Jeffery, Morabia, & Ritenbaugh, 1999). The "prevention paradox" posed by Rose is that population wide approaches, which are designed to create population trends and promote modest changes in a large number of individuals, are difficult to associate with the benefits for any given individual (Rose, 1992). One benefit of whole population approaches is that they permit a focus on producing health, i.e., interventions to facilitate the achievement and maintenance of healthy weights, rather than only on preventing disease. Disease prevention can be interpreted as a minimalistic approach focused only on keeping people below a diagnostic threshold. A population-wide approach is also clearly justified by the nature of the epidemic, which is influenced by a complex set of factors across multiple levels of influence (Figure 1.4).

The whole population includes individuals with higher than average risk and with existing weight problems. Whole populations approaches improve the environment for obesity prevention for everyone, but special attention to high risk populations is part of a population strategy for primary prevention. This concept of complementarity between whole population and high risk approaches is contained in the World Health Organization framework for levels of obesity prevention (World Health Organization, 2000; see Chapter 5). Population wide approaches are termed "universal prevention." The term assigned to prevention efforts directed to high risk individuals and groups is "selective prevention." "Targeted prevention" refers to interventions for those with existing weight problems, e.g., prevention of further weight gain or complications.

High risk groups and individuals may be defined by familial characteristics (e.g., children who are not obese but whose parents are both obese), demographic characteristics (e.g., race/ethnicity or socioeconomic status (see Chapter 3)) or bio-behavioral circumstances (post partum women; post smoking cessation; starting medications that increase appetite or otherwise predispose to weight gain; or limited physical mobility) (Kumanyika & Daniels, 2006; Liou, Pi-Sunyer, & Laferrere, 2005; also see Chapter 21). The advantages of the high-risk approach relate primarily to its specificity—the potential for relative certainty, on all parts, that an appropriate intervention can be selected and is being applied directly to someone who can benefit.

Population by race/ethnicity

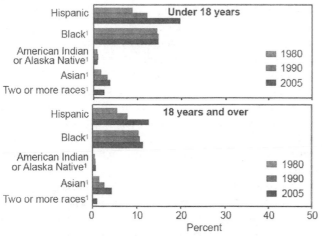

SOURCES: Centers for Disease Control and Prevention, National Center for Health Statistics, *Health, United States, 2006*, Figure 3. Data from the U.S. Census Bureau.

Figure 1.5 U.S. Population by race/ethnicity.

Source: National Center for Health Statistics, 2006.

High Risk Ethnic Minority Populations

As shown in Figure 1.5, ethnic minority populations (populations of color) constitute increasing proportions of the U.S. population. "Minority" populations are already in the majority in some states and cities (U.S. Census Bureau News, 2005). The higher prevalence of obesity in ethnic minority populations (see Tables 1.3 and 1.4) and, in some cases, the faster rate of increase in obesity require focused attention. Some ethnic minority populations are also overrepresented in the low income population (Figure 1.6). In Tables 1.3 and 1.4, prevalence differences by income are not striking in data for the population overall, but living below the poverty line is associated

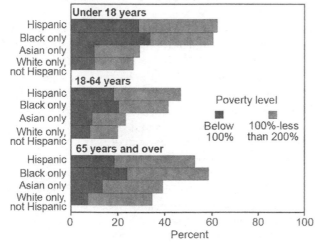

SOURCES: Centers for Disease Control and Prevention, National Center for Health Statistics, *Health, United States, 2006*, Figure 5. Data from the U.S. Census Bureau.

Figure 1.6 U.S. Low income population, 2004, by age and race-ethnicity.

Source: National Center for Health Statistics, 2006.

with higher levels of obesity in some population subgroups (see Chapter 3). In addition, trend analyses in NHANES data suggest that income related disparities in obesity may be increasing for older adolescents (Miech, Kumanyika, Stettler, Link, Phelan J.C., & Chang, 2006). The higher prevalence of obesity in populations of color is associated with an elevated risk of many chronic diseases to which obesity is a contributor (see Table 1.1) and this applies to children as well as adults (Kumanyika & Grier, 2006; Daniels, 2006). For example, cardiovascular diseases are the leading or second highest causes of death in all U.S. ethnic groups (National Center for Health Statistics, 2006). Obesity increases the risk of diabetes, and both obesity and diabetes increase cardiovascular disease risk in ethnic minority populations (Smith, Clark, Cooper, Daniels, Kumanyika, Ofili, Quinones, Sanchez, Saunders, & Tiukinhoy, 2005).

The task of obesity prevention takes on a different, more challenging character within ethnic minority and low income populations. The excess risk may result from an excess prevalence of several of the factors shown in Figure 1.4 (Kumanyika & Grier, 2006; Crawford, Wang, Krathwohl, & Ritchie, 2006; Kumanyika, 2002; Yancey, Kumanyika, Ponce, McCarthy, Fielding, Leslie, & Akbar, 2004). From an individual perspective, ethnocultural and psychobiological factors that are related to food intake or physical activity may predispose to overeating and inactivity. Culturally influenced food and physical activity preferences and attitudes about body weight are often cited as predisposing to positive energy balance in some ethnic minority populations. For example, food preferences and attitudes about physical activity may be especially geared to feasting when food is available, worrying about not having enough to eat, using food to cope with stress, and wanting to rest when not obliged to work, as a personal or culturally-determined response to adverse historical or political circumstances (Kumanyika, 2006). The status assigned to both televisions and automobiles by those seeking upward social mobility may predispose to sedentary behaviors (TV watching) and create a disinclination to follow advice to walk short distances. Higher levels of TV watching are reported in African American, Hispanic, and low income children and youth, in comparison to their white counterparts, and more have TV's in their bedrooms (Roberts, Foehr,Rideout & Brodie, 2004).

A strong orientation toward avoiding hunger may support the view that some excess weight is healthy. Being thin may imply a disease state or to leave insufficient protection against food shortages or unintentional weight loss (Brown & Konner, 1987; Kumanyika, 1993). Also, having very high levels of obesity within a community tends to render this socially normative (e.g., populations such as African American women, in which more than 50% have a BMI of 30 or more (Ogden et al, 2006)). For both these reasons, at a community or social level, the reaction to increasing levels of obesity may be less negative than would be expected based on attitudes in the general population. From an environmental and policy perspective, the circumstances of day-to-day life are also are more likely to promote obesity particularly in low income or minority communities, e.g., less access to healthy foods, more exposure to less healthy foods and lack of access to safe and appealing options for physical activity (Kumanyika, 2002; Kumanyika & Grier, 2006; Yancey et al, 2004; Taylor, Poston, Jones, & Kraft, 2006). These environmental influences may be synergistic with individual predispositions based on ethno-cultural and psy-chobiological factors. For example, ethnically targeted television advertising of high calorie low nutrient foods (Henderson & Kelly, 2006; Tirodkar & Jain, 2003) on television shows with a high African American viewership may interact with the high levels of television watching as well as food and physi-cal activity preferences to promote obesity in African American children (Kumanyika & Grier, 2006).

Behavioral risk factors and exposure to environmental risk factors in ethnic minority populations may be more prevalent in other areas as well. e.g., smok-ing and alcohol use, exposure to allergens, air pollution, environmental tobacco smoke, and less access to health care and preventive and treatment services (U.S. Department of Health & Human Services, 2006; Committee on Environmental Justice, 1999). In addition, socioeconomic factors such as lower income, inade-quate schools, and substandard housing disproportionately affect ethnic minori-ty populations (Gold & Wright, 2005; Lowry, Cann, Collins & Kolbe, 1996; Centers for Disease Control and Prevention, 2004). Taking obesity out of the mix would offer tremendous benefit. However, the ability to intervene effec-tively on obesity in high risk communities may be that much more difficult because multiple issues compete for attention (Kumanyika, 2005; Kumanyika & Morssink, 2006).

Understanding the Process: How will Prevention Work?

We now know that nothing short of a social transformation—however gradual—will change or counteract the many drivers of the chronic excess of energy intake over expenditure that is the proximal cause of high levels of obesity (Economos, Brownson, DeAngelis, Novelli, Foerster, Foreman, Gregson, Kumanyika, & Pate, 2001; Institute of Medicine, 2005). This is not such a radical statement. Not only are social transformations occurring on an ongoing basis, but retrospective analyses of other successes in public health demonstrate that it is possible to bring about such transformations by a set of deliberate and coordinated actions focused on a specific goal (Eriksen, 2005; Kersh & Morone, 2002a; 2002b; Yach, McKee, Lopez, & Novotny, 2005).

The issue of interest is how we can rapidly influence the next generation of social change in ways that will decrease population energy excess and weight levels. Many obesity-related programs and policies are being implemented even while research is just gearing up to build the evidence base about poten-tially effective solutions. It is difficult to know whether current efforts are on track or which set of strategies will create the synergy needed to create and run the course to an ultimate solution. But it is also impossible to "stop the train" with respect to the momentum that has built up in communities and advocacy circles to move an obesity prevention agenda. Moreover, we have to be realis-tic about the types of solutions that will be acceptable in the U.S. culture. Many of the elements that are drivers of the epidemic result from innovations that have been put in place to improve public health and make our lives better. We can't turn back the clock.

Programs and policies are proceeding based on a mix of experience in similar arenas such as tobacco, other efforts to reduce lifestyle risk factors for cancer and cardiovascular disease prevention, and common sense approaches to reversing societal trends that can be readily identified as logically related to the obesity epidemic. These initiatives are going forward within the boundaries of feasibility, which are influenced by various factors such as public opinion, political will, cultural and economic tradeoffs, and the strength of opposition from commercial vested interests. These early experiences, together with potential insights from related research—both positive and negative—are informing concepts and principles to guide future actions

In other words, how can we ensure that obesity prevention efforts succeed and contribute to longterm change? Here the "*we*" refers not just to the health professionals who are usually responsible for treatment programs, but much more broadly to include any professionals, policy makers, and consumer organizations with the ability to generate or implement solutions through the factors in Figure 1.4 (Kumanyika, 2001; see Chapter 5). As explained above, "*success*" means stopping the rise in the occurrence of obesity, e.g., keeping those who are not yet overweight or obese from becoming so, and achieving a downward shift in population average weight to levels that will decrease the incidence of obesity related morbidity and mortality and promote good health and quality of life in both the short and long term (Kumanyika et al., 2002).

How this Handbook will Help

To foster such a social transformation while also attending to the specific obesity prevention needs of individuals and communities is no small challenge. It requires an understanding of the task at hand. It also necessitates an understanding of the big picture in the background for social change, as well as the specific settings and options available for reaching and influencing the eating and physical activity options and behaviors of individuals. The three sections of this handbook follow this line of reasoning.

The next four chapters (Section 1) complete the overview by providing an in-depth understanding of the task by explaining how obesity is defined (Chapter 2), current prevalence and trends (Chapter 3), the costs of obesity (Chapter 4), and key prevention concepts, frameworks, and intervention approaches (Chapter 5).

Section 2 describes the relevant landscape and contextual background. Chapter 6 reviews how obesity is viewed by key consumer constituencies, including the general public and consumer advocacy groups, and considers evidence about stigmatization and bias, and issues of personal responsibility and individual choice. Chapter 7 describes governmental perspectives, including federal agency involvement and organization for combating obesity in policies, programs, and research as well as the relevant jurisdictions of state and local governments. Chapter 8 describes the domain and change mechanisms for city and regional planning as it influences the local infrastructure for food access and physical activity, i.e., "the built environment". Chapter 9 provides a perspective on the food industry as a major influence on and stakeholder in any large scale efforts to prevent obesity. Chapter 10 describes the roles of media and marketing in the context for obesity prevention. Chapter 11 completes the landscape by explaining how the U.S. obesity situation is related to global forces and by highlighting the nature of the epidemic in other countries.

Section 3 includes 10 chapters that focus on intervention considerations and approaches. Part 1 focuses on the how to's of approaching obesity prevention through organizational and systems change, i.e., changing environments and policies rather than only using organizations or settings as locations to reach individuals. A goal of this section is to promote quality and depth in this sphere of intervention, which is generally less well understood and practiced than more individually- and clinically-focused programs. Taking an inclusive view of the types of information and evidence that are relevant, both programmatic examples and formal research studies are included, as available and appropriate. Part 1 begins with a basic 'primer' about characteristics of organizations and systems (Chapter 12), including advice about how to assess organizational characteristics and about theoretical frameworks that can be useful when planning and evaluating programs to foster organizational change. Subsequent chapters are devoted to the main settings in which obesity prevention initiatives are being attempted: community-based settings (Chapter 13), health-care systems and settings (Chapter 14), worksite or occupational settings (Chapter 15), and school or group child care settings (Chapter 16).

Part 2 of Section 3 focuses on the "how to's" for obesity prevention at the individual and family level, i.e., health education or health promotion that involves education and counseling directed toward individuals. This part of the book begins with a primer on the principles of fostering individual behavior change using mass media or social marketing approaches as well as one-to-one interventions and group programs (Chapter 17). Subsequent chapters integrate literature and concepts across a variety of settings where one might reach the audience/age-group in question. Chapter 18 covers obesity prevention from gestation through the first year of life. The remaining chapters cover preschool and school-age years (Chapter 19), pre-adolescents and adolescents (Chapter 20), and adults (Chapter 21).

The concluding chapter of the book touches on several key issues that we believe are among the most pressing and promising areas that will move forward obesity prevention.

References

Antipatis, V. J., Kumanyika, S., Jeffery, R. W., Morabia, A., & Ritenbaugh , C. (1999). Confidence of health professionals in public health approaches to obesity prevention. *International Journal of Obesity and related metabolic disorders, 23*, 1004–1006.

Association of State and Territorial Directors of Health Promotion and Public Health Education (2001). *Policy and environmental change. New directions for Public Health*. Executive summary. Atlanta, GA: U.S. Centers for Disease Control and Prevention.

Booth, S. L., Sallis, J. F., Ritenbaugh, C., Hill, J. O., Birch, L. L., & Frank, L. D. et al. (2001). Environmental and societal factors affect food choice and physical activity rational, influences, and leverage points. *Nutrition reviews, 59*(3 Pt 2), S21–S39.

Bray, G. A., & Champagne, C. M. (2005). Beyond energy balance: There is more to obesity than kilocalories. *Journal of the American Dietetic Association, 105* (5 Suppl 1), S17–S23.

Bray, G. A. (2002). Historical development of scientific and cultural ideas. Chapter 23, In P. Bjorntorp & B. N. Brodoff (Eds.), *Obesity* (pp. 281–293). New York: J.B, Lippincott Company.

Brown, P. J., & Konner, M. (1987). An anthropological perspective on obesity. *Annals of the New York Academy of Science, 499*, 29–46.

Centers for Disease Control and Prevention (CDC). (2004). Health disparities experienced by Hispanics – United States. *MMWR Morbidity and Mortality Weekly Report, 53*, 935–937.

Centers for Disease Control and Prevention (1999). Ten great public health achievements – United States, 1900–1999. *MMWR Morbidity and Mortality Weekly Report, 48*, 241–243.

Comuzzie, A. G. (2002). The emerging pattern of the genetic contribution to human obesity. *Best practice & research: Clinical Endocrinology & Metabolism 16*, 611–621.

Crawford, P. B., Wang, M., Krathwohl, S., & Ritchie, L. Disparities in obesity. (2006). Prevalence, causes, and solutions. *Journal of Hunger and Environmental Nutrition, 1*, 27–48.

Daniels, S. R. (2006). The consequences of childhood overweight and obesity. *The Future of Children, 16*, 47–67.

Dietz, W. H. (2002). Genetic syndromes. Chapter 50, in P. Bjorntorp & B.N. Brodoff (Eds.) , *Obesity* (pp. 589–593). New York: J.B, Lippincott Company.

Dietz, W. H., & Gortmaker, S. L. (2001). Preventing obesity in children and adolescents. *Annual Review of Public Health. 22*, 337–353.

Ebbeling, C. B., Pawlak, D. B., & Ludwig, D. S. (2002). Childhood obesity. Public health crisis, common sense cure. *The Lancet, 360*, 473–482.

Economos, C. D., Brownson, R. C., DeAngelis, M. A., Novelli, P., Foerster, S. B., & Foreman, C. T., et. al., (2001). What lessons have been learned from other attempts to guide social change? *Nutrition Reviews, 59*, S40–S56.

Eriksenn, M. (2005). Lessons learned from public health efforts and their relevance to preventing childhood obesity, Appendix D. In Institute of Medicine, J.P. Koplan, C. T. Liverman, V. I. Kraak, (Eds.)., *Preventing childhood obesity. Health in the balance*, (pp. 405–442). Washington, D.C: National Academy Press.

Flegal, K. M., Carroll, M. D., Kuczmarski, R. J., & Johnson, C. L. (1998). Overweight and obesity in the United States. Prevalence and trends, 1960–1994. *International Journal of Obesity, 22*, 39–47.

French, S. A., Story, M., & Jeffery, R. W. (2001). Environmental influences on eating and physical activity. *Annual Review of Public Health, 22*, 309–335.

Friedman, J. M. (2003). A war on obesity, not the obese. *Science, 299*, 856.

Gold, D. R., & Wright, R. (2005). Population disparities in asthma. *Annual Review of Public Health, 26*, 89–113.

Gortmaker, S. L., Dietz, W. H., Jr., Sobol, A. M., & Wehler, C. A. (1987). Increasing pediatric obesity in the United States. *American Journal of Diseases of Children, 141*, 535–540.

Harris, T. B., Savage, P. J., Tell, G. S., Haan, M., Kumanyika, S., & Lynch, J. C. (1997). Carrying the burden of cardiovascular risk in old age: Associations of weight and weight change with prevalent cardiovascular disease, risk factors, and health status in the Cardiovascular Health Study. *American Journal of Clinical Nutrition, 66*, 837–844.

Henderson, V. R., & Kelly, B. (2005). Food advertising in the age of obesity: Content analysis of food advertising on general market and African American television. *Journal of Nutrition Education and Behavior, 37*, 191–196.

Hill, J. O., Wyatt, H. R., Reed, G. W., & Peters, J. C. (2003). Obesity and the environment: Where do we go from here? *Science, 299*, 853–855.

Hill, J. O., & Peters, J. C. (1998). Environmental contributions to the obesity epidemic. *Science, 280*, 1371–1374.

Institute of Medicine. (1999). Committee on environmental justice. *Toward environmental justice: Research, education, and health policy needs.* Washington, D. C.: National Academies Press.

Institute of Medicine. (2003). *The future of the public's health in the 21st century.* Washington, DC: The National Academies Press.

Institute of Medicine , Koplan, J. P., Liverman, C. T., & Kraak, V. I. (Eds.) (2005). *Preventing childhood obesity, Health in the balance*. Washington, D. C.: National Academy Press, Institute of Medicine.

James, W. P. T. (2006). The challenge of childhood obesity. *International Journal of Pediatric Obestiy*, *1*, 7–10.

Kersh, R., & Morone, J. (2002a). The politics of obesity: Seven steps to government action. *Health Affairs (Millwood)*, *21*, 142–153.

Kersh, R., & Morone, J. (2002b). How the personal becomes the political. Prohibitions, public health, and obesity. *Studies in American Political Development,*. *16*, 162–175.

Kuczmarski, R. J. (1992). Prevalence of overweight and weight gain in the United States. *American Journal of Clinical Nutrition*, *55*, 495S–502S.

Kuczmarski, R. J., Flegal, K. M., Campbell, S. M., & Johnson, C. L. (1994). Increasing prevalence of overweight among U.S. adults. The National Health and Nutrition Examination Surveys, 1960–1991. *Journal of the American Medical Association*, *272*, 205–211.

Kuczmarski, R. J., Ogden, C. L., Grummer-Strawn, L. M., Flegal, K. M., Guo, S. S., & Wei, R. et al. (2000). CDC growth charts: United States. *Advance data*, *8*(314), 1–27.

Kumanyika, S. K. (2001). Minisymposium on obesity: Overview and some strategic considerations. *Annual Review of Public Health*, *22*, 293–308.

Kumanyika, S. K. (2002). Obesity treatment in minorities. In T. A. Wadden, & A. J. Stunkard (Eds.), *Handbook of obesity treatment* (3rd ed. pp. 416–446). New York: Guilford Publications, Inc.,

Kumanyika, S. (2005 September 15). Obesity, health disparities, and prevention paradigms: Hard questions and hard choices. *Preventing Chronic diseases*, *2*(4), A02, Epub.

Kumanyika, S. (2006). Nutrition and chronic disease prevention: Priorities for U.S. minority groups. *Nutrition reviews* *64*(2 Pt 2), S9–S14.

Kumanyika, S., & Grier, S. (2006). Targeting interventions for ethnic minority and low-income populations. *Future of Children*, *16*, 187–207.

Kumanyika, S., Jeffery, R. W., Morabia, A., Ritenbaugh, C., & Antipatis, V. J. (2002). Public Health Approaches to the Prevention of Obesity (PHAPO) Working group of the International Obesity Task Force (IOTF). Obesity prevention: The case for action. *International Journal of Obesity and related metabolic disorders,* *26*, 425–436.

Kumanyika, S. K., & Morssink, C. B. (2006). Bridging domains in efforts to reduce disparities in health and health care. *Health Education Behavior*, *33*, 440–458.

Kumanyika, S. K. (1993). Special issues regarding obesity in minority populations. *Annals of Internal Medicine*, *119*, 650–654.

Kumanyika, S. K., & Daniels, S. R. (2006). Obesity Prevention. In G. A. Bray &, D. H. Ryan (Eds.), *Overweight and the Metabolic Syndrome: From Bench to Bedside* (Endocrine Updates) (pp. 233–254). New York: Springer Verlay.

Lee, C. D., Blair, S. N., & Jackson, A. S. (1999). Cardiorespiratory fitness, body composition, and all-cause and cardiovascular disease mortality in men. *American Journal of Clinical Nutrition*, *69*, 373–380.

Lew, E. A. (1985). Mortality and weight: Insured lives and the American Cancer Society studies. *Annals of Internal Medicine*, *103*(6 Pt 2), 1024–1029.

Lewis, C. E., Jacobs, D. R., Jr., McCreath, H., Kiefe, C. I., Schreiner, P. J., Smith, D. E., & Williams, O. D. (2002). Weight gain continues in the 1990s: 10-year trends in weight and overweight from the CARDIA study. Coronary artery risk development in young adults. *American Journal of Epidemiology.*, *151*, 1172–1181.

Liou, T. H., Pi-Sunyer, F. X., & Laferrere, B. (2005). Physical disability and obesity. *Nutrition reviews*, *63*, 321–331.

Lowry, F. R., Kann, L., Collins, J. L., & Kolbe, L. J. (1996). The effect of socioeconomic status on chronic disease risk behaviors among U.S. adolescents. *Journal of the American Medical Association*, *276*, 792–797.

Miech, R. A., Kumanyika, S. K., Stettler, N., Link, B. G., Phelan, J. C., & Chang, V. W. (2006). Trends in the association of poverty with overweight among U.S. adolescents, 1971–2004. *Journal of the American Medical Association, 295*, 2385–2393.

Mokdad, A. H., Serdula, M. K., Dietz, W. H., Bowman, B. A., Marks, J. S., & Koplan, J. P. (2000). The continuing epidemic of obesity in the United States. *Journal of the American Medical Association, 284*, 1650–1651.

Mokdad, A. H., Serdula, M. K., Dietz, W. H., Bowman, B. A., Marks, J. S., & Koplan, J. P. (1999). The spread of the obesity epidemic in the United States, 1991–1998. *Journal of the American Medical Association, 282*, 1519–1522.

National Center for Health Statistics (2006). *Health, United States, 2006 With Chartbook on Trends in the Health of Americans*, Hyattsville, MD. DHHS Publication number 2006–1232.

National Heart, Lung, and Blood Institute Obesity Education Initiative. (1998). Clinical guidelines on the identification, evaluation, and treatment of overweight and obesity in adults. *Obesity Research. 6*(Suppl. 2).

Ogden, C. L., Carroll, M. D., Curtin, L. R., McDowell, M. A., Tabak, C. J., & Flegal, K. M. (2006). Prevalence of overweight and obesity in the United States, 1999–2004. *Journal of the American Medical Association, 295*, 1549–1555.

Papavramidou, N. S., Papavramidis, S. T., & Christopoulou-Aletra, H. (2004). Galen on obesity: Etiology, effects, and treatment. *World Journal of Surgery, 28*, 631–635.

Roberts, D. F., Foehr, U. G., Rideout, V. J., & Brodie, M. (2004). *Kids and media in America*. New York: Cambridge University Press.

Rose, G. (1992). *The strategy of preventive medicine*. New York: Oxford University Press.

Russell, C. M., Williamson, D. F., & Byers, T. (1995). Can the year 2000 objective for reducing overweight in the United States be reached? A simulation study of the required changes in body weight. *International Journal of Obesity 19*, 149–153.

Sachdev, M. S., Riely, C. A., & Madan, A. K. (2006). Nonalcoholic fatty liver disease of obesity. *Obesity Surgery, 16*, 1412–1419.

Satcher, D. (2006). The prevention challenge and opportunity. *Health Affairs (Millwood), 25*, 1009–1011.

Smedley, B. D., & Syme, S. L. (Eds.). (2000). *Promoting health. Intervention strategies from social and behavioral research*. Washington, D. C.: National Academy Press.

Smith, S. C., Jr., Clark, L. T., Cooper, R. S., Daniels, S. R., Kumanyika, S. K. & Ofili, E. (2005). American heart association obesity, metabolic syndrome, and hypertension writing group. Discovering the full spectrum of cardiovascular disease: Minority health summit 2003: Report of the obesity, metabolic syndrome, and hypertension writing group. *Circulation, 111*(10), e134–e139.

Swinburn, B. A., Caterson, I., Seidell, J. C., & James, W. P. (2004). Diet, nutrition and the prevention of excess weight gain and obesity. *Public Health Nutrition, 7*(Suppl. 1A), 123–146.

Szklo, M. (2001). The evaluation of epidemiologic evidence for policy-making. *American Journal of Epidemiology,154* (Suppl. 12.), S13–S17.

Taylor, W. C., Poston, W. S. C., Jones, L., & Kraft, M. K. (2006). Environmental justice. Obesity, physical activity, and healthy eating. *Journal of Physical Activity and Health*, 3(Suppl. 1), S30–S55.

Tirodkar, M. A., & Jain, A. (2003). Food messages on African American television shows. *American Journal of Public Health*, 93, 439–441.

Troiano, R., Flegal, K. M., Kuczmarski, R. J., Campbell, S. M., & Johnson, C. L. (1995). Overweight prevalence and trends for children and adolescents. The national health and nutrition examination surveys, 1963–1991. *Archives of Pediatric Adolescent Medicine, 149*, 1085–1091.

U.S. Census Bureau News (2005). Texas becomes nation's newest "Majority-Minority" State, Census Bureau Announces, August 11 http://www.census.gov/Press-Release/www/releases/archives/population/005514.html

U.S. Department of Health and Human Services & U.S. Department of Agriculture (2005). *Dietary Guidelines for Americans.* www.healthierus.gov/dietaryguidelines

U.S. Department of Health and Human Services (2001). *The surgeon general's call to action to prevent and decrease overweight and obesity.* Rockville, MD. U.S. Department of health and human services, public health service. Office of the surgeon general. Washington, DC: U.S. Government Printing Office.

U.S. Department of Health and Human Services (2000). *Healthy people 2010.* 2nd ed. *Understanding and improving health and objectives for improving health.* 2 vols. Washington, DC: U.S. Government Printing Office, www.healthypeople.gov

U.S. Department of Health and Human Services (2002). *Healthy people 2010 progress review. Diabetes,* www.healthypeople.gov

U.S. Department of Health and Human Services (2003a). *Healthy people 2010 progress review. Heart disease and stroke.* www.healthypeople.gov

U.S. Department of Health and Human Services (2003b). *Healthy people 2010 progress review. Tobacco use.* www.healthypeople.gov

U.S. Department of Health and Human Services (2004). *Healthy people 2010 progress review. Nutrition and overweight.* www.healthypeople.gov

U.S. Preventive Services Task Force (2003). Screening for obesity in adults. Recommendation and rationale. *Annals of Internal Medicine, 139,* 930–932.

Visscher, T. L., & Seidell, J. C. (2001). The public health impact of obesity. *Annual Review of Public Health, 22,* 355–375.

Wallack, L., & Dorfman, L. (1996). Media advocacy: A strategy for advancing policy and promoting health. *Health Education Quarterly, 23,* 293–317.

Wang, Y., & Lobstein, T. (2006). Worldwide trends in childhood overweight and obesity. *International Journal of Pediatric Obesity, 1,* 11–25.

Wang, Y. C., Gortmaker, S. L., Sobol, A. M., & Kuntz, K. M. (2006). Estimating the energy gap among U.S. children: A counterfactual approach. *Pediatrics, 118,* e1721–e1733.

Wei, M., Kampert, J. B., Barlow, C. E., Nichaman, M. Z., Gibbons, L. W., & Paffenbarger, R. S., Jr., et al. (1999). Relationship between low cardiorespiratory fitness and mortality in normal-weight, overweight, and obese men. *Journal of the American Medical Association, 282,* 1547–1553.

Wetter, A. C., Goldberg, J. P., King, A. C., Sigman-Grant, M., Baer, R., & Crayton, E. et al. (2001). How and why do individuals make food and physical activity choices? *Nutrition Reviews, 59*(3 pt 2), S11–S20.

Whitlock, E. P., Williams, S. B., Gold, R., Smith, P. R., & Shipman, S. A. (2005). Screening and interventions for childhood overweight: A summary of evidence for the U.S. Preventive Services Task Force. *Pediatrics, 116,* e125–e144.

Wing, R. R., & Phelan, S. (2005). Long-term weight loss maintenance. *American Journal of Clinical Nutrition, 82*(Suppl. 1), 222S–225S.

World Health Organization (2000). *Obesity: Preventing and managing the global epidemic.* WHO Technical report series 894. Geneva.

World Health Organization (2003). *Diet, nutrition and the prevention of chronic diseases.* WHO Technical report series 916. Geneva.

Wynder, E. L. (1987). Workshop on guidelines to the epidemiology of weak associations. *Introduction Preventive Medicine, 16,* 139–141.

Yach, D., McKee, M., Lopez, A. D., & Novotny, T. (2005). Improving diet and physical activity: 12 lessons from controlling tobacco smoking. *British Medical Journal, 330,* 898–900.

Yancey, A. K., Kumanyika, S. K., Ponce, N. A., McCarthy, W. J., Fielding, J. E., Leslie, J. P., & Akbar, J. (2004 Jan). Population-based interventions engaging communities of color in healthy eating and active living: A review. *Preventing Chronic diseases, 1*(1), A09.

Chapter 2

What is Obesity? Definitions Matter

Robert J. Kuczmarski

Introduction

The term *obesity* can conjure various mental images that may have subjective or objective connotations, depending upon the knowledge, experience, or background one may have. For trained professionals in the medical, public health, and science fields, whether clinical researchers or health care providers, obesity may indicate a condition that not only can be objectively measured but may also immediately bring to mind a heightened awareness of increased risk for associated adverse health outcomes. To others, *obesity* may bring to the surface social prejudices, biases, or perceptions that often result in preconceived notions of what the obese person's demeanor, tendencies, or abilities might be. This may be reflected for example, in job hiring and promotion practices affecting obese adults at the worksite or in social acceptance or discrimination among obese children on the playground. In such cases, the *definition* of obesity is often loosely based on a visual impression or a preconceived mental attitude about the phenotypic expression or cosmetic appearance of a body size that is considered large.

The term *overweight* is often used interchangeably with obesity, although it sometimes may be construed as a somewhat diluted and therefore less ominous degree of obesity, which also may to some extent reduce the related perceptions, whether they be objectively medically based or subjectively socially based. There are a variety of other lay and professional terms that may be encountered such as *full-figured, heavy, or thick* but these are either not in general use or have limited practical utility for most scientific, clinical, or public health applications.

The term obesity, strictly speaking, means excess adipose tissue or excess body fat beyond a threshold for what is considered a norm or a reference value. More specifically, to quote Villareal et al. (2005), "Obesity is defined as an unhealthy excess of body fat, which increases the risk of medical illness and premature mortality." Although it is possible to have excess adiposity in the presence of reduced muscle mass (sarcopenic obesity) and a concomitant normal weight, in the general population, people who are obese are almost always overweight. The converse, however, does not follow this general pattern; all overweight people are not obese. There may be situations where the amount of body fat is normal, but the amount of muscle mass is large, rendering the classification as overweight but not over-fat.

As will be discussed, the amount of total body fat is important although fat distribution is also highly correlated with adverse health outcomes. So the concept of regional adiposity is one that may come into play when defining obesity, where the specific focus is on the excess deposition of intra-abdominal or visceral adipose tissue which can be sub-divided further into omental, mesenteric, and retroperitoneal fat (Shen et al., 2003). It is possible that in the future, with advancements in imaging capabilities or even with the use of biomarkers, regional obesity may be more highly specified beyond visceral obesity. For example, "omental obesity" conceivably could be a term used more in the future since fatty acids, cytokines, and hormones from omental adipocytes entering the portal circulation may increase risk for glucose intolerance, type 2 diabetes, and other abnormalities (Haslam & James, 2005). Abdominal adiposity is emerging as an active area of research investigation notably among some Asian populations where the outward appearance of obesity may not be apparent, but the internal metabolic disturbances are manifested through the metabolic syndrome and perhaps other chronic conditions and diseases (Steering Committee of the Western Pacific Region of the World Health Organization, International Association for the Study of Obesity, International Obesity Task Force, 2000).

There are various applications and settings in which screening and identification of overweight or obesity are useful. For epidemiological purposes, it is useful to have measures that will permit the assessment of incidence, prevalence, and trends over time. Obesity influences numerous risk factors and disease conditions. Therefore, analytically it is useful to incorporate either continuous or categorical indicators of obesity in their role as correlates, mediators, moderators, confounders, or covariates in analyses that evaluate or control for obesity. In clinical research and office practice, indicators of obesity are used to monitor individuals and track progress of obesity prevention or treatment interventions. Assessment of abdominal obesity is recommended for routine clinical screening although such measurements are not made as routinely as they could be (NHLBI Obesity Education Initiative Expert Panel on the Identification, Evaluation, and Treatment of Overweight and Obesity in Adults, 1998).

Measurements

For screening, identification, and classification of obesity in clinical settings or in epidemiological surveys or surveillance programs, tools and procedures that are simple, quick, inexpensive, valid (accurate), and reliable (reproducible) continue to be highly regarded. Body weight is a measure that meets these criteria. However, because there is variation across individuals in length (for infants) or standing height it is desirable to consider weight adjusted for height. Therefore, weight and height should typically be measured and then used in combination to interpret weight status adjusted for height, in comparison with established references or standards.

Weight-height indices have been in use for a long time. The Quetelet Index (weight/height^2; kg/m^2) was first proposed in 1869 by Adolphe Quetelet

(Weigley, 1989). Over time the Quetelet index has continued to be used, but as proposed by Keys et al. (1972) the Quetelet Index has come to be more commonly known and referred to as the Body Mass Index or BMI. The BMI is now the most commonly used index of weight adjusted for height to define overweight and obesity. There is an earlier body of literature that examined the origin, characteristics, performance, and comparisons of various weight-height indices in more detail (Florey, 1970; Lee et al., 1981; Norgan & Ferro-Luzzi, 1982; Garrow, 1983; Garrow & Webster, 1985). The overall goal when using weight-height indices to define obesity is to assess body weight, adjusting for height, such that the index yields a measure of weight relatively independent of height. This concept led previous investigators to examine wt/ht^p where the value of the exponent p yielded an index that would maximize the correlation with adiposity, given the assumption that adiposity is independent of height (Benn, 1971). However, BMI assessed as weight divided by the square of height, and on the metric scale, has proven to be the most generally useful.

The only direct way to measure total body fat is through chemical analysis of cadavers. All other methods currently available are considered indirect measures. BMI is often referred to as an obesity index because it is moderately to highly correlated with other quantitative estimates of percent body fat. The correlations range from $r = 0.6$ to 0.8, depending on age group, gender, and method used to quantify body fat (Roche, 1996). Using dual emission x-ray absorptiometry (DXA) in adolescents for example, Steinberger et al. (2005) reported a correlation between DXA and BMI of $r = 0.85$ for percent body fat and $r = 0.95$ for fat mass. Consistent with the findings of other investigators and in other age groups, these associations were stronger in heavier persons.

For the majority of people in the general population, higher BMI values will be indicative of higher levels of body fatness. However, there may be exceptions in certain subgroups of the population where higher body mass values are attributable to excess lean mass (muscle) instead of fat, such as in body builders, professional athletes, or military personnel, resulting in an erroneous overestimate of body fatness. Higher BMI values associated with higher lean mass may also apply to certain ethnic groups such as Pacific Islanders, who may have higher than average BMI levels but also higher levels of muscularity for a given BMI level in comparison to other populations (Rush et al., 2004). Similarly, in the elderly who lose muscle mass with advancing age or in persons of any age who lose lean mass as a result of disease or infirmity, BMI may underestimate body fat. It is therefore recommended that users be cognizant of situations or individuals for whom BMI may not be a valid indicator of total body fatness.

There are other methods that can be used either in place of the BMI approach or in addition to it for the purpose of verification of relative fatness. These range from the simple, lower risk, lower burden, and less expensive subcutaneous skinfold measurements through bioelectrical impedance analysis (BIA) and ultrasound, to hydrodensitometry, DXA, magnetic resonance imaging, and computerized tomography (CT) scans (Roche, Heymsfield, & Lohman, 1996) (Table 2.1). These approaches are based on prediction equations for estimating total body fatness indirectly or may only focus on regional estimates of fatness, and rise in complexity of measurement, cost, risk, expense, and general predictive value compared to the simpler weight and height measures that constitute the BMI. The scientific

Table 2.1 Brief descriptions of various methods to estimate body fat.

Skinfolds	Skinfold calipers measure a double fold of skin and subcutaneous adipose tissue at selected sites on the body to estimate percent body fat from prediction equations
Ultrasound	Ultrasound uses high frequency sound waves to image the thickness of fat tissue at selected sites on the body to estimate percent body fat from prediction equations
BIA	Bioelectrical impedance analysis measures total body water, from which lean body mass, total body fat, and percent body fat can be estimated from prediction equations
Hydrodensitometry	Underwater weighing estimates body density from which percent fat and percent body fat can be estimated from prediction equations
DXA	Dual energy x-ray absorptiometry uses low energy x-rays to estimate fat content in bone-free lean tissue
MRI	Magnetic resonance imaging images and estimates subcutaneous and visceral adipose tissue at cross sectional sites on the body
CT	Computerized tomography uses high energy x-rays to image cross-sectional areas of adipose tissue, muscle, and bone.

Source: Roche, Heymsfield, & Lohman (Eds.) (1996). Human Body Composition. Champaign, Il: Human Kinetics.

literature is replete with prediction equations for skinfold measurements and the various other procedures such as ultrasound and BIA, indicating the limitation that prediction equations tend to be specific to the samples of people on which they were developed and often can not be generalized to other groups.

Adults

Interpretation of Measures based on Weight and Height

In research and clinical settings, overweight is defined as weight that exceeds an established criterion threshold value. The threshold may be a statistical cut-off point based either on observed population distributions of measured weight, or on the level of weight beyond which morbidity, other health risk factors, or mortality outcomes increase.

The Metropolitan Life Insurance Company (MLIC) weight-for-height tables were widely used in the U.S. over a 25-year period from approximately 1960 to 1985 in the assessment of weight status for adult men and women. The tables were derived from distributions of weight-for-height associated with minimal mortality among a large group of persons in the United States and Canada at the time they purchased life insurance policies during the period 1935 to 1972. The MLIC tables began to be phased out in the mid-1980s when gender-specific BMI criteria derived from the second National Health and Nutrition Examination Survey (NHANES II) conducted from 1976 to 1980 became available. For approximately the next 15 years from 1985 to 2000 in the U.S., overweight in adults was defined as a BMI ≥27.8 for men and ≥27.3 for women ages 20 years and older. These BMI cutoff points represented the gender-specific 85th percentile values of the BMI distribution for persons aged 20–29 years in NHANES II. The rationale for selecting this age group as the reference population was based on the concept that young adults are relatively lean and the increase in body weight that usually occurs with age is due almost entirely to accretion of excess body fat (Van Itallie, 1985). The limitations of the MLIC height-weight tables and a chronology of the multiple criteria and definitions that led to the current BMI-based classifications of healthy weight, overweight, and obesity have been described in some detail (Kuczmarski & Flegal, 2000).

Following the publication in 1998 of a National Institutes of Health (NIH) report on clinical guidelines for the identification, evaluation, and treatment of overweight and obesity (NHLBI, 1998), from the late 1990s to the present time for all adults, weight categories and corresponding risk have been defined as: healthy weight, BMI = 18.5–24.9 (normal risk); overweight, BMI = 25.0–29.9 (increased risk); obesity BMI ≥30.0 (high to extremely high risk), with subclasses of obesity consistent with those recommended by the World Health Organization (WHO) for international applications and comparisons (class I, BMI 30–34.9; class II, BMI 35.0–39.9; class III, BMI ≥40.0) as indicated in Table 2.2. The World Health Organization (WHO, 1998) classified weight by BMI as follows: normal weight, BMI = 18.5–24.9 (average risk); overweight, BMI ≥25.0; pre-obese, BMI = 25.0–29.9 (increased risk); and class 1, 2, and 3 obesity: BMI = 30.0–34.9 (moderate risk); BMI = 35.0–39.9 (severe risk); and BMI ≥40.0 (very severe risk), respectively. These cutoff points are useful for screening purposes but regardless of which cutoff points are used, when making clinical evaluations for individuals, abdominal circumference, age, ethnicity, gender, clinical history, and presence of other related risk factors should be considered (Bray, 1998a; WHO Expert Consultation, 2004).

Table 2.2 Classification of overweight and obesity by BMI, waist circumference, and associated disease risk[*]

	BMI (kg/m²)	Obesity class	Disease risk[*] Men ≤40 in (≤102 cm) Women ≤35 in (≤88 cm)	>40 in (>102 cm) >35 in (>88 cm)
Underweight	<18.5			
Normal[†]	18.5–24.9			
Overweight	25.0–29.9		Increased	High
Obesity	30.0–34.9	I	High	Very high
	35.0–39.9	II	Very high	Very high
Extreme obesity	≥40.0	III	Extremely high	Extremely high

Source: NHLBI Obesity Education Initiative Expert Panel on the Identification, Evaluation, and Treatment of Overweight and Obesity in Adults (2000).

[*] Relative to normal weight and waist circumference, disease risk for type 2 diabetes, hypertension, and CVD.

[†] Increased waist circumference can also be a marker for increased risk even in persons of normal weight.

Body Fat Ranges

With regard to body fat levels to distinguish normal from abnormal or obese, there is no single cutoff value for percent fat. Instead, body fatness expressed as total body fat as a percentage of body weight is described within ranges. Furthermore, there are gender differences whereby normal body fat can range from approximately 12 to 20% for males and 20 to 30% for females. Understanding that fatness occurs across a range in the population, body fat levels greater than approximately 25% for males or 33% for females generally may be used to indicate obesity (Bray, 1998b).

Gallagher et al. (2000) subsequently confirmed these estimated fat levels in white, African American, and Asian subjects in a study designed to develop percentage body fat ranges that correspond to widely accepted BMI guidelines. Using the criterion of obesity at a BMI ≥ 30.0, the corresponding predicted percentage body fat by age group for white and African American males was 25% at 20–29 years, 28% at 40–59 years, and 30% at 60–79 years. Among women, the percentage body fat corresponding to obesity was 39% at 20–29 years, 40% at 40–59 years, and 42% at 60–79 years. At any BMI level, Asians had a significantly higher percentage body fat than white or African American men and women. As will be discussed, this finding of relatively higher body fat in Asian Americans has implications for the use of cutoff points used to define overweight and obesity.

Regional Obesity

BMI remains the most widely used indicator to define overweight and obesity, based on total body weight adjusted for height as an indictor of total body fatness. However, it is well established that beyond the amount of total adiposity, the distribution of fat on the body is strongly related to health outcomes as well. The distribution of stored fat can be broadly characterized as fat stored peripherally on the extremities (arms and legs) and fat stored centrally on the torso of the body. In the 1940s Jean Vague characterized general fat patterns based on the typical fat distribution observed in men and women. Men tend to have more fat in the abdominal region and this was described as the android or male pattern. In contrast, women tend to have more fat stored in the hip/buttocks region and this was termed the gynoid or female pattern. Vague (1956) subsequently noted increased risk for adverse health outcomes with the male fat distribution pattern. In the 1980s the scientific literature identifying increased risk with abdominal fatness and a host of adverse health outcomes expanded tremendously, further establishing the importance of defining regional obesity (Seidell, Deurenberg, & Hautvast, 1987; Seidell, 1992; Emery et al., 1993).

Abdominal circumference measures are only a surrogate for abdominal adiposity and the more influential visceral fat mass. It appears that the intra-abdominal or visceral fat is the component generally found to be more highly associated with metabolic abnormalities in contrast to subcutaneous abdominal fat. However, the contribution of subcutaneous fat patterning (upper-versus lower-body or truncal/torso versus peripheral/limbs) to the metabolic disturbances associated with upper-body obesity remains uncertain. Variations in findings may be linked with different methodologies to measure fat compartments, including the instrumentation and the site of the fat depot, as well as the outcome variable. For example, in a study of obese women, elevated triglyceride levels were most highly associated with increased visceral fat measured by DXA, whereas insulin resistance was related to increased truncal fat mass measured by skinfold measurements (Albu, Kovera, & Johnson, 2000).

Measurement of the internal visceral fat store is best accomplished with more sophisticated procedures such as magnetic resonance imaging or computerized tomography, although these procedures are more complex and expensive than simpler anthropometric procedures such as circumference measurements. The waist-to-hip circumference ratio (WHR) was used for a period of time and showed increased cardiovascular and type 2 diabetes risk, when defined at a WHR >0.90 cm for men and a WHR >0.80 for women (Albu et al., 1997). It was later shown that a measure of abdominal circumference alone was more predictive of increased risk and could be used as a surrogate marker of visceral adiposity in lieu of WHR (Despres et al., 1989; Lean, Han, & Morrison, 1995). A case-control study of persons with type 2 diabetes and matched controls found that among various measures of central obesity, waist circumference was the strongest predictor of risk (Mamtani & Kulkarni, 2005). Another case-control study of participants from 52 countries showed a higher correlation for waist-to-hip ratio with myocardial infarction risk than did either BMI or waist circumference alone (Yusuf et al., 2005). These investigators suggested that loss of muscle mass in the hip area with decreased physical activity or overall weight reduction may increase risk, although this remains a plausible but insufficiently documented hypothesis. Abdominal circumference is a diagnostic screening tool included as part of a small constellation of measures for assessing the metabolic syndrome (Klein et al., 2004). The International Diabetes Federation (2005) has proposed the use of ethnic-specific waist circumference measures when screening for the metabolic syndrome.

Because abdominal circumference provides an independent prediction of risk beyond that of BMI, in adults with a BMI <35.0 it is a recommended measurement to define abdominal obesity. In persons with a BMI >35, abdominal circumference measurements and BMI are highly correlated and predictive of increased risk for adverse health outcomes associated with obesity. In obese African American men and women with BMI ranging from 30 to 50 kg/m^2, abdominal circumference was reported to predict obesity related co-morbidity risk beyond that obtained by BMI alone (Hope et al., 2005). This study and others suggest that abdominal circumference is an important clinical screening tool in the assessment of obesity health risk. Based on the waist circumference measurement, high-risk abdominal obesity in U.S. adults is defined as a value >102 cm (40 in.) for men and >88 cm (35 in.) for women (NHLBI, 1998). To identify individuals in need of treatment, measurement of abdominal circumference can be an important screening tool for those at a healthy weight (BMI <25.0) and with a large abdominal circumference, although relatively few persons meet this criterion. Among overweight (BMI 25.0–29.9) and obese (BMI ≥30.0) adults, waist circumference appears to add little information beyond BMI alone for identifying individuals in need of weight-loss treatment (Kiernan & Winkleby, 2000) although with increasing BMI and abdominal circumference values, disease risk also increases (Table 2.2).

Defining Obesity Across Racial/Ethnic Groups and in Older Men and Women

There are important racial/ethnic differences that influence both the relative utility of abdominal circumference or BMI as indicators of health risk as well as the definition of obesity using these measures. Studies comparing the association of BMI with percent body fat in Hispanics have been limited. In an investigation of Hispanic Americans, African Americans, and non-Hispanic white Americans, Fernandez et al. (2003) reported no differences in the relation between BMI and percent fat in men from the three ethnic groups, or between black and white women. However, at a BMI <30, Hispanic-American women had more body fat than women of European or African descent, suggesting a potential underestimation in the relative degree of fatness among Hispanic-American women compared to women from the other major race/ethnic groups. However, whereas definitions of obesity based on BMI and abdominal circumference work quite well for white and African American groups, and perhaps generally for most other ethnic groups, substantial evidence suggests that persons of Asian descent may require a different definition of obesity. Characterizations of ethnic differences in obesity prevalence are influenced by these definitional issues, as discussed in chapter 3.

There is evidence that for Asians, obesity should be defined at a considerably lower BMI cutoff point and abdominal circumference may be an equally or more effective indicator of disease risk than BMI (Klatsky & Armstrong, 1991; Fujimoto et al., 1991). Although there are exceptions for some Asian subgroups, in general, at the same age, gender, and BMI level, percentage body fat is higher in Asians than in white persons, or in other words, at a given level of body fat, Asians have lower BMI levels than white persons. The Examination Committee of Criteria for Obesity Disease in Japan of the Japan Society for the Study of Obesity (2002) concluded that at initial screening of Japanese adults, obesity should be defined as a BMI ≥25.0; visceral fat obesity should be defined as a BMI ≥25.0 and a waist circumference ≥85 cm in men or ≥90 cm in women.

The Steering Committee of the Western Pacific Region of the World Health Organization (2000) proposed that overweight in adult Asians be defined as BMI ≥23.0, obesity as BMI ≥25.0, and high risk waist circumference ≥ 90 cm for men and ≥ 80 cm for women. Among Chinese adults, a BMI ≥24.0 was recommended as the cutoff point for overweight, BMI ≥28.0 as the cutoff for obesity, and waist circumference ≥ 85 cm for men and ≥80 cm for women as the cutoff points for central obesity (Bei-Fan & the Cooperative Meta-analysis Group of Working Group on Obesity in China, 2002). Among Asian Indian adults from North India, cardiovascular risk factors are present at even lower cutoff values for waist circumference (78 cm and 72 cm for men and women, respectively) and BMI (>21 kg/m^2) (Misra et al., 2006).

The report of the WHO Expert Consultation (2004) stopped short of selecting cutoff points for overweight and obesity for Asians and instead presented risk categories for determining public health and clinical action based on BMI ranges either for general use or for Asian populations (Table 2.3). Various factors contributed to this conservative recommendation for retaining the widely used WHO BMI cutoff points for Asian populations, including the recognized heterogeneity of Asian populations, differences within Asian populations in the relationships between BMI and body fat, changes in this relationship over time, and the lack of sufficient outcome data that were

Table 2.3 BMI classification for public health action.

	BMI	Risk category
All populations	18.5–27.5	Low to moderate risk
	23.0–33.0	Moderate to high risk
	27.5–37.5	High to very high risk
Many Asian populations	18.5–23.0	Increasing but acceptable risk
	23.0–27.5	Increased risk
	≥27.5	Higher high risk

Source: WHO Expert Consultation (2004).

available to derive cutoff points. These factors suggested it might be premature and inappropriate to recommend new definitions for overweight or obesity, despite the recognition that Asians generally have a higher percentage body fat than white persons of the same age, gender, and BMI, and also have elevated health risk at BMI values below 25 kg/m^2. Compared with Caucasians, Japanese have greater abdominal visceral fat relative to abdominal subcutaneous fat which may partially explain the increased risk for type 2 diabetes and cardiovascular complications among Japanese, even at relatively lower BMI values (Tanaka, Horimai, & Katsukawa, 2003). Clearly there is a need for continuing research on the definition of obesity across various Asian populations. Because inadequate data were available, the WHO panel did not make specific recommendations for Pacific Islanders, although it was noted that Pacific Island populations may have a lower proportion of fat mass to lean mass in comparison with other populations at the same BMI level. This was identified as an area for further research (WHO Expert Consultation, 2004).

In a case-control study of 52 countries representing several major ethnic groups from Asia, Europe, the middle east, Africa, Australia, North America, and South America, Yusuf et al. (2005) examined the association of various indicators of obesity (BMI, waist circumference, WHR) with myocardial infarction (MI) risk in more than 12,000 cases with MI and 14,000 control subjects. BMI had the weakest association with MI risk in all ethnic groups and no significant relation is south Asians, Arabs, and mixed-race Africans. Waist circumference was the strongest predictor of MI in Chinese and black Africans, but intermediate in most other ethnic groups. These investigators concluded that WHR had the strongest relation with MI risk worldwide suggesting that it is the best predictor of MI in most populations, and a redefinition of obesity based on WHR instead of BMI may increase the estimate of MI attributable to obesity in most ethnic groups. The findings of this study raise the question of whether waist circumference or WHR may be superior to BMI in defining obesity, at least with regard to the association of obesity with cardiovascular disease and in particular MI (Kragelund & Omland, 2005).

· BMI is a surrogate marker for the relative level of total body fat. Waist circumference and WHR are surrogate markers for the relative amount of visceral fat or the ratio of visceral to gluteal-femoral fat mass. These measures and the associated definitions of total or central adiposity based on these measures are important because they allow estimates of increased risk.

As total body fat increases, BMI becomes a better indicator of total body fat. In older adults, lean body mass decreases, total body fat increases, and there is a redistribution of body fat to the higher risk intra-abdominal area

(Gallagher, 1996). However, changes in body composition (loss of muscle mass) and height (due to vertebral compression) in older adults can diminish the association between BMI and percentage body fat, such that loss of lean mass can tend to underestimate fatness and loss of height can tend to overestimate fatness (Villareal et al., 2005). Nevertheless, in older persons Harris et al. (2000) concluded that BMI and waist circumference were more highly correlated with total fat than with visceral fat, and visceral obesity is not well measured by waist circumference at ages 70–79 years.

Children

From the late 1970s to 2000, weight status of infants and children was most often assessed using age- and gender-specific weight-for-length (ages birth to 2 years) or weight-for-height (ages 2–11.5 years for boys and 2–10.0 years for girls) growth references from the 1977 NCHS pediatric growth charts (Hamill et al., 1977). The weight-for-height growth references were developed for pre-pubescent children and did not extend through the adolescent ages. BMI cutoff points derived from national reference data were available for children and adolescents aged ≥2 years, but did not receive widespread use (Must, Dallal, & Dietz, 1991). Others used data for distributions of skinfold measures to define obesity in youths, based on statistical cutoff points unrelated to health outcomes (Gortmaker et al., 1987).

In 2000, with the release of age- and gender-specific BMI-for-age growth charts for ages 2 to 20 years (Kuczmarski et al., 2000), it became possible to use smoothed percentile curves and z-scores based on reference data for U.S. children to assess and track children who are at-risk-for-overweight (BMI 85th to 95th percentile) or overweight (BMI ≥95th percentile), as defined earlier by an expert committee (Himes & Dietz, 1994). Below two years of age, the weight-for-length growth charts are available and may be used in analogous fashion, although percentile cutoff criteria to identify overweight in this age range have not received widespread endorsement. In clinical assessment, a transition from the weight-for-length to the BMI-for-age charts from 24 to 36 months of age becomes possible when children can stand unassisted and adequately follow directions to assume the correct posture for a height measurement. Even though BMI growth charts identify overweight better than height and weight charts, most pediatricians still do not report using this tool regularly (Perrin, Flower, & Ammerman, 2004).

BMI increases rapidly from birth to approximately 8 months of age, then decreases until approximately age 6 years when it reaches its nadir before rebounding or increasing once again (Rolland-Cachera, et al. 1984). This has been termed the *adiposity rebound* because it is believed to be the point when body fatness begins to increase after reaching a minimum. When the BMI curve reaches its nadir at younger ages, the likelihood that the level of adiposity will be higher in adolescence and early adulthood is greater (Rolland-Cachera, 1993; Siervogel et al., 1991; Whitaker et al., 1998). Children at higher percentiles for BMI tend to achieve adiposity rebound at younger ages. These children have a greater likelihood to track at a higher BMI percentile with increasing age. There is a need for further research to determine the predictive value of adiposity rebound as a measure to define current overweight status or as an indicator of future obesity, although it appears to have utility as a potential predictor of future risk. One limitation is that assessment of adiposity rebound requires accurate serial measurements at frequent intervals. On a related theme, there is evidence to suggest that rapid weight gain from birth to two years and through 11 years of age, as indicated by progressive increase in BMI z-score, is more predictive of subsequent coronary risk than is obesity defined at any particular age (Barker et al., 2005).

Percentiles are the most commonly used clinical indicator to assess the size and growth patterns of individual children in the United States. Percentiles rank the position of an individual by indicating what percent of the reference population the individual would equal or exceed. The 2000 CDC growth charts are age and gender specific and include nine major percentile curves ranging from the 5th to 95th or the 3rd to 97th percentiles (Figures 2.1 and 2.2). As an example, a girl age 10 years with a BMI of 21.0 kg/m² would be at the

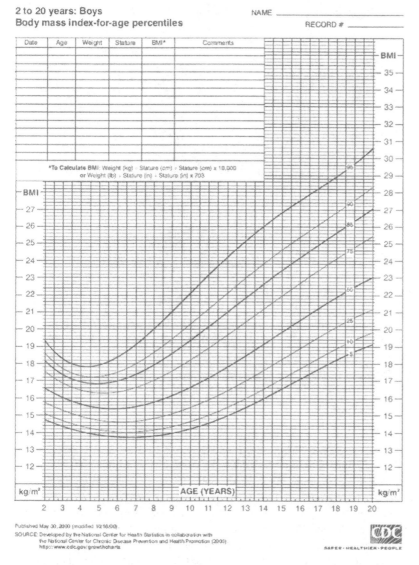

Figure 2.1 2000 CDC body mass index-for-age growth chart.

Source: http://www.cdc.gov/growthcharts/ (Last accessed April 11, 2006).

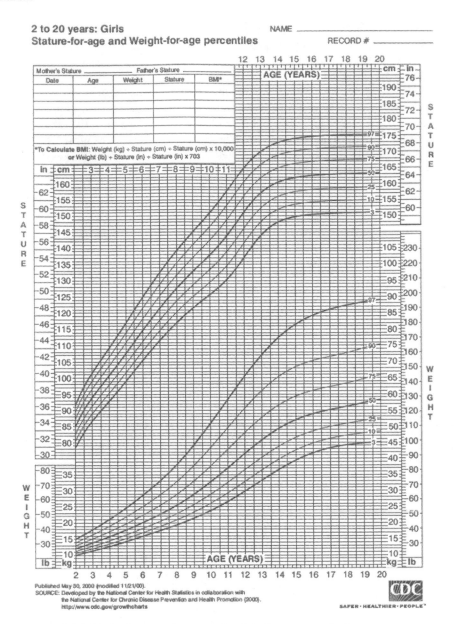

Figure 2.2 2000 CDC stature-for-age and weight-for-age growth chart.

Source: http://www.cdc.gov/growthcharts/-(Last accessed April 11, 2006).

90th percentile, indicating that 90% of girls in the reference population would have a BMI value equal to or lower than 21.0 and 10% of girls this age in the reference population would have a higher BMI value.

The 2000 CDC growth charts were constructed using pooled data from the National Health and Nutrition Examination Surveys from 1963–1994. However, in the construction of these charts, population increases in body weight that occurred in recent years led to a decision to exclude survey data from the 1988–1994 time period for weight and BMI data for ages 6 years and older. In brief, this decision was made because inclusion of the 1988–1994 survey data resulted in an upward shift of the higher 85th and 95th percentile curves which are used as cutoff criteria to identify risk-of overweight and overweight. Although an increase in overweight happened because of environmental influences, that is, shifts in dietary intake and physical activity patterns, it is not what is believed to be biologically or medically desirable. Because these references are based on data from an earlier time period, when the 95th percentile for BMI is used to calculate overweight prevalence, it is possible to obtain estimates that exceed 5% over the threshold. More thorough discussions are presented elsewhere (Kuczmarski et al., 2000; Ogden et al., 2002). A major use of the BMI growth charts is as a clinical screening tool, although they are not intended to be the sole diagnostic criterion for overweight. When used properly, plotting points over time on BMI growth charts can monitor BMI trends and identify individuals with unusual growth patterns. Large deviations exemplified by data points that cross over two or more of the major percentile lines on growth charts, known as decanalization, can be utilized to identify children who are potentially on a growth trajectory that might require increased attention and possibly intervention (Kuczmarski, Kuczmarski, & Roche, 2002).

The BMI standard deviation score (z-score) is the deviation of the value for an individual from the mean BMI value of the reference population divided by the standard deviation for the reference population. Z-scores and percentiles are interchangeable. Which one is used is based primarily on convention or preference. In certain population-based applications, such as research settings and surveillance systems, the mean and standard deviation are often calculated for a group of z-scores (WHO Working Group on Infant Growth, 1995). In selected clinical situations where monitoring of growth is an important evaluation tool and greater measurement precision is necessary, z-scores or exact percentiles may be preferred (Kuczmarski et al., 2000). Cole et al. (2005) reported that change in BMI units is the preferred measure to quantify short-term changes in adiposity. When ranking children, BMI values, BMI percentiles, and BMI z-scores have correlation coefficients with percentage body fat that are almost identical (Field et al., 2003).

For children of all ages, The Centers for Disease Control and Prevention has recommended use of the term overweight rather than obesity. Cautious and limited use of the term *obesity* is urged when only BMI screening data are available, especially in the absence of additional measures of body fat. Because children are still growing linearly, a child who appears to be overweight at one point in time may subsequently achieve a body weight that is appropriate for height with a BMI in the normal range. There may be social stigma concerns associated with prematurely or inaccurately labeling a child as obese that could lead to unwarranted social discrimination by peers or inappropriate behaviors by the overweight child potentially resulting in exacerbation of the condition. Nevertheless, "childhood obesity" is the term in common usage in the larger public health and policy arena, to highlight attention to the problem and avoid the confusion that might be caused by the difference in the way overweight is used in children and adults (Committee on Prevention of Obesity in Children and Youth, 2005). As previously mentioned, the gender specific 2000 CDC BMI-for age growth charts allow the classification of overweight (BMI ≥95th percentile) and at-risk-of-overweight (BMI ≥85th percentile to <95th percentile). The at-risk-of-overweight category is intended to identify and clinically monitor youths with BMI values in a range that may subsequently progress over the threshold to the overweight category. However, readers should be aware that some authors have taken the liberty of publishing reports that define overweight (BMI ≥85th to 95th percentile) and obese (>BMI ≥95th percentile). Since most obese youths are also overweight, such an approach sometimes dramatically inflates the prevalence of overweight in children and adolescents. This reflects the multiple uses that the CDC BMI growth charts receive in diverse clinical and epidemiological applications.

Definitions Matter

From the perspective of policy development and setting public health priorities, the BMI cutoff points for overweight and obesity are not a trivial issue because of the absolute proportion of the population that may be defined as overweight or obese and also because changes in BMI cutoff points can drastically change prevalence estimates. The impact of changes in BMI cutoff points became evident when the switch was made from use of the NHANES II BMI cutoff values (27.8 for men and 27.3 for women) to a BMI ≥25.0 for estimating the prevalence of overweight and obesity in the U.S. The prevalence of overweight among U.S. adults in NHANES III (1988–1994) was 33.3 and 36.4% for men and women respectively using the NHANES II definition of overweight. For the exact same data set, using the overweight definition of BMI ≥25.0, the prevalence of overweight increased to 59.4 and 50.7% for men and women respectively (Kuczmarski et al., 1997). This was an increase in the national prevalence of overweight from 1/3 to 1/2 of the population simply by changing the BMI cutoff point at which overweight was defined. Similarly, the prevalence of obesity, previously termed "severe overweight" at a BMI ≥31.1 and 32.3 for adult men and women respectively, increased when these cutoff points were shifted downward to a BMI ≥30.0 (Kuczmarski & Flegal, 2000). The change in BMI cutoff points used to define overweight was a seemingly minor transition that had a dramatic effect on estimates of the number of overweight people in the U.S. and raised considerable interest in the topic from various sectors, including the news media.

In the above example, the switch to a lower BMI cutoff value at which overweight is defined not only changed the magnitude of overweight prevalence, but also indicated that men now had a higher prevalence of overweight than women. This raises the issue of potential misclassification for overweight near a BMI of 25 and especially among men who may appear to be overweight near this threshold because of an accumulation of lean body mass. A study from Australia, where, as in the United States more than half of all adult men are overweight or obese (BMI ≥25.0), reported that a significant proportion of men did not consider themselves to be overweight, when in fact they had BMI values ≥25.0. At all adult ages, the men in this study indicated their perception that overweight begins at body weights corresponding to BMI values closer to approximately 26–27 (Crawford & Campbell, 1999). The extent to which men in the BMI range of approximately 25–27 may be incorrectly classified as overweight, attributable to more lean body mass, may be an area for further research. Regardless of which BMI cutoff points are used to determine the prevalence of overweight, among adults in the U.S., when compared to NHANES II data, the NHANES III data revealed that the entire BMI distribution had shifted upward and has become more skewed at higher BMI levels, indicating that changes in the BMI distribution are most marked at the upper end of the distribution (Flegal & Troiano, 2000). These elevated obesity patterns have remained through the 2004 NHANES (Ogden et al., 2006).

When considering recommendations for BMI among Asian populations, the aforementioned WHO Expert Panel concluded that the WHO BMI cutoff point classification should be retained to facilitate international classification and comparisons (WHO Expert Consultation, 2004). However, recognizing that health risk increases along the BMI continuum, this Panel also recommended that additional BMI cut-off points for public health action among Asian populations be considered (23.0, 27.5, 32.5, and 37.5 kg/m^2).

At low to moderate BMI values, BMI and fatness may have a low sensitivity although at high values for percent body fat, BMI has high specificity as a screening tool (Roche, 1996). Sensitivity is the extent to which BMI correctly classifies persons who are overweight or obese. Specificity is the extent to which BMI correctly classifies persons who are not overweight or obese. In any event, BMI tends to be predictive of common health risks such as hypertension and dyslipidemias and at BMI ≥25.0 there is evidence of increased risk for coronary heart disease, type 2-diabetes, and premature mortality (Willett, Dietz, & Colditz, 1999; NHLBI Obesity Education Initiative Expert Panel, 1998). The exact impact of obesity on population mortality remains controversial. Earlier estimates indicated that approximately 300,000 excess deaths annually were associated with obesity (Allison et al., 1999). A subsequent report that used estimation methods believed to better account for selective confounding and effect modification by age, reported that in 2000 obesity (BMI ≥30.0) was associated with approximately 112,000 excess deaths in the U.S., although overweight (BMI 25.0–29.9) was not associated with excess mortality (Flegal et al., 2005). The data for excess deaths were based on BMI definitions of overweight instead of measures of fatness derived from body composition. The associations do not confirm causality, the cross-sectional data do not consider previous health status, and the role of additional confounders was not fully explored. These studies have led others to question how obesity is defined and how obesity statistics are derived and interpreted (Gibbs, 2005). Clearly there are other aspects that must be critically factored in when analyzing obesity data and drawing conclusions.

Nationally representative trend data for prevalence of overweight and obesity based on measured height and weight are available from the National Health Examination Surveys beginning in 1960. BMI trend analyses in which overweight was defined at a BMI 25.0–29.9 indicate that from 1960 to 2002 overweight (but not obese) has remained fairly constant at approximately 40% among adult men and approximately 25% among adult women (National Center for Health Statistics, 2005). However, at higher BMI cutoff levels (≥30.0) increases in the prevalence of obesity become more apparent. At a BMI ≥30.0, from 1960 to 2002, the prevalence of obesity nearly tripled from 10.7 to 28.1% among adult men and more than doubled from 15.7 to 34.0% among adult women. Thus, BMI cutoff values to define overweight and obesity can have a considerable impact on identification of these conditions and this applies regardless of whether BMI is treated as a continuous or categorical variable in epidemiological analyses.

Theoretically, it would be possible to set the prevalence of overweight anywhere from zero to 100% simply by shifting the cutoff point in one direction or the other. The cutoff points in current use are not at all this arbitrary although there clearly is some rounding to facilitate ease of use. BMI, waist circumference, or other indicators for the definition of obesity are used because at increasing values for these measures health risk increases in populations. However, for any given individual the strength of the relationship between measures of obesity and health outcomes can vary considerably. Other considerations may pertain to the quality of measurements. Self-reported values as recorded in various interview surveys for example, are known to over-estimate height and under-estimate weight in some groups. Among persons ages 60 years or older, self-reported height and weight can result in misclassification of overweight status because the person reporting may not have taken into account aging related decreases in height. For persons 70 years and older, BMI calculated from self-reported measures can be one unit lower than when height and weight are measured (Kuczmarski, Kuczmarski, & Najjar, 2001). Comparisons of surveillance and survey data indicate that self-reported weight and height have also been found to yield disproportionate underestimates for the prevalence of overweight and obesity across gender, race, age, and education subgroups in the U.S. (Yun et al., 2006). Inconsistent anthropometric measurement procedures can also contribute to misclassification. Standardized procedures are recommended, and both text (Lohman, Roche, & Martorell, 1988) and video (Kuczmarski, 2005) reference procedures can facilitate standardization.

In summary, the BMI-based classification scheme is the most frequently used approach to define overweight and obesity for both clinical and public health purposes. However, BMI remains a screening tool and should not be used as the sole clinical diagnostic criterion for the assessment of obesity. BMI is useful for adults because the BMI levels used to define overweight and obesity are associated with increased risk for numerous chronic health conditions. Chronic diseases are comparatively less common among children and adolescents than among adults so the high risk BMI cutoff points for children are not as well known. Nevertheless, the recommended 85th and 95th age- and gender-specific percentile values in late adolescence appear to be fairly consistent with the adult BMI cutoff values ≥ 25 used to define overweight and ≥ 30 to define obesity (Cole et al., 2000). These adult values are known to be associated with increased health risk. Given that BMI tends to track from late childhood and especially from adolescence into early adulthood and beyond (Whitaker et al., 1997), consistent with current knowledge and technology, BMI remains a most useful tool for screening, identification, and classification of overweight and obesity in clinical and public health applications for most groups. Emerging evidence suggests that selected Asian groups may be a notable exception. BMI is still an extremely useful tool in these groups although the cutoff points may need to be shifted downward and abdominal circumference may hold greater importance in defining increased risk for obesity.

References

Albu, J. B., Kovera, A. J., & Johnson, J. A. (2000). Fat distribution and health in obesity. *Annals of the New York Academy of Sciences, 904*, 491–501.

Albu, J. B., Murphy, L., Frager, D. H., Johnson, J. A., & Pi-Sunyer, F. X. (1997). Visceral fat and race-dependent health risks in obese non-diabetic pre-menopausal women. *Diabetes, 46*, 456–462.

Allison, D. B., Fontaine, K. R., Manson, J. E. Stevens, J., & Van Itallie, T. B. (1999). Annual deaths attributable to obesity in the United States. *Journal of the American Medical Association, 282*, 1530–1538.

Barker, D. J. P., Osmond, C., Forsen, T. J., Kajantie, E., & Eriksson, J. G. (2005). Trajectories of growth among children who have coronary events as adults. *New England Journal of Medicine, 353*, 1802–1809.

Bei-Fan, Z. And the Cooperative Meta-analysis Group of Working Group on Obesity in China (2002). Predictive values of body mass index and waist circumference for risk factors of certain related diseases in Chinese adults: Study on optimal cut-off points of body mass index and waist circumference in Chinese adults. *Asia Pacific Journal of Clinical Nutrition, 11*(Suppl. 8), S685–S693.

Benn, R. J. (1971). Some mathematical properties of weight for height indices used as measures of adiposity. *British Journal of Preventive and Social Medicine, 25*, 42–50.

Bray, G. A. (1998a). In defense of a body mass index of 25 as the cut-off point for defining overweight. *Obesity Research, 6*, 461–462.

Bray, G. A. (1998b). *Contemporary diagnosis and management of obesity.* Newtown, PA: Handbooks in Health Care Co.

Cole, T. J., Bellizzi, M. C., Flegal, K. M., & Dietz, W. H. (2000). Establishing a standard definition for child overweight and obesity worldwide: International survey. *British Medical Journal, 320*, 1240–1243.

Cole, T. J., Faith, M. S., Pietrobelli, A., & Heo, M. (2005). What is the best measure of adiposity change in growing children: BMI, BMI%, BMI z-score or BMI centile? *European Journal of Clinical Nutrition, 59*, 419–425.

Committee on Prevention of Obesity in Childhood and Youth (2005). *Preventing childhood obesity: Health in the balance.* Washington, DC: National Academies Press.

Crawford, D., & Campbell, K. (1999). Lay definitions of ideal weight and overweight. *International Journal of Obesity and Related Metabolic Disorders, 23*, 738–745.

Despres, J. P., Nadeau, A., Tremblay, A., Ferland, M., Moorjani, S., & Lupien, P. J. et al. (1989). Role of deep abdominal fat in the association between regional adipose tissue distribution and glucose tolerance in obese women. *Diabetes, 38*, 304–309.

Emery, E. M., Schmid, T. L., Kahn, H. S., & Filozof, P. P. (1993). A review of the association between abdominal fat distribution, health outcome measures, and modifiable risk factors. *American Journal of Health Promotion, 7*, 342–353.

Examination Committee of Criteria for Obesity Disease in Japan, Japan Society for the Study of Obesity (2002). New criteria for obesity disease in Japan. *Circulation Journal, 66*, 987–992.

Fernandez, J. R., Heo, M., Heymsfield, S. B., Pierson, R. N., Pi-Sunyer, F. X., & Wang, Z. M. et al. (2003). Is percentage body fat differentially related to body mass index in Hispanic Americans, African Americans, and European Americans? *American Journal of Clinical Nutrition, 77*, 71–75.

Field, A. E., Laird, N., Steinberg, E., Fallon, E., Semega-Janneh, M., & Yanovski, J. A. (2003). Which metric of relative weight best captures body fatness in children? *Obesity Research, 11*, 1345–1352.

Flegal, K. M., Graubard, B. I., Williamson, D. F., & Gail, M. H. (2005). Excess deaths associated with underweight, overweight, and obesity. *Journal of the American Medical Association, 293*, 1861–1867.

Flegal, K. M., & Troiano, R. P. (2000). Changes in the distribution of body mass index of adults and children in the U.S. population. *International Journal of Obesity, 24*, 807–818.

Florey, C. V. (1970). The use and interpretation of ponderal index and other weight-height ratios in epidemiological studies. *Journal of Chronic Disease, 23*, 93–103.

Fujimoto, W. Y., Newell-Morris, L. L., Grote, M., Bergstrom, R. W., & Shuman, W. P. (1991). Visceral fat obesity and morbidity: NIDDM and atherogenic risk in Japanese-American men and women. *International Journal of Obesity, 15*(Suppl. 2), 41–44.

Gallagher, D., Heymsfield, S. B., Heo, M., Jebb, S. A., Murgatroyd, P. R., & Sakamoto, Y. (2000). Healthy percentage body fat ranges: an approach for developing guidelines based on body mass index. *American Journal of Clinical Nutrition, 72*, 694–701.

Gallagher, D., Visser, M., Sepulveda, D., Pierson, R. N., Harris, T., & Heymsfield, S. B. (1996). How useful is body mass index for comparison of body fatness across age, sex, and ethnic groups? *American Journal of Epidemiology, 3*, 228–239.

Garrow, J. S. (1983). Indices of adiposity. *Nutrition Abstracts and Reviews, 53*, 697–708.

Garrow, J. S., & Webster, J. (1985). Quetelet's index (W/H²) as a measure of fatness. *International Journal of Obesity, 9*, 147–153.

Gibbs, W. W. (2005). Obesity: An overblown epidemic? *Scientific American, 292*, 70–77.

Gortmaker, S. L., Dietz, W. H., Sobol, A. M., & Wehler, C. A. (1987). Increasing pediatric obesity in the United States. *American Journal of Diseases in Children, 141*, 535–540.

Hamill, P., Drizd, T., Johnson, C., Reed, R., & Roche, A. (1977). *NCHS growth curves for children, birth-18 years, United States. Vital and Health Statistics, Series 11, no. 165*. Washington, DC: U. S. Department of Health, Education, and Welfare.

Harris, T. B., Visser, M., Everhart, J., Cauley, J., Tylavsky, F., & Fuerst, T. (2000). Waist circumference and sagittal diameter reflect total body fat better than visceral fat in older men and women: The health, aging, and body composition study. *Annals of the New York Academy of Sciences, 904*, 462–473.

Haslam, D. W., & James, W. P. T. (2005). Obesity. *Lancet, 366*, 1197–1209.

Himes, J. H., & Dietz, W. H. (1994). Guidelines for overweight in adolescent preventive services: Recommendations from an expert committee. *American Journal of Clinical Nutrition, 59*, 307–316.

Hope, A. A., Kumanyika, S. K., Whitt, M. C., & Shults, J. (2005). Obesity-related comorbidities in obese African Americans in an outpatient weight loss program. *Obesity Research, 13*, 772–779.

International Diabetes Federation. (2005). Worldwide definition of the metabolic syndrome. http://www.idf.org (Last accessed April 11, 2006).

Keys, A., Fidanza, F., Karvonen, M. J., Kimura, N., & Taylor, H. L. (1972). Indices of relative weight and obesity. *Journal of Chronic Diseases, 25*, 329–343.

Kiernan, M., & Winkleby, M. A. (2000). Identifying patients for weight-loss treatment: An empirical evaluation of the NHLBI obesity evaluation initiative expert panel treatment recommendations. *Archives of Internal Medicine, 160*, 2169–2176.

Klatsky, A. L., & Armstrong, M. A. (1991). Cardiovascular risk factors among Asian Americans living in northern California. *American Journal of Public Health, 81*, 1423–1428.

Klein, S., Burke, L. E., Bray, G. A., Blair, S., Allison, D. B., & Pi-Sunyer, X. et al. (2004). Clinical implications of obesity with specific focus on cardiovascular disease. *Circulation, 110*, 2952–2967.

Kragelund, C., & Omland, T. (2005). A farewell to body mass index? *Lancet, 366*, 1589–1591.

Kuczmarski, M. F., Kuczmarski, R. J., & Najjar, M. F. (2001). Effects of age on validity of self-reported height, weight, and body mass index: Findings from the third National Health and Nutrition Examination Survey, 1988–1994. *Journal of the American Dietetic Association, 101*, 28–34.

Kuczmarski, R. J. (2005). NHANES III anthropometric procedures video. http://www.cdc.gov/nchs/about/major/nhanes/avideo.htm (Last accessed April 11, 2006).

Kuczmarski, R. J., Carroll, M. D., Flegal, K. M., & Troiano, R. P. (1997). Varying body mass index cutoff points to describe overweight prevalence among U.S. adults: NHANES III (1998 to 1994). *Obesity Research, 5*, 542–548.

Kuczmarski, R. J., & Flegal, K. M. (2000). Criteria for definition of overweight in transition: Background and recommendations for the United States. *American Journal of Clinical Nutrition, 72*, 1074–1081.

Kuczmarski, R. J., Kuczmarski, M. F., & Roche, A. F. (2002). CDC growth charts: Background for clinical application. *Topics in Clinical Nutrition, 17*, 15–26.

Kuczmarski, R. J., Ogden, C. L., Guo, S. S., Grummer-Strawn, L. M., Flegal, K. M., & Mei, Z. et al. (2000). CDC growth charts for the United States: methods and development. *Vital and Health Statistics, Series 11, No. 246*. http://www.cdc.gov/growthcharts/ (Last accessed April 11, 2006).

Lean, M. E., Han, T. S., & Morrison, C. E. (1995). Waist circumference as a measure for indicating need for weight management. *British Medical Journal, 311*, 158–161.

Lee, J., Kolonel, L. N., & Hinds, M. W. (1981). Relative merits of the weight-corrected-for height indices. *American Journal of Clinical Nutrition, 34*, 2521–2529.

Lohman, T. G., Roche, A. F., & Martorell, R. (1988). *Anthropometric standardization reference manual*. Champaign, IL: Human Kinetics.

Mamtani, M. R., & Kulkarni, H. R. (2005). Predictive performance of anthropometric indices of central obesity for the risk of type 2 diabetes. *Archives of Medical Research, 36*, 581–589.

Misra, A., Vikram, N. K., Gupta, R., Pandey, R. M., Wasir, J. S., & Gupta, V. P. (2006). Waist dircumference cutoff points and action levels for Asian Indians for identification of abdominal obesity. *International Journal of Obesity, 30*, 106–111.

Must, A., Dallal, G. E., & Dietz, W. H. (1991). Reference data for obesity: 85th and 95th percentiles of body mass index (wt/ht^2) and triceps skinfold thickness. American Journal of Clinical Nutrition 53, 839–846. Erratum in: *American Journal of Clinical Nutrition 54*, 773.

National Center for Health Statistics (2005). *Health United States, 2005 with chartbook on trends in the health of Americans*. Hyattsville, MD.

NHLBI Obesity Education Initiative Expert Panel on the Identification, Evaluation, and Treatment of Overweight and Obesity in Adults (1998). Clinical guidelines on the identification, evaluation, and treatment of overweight and obesity in adults—the evidence report. *Obesity Research, 6*, 51S–209S.

NHLBI Obesity Education Initiative Expert Panel on the Identification, Evaluation, and Treatment of Overweight and Obesity in Adults (2000). The practical guide: Identification, evaluation, and treatment of overweight and obesity in adults. NIH publication No. 00-4084. http://www.nhlbi.nih.gov/guidelines/obesity/ob_home.htm (Last accessed April 11, 2006).

Norgan, N. G., & Ferro-Luzzi, A. (1982). Weight-height indices as estimators of fatness in men. *Human Nutrition: Clinical Nutrition, 36C*, 363–372.

Ogden, C. L., Carroll, M. D., Curtin, L. R., McDowell, M. A., Tabak, C. J., & Flegal, K. M. (2006). Prevalence of overweight and obesity in the United States, 1999–2004. *Journal of the American Medical Association, 295*, 1549–1555.

Ogden, C. L., Kuczmarski, R. J., Flegal, K. M., Mei, Z., Guo, S., & Wei, R., et al. (2002). Centers for Disease Control and Prevention 2000 growth charts for the United States: improvements to the National Center for Health Statistics version. *Pediatrics, 109*, 45–60.

Perrin, E. M., Flower, K. B., & Ammerman, A. S., (2004). Body mass index charts: useful yet underused. *Journal of Pediatrics, 144*, 455–460.

Roche, A. F. (1996). Anthropometry and ultrasound. In A. F. Roche, S. B. Heymsfield, & T. G. Lohman (Eds.), *Human body composition* (pp. 167–189). Champaign, IL: Human Kinetics.

Roche, A. F., Heymsfield, S. B., & Lohman, T. G. (Eds.). (1996). *Human body composition*. Champaign, IL: Human Kinetics.

Rolland-Cachera, M. F. (1993). Onset of obesity assessed from the weight/height^2 curve in children: The need for a clear definition. *International Journal of Obesity and Related Metabolic Disorders, 17*, 245–246.

Rolland-Cachera, M. F., Deheeger, M., Belllisle, F., Sempe, M., Guilloud-Bataille, M., & Patios, E. (1984). Adiposity rebound in children: A simple indicator for predicting obesity. *American Journal of Clinical Nutrition, 39*, 129–135.

Rush, E., Plank, L., Chandu, V., Laulu, M., Simmons, D., Swinburn, B., & Yajnik, C. (2004). Body size, body composition, and fat distribution: A comparison of young New Zealand men of European, Pacific Island, and Asian Indian ethnicities. *The New Zealand Medical Journal, 117*, 1–9.

Seidell, J. C., (1992). Regional obesity and health. *International Journal of Obesity, 16*(Suppl. 2), S31–S34.

Seidell, J. C., Deurenberg, P., & Hautvast, J. G. (1987). Obesity and fat distribution in relation to health: Current insights and recommendations. *World Review of Nutrition and Dietetics, 50,* 57–91.

Shen, W., Wang, Z., Punyanita, M., Lei, J., Sinav, A., & Kral, J. G. et al. (2003). Adipose tissue quantification by imaging methods: A proposed classification. *Obesity Research, 11,* 5–16.

Siervogel, R. M., Roche, A. F., Guo, S. S., Mukherjee, D., & Chumlea, W. C. (1991). Patterns of change in weight/height² from 2 to 18 years: Findings from long-term serial data for children in the Fels Longitudinal Study. *International Journal of Obesity, 15,* 479–485.

Steering Committee of the Western Pacific Region of the World Health Organization, International Association for the Study of Obesity, & International Obesity Task Force (2000). *The Asia-Pacific perspective: Redefining obesity and its treatment.* Sydney, Australia: Health Communications Australia Pty Limited. http://www.vepachedu.org/TSJ/BMI-Guidelines.pdf (Last accessed April 11, 2006).

Steinberger, J., Jacobs, D. R., Moran, A., Hong, C.-P., & Sinaiko, A. R. (2005). Comparison of body fatness measurements by BMI and skinfold measurements vs dual energy X-ray absorptiometry and their relation to cardiovascular risk factors in adolescents. *International Journal of Obesity, 29,* 1346–1352.

Tanaka, S., Horimai, C., & Katsukawa, F. (2003). Ethnic differences in abdominal visceral fat accumulation between Japanese, African-Americans, and Caucasians: A meta-analysis. *Acta Diabetol, 40,* S302–S304.

Vague, J. (1956). The degree of masculine differentiation of obesities: A fact for determining predisposition to diabetes, atherosclerosis, gout and uric calculus disease. *American Journal of Clinical Nutrition, 4,* 20–34.

Van Itallie, T. B. (1985). Health implications of overweight and obesity in the United States. *Annals of Internal Medicine, 103,* 983–988.

Villareal, D. T., Apovian, C. M., Kushner, R. F., & Klein, S. (2005). Obesity in older adults: Technical review and position statement of the American Society for Nutrition and NAASO, the Obesity Society. *American Journal of Clinical Nutrition, 82,* 923–934.

Weigley, E. S. (1989). Adolphe Quetelet (1796–1874): Pioneer anthropometrist. *Nutrition Today, 24,* 12–16.

Whitaker, R. C., Pepe, M. S., Wright, J. A. Seidel, K. D., & Dietz, W. H. (1998). Early adiposity rebound and the risk of adult obesity. *Pediatrics, 101*(3):e5. URL: http://www.pediatrics.org/cgi/content/full/101/3/e5 (Last accessed April 11, 2006).

Whitaker, R. C., Wright, J. A., Pepe, M. S., Seidel, K. D., & Dietz, W. H. (1997). Predicting obesity in young adulthood from childhood and parental obesity. *New England Journal of Medicine, 337,* 869–873.

Willett, W. C., Dietz, W. H., & Colditz, G. A. (1999). Guidelines for healthy weight. *New England Journal of Medicine, 341,* 427–434.

World Health Organization (1998). *Report of a WHO consultation on obesity. Obesity: preventing and managing the global epidemic.* Geneva: World Health Organization.

WHO Expert Consultation (2004). Appropriate body-mass index for Asian populations and its implications for policy and intervention strategies. *Lancet, 363,* 157–163.

WHO Working Group on Infant Growth (1995). An evaluation of infant growth: The use and interpretation of anthropometry in infants. *Bulletin of the World Health Organization, 73,* 165–174.

Yun, S., Zhu, B.-P., Black, W., & Brownson, R. C. (2006). A comparison of national estimates of obesity prevalence from the behavioral risk factor surveillance system and the national health and nutrition examination survey. *International Journal of Obesity, 30,* 164–170.

Yusuf, S., Hawken, S., Ounpuu, S., Bautista, L., Franzosi, M. G., & Commerford, P., et al. (2005). Obesity and the risk of myocardial infarction in 27000 participants from 52 countries: A case-control study. *Lancet, 366,* 1640–1649.

Chapter 3

Descriptive Epidemiology of Obesity in the United States

Youfa Wang and Shiriki Kumanyika

Introduction

This chapter provides an overview of the descriptive epidemiology of overweight and obesity among U.S. adults, children and adolescents with respect to prevalence and trends based on recent, nationally representative data. Analytic data that link obesity prevalence data to data on characteristics of environments, population groups or individuals can suggest what needs to be done to address the problem and inform the development of interventions (Swinburn et al, 2005). This type of evidence is reviewed in chapters throughout this book. Reviews of current knowledge of the overall etiology of obesity are available elsewhere in the epidemiologic literature (WHO, 2000; French et al, 2001; Ebbeling et al, 2002; NHLBI, 2004; Brug and Van Lenthe, 2005)

The scope and nature of the obesity epidemic are typically described with statistics on the prevalence (percent) of obesity in the population as a whole and also within demographic groups. Age, gender, race/ethnicity, socioeconomic status and rural/urban residence are usually the main demographic variables of interest nationally and at state and local levels. Questions that can potentially be answered by these types of data include: "How many people are affected by the problem?" Which demographic groups are more affected than others, i.e., are the "high risk" or "high need" populations with respect to obesity intervention, and "How is the prevalence of the problem changing over time?" Such descriptive data are useful to justify the need for action, to indicate where interventions are most needed, and to track progress. Demographic categories used at the state and local level are, ideally, more specific than the broad aggregations used nationally and are tailored to the population characteristics (e.g., breaking down an ethnic group into specific sub-ethnic groups or identifying recent immigrants separately; tabulating prevalence by neighborhood within an urban area).

We highlight key demographic differences such as the higher than average prevalence of obesity in many ethnic minority populations and among lower socioeconomic status (SES) groups, and examine trends from the 1960s to the present. Estimates of the prevalence and trends in overweight and obesity are affected by the definition used (Troiano and Flegal, 1999; Wang and Wang, 2002) and, several definitions are applied both in the United States and internationally (Guillaume, 1999; Cole et al, 2000; Wang, 2004; WHO, 1995). Prevalence estimates and the validity of comparisons among groups and over time are also influenced by the quality and standardization of measurement as well as the representativeness of the sample on which the estimates are based. For example, estimates based on program data used for surveillance will differ from estimates based on probability samples. Estimates based on self-reported weight and height will differ from and be potentially biased compared to estimates based on objective measurements (Gillum and Sempos, 2005; Yun et al, 2006). Assessment of overweight and obesity are discussed in Chapter 2, but key issues are also reviewed here to facilitate the understanding of the information within this chapter.

Background

Data Sources

To permit valid comparisons of overweight and obesity prevalence over time and across groups, most of the data presented in the chapter are drawn from the National Health and Nutrition Examination Surveys (NHANES). The NHANES are a well-established series of cross-sectional, nationally representative examination surveys that have been conducted by the National Center for Health Statistics (NCHS) of the Centers for Disease Control and Prevention (CDC) since the 1960s and for which comparability over time in sampling and measurement methods is a main consideration.

These surveys were designed using stratified multistage probability samples. Beginning in 1999, NHANES became a continuous survey. NHANES III (1988–94) and NHANES 1999–2002 were designed to over-sample Mexican Americans, African Americans, and adolescents to improve estimates for these groups (see Chapter 2). In each survey, standardized protocols were used for all interviews and examinations. Weight and height measurements were collected for each individual through direct physical examination in a mobile examination center. Recumbent length was measured in children younger than 4 years and stature was measured in children 2 years and older. Details regarding the study design and data collection of NHANES have been provided elsewhere (CDC, 1996, 2004; McDowell et al, 1981; NCHS, 1973).

The NHANES data provide national estimates of overweight from infancy through old age and also other demographic information that can be used for subgroup estimates. Sample sizes for subgroups depend on the sampling strategy, which has changed over time with respect to what groups are over sampled to increase the ability to produce statistically reliable subgroup estimates. With respect to race/ethnicity, current NHANES data provide national estimates for three racial/ethnic groups: whites, blacks/African Americans, and Mexican Americans in the U.S. population, an improvement relative to the earlier surveys. However, there are many other ethnic minority populations for which data on obesity prevalence are of interest, who have an excess of obesity or of obesity related diseases relative to whites, and whose profiles may differ substantially from those of the populations covered by NHANES (Kumanyika, 1993, 1994; Crawford et al, 2001).These populations include: Hispanic populations overall and in subgroups other than Mexican American; American Indians and Alaska Natives; Native Hawiians; Pacific Islanders; and Asian Americans.

Even for whites and African Americans, there have been changes over time in how race is ascertained (e.g., initially by the interviewer's observation and more recently based on self-report), and the designation of Hispanic ethnicity was not collected in the earlier data sets. Therefore, the currently recommended NHANES categorizations of "non-Hispanic black or "non-Hispanic white" cannot be uniformly applied to trend analyses over all years for which survey data are otherwise available. Hispanic ancestry is ascertained separately from the 'racial' categories, and Hispanics can be of any race in the Census Bureau classification scheme (Grieco and Cassidy, 2001). However, reporting Hispanic ancestry effectively supersedes racial classification in data reporting schemes. That is, people who are not-Hispanic are classified as white, black, American Indian/Alaska Native, Asian, Pacific Islander, or perhaps Native Hawaiian (which is a sometimes a separate designation) but those who report Hispanic ancestry are classified as Hispanic or according to a specific Hispanic subgroup (e.g., Mexican American), without specification of a racial category.

Interview surveys are resources for estimating obesity prevalence including: (1) the National Health Interview Survey (NHIS), which is national level only and (2) the Behavioral Risk Factor Surveillance System (BRFSS), which is a state-based surveillance system but can provide national estimates when data are properly weighted. Prevalence estimates based on self-reported height and weight are substantially lower than those from NHANES (Gillum and Sempos, 2001; Yun et al, 2006). Overall prevalence patterns may be similar in self-reported and measured data, e.g., comparisons of ethnic groups or age or gender differences. However, the degree of underreporting differs by ethnicity, gender, and socioeconomic status and in some cases may suggest associations that are not present or that are different from those based on height and weight measurements.

Some obesity prevalence data come from school-based nutrition data (Thorpe et al, 2004), research studies or special surveys, e.g., in specific populations such as American Indians (Caballero et al, 2003; Eisenmann et al, 2000; Zephier et al, 1999). Surveillance data based on height and weight measurements collected in populations served by health centers or nutrition programs such as the Supplemental Nutrition Program for Women, Infants, and Children (WIC) (e.g., the Pediatric Nutrition Surveillance System (Sherry et al, 2004)) should be interpreted with the recognition that they are not based on representative samples of the population at large. With this caveat, these data may be very useful for describing the relevant reference populations and have the potential for direct links to state and local policies and programs. Such direct links are not possible with NHANES or NHIS data. In this chapter, data sources other than NHANES, when cited, were felt to provide, within acknowledged limitations, a sufficiently useful picture for specific populations or for cross-population comparisons to be preferable to providing no data at all for the populations in question.

The meaning of commonly used racial/ethnic designations is highly debated as to how much of any associated health status differences are due to genes or environment. It is relatively clear that these categories—which follow Census Bureau policies and are primarily based on sociopolitical factors—are "real" in the sense that they reflect differences in health status and other aspects of life experiences within the United States (Smelser et al, 2001). What is at issue is whether the racial/ethnic categories coincide sufficiently with genetically based biological variations to represent separate "races" or whether they are not, in fact, really groupings constructed on the basis of socio-political history or status. In fact, there has been decreasing support for the entire concept of designating racial divisions within the human race. There is not a rule of thumb with respect to how differences across these categories can be interpreted. These issues, although worthwhile noting here as background for considering the implications of prevalence and trend data for obesity prevention, are complex and far beyond the scope or intent of this chapter but are well covered, for example, by an Institute of Medicine report on this topic (Smelser et al, 2001).

Definitions and assessment of overweight and obesity

According to the World Health Organization (WHO), obesity is a disease, and it is defined as the condition of excess body fat to the extent that health is impaired (WHO, 2000). The CDC defines overweight and obesity as ranges of weight that have been shown to increase the likelihood of certain diseases and other health problems (CDC, 2005). For practical purposes, obesity is often defined as excess body weight rather than as excess fat. In population-based studies, body mass index (BMI = weight (kg)/height (m)^2) has been widely used for both children and adults during recent years.

Adults

For adults, the WHO recommends defining overweight and obesity using BMI cut points of 25 and 30 kg/m^2, respectively (WHO, 1995, 2000). BMI is used because it correlates with amount of body fat and obesity-related health consequences. An adult who has a BMI between 25 and 29.9 is considered overweight, a BMI of 30 or higher is considered obese. These cut offs were also recommended by a National Heart, Lung, and Blood Institute (NHLBI) expert panel (NHLBI, 1998). Different measures such as ideal body weight (a body weight less than 20% above the midpoint of the weight range) and BMI cut points such as ≥27.8 for men and ≥27.3 for women have been used previously in the United States. In addition, the NHLBI guidelines also recommend using waist circumference cut points of 40 in. (102 cm) in men and 35 in. (88 cm) in women to define central obesity. In this chapter, all reported prevalence in adults is based on the BMI 25 and 30 cutoff points.

Children and Adolescents

For adults, the currently used definitions of overweight and obesity are related to health consequences including mortality and morbidity. They are based on fixed values of BMI for all ages and are the same for men and women. Given the latency before some effects of childhood overweight and obesity emerge, BMI definitions in children and adolescents cannot be referenced directly to morbidity and mortality. In addition, BMI changes with age during development, with different patterns by gender. Thus, BMI cut points for the classification of overweight and obesity in childhood vary by gender and age.

Two slightly different sets of BMI percentile references for children have been used in the United States. The "old" BMI reference consists of gender-specific percentiles for a single year of age from 6 to 19 years based on

NHANES I data collected in 1971–74 (Must et al, 1991). The Committee on Clinical Guidelines for Overweight in Adolescent Preventive Services has recommended using the 85th and 95th BMI percentiles for screening of overweight in adolescents (Himes and Dietz, 1994), and similar expert committee recommendations were made subsequently for younger children (Barlow and Dietz, 1998). Thus, "overweight" among individuals 2–19 years old is defined as BMI greater than or equal to the sex-age-specific 95th BMI percentile, and "at risk for overweight," is BMI greater than or equal to the 85th but less than the 95th percentile. Recently the 2000 CDC growth charts (Kuczmarski et al, 2000) were developed based on data collected from five national data sets: the National Health Examination Surveys (NHES II and III) in the 1960s, the NHANES I, II and III between 1971 and 1994. The 2000 CDC growth charts were created for all children in the United States, because all children have similar growth potential. The "new" sex-age-specific BMI 85th and 95th percentiles, based on this reference, are recommended for screening of overweight children and youth ages 2 to 19. For children younger than 2 years there is no BMI-for-age reference on which to recommend the definition of overweight. The weight-for-length 95th percentiles have, therefore, been used to define overweight in this age group (e.g., Black et al, 2004).

Different references can give different prevalence estimates (Wang, 2004; Wang and Wang, 2002). In this chapter, the majority of the reported figures are based on the 2000 CDC growth charts. References used within the United States for epidemiological and clinical purposes may differ from references used to compare across countries, for example. Countries may use different anthropometric measures or/and BMI cut points to classify overweight and obesity (Wang, 2004). Weight-for-height was previously recommended to assess children's nutritional status and may still be used (Guillaume, 1999; WHO, 1995). The International Obesity Taskforce (IOTF) recommends using a set of smoothed BMI percentiles developed by Cole et al (2000) based on data from six different countries, including the United States, to define overweight and obesity for children and adolescents aged 2–18 years. These percentile cutoff points were derived based on sex-specific BMI-age curves that match the adult cutoffs of a BMI of 25 and 30 at age 18 years, respectively.

Ethnic Groups

BMI is usually interpreted without regard to ethnicity. However, there is ongoing research about the possible need to adjust references or cut off points used to denote overweight and obesity to account for differences in body composition and conformation, on average, at the same level of BMI among people in different ethnic groups (see Chapter 2). This issue has been raised primarily with respect to comparisons of Asian descent populations vs. other groups, and Pacific Islander populations vs. other groups (WHO Expert Consultation, 2004).Where the expectation is lower percent body fat and more lean tissue than the reference population (e.g. Pacific Islanders), the usual cutoffs may overestimate obesity. Underestimation of obesity using the typical cutoffs would occur for populations who have, on average, more body fat than the reference population. Some prevalence data for Asian Americans have been reported using lower cut offs than BMI 25 and 30, following recommendations of various expert groups. However it is still not clear under what circumstances these lower cutoffs would be routinely applicable. Data for Asian populations globally in which

BMI is related to mortality do not consistently suggest a single cut off point for all Asian populations (Stevens and Nowicki, 2003). Also, the extent to which this applies to children has not been determined. The current consensus is to a universal reference for all ethnic groups in the United States (NHLBI, 1998).

Obesity Prevalence

Adults

Since NHANES is now continuous, updated estimates are available every two or three years. Table 3.1 shows estimates for the combined prevalence, in 2003–2004, of overweight (BMI ≥ 25) or obesity (BMI ≥ 30) and for obesity separately, overall, by gender, and by race-ethnicity for whites, blacks, and Mexican Americans (Ogden et al, 2006). Among adults aged 20 years and over, overall approximately two-thirds (66.3%) were overweight or obese and approximately one third (32.2%) were obese. Subclasses of obesity have been identified within the category of BMI ≥ 30, to enable tracking of obesity by severity. The prevalence of extreme obesity (BMI ≥ 40) among U.S. adults was 4.8% in the 2003–2004 NHANES data. Extreme obesity is associated with very high risk of disease and disability (Kuczmarski et al, 2000; NHLBI, 1998).

Age and gender: As shown in Table 3.1, overweight and obesity are more prevalent among middle aged and older adults (40 to 59 years or 60+) compared to the 20 to 39 year old group. This is true for both men and women and across ethnicity. Whether these age-differences in prevalence reflect weight gains with age or differences across generations (sometimes called "birth cohort effects") cannot be determined directly from cross-sectional data. Longitudinal data suggest gradual weight gain with age during young adulthood (Williamson, 1993; Lewis et al, 2000), which is consistent with the finding of higher obesity prevalence after age 40. Weight losses at older ages, related to illness, for example, or mortality among obese people may result in lower obesity prevalence at older ages, particularly among the oldest old (e.g., at ages 80 and over) (Williamson, 1993; Ogden et al, 2006). However, lower prevalence of obesity in older age groups may also reflect the fact that prior generations did not experience the recent obesity epidemic and may, therefore, have entered the older ages with lower BMI levels.

Although obesity is often thought to be more common in women, in the overall U.S. population data for 2003–2004, the prevalence of obesity assessed by BMI criteria was similar and not statistically different in men and women (31.1% and 33.2%, respectively, with BMI of 30 or more) (Ogden et al, 2006) (Table 3.1). Data on the combined prevalence of overweight and obesity show higher figures for men than women (70.8% vs. 61.8%, respectively), i.e., men are more likely than women to be in the overweight part of the range. At the other end of the continuum, the prevalence of extreme obesity is higher in women (6.9%) than in men (2.8%).

Ethnic differences: Ethnic differences in overweight and obesity prevalence are substantial for women but not for men (Table 3.1). Non-Hispanic black women and Mexican American women are more likely than non-Hispanic white women to have a BMI of 25 or more and of 30 or more. More than four-fifths of black women are classified as overweight or obese and more than half are classified as obese. Levels for Mexican American women are intermediate. The range for

Table 3.1 Prevalence of overweight and obesity in American adults: NHANES 2003–2004.

Age, y	Overweight or Obesity (BMI ≥25)				Obesity (BMI ≥30)			
	All	Non-Hispanic White	Non-Hispanic Black	Mexican American	All	Non-Hispanic White	Non-Hispanic Black	Mexican American
Both sexes								
≥20	66.3	64.2	76.1	75.8	32.2	30.6	45.0	36.8
20–39	57.1	52.5	69.7	71.2	28.5	25.5	41.9	34.0
40–59	73.1	72.5	81.2	79.4	36.9	36.7	48.4	39.8
≥60	71.0	71.1	78.8	78.1	31.0	29.7	44.9	36.9
Men								
≥20	70.8	70.6	69.1	76.1	31.1	31.1	34.0	31.6
20–39	62.2	59.3	65.0	72.6	28.0	27.2	32.3	32.7
40–59	78.2	79.6	73.1	79.1	34.8	35.6	37.6	31.8
≥60	73.7	75.4	69.8	77.2	30.4	30.6	31.1	29.5
Women								
≥20	61.8	58.0	81.6	75.4	33.2	30.2	53.9	42.3
20–39	51.7	45.6	73.7	69.3	28.9	23.8	50.3	35.7
40–59	68.1	65.3	88.0	79.7	38.8	37.8	57.5	48.3
≥60	68.9	67.6	84.8	78.9	31.5	28.9	54.0	43.8

Source: Adapted from Ogden et al, 2006.

extreme obesity (BMI of 40 or more) among women ages 20 and over shows a similar pattern: highest in non-Hispanic blacks (14.7%), lowest in whites (5.8%), and intermediate in Mexican Americans (7.8%). Ethnic differences in overweight and obesity in men were smaller and less consistent than in women (see Table 3.1) and not statistically significant in the NHANES 2003–2004 data.

Table 3.1 also allows comparisons by gender within the racial/ethnic groups. Obesity or overweight and obesity combined are more prevalent among women than men for non-Hispanic blacks at all ages. Obesity is more prevalent among women than men among Mexican Americans.

Overweight and obesity prevalence have been reported for a broader set of racial/ethnic groups from both the 2001 National Health Interview Survey (NHIS) (for ages 18 and over) and the Behavioral Risk Factor Surveillance System (BRFSS) data (for ages 30 and over) (McNeely and Boyko, 2004; Lucas et al, 2004). These two data sources give a similar impression of the status of groups not covered in NHANES, relative to whites, Blacks and Mexican Americans, although neither source presents subgroup data for age and gender within race/ethnicity. The NHIS data have been plotted in Figure 3.1. The age range and age categories are not identical to those in Table 3.1, however. The prevalence is lower than that from NHANES, as commonly observed in self-reported data. For example, adding the percent overweight and obese for adults 18 years and older gives a combined prevalence of 58.1%, compared to 66.3% for adults ages 20 years and older in NHANES.

The difference in obesity prevalence may be larger than that for overweight, i.e., underreporting of weight may increase as weight increases. For example, obesity prevalence for African Americans is 32.3% in Figure 3.1, compared to 45% for both sexes in NHANES (Table 3.1). The ranking by age (more overweight and obesity in the middle aged and older population) and by ethnicity (more obesity in blacks and Mexican Americans than in non-Hispanic whites)

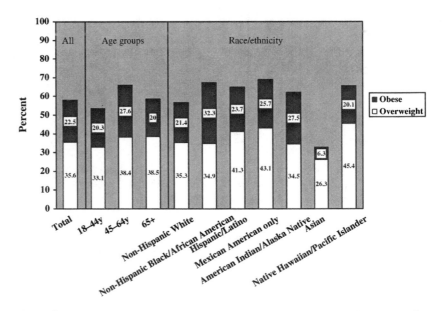

Figure 3.1 Prevalence (%) of overweight and obesity in adults by ethnicity ages 18 years and older from the 2001 (National Health Interview Survey data).

is the same in both the NHANES and NHIS data. The high prevalence of obesity in American Indians and Alaska Natives and in Native Hawaiians or Pacific Islanders in comparison to whites is consistent with the impression from other data sources (Kumanyika, 1994; NHLBI, 1998; Davis et al, 2004). The relatively low prevalence of overweight and obesity in Asian Americans in Figure 3.1 is also consistent with data from other sources (Lauderdale and Rathouz, 2000) and may be affected by the definitional issues discussed previously (WHO Expert Consultation, 2004). That is, lowering the cutoffs used to estimate prevalence in Asian Americans would result in a higher prevalence and could be more reflective of the risk status of Asian American populations with respect to comorbidities.

Within-group diversity may relate to country or region of origin and nativity, including whether the person or his or her parents were born in the United States or how recently they immigrated, and to the degree of acculturation to the U.S. mainstream way of life. People grouped as "Hispanic" may have origins in Mexico, Puerto Rico, Cuba, Central America, or other Spanish Speaking countries. American Indian and Alaska Native groups originate in various U.S. regions, and there are several different ethnic groups within Pacific Islander populations. Representative within-group data are difficult to identify, although some older data illustrate the nature of differences that might be observed:

- The 1982–84 Hispanic Health and Nutrition Examination Survey (HHANES), which sampled Puerto Ricans and Cuban Americans in addition to Mexican Americans, suggests the nature of differences among these Hispanic subgroups. For example, the prevalence of overweight (at the time defined as a BMI ≥ 27.8 for men and ≥ 27.3 for women; based on height and weight measurements) was similar in Mexican American and Puerto Rican women (41.8% and 40.0% respectively) but relatively lower (31.4%) in Cuban American women (Crespo et al, 1996).

- An analysis of BRFSS data for 1985 through 1996 illustrates differences in overweight prevalence (also using BMI ≥ 27.8 for men and ≥ 27.3 for women; based on self-reported height and weight) among American Indians. Prevalence among men was 45.3% in North Dakota and South Dakota; 33.5% in Washington and Oregon; 39.3 % in Oklahoma; and 33.4% in New Mexico and Arizona. Prevalence among women was 46.4% in North Dakota and South Dakota; 43.2% in Washington and Oregon; 35.8% in Oklahoma; and 34.5% in New Mexico and Arizona. This analysis also shows the differences that may occur across age in populations experiencing marked economic and nutrition transitions that result in upward secular trends in obesity (Kumanyika 1994). The *highest* prevalence of overweight in these American Indian samples was among those 18 to 44 years of age—ranging from 44% to 73% in men and from 56 to 65% in women. The prevalence among those over 65 was lowest—less than 10% for older men in three of the four areas; 10 to 19% for the older women.

- An analysis of the 1992–95 National Health Interview Survey (NHIS) illustrates variation in overweight and obesity prevalence among men and women in the six largest Asian American ethnic groups (Chinese, Filipino, Asian Indian, Japanese, Korean, Vietnamese) with comparison data for all NHIS respondents (e.g., including whites and blacks) (Lauderdale, Rathouz, 1999, 2000) (see Figure 3.2). This study also highlighted the effects of nativity and duration of U.S. residence: U.S. born Asian Americans were four times more

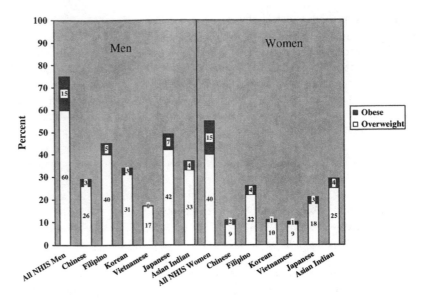

Figure 3.2 Prevalence (%) of overweight and obesity among adults in Asian American ethnic groups, the 2001 (National Health Interview Survey).

likely to be obese than those who were foreign-born. Among the foreign-born, more years in the United States were associated with higher risk of being overweight or obese. The finding of increased obesity with increased duration of U.S. residence applies generally, i.e., not only to Asian Americans (Goel et al, 2004; Kaplan et al, 2004).

Socioeconomic status (SES) differences: The relationship between SES and obesity has been difficult to describe because it differs for men and women and also varies across populations, over time within the same population, depending on the SES indicators and categories used, and also depending on the type of obesity data (which cut off points, or whether self-reported) (Sobal and Stunkard, 1989; Molarius et al, 2000; Leigh et al, 1992; Zhang and Wang, 2004a and 2004b; Chang and Christakis, 2005; Yun et al, 2006). Historically, the impression that there is an inverse association of obesity with SES has been most valid for white females in affluent countries, with no association, direct associations, or curvilinear associations among men and in lower income populations or population subgroups (Sobal and Stunkard, 1989; Leigh et al, 1992). Within the United States, the size of the differential by education has been decreasing over time. Results of analyses in 1999–2000 NHANES data are in Table 3.2 (From Zhang and Wang, 2004b). Using 9th grade or less to define the lowest education category, those with less than high school education have a higher prevalence of obesity than their more educated counterparts, with the exception of black women (Table 3.2), for whom an inverted U-shaped association is suggested, with the highest prevalence among those with a 10th to 12th grade education. Mokdad et al (2003) reported a clear inverse gradient in obesity prevalence by education in the 2001 BRFSS data: 27.4%, 23.2%, and 21.0%, and 15.7% in people with less than high school, high school degree, some college, and college or above. However, a comparison of NHANES and BRFSS data for 1999–2000 found discrepancies in the association with education between these two data sets

Table 3.2 Prevalence of obesity (BMI ≥30, %) in American adults ages 20 to 60 years, by ethnicity and education, NHANES 1999–2000

	Women	Men
All		
<9th grade or less	37.8	26.7
10–12th grade	34.5	29.4
College or higher	29.9	23.6
Non-Hispanic White		
<9th grade or less	36.3	27.7
10–12th grade	31.9	28.3
College or higher	26.6	23.9
Non-Hispanic Black		
<9th grade or less	44.3	32.8
10–12th grade	54.4	22.6
College or higher	51.5	24.8

Data source: Zhang and Wang, 2004b.

(Yun et al, 2006). Particularly noteworthy was the finding of an inverse association of obesity prevalence with education among black women in the BRFSS but not in NHANES. In NHANES, the association was an inverted U-shaped association similar to that shown in Table 3.2: 45.7%, 55.4%, and 49.6%, respectively, among black women with less than high school, high school, or more than high school education.

Region and degree of urbanization: The state-level BRFSS data have highlighted geographic variation in obesity, suggesting that some areas are at higher or lower risk than the country as a whole. Identifying the factors responsible for these differences may provide important clues to obesity prevention overall, particularly in those cases where state rankings have improved or worsened over time (see Figure 3.3). A cluster of Southern, mid-western states (Alabama, Arkansas, Kentucky, Louisiana, Mississippi, Tennessee, Texas, and West Virginia) and the State of Michigan stand out as having the highest obesity prevalence in 2004; Colorado, Montana, Utah, and several New England States stand out as having lower than average obesity prevalence. Consistent with the impression from the BRFSS maps, NHIS data for 2001 suggest lower prevalence of obesity in the West (18.9%), and Northeast (20.3%) compared to the Midwest and South (24.2% and 24.3%, respectively) (Lucas et al, 2004).

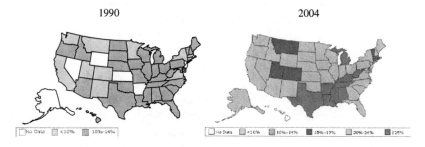

Figure 3.3 Regional differences in the prevalence (%) of obesity in the U.S.: trends based on 1990 and 2001 (BRFSS data).

In the NHIS data, obesity prevalence is lower in large (population of one million or more) vs. small (population less than one million) metropolitan statistical areas—20.0% vs. 23.9%, respectively) and higher still in non-metropolitan areas (25.7%) (Lucas et al, 2004). Prior reports of obesity by urbanization suggest different effects in men and women, also with variation by region. In 1997–98 NHIS data, women living in metropolitan fringe counties (e.g., suburbs) had lower obesity prevalence than women in large or small metropolitan areas (Eberhardt et al, 2001). Women in non-metropolitan areas had the highest obesity prevalence in the Northeast and South. In the Midwest, the highest obesity prevalence was observed among women living in central counties of the large metropolitan areas. Little variation by urbanization level was observed in men.

Children and adolescents

The 2003–2004 NHANES estimates of the prevalence of overweight (BMI 95th percentile) and at risk of overweight (BMI 85th percentile) or overweight are shown in Table 3.3 for children and adolescents ages 2 through 19 years. A third (33.6%) are at risk for overweight or overweight and 17% are overweight. Age, gender, and race-ethnicity data are discussed below.

Age and gender: The age-specific data in Table 3.3 show a substantial prevalence of obesity between the ages of 2 and 5 years, but a marked increase after age 5, with the highest prevalence among children in the 6 to 11 year age range. The prevalence of being at risk for overweight is also somewhat higher among 6 to 11 year olds than in 12 to 19 year olds.

Ethnic differences: African American boys have the lowest percent at risk of overweight or overweight at all ages, except for overweight among 12 to 19 year olds, where ethnic differences are minimal. Mexican American boys have the highest percent in both categories between the ages of 2 and 11 years, with approximately one-fourth in the overweight category at these ages. Among girls, the overall prevalence of being at risk for overweight or overweight is notably higher for African American girls except for at risk of overweight at ages 2 through 5. More than one in four African American girls ages 6 years and older are overweight. Mexican American girls ages 2 through 11 are more likely to be overweight than non-Hispanic white girls.

Obesity prevalence among children in other ethnic groups generally follows patterns similar to those described for adults, e.g., American Indian children and Pacific Islander children have a higher prevalence than the national average. For example:

• Data collected in the PATHWAYS study from 1704 schoolchildren (in 2nd and 3rd grade) in 41 schools from 7 American Indian communities show that half of the children were at risk for overweight or overweight (51.5% in girls vs. 46.5% in boys); and 30.5% of girls and 26.8% of boys were overweight. Although there was a wide range in BMI across study sites, the prevalence was consistently higher than the national averages in all 7 communities and in both girls and boys (Caballero et al, 2003).
• Nationally representative data collected in 1996 from 13,113 U.S. adolescents enrolled in the National Longitudinal Study of Adolescent Health suggest that Asian adolescents had a lower prevalence compared to the national average and to the other ethnic groups. The prevalence of at risk for overweight was 22.8% and 10.4% in Asian American adolescent boys and girls, respectively, compared to 26.5% and 22.2% in white adolescent

Table 3.3 Prevalence of at risk for overweight and overweight in American children and adolescents: NHANES 2003–2004.

	Age, y	At risk for overweight or overweight (BMI ≥85th Percentile)				Overweight (BMI ≥95th Percentile)			
		All	Non-Hispanic White	Non-Hispanic Black	Mexican American	All	Non-Hispanic White	Non-Hispanic Black	Mexican American
Both sexes	2–19	33.6	33.5	35.1	37.0	17.1	16.3	20.0	19.2
	2–5	26.2	25.0	24.0	32.6	13.9	11.5	13.0	19.2
	6–11	37.2	36.9	40.0	42.9	18.8	17.7	22.0	22.5
	12–19	34.3	34.7	36.5	34.3	17.4	17.3	21.8	16.3
Boys	2–19	34.8	35.4	30.4	41.4	18.2	17.8	16.4	22.0
	2–5	27.3	26.6	21.0	38.3	15.1	13.0	9.7	23.2
	6–11	36.5	35.6	34.5	47.9	19.9	18.5	17.5	25.3
	12–19	36.8	38.7	31.4	37.3	18.3	19.1	18.5	18.3
Girls	2–19	32.4	31.5	40.0	32.2	16.0	14.8	23.8	16.2
	2–5	25.2	23.5	27.0	26.7	12.6	10.0	16.3	15.2
	6–11	38.0	38.2	45.6	37.4	17.6	16.9	26.5	19.4
	12–19	31.7	30.4	42.1	31.1	16.4	15.4	25.4	14.1

Source: Adapted from Ogden et al, 2006.

boys and girls, respectively (Gordon-Larsen et al, 2003). Overweight prevalence (i.e., at the 95th percentile) was not reported.

- Based on data collected from 21,911 preschool children aged 12–59 months who participated in the Hawaii Women, Infants, and Children (WIC) program in 1997–98, Baruffi and colleagues reported large ethnic differences in the prevalence of overweight (Baruffi et al, 2004). Among the 8 ethnic groups (white, black, Asian, Filipino, Hawaiian, Hispanic, Samoan, and other), Samoan children had the highest prevalence (17.5% in one-year olds and 27.0% in 2–4 years old), while Asian one-year olds (2.3%) and black 2 to 4 year old children (7.3%) had the lowest rate. The overall prevalence was 5.9% in one-year olds and 11.4% in the 2 to 4 year olds.

Socioeconomic Status (SES) differences: SES associations with overweight are much less clear in children and adolescents than in adults, but—as in adults—are also changing over time (Troiano and Flegal, 1998; Wang and Zhang, 2006; Zhang and Wang, 2004b). Results of NHANES analyses of differences in overweight among children up to age 19 by level of family income are shown in Table 3.4 for two time periods (Wang, 2001; Wang and Zhang, 2006). Relationships are inconsistent across gender and age, although the highest income group has the lowest prevalence in several strata. Among adolescents there is no consistent association between SES and overweight in boys; but low-SES adolescent girls had a much higher prevalence than their low- and medium-SES counterparts (the prevalence was, respectively, 20.0%, 14.2%, and 12.9% in the low-, medium-, and high SES strata). This is mainly due the strong inverse association between SES and overweight in white adolescent girls (Wang and Zhang, 2006). In fact, high-SES black adolescent girls were at increased risk (38.0% prevalence) relative to their lower-SES counterparts 24.5% and 18.7% prevalence, respectively for medium- and low-SES.

Region and degree of urbanization: Rural–urban differences in the prevalence of overweight in U.S. children and adolescents appear small and variable by age groups (Wang, 2001; Wang et al, 2002). In children aged 6–9 years, the

Table 3.4 Prevalence of overweight (≥95th percentile, %) in American children and adolescents, by sex and SES, NHANES 1988–94 and 1999–2002[*].

| | NHANES III (1988–94)[**] | NHANES 1999–2002 | |
	Boys and girls	Boys	Girls
Children[*]			
Low-SES	12.1	17.4	11.9
Medium-SES	11.1	15.0	14.7
High-SES	13.2	9.7	11.4
Adolescents (10–18 y)			
Low-SES	14.0	17.3	20.0
Medium-SES	11.9	18.8	14.2
High-SES	5.5	15.9	12.9

[*] Per capita family income tertiles were used to indicate low-, medium-, and high-SES. Children aged 6–9 years were included in the analysis of NHANES III; and for the NHANES 1999–2002 analysis children aged 2–9 years were included.
[**] Defined at the 95th BMI percentile based on NHANES I data developed by Must et al (1991) before the release of CDC 2000 Growth Chart.
Data sources: Wang 2001; Wang and Zhang 2006

combined prevalence of at risk for overweight and overweight was higher in urban than in rural areas (26.1% vs. 22.8%), but the prevalence of overweight (BMI ≥95th percentile) was almost the same (11.9% vs. 12.1%). In adolescents aged 10–18 years, the combined prevalence of at risk for overweight and overweight was slightly higher in rural than in urban areas (27.2% vs. 24.4%). The prevalence of overweight was similar, 11.2% vs 10.2%.

Tracking of BMI and obesity from childhood to adulthood: A large number of studies have shown the tracking of BMI and obesity status from childhood to adulthood (e.g., Freedman et al, 2005; Guo, Chumlea, 1999; Lack et al, 1997; Mossberg, 1989; Rolland-Cachera et al, 1989; Whitaker et al, 1997), which provides additional support for early prevention. Overall, it is estimated that about one-third of obese preschool children and about half of obese school-age children become obese adults, although findings from different studies vary considerably. Most recently, using longitudinal data collected from 2392 children (initially aged 5–14 years) over 17 years from childhood to adulthood, Freedman et al (2005) found that the tracking of childhood BMI differed between whites and blacks, i.e., the tracking was stronger in blacks. Among overweight children, 65% of white girls vs. 84% of black girls became obese adults; among boys, the figures were 71% in whites vs. 82% in blacks.

Trends in Overweight and Obesity in the United States

The sense of an "epidemic" of obesity comes from trends of marked increases in obesity prevalence over time, in both adults and children and affecting all demographic groups in the U.S. population. These trends, shown in Table 3.5

Table 3.5 Trends in the prevalence of obesity (BMI ≥30, %) in American adults by gender and age: 1960–2002.

	NHES I 1960–62 (N = 6,126)	NHANES I 1971–74 (N = 12,911)	NHANES II 1976–80 (N = 11,765)	NHANES III 1988–94 (N = 14,468)	NHANES 1999–2002 (N = 8,505)
All					
20–74 y[*]	13.4	14.5	15.1	23.3	30.4
Men					
20–74 y[*]	10.7	12.1	12.7	20.6	27.6
20–39 y	9.8	10.2	9.8	14.9	23.0
40–59 y	12.6	14.7	15.4	25.4	30.7
60–74 y	8.4	10.5	13.5	23.8	30.5
Women					
20–74 y[*]	15.8	16.6	17.0	25.9	33.2
20–39 y	9.3	11.2	12.3	20.6	29.1
40–59 y	18.5	19.7	20.4	30.4	36.7
60–74 y	26.2	23.4	21.3	28.6	34.7

[*]Before 1988, the surveys included individuals aged up through 74 years; after 1988, there was no upper age limit.
Data sources: CDC 2003; Hedley et al, 2004; Ogden et al, 2003

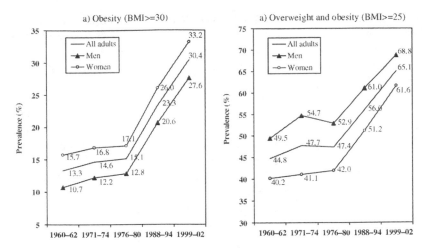

Figure 3.4 Trends in prevalence (%) of obesity in American adults, by sex: 1960–2002.

and Figures 3.4 through 3.6 for adults and in Table 3.6 and Figures 3.7 and 3.8 for children and adolescents, are reviewed below.

Adults

The trends in American adults through 2002 are shown in Table 3.5 and Figures 3.3 through 3.5. Before 1988, the surveys included individuals aged up through 74 years; after 1988, there was no upper age limit. During 1960–80, the increase in the prevalence was slow, but since NHANES II (1976–80), the prevalence has increased dramatically at an average annual rate of approximately one percentage point per year (see Figure 3.5 and Table 3.4). The prevalence of obesity doubled between NHANES II and the 1999–2002 NHANES, an increase from 15.1% to 30.4%, with similar trajectories in men and women. The combined prevalence of overweight and obesity increased at a lower rate, by about one-third, from 52.9% to

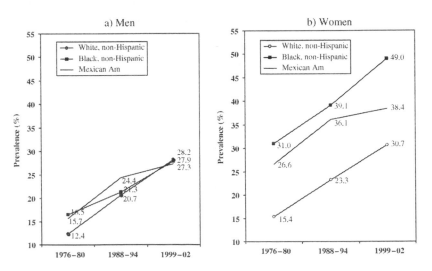

Figure 3.5 Trends in the prevalence (%) of obesity in American adults, by sex and ethnicity: 1976–2002.

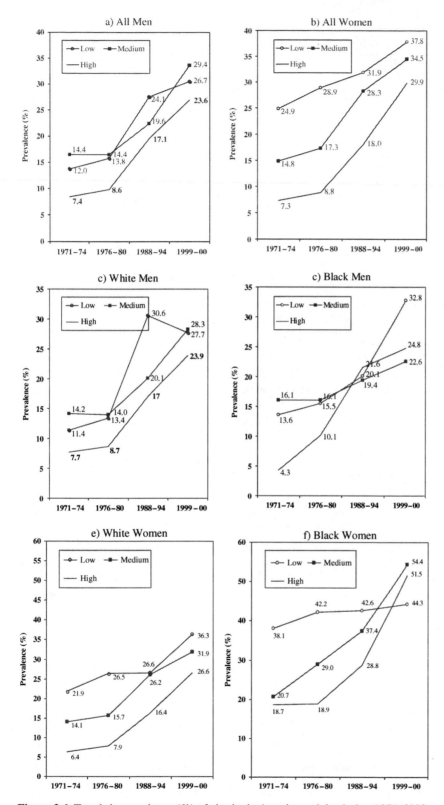

Figure 3.6 Trends in prevalence (%) of obesity in American adults during 1971–2002, by sex, ethnicity and SES.

Table 3.6 Trends in the prevalence of overweight (≥95th percentile, %) in American children and adolescents by gender and age: 1960s–2002.

	NHES II 1963–65 (N = 7,047) and NHES III 1966–70 (N = 6,768)	NHANES I 1971–74 (N = 7,041)	NHANES II 1976–80 (N = 7,904)	NHANES III 1988–94 (N = 13,219)	NHANES 1999–2002 (N = 8,276)
Boys					
6–23 mo	—	—	8.2	9.9	—
2–5 y	—	5.0	4.7	6.1	9.9
6–11 y	4.0	4.3	6.6	11.6	16.9
12–19 y	4.5	6.1	4.8	11.3	16.7
Girls					
6–23 mo	—	—	6.1	7.9	—
2–5 y	—	4.9	5.3	8.2	10.7
6–11 y	4.5	3.6	6.4	11.0	14.7
12–19 y	4.7	6.2	5.3	9.7	15.4

Data sources: CDC 2003; Hedley et al, 2004; Ogden et al, 2003

68.8%. The rate of increase was similar across age groups among men but greater among the 20–39 year old group in women (Table 3.5).

Ethnic differences: In general, notwithstanding some differences in prevalence, particularly among women, the rate of increase has been similar across ethnic groups in both men and women over the past three decades. However,

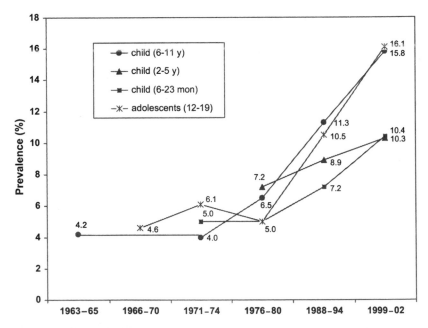

Figure 3.7 Trends in the prevalence (%) of overweight in American children and adolescents: 1960–2002.

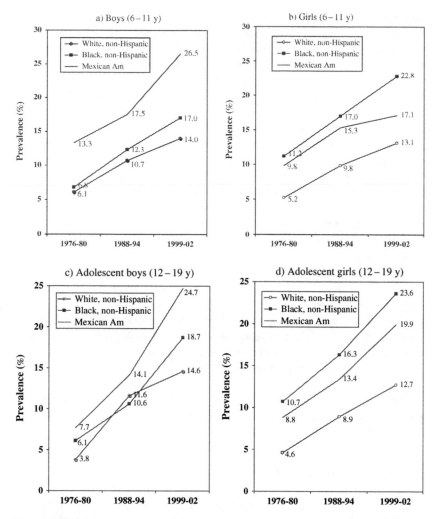

Figure 3.8 Trends in the prevalence (%) of overweight in American children and adolescents during 1976–2002, by sex and ethnicity.

between 1988–94 and 1999–2002, the increase was slower in Mexican American than white and black women (Figure 3.5).

SES differences: Obesity has increased in all SES groups in men and women since the 1970s, but the pattern of trends in SES differences in obesity is changing (Zhang and Wang, 2004b), as noted previously. Age-, gender-, and ethnic differences are shown in Figure 3.6. In white men, the prevalence of obesity in the low-SES group decreased between 1988–94 and 1999–2002, whereas the prevalence in low-SES black men increased at much higher rate than in other SES groups. In black women, obesity increased at a higher rate in the high- and medium-SES group than in low-SES group between 1976–80 and 1999–2002.

Children and Adolescents

The trends in the prevalence of overweight in American children and adolescents are shown in Table 3.6 and Figures 3.7 and 3.8. In all age groups, the prevalence of overweight has increased since the 1960s, more rapidly since NHANES II

(1976–80). Between NHANES II and 1999–2002, the average annual increase rate was approximately 0.5 percentage points in children and adolescents ages 6 years and over. The rate of increase appears to be greater at successive ages. The prevalence of overweight in children aged 2–5 years increased from 7.2% to 10.3%; in children aged 6–11, it almost tripled (increased from 6.5% to 15.8%). In adolescents aged 12–19, it more than tripled (increased from 5.0% to 16.1%) (See Figure 3.7).

Ethnic differences: Available data allow comparisons of trends in non-Hispanic white, non-Hispanic black, and Mexican American children and adolescents from NHANES II (1976–80), although the sample size was small for Mexican Americans in NHANES II (see Figure 3.8). Overweight increased in all ethnic groups. In girls 6 to 11 the rate of increase appears somewhat slower in Mexican Americans. In boys 12 to 19, the rate of increase was slower in whites compared to the other two groups.

Socioeconomic status (SES) differences: Analysis of NHANES data collected between 1971 and 2002 show that overweight increased in all SES groups in all age-sex groups, and in all sex-age-ethnic groups (non-Hispanic white, non-Hispanic black, Mexican American) except for low-SES Mexican American girls aged 2–9 years (Zhang and Wang, 2006). Family per capita income tertiles were used to define low-, medium-, and high-SES groups. There were no consistent patterns regarding SES-differences in the rate of increase. Between NHANES II (1976–80) and 1999–2002, in young boys and girls aged 2–9 and adolescent boys and girls aged 10–18, the prevalence (%) increased from 5.1% to 17.4%, 7.0% to 11.9%, 5.7% to 17.3%, and 8.7% to 30.0%, respectively in low-SES groups. In high-SES groups, overweight prevalence increased from 6.5% to 9.7%, 3.6% to 11.4%, 3.9% to 15.9%, and 3.1% to 12.9%.

Summary and Conclusions

As of 2003–2004, nearly two-thirds of American adults and approximately one-third of American children and adolescents were overweight or obese (labeling the "at risk of overweight" and "overweight" categories for children and youth as "overweight" and "obese" in this context). The prevalence of overweight and obesity among American children and adults has more than doubled since the 1970s and the rate has continues to rise (Ogden et al, 2006). Numerous studies have shown that obesity increases morbidity and mortality (WHO, 2000). Obesity has become the second leading preventable cause of disease and death in the United States, second only to tobacco use (USDHHS, 2001). Obesity is likely to continue to increase and become the leading cause soon if no effective approaches to controlling it can be implemented.

There are large ethnic differences in overweight and obesity in women and children and adolescents in the United States. Some minority and low-SES groups such as non-Hispanic black women and children, Mexican American women and children, low-SES black men and white women and children, Native Americans and Pacific Islanders are disproportionately affected. Asian Americans have a lower prevalence of obesity using the current definitions. However, evidence both within the United States and globally suggests that obesity related risks may emerge among populations of Asian descent at relatively lower BMI levels than would be expected from data based on other populations (McNeely and Boyko, 2004; WHO Expert Consultation, 2004; Smith et al, 2005). Obesity prevalence is currently defined by BMI levels, although waist circumference and other indices of abdominal obesity have been suggested for use to further specify risk levels in general (NHLBI, 1998) and particularly for Asian descent populations (WHO Expert Consultation, 2004; Smith et al, 2005)

The dramatic increase in the prevalence of overweight and obesity across all population groups and declining disparity of obesity across SES groups in the United States suggests that that individual characteristics are not the dominant factor that has contributed to the rising obesity epidemic over the past two decades. The probable social environmental factors contributing to the risk of obesity have been identified across the spectrum of societal sectors and at levels from neighborhoods to national and global (French et al, 2001; Kumanyika, 2001; Kumanyika et al, 2002; Koplan et al, 2005) In addition to the relatively steep increases in prevalence within the same overall population gene pool, the importance of environmental factors driven by societal changes—overall and within high risk ethnic groups—is evident from data on migrants (e.g., the earlier cited increases in obesity with duration of U.S. residence), and by comparing populations of similar ancestry living in different environments (Luke et al, 2001; Schulz et al, 2006). Misconceptions about the tolerance for obesity in ethnic minority populations with high rates of obesity, perhaps based on observations during nutrition and health transitions, have been dispelled by strong evidence of obesity-related comorbidities in these populations (Kumanyika, 1994; Smith et al, 2005).

Without developing effective strategies to modify the current "obesogenic" environment in the United States, it is likely that the obesity epidemic will continue, which implies that there will be a greater burden of obesity-associated chronic disease such as cardiovascular disease and type 2 diabetes to contend with in the future. Government agencies, industry, public health workers, and individuals all need to play an active role in the growing national efforts to combat the obesity epidemic. As discussed throughout this book, population-based policies and programs that emphasize environmental changes are critical for addressing the obesity epidemic—to improve the landscape for successful efforts oriented toward individuals. Such strategies are particularly important to level the playing field for high risk populations. Not only are options and perceived options for individual choices more limited in minority and low income communities (Power, 2004; Cockerham et al, 1997; Yancey et al, 2004; Koplan et al, 2007) but adverse influences such as targeted marketing of low nutrition foods are also more prevalent in these communities (Kumanyika and Grier, 2006). Strategies to address ethnic and SES disparities should also be sensitive to cultural variables that influence attitudes and perceptions related to body weight, food preparation, eating practices, physical activity and inactivity patterns, child-feeding and child-rearing practices.

Ongoing national surveys and surveillance systems provide good data about overweight and obesity measures and some related risk factors such as selected dietary intake and physical activity variables. Greater efforts are needed to study underserved population groups such as minority groups other than African Americans and Mexican Americans. Intervention programs and policies tailored for specific ethnicity and age groups are needed for the primary and secondary prevention of obesity. Childhood and adolescence are key times for individuals to form lifelong eating and physical activity habits, and overweight children are likely to remain obese as adults. Obesity prevention in children and adolescents is a particular public health priority given the dependence of children and youth on environments controlled by adults (Koplan et al, 2005). However, obesity prevention in adults also has a very strong rationale with respect to the potential for immediate benefits in reduction of morbidities that usually occur during middle and older adult years (Seidell et al, 2005).

Acknowledgements This work was supported in part by Dr. Wang's research grants from the National Institutes of Health (NIH)/National Institute of Diabetes & Digestive & Kidney Diseases (NIDDK) (R01 DK63383) and United States Department of Agriculture (USDA, 2044–05322) and by Dr. Kumanyika's Center of Excellence grant from the National Center for Minority Health and Health Disparities at the National Institutes of Health (P60 MD000209).

References

Barlow, S. E. & Dietz, W. H. (1998). Obesity evaluation and treatment: Expert committee recommendations. The maternal and child health bureau, health resources and services administration, and the department of health and human services. *Pediatrics, 102,* E29

Baruffi, G., Hardy, C. J., Waslien, C. I., Uyehara, S. J., & Krupitsky, D. (2004). Ethnic differences in the prevalence of overweight among young children in Hawaii. *Journal of the American Dietetic Association, 104,* 1701–1707.

Black, M. M., Cutts, D. B., & Frank, D. A. et al. (2004). Children's sentinel nutritional assessment program study group. Special supplemental nutrition program for women. Infants, and children participation and infants' growth and health: A multisite surveillance study. *Pediatrics, 114,* 169–176.

Brug, J., & van Lenthe, F. (2005). *Environmental determinants and interventions for physical activity, nutrition, and smoking: A review.* Rotterdam: Ikenweij.

Caballero, B., Himes, J. H., Lohman, T., Davis, S. M., Stevens, J., & Evans, M. et al. (2003). Pathways Study Research Group. Body composition and overweight prevalence in 1704 schoolchildren from 7 American Indian communities. *American Journal of Clinical Nutrition, 78,* 308–312.

Centers for Disease Control and Prevention (CDC). (2004). NHANES 1999–2002 data files: Data, Docs, Codebooks, SAS Code, http://www.cdc.gov/nchs/about/major/nhanes/NHANES99_02.htm (accessed December 2, 2004).

Centers for Disease Control and Prevention (CDC). Table70 (page 1 of 2). Healthy weight, overweight, and obesity among persons 20 years of age and over, according to sex, age, race, and Hispanic origin:United States, 1960–1962, 1971–1974, 1976–1980, 1988–1994, and 1999–2000. http://www.cdc.gov/nchs/data/hus/tables/2002/02hus070.pdf#search='overweight%20and%2020%20years%20and%20over%20and%20CDC' Table 71. Overweight children and adolescents 6–19 years of age, according to sex, age, race, and Hispanic origin: United States, selected years 1963–1965 through 1999–2000 http://www.cdc.gov/nchs/data/hus/tables/2002/02hus071.pdf#search='Table%2071. %20Overweight%20children%20and%20adolescents%206%E2%80%9319%20years %20of%20age%2C' (Access date: September 5th, 2004: CDC, 2002).

Centers for Disease Control and Prevention (CDC). (2005). Overweight and obesity: Defining overweight and obesity, http://www.cdc.gov/nccdphp/dnpa/obesity/defining.htm (assessed November 10, 2005).

Centers for Disease Control and Prevention (CDC). (2005). Overweight and obesity: Obesity trends: U.S. obesity trends 1985–2004, http://www.cdc.gov/nccdphp/dnpa/obesity/trend/maps/index.htm (assessed December 4, 2005).

Centers for Disease Control and Prevention (CDC). Health, United States, 2002, with Chartbook on Trends in the Health of Americans, http://www.cdc.gov/nchs/data/hus/hus02.pdf (accessed April 27, 2007)

Centers for Disease Control and Prevention (1996). The Third National Health and Nutrition Examination Survey (NHANES III 1988–1994) Reference Manuals and Reports (CD-ROM) Centers for Disease Control and Prevention Bethesda, MD.

Chang, V. W., & Christakis, N. A. (2005). Income inequality and weight status in U.S. metropolitan areas. *Social Science and Medicine, 61,* 83–96.

Cockerham, W. C., Rütten, A., & Abel, T. (1997). Conceptualizing contemporary health lifestyles: Moving beyond Weber. *The Sociological Quarterly, 38*(2), 321–342.

Cole, T. J., Bellizzi, M. C., Flegal, K. M., & Dietz, W. H. (2000). Establishing a standard definition for child overweight and obesity worldwide: International survey. *British Medical Journal, 320,* 1240–1243.

Crawford, P. B., Story, M., Wang, M. C., Ritchie, L. D., & Sabry, Z. I. (2001). Ethnic issues in the epidemiology of childhood obesity: Review (August). *Pediatric Clinical of North America, 48*(4), 855–878.

Crespo, C. J., Loria, C. M., & Burt, V. L. (1996). Hypertension and other cardiovascular disease risk factors among Mexican Americans, Cuban Americans, and Puerto Ricans from the Hispanic Health and Nutrition Examination Survey. *Public Health Reports, 111*(Suppl. 2), 7–10.

Davis, J., Busch, J., Hammatt, Z., Novotny, R., Harrigan, R., Grandinetti, A., & Easa, D. (2004). The relationship between ethnicity and obesity in Asian and Pacific Islander populations: A literature review. *Ethnicity and Disease, 14*(1), 111–118.

Ebbeling, C. B., Pawlak, D. B., & Ludwig, D. S. (2002 August 10). Childhood obesity: Public-health crisis, common sense cure. *Lancet, 360*(9331), 473–482.

Eberhardt, M. S., Ingram, D. D., Makuc, D. M., Pamuk, E. R., Freid, V. M., Harper, S. B., Schoemorn, C. A., & Xia, H. (2001) *Urban and rural health chartbook.* Health, United States. Hyattsville, MD: National Center for Health Statistics.

Eisenmann, J. C., Katzmarzyk, P. T., Arnall, D. A., Kanuho, V., Interpreter, C., & Malina, R. M. (2000). Growth and overweight of Navajo youth: Secular changes from 1955–1997. *International Journal of Obesity and Related Metabolic Disorders, 24*(2), 211–218.

Freedman, D. S., Khan, L. K., Serdula, M. K., Dietz, W. H., Srinivasan, S. R., & Berenson, G. S. (2005). Racial differences in the tracking of childhood BMI to adulthood. *Obesity Research, 13,* 928–935.

French, S. A., Story, M., & Jeffery, R. W. (2001). Environmental influences on eating and physical activity. *Annual Review of Public Health, 22,* 309–335.

Gillum, R. F., & Sempos, C. T. (2005). Ethnic variation in validity of classification of overweight and obesity using self-reported weight and height in American women and men: The Third National Health and Nutrition Examination Survey. *Nutrition Journal, 4,* 27.

Goel, M. S., McCarthy, E. P., Phillips, R. S., & Wee, C. C. (2004). Obesity among U.S. immigrant subgroups by duration of residence. *Journal of the American Medical Association, 292*(23), 2860–2867.

Gordon-Larsen, P., Adair, L. S., & Popkin, B. M. (2003). The relationship of ethnicity, socioeconomic factors, and overweight in U.S. adolescents. *Obesity Research, 11,* 121–129.

Grieco, E. M., & Cassidy, R. C. (2001). Overview of race and Hispanic origin: 2000 (U.S. Census Bureau, Census 2000 Brief, C2KBR/01-1). Washington, DC: Government Printing Office. Retrieved January 29, 2006, from http://www.census.gov/prod/2001pubs/cenbr01-1.pdf

Guillaume, M. (1999). Defining obesity in childhood: Current practice. *American Journal of Clinical Nutrition, 70,* 126S130S.

Guo, S. S., & Chumlea, W. C. (1999). Tracking of body mass index in children in relation to overweight in adulthood. *American Journal of Clinical Nutrition, 70,* 145S–148S.

Hedley, A. A., Ogden, C. L., Johnson, C. L., Carroll, M. D., Curtin, L. R., & Flegal, K. M. (2004). Overweight and obesity among U.S. children, adolescents, and adults, 1999–2002. *Journal of the American Medical Association, 291,* 2847–2850.

Himes, J. H., & Dietz, W. H. (1994). Guidelines for overweight in adolescent preventive services: Recommendations from an expert committee. The expert committee on clinical guidelines for overweight in adolescent preventive services. *American Journal of Clinical Nutrition, 59,* 307–316.

Kaplan, M. S., Huguet, N., Newsom, J. T., & McFarland, B. H. (2004). The association between length of residence and obesity among Hispanic immigrants. *American Journal of Preventive Medicine, 27*(4), 323–326.

Koplan, J. P., Liverman, C. T., & Kraak, V. I., (Eds.). (2005). Preventing childhood obesity. Health in the balance. Washington, DC: National Academy Press, Institute of Medicine.

Koplan, J. P., Liverman, C. T., Kraak, V. I., & Wisham, S. L. (Eds.). (2007). *Progress in preventing childhood obesity. How do we measure up?* Washington, DC: National Academy Press, Institute of Medicine.

Kuczmarski, R. J., Ogden, C. L., Guo, S. S., Grummer-Strawn, L. M., Flegal, K. M., Mei, Z., Wei, R., Curtin, L. R., Roche, A. F., & Johnson, C. L. (2000). CDC growth charts: United States. Advance Data. No. 314.

Kumanyika, S. (1993 October 29). Ethnicity and obesity development in children. *Annals of the New York Academy of Science, 699,* 81–92.

Kumanyika, S., & Grier, S. (2006). Targeting interventions for ethnic minority and low-income populations. *Future of Children, 16,* 187–207.

Kumanyika, S., Jeffery, R. W., Morabia, A., Ritenbaugh, C., & Antipatis, V. J. (2002). Public Health Approaches to the Prevention of Obesity (PHAPO) Working Group of the International Obesity Task Force (IOTF). Obesity prevention: The case for action. *International Journal of Obesity and Related Metabolic Disorders 26*(3), 425–436.

Kumanyika, S. K. (2001). Minisymposium on obesity: Overview and some strategic considerations. *Annual Review of Public Health. 22,* 293–308.

Kumanyika, S. K. (1994). Obesity in minority populations: An epidemiologic assessment. *Obesity Research 2*(2), 166–182.

Lauderdale, D. S., & Rathouz, P. J. (1999). Body mass index and Asian Americans: The effect of nativity and years in the U.S. *American Journal of Epidemiology, 149,* S73.

Lauderdale, D. S., & Rathouz, P. J. (2000). Body mass index in a U.S. national sample of Asian Americans: Effects of nativity, years since immigration and socioeconomic status. *International Journal of Obesity and Related Metabolic Disorders, 24,* 1188–1194.

Lewis, C. E., Jacobs, D. R., Jr., McCreath, H., Kiefe, C. I., Schreiner, P. J., Smith, D. E., et al. (2000). Weight gain continues in the 1990s: 10-year trends in weight and overweight from the CARDIA study. Coronary artery risk development in young adults. *American Journal of Epidemiology, 151*(12), 1172–1181.

Lucas, J. W., Schiller, J. S., & Benson, V. (2004). Summary health statistics for U.S. Adults: National Health Interview Survey, 2001. National Center for Health Statistics. *Vital & Health Statistics, 10*(218).

Luke, A., Cooper, R. S., Prewitt, T. E., Adeyemo, A. A., & Forrester, T. E. (2001). Nutritional consequences of the African diaspora. *Annual Review of Nutrition, 21,* 47–71.

McDowell, A., Engle, A., Massey, J., & Maurer, K. (1981). Plan and operation of the Second National Health and Nutrition Examination Survey, 1976–1980. *Vital & Health Statistics, 1*(15), 1–144.

McNeely, M. J., & Boyko, E. J. (2004). Type 2 diabetes prevalence in Asian Americans: results of a national health survey. *Diabetes Care, 27*(1), 66–69.

Mokdad, A. H., Ford, E. S., Bowman, B. A., Dietz, W. H., Vinicor, F., Bales, V. S., et al. (2003). Prevalence of obesity, diabetes, and obesity-related health risk factors, 2001. *Journal of the American Medical Association, 289,* 76–79.

Molarius, A., Seidell, J. C., Sans, S., Tuomilehto, J., Kuulasmaa, K. (2000). Educational level, relative body weight, and changes in their association over 10 years: An international perspective from the WHO MONICA Project. *American Journal of Public Health, 90*(8), 1260–1268.

Mossberg, H. O. (1989). 40-year follow-up of overweight children. *Lancet., 2,* 491–493.

Must, A., Dallal, G. E., & Dietz, W. H. (1991). Reference data for obesity: 85th and 95th percentiles of body mass index (wt/ht2) and triceps skinfold thickness. *American Journal of Clinical Nutrition, 53,* 839–846.

National Center for Health Statistics. (1973). Plan and operation of the health and nutrition examination survey, United States 1971–1973. *Vital & Health Statistics, 1*(10), 1–46.

National Heart, Lung, and Blood Institute (NHLBI) (September 1998). Expert Panel on the Identification, Evaluation, and Treatment of Overweight and Obesity in Adults. Clinical guidelines on the identification, evaluation, and treatment of obesity in adults. *Obesity Research* (Suppl.).

National Heart, Lung, and Blood Institute. (2004). Think Tank on Enhancing Obesity Research at the National Heart, Lung, and Blood Institute. U.S. Department of Health and Human Services. National Institutes of Health. Washington, DC: U.S. Government Printing Office. NIH Publication No. 04-5249. (August). Available at http://www.nhlbi.nih.gov/health/prof/heart/obesity/ob_res_exsum/obesity_tt.pdf

Ogden, C. L., Carroll, M. D., Curtin, L. R., McDowell, M. A., Tabak, C. J., Flegal, K. M. (2006). Prevalence of overweight and obesity in the United States, 1999–2004. *Journal of the American Medical Association, 295,* 1549–1555.

Ogden, C. L., Carroll, M. D., & Flegal, K. M. (2003). Epidemiologic trends in over-weight and obesity. *Endocrinology and Metabolic Clinics of North America, 32,* 741–760.

Ogden, C. L., Flegal, K. M., Carroll, M. D., & Johnson, C. L. (2002). Prevalence and trends in overweight among U.S. children and adolescents, 1999–2000. *Journal of the American Medical Association, 288,* 1728–1732.

Power, E. M. (2004). The determinants of healthy eating among low-income Canadians. Scoping paper for the Office of Nutrition Policy and Promotion, Health Canada.

Rolland-Cachera, M. F., Bellisle, F., & Sempe, M. (1989). The prediction in boys and girls of the weight/height index and various skinfold measurements in adults: A two-decade follow-up study. *International Journal of Obesity, 13,* 305–311.

Schulz, L. O., Bennett, P. H., Ravussin, E., Kidd, J. R., Kidd, K. K., Esparza, J., & Valencia, M. E. (2006). Effects of traditional and western environments on preva-lence of type 2 diabetes in Pima Indians in Mexico and the U.S. *Diabetes Care, 29*(8), 1866–1871.

Seidell, J. C., Nooyens, A. J., & Visscher, T. L. (2005). Cost-effective measures to prevent obesity: Epidemiological basis and appropriate target groups. *Proceedings of the Nutrition Society, 64*(1), 1–5.

Sherry, B., Mei, Z., Scanlon, K. S., Mokdad, A. H., & Grummer-Strawn, L. M. (2004 December). Trends in state-specific prevalence of overweight and underweight in 2- through 4-year-old children from low-income families from 1989 through 2000. *Archives of Pediatric and Adolescent Medicine, 158*(12), 1116–1124.

Smelser, J. N., Wilson, W. J., & Mitchell, F. (Eds.). (2001). *America becoming: Racial trends and their consequences* (Vol. 1). Washington, DC: National Academy Press.

Smith, S. C. Jr., Clark, L. T., Cooper, R. S., Daniels, S. R., Kumanyika, S. K., & Ofili, E. et al. (2005 March 15). American Heart Association Obesity, Metabolic Syndrome, and Hypertension Writing Group. Discovering the full spectrum of cardiovascular disease: Minority Health Summit 2003: Report of the Obesity, Metabolic Syndrome, and Hypertension Writing Group. *Circulation, 111*(10), e134–e139.

Sobal, J., & Stunkard, A. J. (1989). Socioeconomic status and obesity: A review of the literature. *Psychological Bulletin, 105,* 260–275.

Stevens, J., & Nowicki, E. M. (2003). Body mass index and mortality in Asian populations: Implications for obesity cut-points. *Nutrition Reviews, 61*(3), 104–107.

Swinburn, B., Gill, T., & Kumanyika, S. (2005). Obesity prevention: A proposed framework for translating evidence into action. *Obesity Review, 6*(1), 23–33.

Thorpe, L. E., List, D. G., Marx, T., May, L., Helgerson, S. D., & Frieden, T. R. (2004 September). Childhood obesity in New York City elementary school students. *American Journal of Public Health, 94*(9), 1496–1500.

Troiano, R. P., & Flegal, K. M. (1998). Overweight children and adolescents: Description, epidemiology, and demographics. *Pediatrics, 101*(3, Pt. 2), 497–504.

Troiano, R. P., & Flegal, K. M. (1999). Overweight prevalence among youth in the United States: Why so many different numbers? *International Journal of Obesity and Related Metabolic Disorders, 23,* S22–S27.

U.S. Dept. of Health and Human Services, Public Health Service. (2001). The surgeon general's call to action to prevent and decrease overweight and obesity. Rockville, MD: Office of the Surgeon General.

Wang, Y. & Zhang, Q. (2006). Are low-socioeconomic-status American children and adolescents at increased risk of obesity? Changes in the association between overweight and family income between 1971 and 2002. *American Journal of Clinical Nutrition, 84*(4), 707–716.

Wang, Y., Monteiro, C., & Popkin, B. M. (2002). Trends of obesity and underweight in older children and adolescents in the United States, Brazil, China, and Russia. *American Journal of Clinical Nutrition, 75,* 971–977.

Wang, Y., & Wang, J. Q. (2002). A comparison of international references for the assessment of child and adolescent overweight and obesity in different populations. *European Journal of Clinical Nutrition, 56,* 973–982.

Wang, Y. (2001). Cross-national comparison of childhood obesity: The epidemic and the relationship between obesity and socioeconomic status. *International Journal of Epidemiology, 30,* 1129–1136.

Wang, Y. (2004). Epidemiology of childhood obesity—methodological aspects and guidelines: What is new? *International Journal of Obesity and Related Metabolic Disorders, 28,* S21–S28.

Whitaker, R. C., Wright, J. A., Pepe, M. S., Seidel, K. D., & Dietz, W. H. (1997). Predicting obesity in young adulthood from childhood and parental obesity. *New England Journal of Medicine, 337,* 869–873.

WHO Expert Committee. (1995). Physical status, the use and interpretation of anthropometry. WHO Technical Report Series No. 854. Geneva: WHO.

WHO Expert Consultation. (2004). Appropriate body-mass index for Asian populations and its implications for policy and intervention strategies. *Lancet, 363*(9403), 157–163. Erratum in: *Lancet, 363*(9412), 902.

Williamson, D. F., Madans, J., Anda, R. F., Kleinman, J. C., Kahn, H. S., Byers, T. (1993). Recreational physical activity and ten-year weight change in a U.S. national cohort. *International Journal of Obesity and Related Metabolic Disorders, 17,* 279–286.

World Health Organization (WHO). (2000). Obesity: Preventing and managing the global epidemic Report of a WHO consultation. WHO Technical Report Series, No. 894, Geneva: WHO.

Yancey, A. K., Kumanyika, S. K., Ponce, N. A., McCarthy, W. J., Fielding, J. E., Leslie, J. P., & Akbar, J. (2004). Population-based interventions engaging communities of color in healthy eating and active living: A review. *Preventing Chronic Diseases* (January), *1*(1), A09.

Yun, S., Zhu, B. P., Black, W., & Brownson, R. C. (2006). A comparison of national estimates of obesity prevalence from the behavioral risk factor surveillance system and the National Health and Nutrition Examination Survey. *International Journal of Obesity, 30*(1), 164–170.

Zephier, E., Himes, J. H., Story, M. (1999). Prevalence of overweight and obesity in American Indian school children and adolescents in the Aberdeen area: A population study. *International Journal of Obesity and Related Metabolic Disorders, 23*(Suppl. 2), S28–S30.

Zephier, E., Himes, J. H., Story, M., & Zhou, X. (2006). Increasing prevalences of overweight and obesity in Northern Plains American Indian children. *Archives of Pediatric and Adolescent Medicine, 160*(1), 34–39.

Zhang, Q., & Wang, Y. (2004a). Socioeconomic inequality of obesity in the United States: Do gender, age, and ethnicity matter? *Social Science and Medicine, 58,* 1171–1180.

Zhang, Q., & Wang, Y. (2004b). Trends in the association between obesity and socioeconomic status in U.S. adults: 1971 to 2000. *Obesity Research, 12,* 1622–1632.

Chapter 4

Costs of Obesity

Graham A. Colditz and Cynthia Stein

As the prevalence of overweight and obesity continues to climb, the challenge of quantifying the impact of this epidemic also grows. There are many different measures that can be used to evaluate the costs of obesity for the individual and for society, and the objective of this chapter is to discuss some of these costs, including the disease burden, the psychosocial toll, and the financial costs.

Disease Burden

The majority of the U.S. adult population is now overweight or obese (Flegal, Carroll et al. 2002; Hedley, Ogden, et al. 2004), and as the number of overweight children and adults continues to grow, we can expect to see a corresponding increase in obesity-related disease; even small changes in weight across a population can translate into large shifts in disease prevalence and a tremendous public health impact.

Excess weight causes many negative health consequences (U.S. Department of Health and Human Services 2001), including cardiovascular disease (Rimm, Stampfer et al. 1995), type 2 diabetes(Chan, Rimm et al. 1994), cancer (Huang, Hankinson et al. 1997), and premature death (Hu, Willett et al. 2004). Overweight and obesity exacerbate conditions such as hypertension, high cholesterol, and osteoarthritis (National Heart Lung and Blood Institute 1998). Excess weight is also associated with an increased risk of sleep apnea, asthma (U.S. Department of Health and Human Services 2001) cataracts (Hiller, Podgor et al. 1998; Schaumberg, Glynn et al. 2000; Weintraub, Willett et al. 2002), benign prostatic hypertrophy (Giovannucci, Rimm et al. 1994) gallstones (Field, Coakley et al. 2001), menstrual irregularities, infertility (Rich-Edwards, Goldman et al. 1994) and pregnancy complications (U.S. Department of Health and Human Services 2001). Furthermore, health risks do not occur only in those individuals classified as overweight and obese; for some conditions, increase in risk is seen even at the upper end of the normal range of body mass index (Field, Coakley et al. 2001).

In addition to the vast number of obesity related diseases seen in adults, weight-related conditions, such as type 2 diabetes, are being seen more commonly at younger ages, even in pediatric and adolescent populations

(Slyper 1998; Must and Strauss 1999). If the current trends in childhood over-weight and obesity continue, it is probable that complications and lifetime expenditures related to these conditions will also continue to grow.

One measure frequently used to quantify the health effect of obesity is premature mortality. Estimates of the number of obesity-related deaths vary widely, ranging from approximately 112,000 (Flegal, Graubard et al. 2005) to 365,000 per year (Mokdad, Marks et al. 2005). Despite ongoing controversy over the exact number of associated deaths, obesity is clearly associated with increased mortality (McGinnis and Foege 1993; Hu, Willett et al. 2004) and remains a major preventable cause of death in this country. Although mortality is an important measure, it alone cannot give an adequate accounting of disease burden because it omits the morbidity associated with chronic conditions as well as the negative impact of obesity on quality of life and productivity.

Psychosocial Toll

In addition to the large number of physical conditions associated with excess weight, obesity also has severe psychosocial consequences. For example, obesity increases the risk of depression (U.S. Department of Health and Human Services 2001). It also negatively affects vitality (Coakley, Kawachi et al. 1998) and general health-related quality of life (Fine, Colditz et al. 1999; Fallon, Tanofsky-Kraff et al. 2005). In addition, obesity increases the risk social discrimination (U.S. Department of Health and Human Services 2001), and such discrimination may lead to poor quality of life and downward social mobility (Sarlio-Lahteenkorva, Stunkard et al. 1995) (see Chapter 6). Through a prospective analysis, Gortmaker et al. found that women who were over-weight in adolescence had delay in marriage and lower household income than women with weight within the normal range (Gortmaker, Must et al. 1993). Several other studies have evaluated salary according to level of obesity and have concluded that in general more obese individuals have lower wages (Baum and Ford 2004; Finkelstein, Ruhm et al. 2005). The impact of obesity on wages and occupational choice is variable; it has been seen more among women than men, and differs by race, affecting white women more than Black women (Averett and Korenman 1999; Finkelstein, Ruhm et al. 2005). It is not well understood whether this "wage penalty" is a consequence of dis-crimination, poor health, and/or personal characteristics that result in both excess weight and limited earnings.

While the prevalence of overweight and obesity has risen in all segments of our population, certain groups experience a higher burden than others. For example, in our society, body weight tends to increase with advancing age (Field, Wing et al. 2001); the prevalence of obesity is also higher in women than in men and is higher in African Americans than in Whites. National data for 1988–1994 showed that the prevalence of obesity was approximately 15% higher among non-Hispanic Black women and Mexican American women than among white women. Among men, large difference in obesity rates were not noted, but the prevalence of overweight was greater among Mexican American men than among non-Hispanic white and non-Hispanic black men (Flegal, Carroll et al. 1998). See Figure 4.1. These inequalities in obesity rates and the associated physical and psychosocial consequences are likely to

Prevalence of Obesity, by Gender and Race/Ethnicity (adults, aged 20 and older)

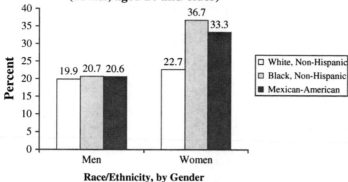

Figure 4.1 Prevalence of Obesity by Gender and Race/Ethnicity (adults, aged 20 and older).

translate into greater disparities in our society, particularly given that obesity has increased since that time and the ethnic disparity also has increased (Hedley et al. 2004) (see Chapter 3).

Financial Cost

Assessing economic cost is another method of quantifying the far-reaching impact of obesity. It has been estimated that obesity costs the United States $117 billion each year (U.S. Department of Health and Human Services 2001). This estimate includes both direct costs (related to diagnosis and treatment of illness) and indirect costs (resulting from lost productivity) (Wolf 1998; U.S. Department of Health and Human Services 2001).

Direct costs

The direct medical costs of obesity include increased utilization of office visits, hospitalizations, nursing home care, treatments and medications. Thompson et al. found that obese individuals have more primary care visits, hospitalizations, and prescriptions than their non-obese counterparts. (Thompson, Brown et al. 2001) Quesenberry et al. looked at similar measures in moderately obese (BMI of 30–34.9) and severely obese (BMI of 35 or more) individuals. They found that, compared to people with a BMI less than 25, moderately obese people had a 17% higher outpatient visit rate and 34% more inpatient days, while severely obese people had a 24% higher outpatient visit rate and 74% more inpatient days (Quesenberry, Caan et al. 1998). In total, obese adults have over 35% higher medical expenditures than their non-obese peers (Sturm 2002; Finkelstein, Fiebelkorn et al. 2003).

To calculate a sum of these direct costs of obesity, many studies have used a prevalence-based approach. This approach reported by Colditz (Colditz 1992) calculates expenditures using the prevalence of a specific disease, the associated annual costs of care, and the estimated proportion of that disease attributable to obesity. To derive the population attributable risk of disease due to obesity,

Table 4.1 Costs ($ billions) of obesity (BMI >30) in the United States, 1995.

Condition	Relative risk	PAR (%)	Direct costs
Type 2 diabetes	11	69	36.6
CHD	4	40	16.2
Hypertension	4	40	7.6
Gall bladder disease	5.5	50	4.3
Cancer			
Breast	1.3	7	.53
Endometrium	2.5	27	.23
Colon	1.5	10	0.89
Osteoarthritis	2.1	20	3.6
Total			70 billion

Uses prevalence of obesity = 22.5% as reported in NHANES III and for breast and endometrial cancer uses prevalence of 24.9% as reported by Flegal et al. 1998.

relative risks are determined from prospective studies, and the prevalence of overweight and obesity are taken from national estimates. Costs of illness are taken from medical expenditure data (Hodgson 1994).

Using this prevalence-based approach, Wolf and Colditz calculated the proportion of disease attributable to obesity and the associated costs (Wolf and Colditz 1994). They included type 2 diabetes, cardiovascular disease, hypertension, gallbladder disease, postmenopausal breast cancer, endometrial cancer, colon cancer and osteoarthritis in their analysis. Using prevalences from NHANES III (22.4% overall obesity in the USA and 24.9% among women for breast and endometrial cancers) Colditz updated the costs attributable to obesity (Colditz 1999). Overall the direct health care costs of obesity were approximately 70 billion dollars or 7% of total health care costs in 1995 (see Table 4.1). Other studies have had similar results, estimating that obesity related health care costs total 5–7% of annual U.S. health care costs (Finkelstein, Ruhm et al. 2005).

Of note, these cost assessments are likely to be underestimates given the limited range of health conditions examined. Considerable evidence now indicates that many other conditions should be included. For example, increased abdominal adiposity causes benign prostatic hypertrophy (Giovannucci, Rimm et al. 1994), and infertility is clearly related in prospective studies to higher BMI categories among young women (Rich-Edwards, Garland et al. 1998). Asthma risk is directly related to adiposity among children (Camargo, Wentowski et al. 2003) and may also be increased by obesity among adults (Camargo, Weiss et al. 1999). Sleep apnea is also directly related to adiposity (Rossner, Lagerstrand et al. 1991).

The selection of cancers to include in cost estimates has also evolved over time. The most recent review by the International Agency for Research on Cancer concluded that overweight and obesity cause cancer of the colon, postmenopausal breast, esophagus (adenocarcinoma), kidney, and endometrium (International Agency for Research on Cancer 2002). Based on the European estimates overweight and obesity account for approximately 5% of all cancer diagnoses (Bergström, Pisani et al. 2001). Subsequent data from the American

Cancer Society Cancer Prevention Study II suggest that an even broader range of cancers is directly related to obesity and may account for 14 to 20% of cancer mortality (Calle, Rodriguez et al. 2003). Recent prospective cohort data for incidence (new cases of disease in a specified time period) support the ACS mortality findings indicating that NHL, multiple myeloma (Blair, Cerhan et al. 2005) and pancreatic cancer (Michaud, Giovannucci et al. 2001; Patel, Rodriguez et al. 2005) are also caused by overweight and obesity, further increasing the proportion of cancer due to overweight and obesity to approximately 10%.

Based on this evidence, many of the previous cost estimates of obesity have substantially underestimated the total direct costs of excess weight. In addition, many of the recent estimates examined the effect of excess weight using the current WHO recommended definition of obesity (BMI of 30 kg/m^2 or greater) thus omitting the substantial weight-related expenditures among those who are overweight (BMI 25 to 29.9 kg/m^2) but not obese (Willett, Dietz et al. 1999).

Another area of growing cost is in obesity-related expenditures in children and adolescents. Wang and Dietz compared national data on hospital discharges from 1979–1981 and 1997–1999 for children between 6 and 17 years of age. Looking at diagnoses at discharge, they found almost twice the amount of diabetes, three times as much obesity and gallbladder disease, and over five times the number of sleep apnea diagnoses. They calculated that the cost of these obesity related hospitalizations more than tripled from $35 million in 1979–1981 to $127 million in 1997–1999 (2001 dollars) (Wang and Dietz 2002).

Internationally, cost analyses have varied by definition of obesity and associated conditions. Using the same approach as Colditz, Levy (Levy, Levy et al. 1995) estimated that the costs of obesity in France was approximately 2% of health care costs in 1992. In the Netherlands, Seidell estimates that the cost was 4% (Seidell 1995), and Segal estimated that obesity is responsible for 2% of health care costs in Australia (Segal, Carter et al. 1994). The definition of obesity, the conditions included in cost estimates, and the findings from these studies are summarized in Table 4.2.

Indirect costs

Not included in the direct cost estimates above are the significant indirect costs, which refer to lost wages and productivity due to illness or premature death; these include sick days, restriction of activities, early retirement, and disability pensions. Narbro et al. (Narbro, Jonsson et al. 1996) estimate that for Sweden, obese subjects are 1.5 to 1.9 times more likely to take sick leave and that 12% of obese women had disability pensions attributable to obesity, costing the equivalent of some 300 million U.S. dollars for every 1 million adult females in the population. Overall approximately 10% of sick leave and disability pensions in women may be related to obesity and obesity-related conditions (Narbro, Jonsson et al. 1996).

In addition to early retirement and disability payments, indirect costs include other measures of lost productivity, such as lost income from sick days and forgone wages due to premature mortality. Future earnings after death are translated into current monetary value using an inflation or discount factor, usually 3% (Gold, Siegel et al. 1996). Lower wages and reduced household income associated with overweight and obesity are additional indirect costs of this epidemic (Gortmaker, Must et al. 1993).

Table 4.2 Cost of obesity from different countries.

Author	Country, Year ($)	Definition of obesity	Conditions included	% total	Comment
Wolf and Colditz (Wolf and Colditz, 1998)	U.S., 1995	29	Type 2 DB, CHD, hypertension, gallbladder, breast, endometrial, and colon ca, osteoarthritis	5%	
Levy (Levy, Levy et al. 1995)	France, 1992	27	Hypertension, MI, angina, stroke, venous thrombosis, NIDDM, hyperlipidemia, gout, osteoarthritis, gallbladder disease, colorectal cancer, breast cancer, genitourinary ca, hip fracture	2%	
Seidell (Seidell, 1995)	Netherlands, 1991	25		4%	Costs of overweight greater than that of obesity
Segal (Segal, Carter et al. 1994)	Australia, 1989	30	NIDDM, gallstones, hypertension, CHD, breast cancer, colon cancer	2%	Comparable to cost of alcohol related conditions in Australia

Colditz estimated that the indirect costs attributable to obesity in the United States amounted to at least 48 billion dollars in 1995 (Colditz 1999). The major contributor to these costs is coronary heart disease (48%), which accounts for the large portion of premature mortality. Other indirect costs were type 2 diabetes (17.5%), and osteoarthritis (17.1%); the latter largely due to excess bed days, work-days lost and restricted activity days. As Colditz noted, his estimate is the lower bound of the health care cost since there are adverse health affects associated with overweight below a BMI of 30 (U. S. Department of Agriculture and U. S. Department of Health and Human Services 1995; NHLBI Obesity Education Initiative Expert Panel on the Identification, Evaluation et al. 1998), and therefore, there are substantial additional costs incurred among those who are overweight but not obese.

Incidence-based approach

Another method of determining cost involves an incidence-based approach to estimating lifetime expenditures. This approach models disease incidence in a hypothetical cohort and estimates the associated costs of care. Future costs are discounted to current dollar values in order to determine the sum of the costs over the life course. Gorsky et al. simulated three hypothetical cohorts and estimated that 16 billion additional dollars will be spent over the next 25 years treating obesity-related illness among middle-aged women (Gorsky, Pamuk et al. 1996). Thompson et al. (Thompson, Edelsberg et al. 1999) estimated the excess costs of health services due to high blood pressure, high cholesterol, diabetes, coronary heart disease and stroke according to level of obesity. Using their model, which did not include any future weight gain, they calculated that the per person costs for obesity comparable to those for smoking. Given the substantial increase in obesity in recent years, this approach appears overly conservative.

It has been postulated that despite higher annual expenditures, obese individuals may have lower lifetime medical costs due to shorter life expectancies. However, the data do not support this theory (Finkelstein, Ruhm et al. 2005).

Summary and Areas of Future Research

The evidence is overwhelming that excess weight is associated with increased morbidity and mortality. Current estimates of expenses related to excess weight clearly underestimate the true costs because these estimates have evaluated only a narrow range of overweight- and obesity-related illness; they have not included factors, such as the impact of reduced physical functioning (Fontaine, Cheskin et al. 1996; Coakley, Kawachi et al. 1998; Fine, Colditz et al. 1999); and many have not accounted for the effects on those who are classified as overweight but not obese. Future studies should also consider the impact of obesity on increased health care costs (Thorpe et al. 2004) as well as in less obvious areas such as cost implications for the airline industry (Dannenberg et al. 2004).

With the rising prevalence of overweight and obesity, we will continue to see growing effects and mounting to costs on the individual, our communities, and our society as a whole. The health consequences and financial costs of this epidemic have moved far beyond the point that can be addressed at the individual level alone. This multidimensional problem requires multilevel interventions, including those that work through individuals, community programs, health care systems, schools, employers, and all levels of government.

Acknowledgment. The authors would like to thank Rebekka Lee for her valuable research assistance.

References

Averett, S., & Korenman, S. (1999). Black-white differences in social and economic consequences of obesity. *International Journal of Obesity and Related Metabolic Disorders, 23*(2): 166–173.

Baum, C. L., II., & Ford, W. F. (2004). The wage effects of obesity: A longitudinal study. *Health Economics, 13*(9): 885–899.

Bergström, A., Pisani, P., Tenet, V., Wolk, A., & Adami, H. O. (2001). Overweight as an avoidable cause of cancer in Europe. *International Journal of Cancer, 91*: 421–430.

Blair, C. K., Cerhan, J. R., Folsom, A. R., & Ross, J. A. (2005). Anthropometric characteristics and risk of multiple myeloma. *Epidemiology, 16*(5): 691–694.

Calle, E. E., Rodriguez, C., Walker-Thurmond, K., & Thun, M. J. (2003). Overweight, obesity, and mortality from cancer in a prospectively studied cohort of U.S. adults. *New England Journal of Medicine, 348*(17): 1625–1638.

Camargo, C. A., Jr., Weiss, S. T., Zhang, S., Willett, W. C., & Speizer, F. E. (1999). Prospective study of body mass index, weight change, and risk of adult-onset asthma in women. *Archives of Internal Medicine, 159*(21): 2582–2588.

Camargo, C. A., Wentowski, C. C., Field, A. E., Gillman, M. W., Frazier, A. L., & Colditz, G. A. (2003). Prospective cohort study of body mass index and risk of asthma in children. *Annals of Epidemiology, 13*(8): 565.

Chan, J. M., Rimm, E. B., Colditz, G. A., Stampfer, M. J., & Willett, W. C. (1994). Obesity, fat distribution, and weight gain as risk factors for clinical diabetes in men. *Diabetes Care, 17*(9): 961–969.

Coakley, E., Kawachi, I., Manson, J. E., Speizer, F. E., Willet, W. C., & Colditz, G. A. (1998). Lower levels of physical functioning are associated with higher body weight among middle-aged and older women. *International Journal of Obesity, 22*: 958–996.

Coakley, E., Kawachi, I., Manson, J. E., Speizer, F. E., Willet, W. C., & Colditz, G. A. (1998). Lower levels of physical functioning are associated with higher body weight among middle-aged and older women. *International Journal of Obesity and related metabolic disorders, 22*(10): 958–965.

Colditz, G. (1992). Economic costs of obesity. *American Journal of Clinical Nutrition, 55*: 503S–507S.

Colditz, G. (1999). Economic costs of obesity and inactivity. *Medicine and Science in Sports and Exercise, 31*: S663–S667.

Dannenberg, A. L., Burton, D. C., & Jackson, R. J. (2004 Oct) Economic and environmental costs of obesity: The impact on airlines. *American Journal of Preventive Medicine, 27*(3) 264.

Fallon, E. M., Tanofsky-Kraff M., Norman, A. C., McDuffie, J. R., Taylor, E. D., Cohen, M. L., Young-Hyman, D., Keil, M., Kolotkin, R. L., & Yanovski, J. A. (2005). Health-related quality of life in overweight and nonoverweight black and white adolescents. *Journal of Pediatrics, 147*(4): 443–450.

Field, A. E., Coakley, E. H., Must. A,, Spadano, J. L., Laird, N., Dietz, W. H., Rimm. E., & Colditz, G. A. (2001). Impact of overweight on the risk of developing common chronic diseases during a 10-year period. *Archives of Internal Medicine, 161*(13): 1581–1586.

Field, A. E., Wing, R. R., Manson, J. E., Spiegelman, D. L., & Willett, W. C. (2001). Relationship of a large weight loss to long-term weight change among young and middle-aged U.S. women. *International Journal of Obesity and related metabolic disorders, 25*(8): 1113–1121.

Fine, J. T., Colditz, G. A., Coakley, E. H., Moseley, G., Manson, J. E., Willett, W. C., & Kawachi, I. (1999). A prospective study of weight change and health-related quality of life in women. *Journal of the American Medical Association, 282*: 2136–2142.

Fine, J. T., Colditz, G. A., Coakley, E. H., Moseley, G., Manson, J. E., Willett, W. C., & Kawachi, I. (1999). A prospective study of weight change and health-related quality of life in women. *Journal of the American Medical Association, 282*(22): 2136–2142.

Finkelstein, E. A., Fiebelkorn, I. C., & Wang, G. (2003). National medical spending attributable to overweight and obesity: How much, and who's paying? *Health Affairs (Millwood) Suppl Web Exclusives*, W3, 219–226.

Finkelstein, E. A., Ruhm, C. J., Kosa, K. M. (2005). Economic causes and consequences of obesity. *Annual Review of Public Health, 26*: 239–257.

Flegal, K. M., Carroll, M. D., Kuczmarski, R. J., & Johnson, C. L. (1998). Overweight and obesity in the United States: Prevalence and trends, 1960–1994. *International Journal of Obesity, 22*: 39–47.

Flegal, K. M., Carroll, M. D., Ogden, C. L., & Johnson, C. L. (2002). Prevalence and trends in obesity among U.S. adults, 1999–2000. *Journal of the American Medical Association, 288*(14): 1723–1727.

Flegal, K. M., Graubard, B. I., Williamson, D.F., & Gail, M. H. (2005). Excess deaths associated with underweight, overweight, and obesity. *Journal of the American Medical Association, 293*(15): 1861–1867.

Fontaine, K. R., Cheskin, L. J., & Barofsky, I. (1996). Health-related quality of life in obese persons seeking treatment. *Journal of Family Practice, 43*: 265–270.

Giovannucci, E., Rimm, E. B., Chute, C. G., Kawachi, I., Colditz, G. A., Stampfer, M. J., & Willett, W. C. (1994). Obesity and benign prostatic hyperplasia. *American Journal of Epidemiology, 140*(11): 989–1002.

Gold, M. R., Siegel, J. E., Russell, L. B., & Weinstein, M. C. (1996). Cost-effectiveness in health and medicine. New York, Oxford University Press.

Gorsky, R. D., Pamuk, E., Williamson, D. F., Shaffer, P. A., & Koplan, J. P. (1996). The 25-year health care costs of women who remain overweight after 40 years of age. *American Journal of Preventive Medicine, 12*, 388–394.

Gortmaker, S. L., Must, A., Perrin, J. M., Sobol, A. M., & Dietz, W. H. (1993). Social and economic consequences of overweight in adolescence and young adulthood. *New England Journal of Medicine, 329*(14): 1008–1012.

Hedley, A. A., Ogden, C. L., Johnson, C. L., Carroll, M. D., Curtin, L. R., & Flegal, K. M. (2004 Jun 16) Prevalence of overweight and obesity among U.S. children, adolescents, and adults, 1999–2002. *Journal of the American Medical Association, 291*(23): 2847–2850.

Hiller, R., Podgor, M. J., Sperduto, R. D., Nowroozi, L., Wilson, P. W., D'Agostino, R.B., & Colton, T. (1998). A longitudinal study of body mass index and lens opacities. The Framingham Studies. *Ophthalmology, 105*(7): 1244–1250.

Hodgson, T. A. (1994). Costs of illness in cost-effectiveness analysis. A review of the methodology. *Pharmacoeconomics, 6*(6): 536–552.

Hu, F. B., Willett, W. C., Li, T., Stampfer, M. J., Colditz, G. A., & Manson, J. E. (2004). Adiposity as compared with physical activity in predicting mortality among women. *New England Journal of Medicine 351*(26): 2694–2703.

Huang, Z., Hankinson, S. E., Colditz, G. A., Stampfer, M. J., Hunter, D. J., Manson, J. E., Hennekens, C. H., Rosner, B., Speizer, F. E., & Willett, W. C. (1997). Dual effects of weight and weight gain on breast cancer risk. *Journal of the American Medical Association, 278*(17): 1407–1411.

International Agency for Research on Cancer (2002). Weight Control and Physical Activity. Lyon, International Agency for Research on Cancer.

Levy, E., Levy, P., Le Pen, C., & Basdevant, A. (1995). The economic cost of obesity: The French situation. *International Journal of Obesity and Related Metabolic Disorders, 19*(11): 788–792.

McGinnis, J. M., & Foege, W. H. (1993). Actual causes of death in the United States. *Journal of the American Medical Association, 270*(18): 2207–2212.

Michaud, D. S., Giovannucci, E., Willett, W. C., Colditz, G. A., Stampfer, M. J., & Fuchs, C. S. (2001). Physical activity, obesity, height, and the risk of pancreatic cancer. *Journal of the American Medical Association, 286*(8): 921–929.

Mokdad, A. H., Marks, J. S., Stroup, D. J., & Gerberding, J. L. (2005). Correction: actual causes of death in the United States, 2000. *Journal of the American Medical Association, 293*(3): 293–294.

Must, A., & Strauss, R. S. (1999). Risks and consequences of childhood and adolescent obesity. *International Journal of Obesity and Related Metabolic Disorders, 23*(Suppl. 2): S2–S11.

Narbro, K., Jonsson, E., Larsson, B., Waaler, H., Wedel, H., & Sjöström, L. (1996). Economic consequences of sick-leave and early retirement in obese Swedish women. *International Journal of Obesity and related metabolic disorders, 20*(10): 895–903.

National Heart Lung and Blood Institute (1998). Clinical guidelines on the identification, evaluation, and treatment of overweight and obesity in adults – The Evidence Report. National Institutes of Health. *Obesity Research, 6*(Suppl. 2): 51S–209S.

NHLBI Obesity Education Initiative Expert Panel on the Identification, Evaluation, (1998). Clinical Guidelines on the identification, evaluation and treatment of overweight and obesity in adults. Bethesda, MD, National Heart, Lung, and Blood Institute, National Institutes of Health, 228.

Patel, A. V., Rodriguez, C., Bernstein, L., Chao, A., Thun, M. J., & Calle, E. E. (2005). Obesity, recreational physical activity, and risk of pancreatic cancer in a large U.S. Cohort. *Cancer Epidemiology, Biomarkers & Prevention, 14*(2): 459–466.

Quesenberry, C. P., Jr., Caan, B., & Jacobson, A. (1998). Obesity, health services use, and health care costs among members of a health maintenance organization. *Archives of Internal Medicine, 158*(5): 466–472.

Rich-Edwards, J. W., Spiegelman, D., Garland, M., Hertzmark, E., Hunter, D. J., Colditz, G. A., Willett, W. C., Wand, H., & Manson, J. E. (2002). Physical activity, body mass index, and ovulatory disorder infertility (abstract). *American Journal of Epidemiology, 13*(2): 184–190.

Rich-Edwards, J. W., Goldman, M. B., Willett, W. C., Hunter, D. J., Stampfer, M. J., Colditz, G. A., & Manson, J. E. (1994). Adolescent body mass index and infertility caused by ovulatory disorder. *American Journal of Obstetrics and Gynecology, 171*(1): 171–177.

Rimm, E. B., Stampfer, M. J., Giovannucci, E., Ascherio, A., Spiegelman, D., Colditz, G. A., & Willett, W. C. (1995). Body size and fat distribution as predictors of coronary heart disease among middle-aged and older U.S. men. *American Journal of Epidemiology, 141*(12): 1117–1127.

Rossner, S., Lagerstrand, L., Persson, H. E., & Sachs, C. (1991). The sleep apnoea syndrome in obesity: Risk of sudden death. *Journal of Internal Medicine, 230*(2): 135–141.

Sarlio-Lahteenkorva, S., Stunkard, A., & Rissanen, A. (1995). Psychosocial factors and quality of life in obesity. *International Journal of Obesity and related metabolic disorders, 19*(Suppl. 6): S1–S5.

Schaumberg, D. A., Glynn, R. J., Christen, W. G., Hankinson, S. E., & Hennekens, C. H. (2000). Relations of body fat distribution and height with cataract in men. *American Journal of Clinical Nutrition, 72*(6): 1495–1502.

Segal, L., Carter, R., & Zimmet, P. (1994). The cost of obesity. The Australian perspective. *PharmacoEconomics, 5*(Suppl. 1): 45–52.

Seidell, J. C. (1995). The impact of obesity on health status – some implications for health care costs. *International Journal of Obesity, 19*(Suppl. 6): S13–S16.

Slyper, A. H. (1998). Childhood obesity, adipose tissue distribution, and the pediatric practitioner. *Pediatrics, 102*(1): e4.

Sturm, R. (2002). The effects of obesity, smoking, and drinking on medical problems and costs. *Health Affairs (Millwood), 21*(2): 245–253.

Thompson, D., Brown, J. B., Nichols, G. A., Elmer, P. J., & Oster, G. (2001). Body mass index and future healthcare costs: A retrospective cohort study. *Obesity Research 9*(3): 210–218.

Thompson, D., Edelsberg, J., Colditz, G. A., Bird, A. P., & Oster, G. (1999). Lifetime health and economic consequences of obesity. *Archives of Internal Medicine, 159*: 2177–2183.

Thorpe, K. E., Florence, C. S., Howard, D. H., & Joski, P. (2004) The impact of obesity on rising medical spending. *Health Affairs (Millwood).* Jul–Dec;Suppl Web Exclusives:W4, 480–486.

U.S. Department of Agriculture and U.S. Department of Health and Human Services (1995). Nutrition and Your Health: Dietary Guidelines for Americans, 4th ed. Washington, DC: U.S. Government Printing Office.

U.S. Department of Health and Human Services (2001). The Surgeon General's call to action to prevent and decrease overweight and obesity. Rockville, MD, U.S. Department of Health and Human Services, Public Health Service, Office of the Surgeon General.

Wang, G., & Dietz, W. H. (2002). Economic burden of obesity in youths aged 6 to 17 years: 1979–1999. *Pediatrics, 109*(5): E81–E86.

Weintraub, J. M., Willett, W. C., Rosner, B., Colditz, G.A., Seddon, J.M., & Hankinson, S.E. (2002). A prospective study of the relationship between body mass index and cataract extraction among U.S. women and men. *International Journal of Obesity and related metabolic disorders*, *26*(12): 1588–1595.

Willett, W., Dietz, W. & Colditz, G. A. (1999). Guidelines for healthy weight. *New England Journal of Medicine*, *341*: 427–434.

Wolf, A., & Colditz, G. (1998). Current estimates of the economic cost of obesity in the United States. *Obesity Research*, *6*: 97–106.

Wolf, A. M. (1998). What is the economic case for treating obesity? *Obes Research*, *6*(Suppl. 1): 2S–7S.

Wolf, A. M., & Colditz, G. A. (1994). The cost of obesity: the U.S. perspective. *Pharmacoeconomics*, *5*(Suppl. 1): 34–37.

Chapter 5

Obesity Prevention Concepts and Frameworks

Shiriki Kumanyika

Introduction

In 2001, former Surgeon General David Satcher's *Call to Action to Prevent and Decrease Overweight and Obesity* (U.S. Department of Health and Human Services, 2001) gave prominence to the need for public attention to the obesity epidemic with the United States. The Call to Action defined the field of obesity prevention as not only a public health issue but also a societal problem to be addressed through actions that involve many sectors not traditionally identified with health. Five overarching principles were set forth in this call (from page v):

– Promote the recognition of overweight and obesity as major public health problems.
– Assist Americans in balancing healthful eating with regular physical activity to achieve and maintain a healthy or healthier body weight.
– Identify effective and culturally appropriate interventions to prevent and treat overweight and obesity.
– Encourage environmental changes that help prevent overweight and obesity.
– Develop and enhance public-private partnerships to help implement this vision.

Since the Surgeon General's call there have been numerous initiatives within the federal government (see Chapter 7), in states and localities and in the nonprofit, private, and philanthropic sectors (Alliance for a Healthier Generation, 2006; Action for Healthy Kids, 2007; Institute of Medicine, 2005; Institute of Medicine, 2007; Robert Wood Johnson Foundation, 2006; Sallis, Moudon, Linton, & Powell, 2005; Ryan, Card-Higginson, McCarthy Justus, & Thompson, 2006; The California Endowment, 2004). Initiatives to address obesity in children have generated the most widespread support for several reasons: the vulnerability of children and greater clarity of the need to protect them from adverse environments; the intuitive sensibility of intervening early to prevent obesity development rather than depend on treatment (see Chapter 1); and the sheer social shock associated with observations of type 2 diabetes (i.e., the type of diabetes formerly named for its adult onset) with onset in childhood. The diabetes issue has been effectively dramatized to emphasize the seriousness of the obesity epidemic. A national action plan to prevent childhood obesity was developed by an Institute of Medicine Committee at the request of the U.S. Congress (Institute of Medicine, 2005). Prior to and concurrent with these U.S. initiatives, similar and even more far reaching calls to action have been issued by other countries and by the World Health Organization and Food and Agriculture Organization (National Obesity Task Force, 2003; Waxman, 2003; World Health Organization, 2000; 2003) and through the International Obesity Task Force (IOTF; see www.iotf.org) (Kumanyika, Jeffery, Morabia, Ritenbaugh, & Antipatis, 2002). Because of the close association of obesity with diabetes, cardiovascular diseases, and other chronic diseases, many of these initiatives are being undertaken in collaboration with the more longstanding efforts to reduce the global burden of these diseases.

To undertake obesity prevention requires familiarity with several key concepts and frameworks. Obesity prevention means different things to different audiences. There are various ways of understanding and describing prevention via multiple frameworks or models. The utility of these prevention frameworks with respect to obesity depends upon the perspective and the purpose. Some frameworks are broadly conceptual and may be most useful for understanding the scope and nature of the task of obesity prevention, how it relates to broader public health concepts and how it is similar to or different from obesity treatment. Other frameworks are particularly informative for planning, i.e., identifying and selecting targets and strategies for action and for seeing how different types of actions fit together as well as the knowledge and skills needed to take the identified actions. Some ways of conceptualizing obesity prevention are relevant to clinical settings or interpersonal interventions, whereas others are more useful when framing issues for action through community mobilization or public policy.

This chapter provides background and an overview of key concepts related to obesity prevention and describes the emergence of obesity prevention as a specific field. The rationale for a paradigm shift away from obesity treatment and toward health promotion and public health approaches to obesity prevention, introduced in Chapter 1, is further elaborated, and some challenges and controversies associated with making this shift are highlighted. Several guiding frameworks are presented with respect to levels of prevention, levels of influence on the problem, and developing action strategies, followed by comments on evaluation of obesity prevention.

Background

The Role of Obesity Prevention Research

Emergence of the Field

Prevention research involves the "direct and immediate application of effective strategies to benefit the public's health," (Stoto, Green, & Bailey, 1997, p. 93) representing a continuum from basic research, to hypothesis testing in controlled settings, to application of interventions in large populations. Within this category, obesity prevention research is still emerging as a specific field of scientific endeavor within the larger field of obesity research. Broad awareness of the need for obesity prevention began to develop in the mid-1990s, with publication of an article indicating increasing prevalence of overweight in U.S. adults (Kuczmarski, Flegal, Campbell, & Johnson, 1994; The National

Task Force on Prevention and Treatment of Obesity, 1994). Reviews of the obesity literature typically offered a vast number of studies on obesity treatment but relatively few on prevention (Glenny, O'Meara, Melville, Sheldon, & Wilson, 1997), even when weight-related cardiovascular disease (CVD) prevention studies were counted (Schmitz & Jeffery, 2000). The field of CVD prevention was already well established and included concerns related to dietary composition (e.g., percent of calories from saturated fat, or amount of salt), levels of physical activity, and overweight or obesity as important CVD risk factors. For example, these variables were the focus of three large scale community-intervention studies to reduce CVD risk factors—involving 12 cities—funded by the National Heart, Lung, and Blood Institute: the Stanford Five City Project, the Pawtucket Heart Health Program, and the Minnesota Heart Health Program (Winkleby, Feldman & Murray, 1997).

When the National Institutes of Health (NIH) called for pilot studies of obesity prevention in 1998, only three studies of obesity prevention in adults, two small pilot studies in children, three school-based studies in children, and one additional study in progress could be identified in the English-language published literature (Kumanyika & Obarzanek, 2003). A 2000 review of obesity prevention studies identified 9 distinct interventions (including two from outside of the United States), and a taxonomy was developed for classifying these interventions according to the underlying model, behavior change methods and modes of delivery (Hardeman, Griffin, Johnston, Kinmonth, & Wareham, 2000). All nine studies used information and common behavior change methods such as self-monitoring, incentives, increasing skills, and goal setting. The authors identified only one intervention—conducted within a school setting—as having made direct environmental changes. Otherwise environmental issues were addressed as part of individual or group counseling or with staff (e.g., school food service staff). These studies showed mixed effectiveness, with only one of the five identified randomized trials reporting a statistically significant effect on weight within the time frame of the study.

Similarly, the pilot studies funded in response to the 1998 NIH initiative relied primarily on nutrition education or behavioral treatment of overweight or early obesity, involving education and counseling about how to maintain energy balance in order to avoid gaining excess weight (Kumanyika & Obarzanek, 2003). Approaches for children were oriented toward putting eating and physical activity behaviors on a trajectory conducive to healthy weight, through working with parents or direct interventions with children. In some cases these approaches were applied to populations irrespective of weight, e.g., children at day care centers, in the client populations of WIC programs[1], or reached through churches or schools. Settings were often selected to reach children in high risk population groups defined by ethnicity or low income. In other cases these approaches were applied to individuals selected to be high risk on the basis of behavioral/physiological circumstances that predispose to excess weight gain (e.g., pregnant women, postpartum women, or smokers who have quit).

---

[1] Supplemental Nutrition Program for Women, Infants, and Children, a program that serves low income families.

Limitations of the Treatment Research Paradigm

The limitations of approaching obesity prevention with treatment-oriented paradigms became evident during two workshops held in 2001 and 2002 with the NIH-funded pilot study investigators (Kumanyika & Obarzanek, 2003; Kuczmarski, 2002). Problems related to behavioral difficulty, motivation, settings, sustainability, and comprehensiveness of preventive interventions, as follows.

Behavioral counseling for prevention presumably targets smaller behavioral changes than in treatment situations, because the goal is not to create a caloric deficit as such. The goal is usually small daily adjustments to caloric intake and expenditure, to be maintained indefinitely vs. more drastic changes to be implemented for a limited time period, as in weight loss. Making smaller changes sounds easier in the sense that people don't have to make as much effort or give up as much. However, such small changes are actually more difficult to observe and track than the larger changes needed to lose weight. The only way to be sure that these small behavior changes are working is, in fact, if they are not working, i.e., if weight gain occurs. Moreover, whereas observing pounds come off is intrinsically motivating to people who are attempting to lose weight, there is no such cognitive reward for not gaining (Rothman, 2000). People who are not overweight might be relatively unmotivated to go through the rather intensive processes involved in cognitive behavioral counseling for weight loss with no immediate rewards attached.

The issue of motivation was also mentioned with respect to the types of people likely to avail themselves of counseling for weight gain prevention. Based on the NIH pilot studies, participants were more likely to be health conscious people who might have attended to weight gain prevention information with minimal or no intervention. People who really need counseling about how to maintain their weight would not necessarily be the ones to seek it out. Furthermore, people who are overweight or obese may not be satisfied with mere avoidance of weight gain as a goal or an outcome (Kumanyika & Obarzanek, 2003).

Many of the pilot studies were conducted in "natural" social settings, including churches, community centers, schools, and worksites. These settings were advantageous with respect to the potential for sustaining the intervention program or reinforcing outcomes achieved after the program was discontinued. However, such settings were not always conducive to delivering intensive counseling programs. Stability of staff, availability of space, and competition with other programs were among the challenges encountered. This suggested the need for more attention to the characteristics of settings and their operational issues, from both theoretical and practical perspectives (see Chapter 12). In addition, it seemed that the programs offered might be a better fit if generated from within rather than imposed upon the setting (see Chapter 13). Such approaches are more characteristics of participatory, community health initiatives than of clinical approaches. Clinical programs tend to ignore or attempt to work around the social context, focusing primarily on the individual. However, the influence of the environment (i.e., the circumstances and options surrounding individual choices) on what people do is evident. The ability of narrowly focused interventions to address only one or two aspects of a much more complex constellation of influences on obesity was seen as problematic,

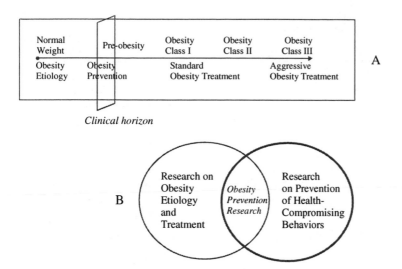

Figure 5.1. View of obesity and obesity prevention research.

Source: Kumanyika & Obarzanek (2003). Pathways to obesity prevention. Report of an NIH workshop. *Obesity Research* 11: 1263–74.

and multilevel interventions involving environmental and policy changes were recommended (Kuczmarski, 2002)

Shifting the Emphasis toward Health Promotion and Public Health

Ultimately, the question was posed as to whether the emphasis should be more on "obesity" or "prevention" (Kuczmarski, 2002; Kumanyika & Obarzanek, 2003) The concept of obesity prevention as a type of *prevention,* with the attendant implications for research and action, had also been raised in the concurrently emerging dialogue on "prevention science". For example, an NIH conference on preventive intervention research identified several common themes in prevention research across a range of topics such as AIDS, smoking, depression, drug abuse, suicide, homicide, child abuse, and obesity (Persons, 1998). Taking a prevention framework would suggest drawing from the theories and interventions in the fields of health promotion and public health (see Figure 5.1). This is consistent with the progression of knowledge and strategies across "generations" of prevention research more generally (Eriksson, 2000) (see Table 5.1).

Clinically oriented approaches to prevention, i.e., framed as intervention earlier in the spectrum of disease emergence to prevent complications and death, may be highly applicable to *targeted prevention,* as defined in Chapter 1 and discussed later in this chapter, which is essentially treatment of individuals with an existing weight problem. Health promotion and public health approaches to risk reduction are more applicable to prevention in the population at large. These approaches span a continuum that includes individually-oriented strategies at one extreme (e.g., health education and counseling) and policy change to improve environments for individual behavior change at the other extreme (e.g., to foster enabling environments for health)—motivating people to seek health and educating them about the behaviors that promote health but also making it easier for people to act in a way that is conducive to good health

Table 5.1 Four generations of cardiovascular prevention.

Generation and basic approach	Knowledge base	Expanded knowledge base and approach
I. Clinical	Medical knowledge	+ Patient-physician psychology
– high-risk, single factor – medical science		+ Information, education, and communication strategies
II. Bioepidemiological	Behavioral change	+ Diffusion theory, media theory
– multiple risk factors – preventive medicine	Social learning theory	+ Population approach, health education
III. Socioepidemiological	Organizational theory	+ Mobilization theory
– Local prevention – Public health actions	Public health sciences	+ Community development, mobilization strategies
IV. Environment & policy oriented	Theory of society	+ Systems theory
– Health sector policy – Health promotion		+ Inter-sectoral action, policy analysis

Source: Adapted from Tables 1 and 2 in Eriksson, C. (2000) *Scandinavian Journal of Public Health*, 28, 298–308.

without necessarily having to think about it. Ideally, many behaviors conducive to health can be incidental to other aspects of daily routines.

The ability to render prevention unobtrusive in daily life is particularly relevant to obesity prevention. A nation preoccupied with calorie counting or "sweating it out" in the gym is not really the goal. In fact, both casual observation and national data demonstrate that dieting does not necessarily result in effective weight control (Serdula, Mokdad, Williamson, Galuska, Mendlein, & Heath, 1999). The obesity epidemic occurred while a majority of the population was attempting to lose or maintain weight. Therefore, many obesity prevention strategies will now work "upstream" (discussed below) to target factors that are beyond individual control but where changes can affect many individuals at once. The most familiar examples come from the field of tobacco control (Mercer, Green, Rosenthal, Husten, Khan, & Dietz, 2003). One policy change, e.g., prohibiting smoking in workplaces or restaurants, greatly reduces the likelihood that nonsmoking individuals will be exposed to secondhand smoke and increases the likelihood that smokers working in these settings will quit.

Subsequent NIH calls for research, as well as research initiatives from the Centers for Disease Control, embraced the need to develop and evaluate obesity prevention approaches geared to policy and environmental changes (Kuczmarski, 2004; League & Dearry, 2004). Private funders have become engaged in this area as well. The Robert Wood Johnson Foundation-funded Active Living Research Program has become a critical contributor to research that integrates expertise and insights from a broad range of disciplines to inform environmental and policy approaches to increase physical activity (Sallis, Cervero, Ascher, Henderson, Kraft, & Kerr, 2006). The Robert Wood Johnson Foundation has also initiated a similar program to build the field of environmental and policy approaches to healthy eating (Story & Orleans, 2006).

Evidence Base

Issues related to the type of evidence needed to support obesity prevention are a major focus of current attention. These issues fall within the general area of evidence-based public health (Brownson, Baker, Leet, & Gillespie, 2003; Rychetnik, Frommer, Hawe, & Shiell, 2002; Rychetnik, Hawe, Waters, Barratt, & Frommer, 2004), developed in parallel and somewhat in contrast to guidelines developed under the rubric of evidence-based medicine. Evidence-based medicine uses a hierarchical approach in which randomized controlled trials (RCTs) and synthetic reviews of sets of RCTs are considered the "gold standard", providing the very best type of evidence. "Best" in this case means most valid with respect to concluding that a particular intervention yielded a particular result, where validity refers only to conditions within the study itself (internal validity). *External* validity, e.g., applicability in the "real world", is not a criterion of rigor for a randomized controlled trial. The conditions that would influence the intervention effectiveness in the real world may have been "designed out" of the study in order to achieve a clearly interpretable *internal* comparison. The actual applicability of the results of randomized controlled trials in natural settings may be questionable, or at least cannot be assumed. Studies that give priority to testing interventions in the natural context are needed—using methods of program evaluation where appropriate.

Other problems with applying the traditional evidence-based medicine approach relate to the types of questions that need to be asked—for which trials of any type might not be suitable research approaches—and the limitations on the ability to study multiple levels of systems of effect that work together to determine an outcome. The need to incorporate systems is relevant to the issue of external validity. Factors that are related in reality cannot be experienced independently. The call for 'practice-based evidence' has emphasized the importance of studying complex problems such as obesity in the context in which the results of the research will be used (Green & Glasgow, 2006).

Swinburn, Gill, and Kumanyika (2005) have developed a framework for thinking through evidence needs for obesity prevention (see Table 5.2). This framework differentiates evidence needs according to the policy objective or question: documenting that a problem exists and the extent of the associated burden; identifying potentially modifiable determinants or pathways in which one might intervene; developing frameworks for taking action; identifying possible actions; and choosing a specific mix of actions to undertake. Accompanying this framework is a broadening of the definition of "evidence" to value—for certain purposes—types of information that are not included on typical evidence hierarchies. These types of information, which are used extensively outside of the health field, include simulation, case histories, and logic modeling (Swinburn et al., 2005). Inherent in this approach is an understanding that action must be taken to address the problem of obesity regardless of the amount of traditional evidence that is available— requiring a systematic approach to using the "best available evidence" to answer the question at hand. The ultimate dilemma in policy making is reduction, not elimination, of uncertainty. Reviews by McKinlay (1992) and by Petticrew & Roberts (2003) and methods papers by Briss and colleagues (Briss, Zaza, Pappaioanou, Fielding, Wright-De Aguero, Truman, Hopkins,

Table 5.2 Examples of proposed components of evidence-based obesity prevention.

Issue (implied question)	Policy/program relevance	Relevant evidence and information	Examples of outputs
1. Building a case for action on obesity (*Why should we do something about obesity?*)	• Show urgency of taking action • Address prioritization of obesity over other issues • Identify populations of special interest • Set benchmarks for goal setting	• Monitoring & surveillance data • Observational studies • Economic analyses • Informed opinion (e.g., assumptions for modelling)	• Prevalence and trend estimates • Cost estimates • Estimated reductions in health burden after interventions
2. Identifying the contributing factors and points of intervention (*What are the causative and protective factors that could potentially be targeted by interventions?*)	• Identify targets for intervening • Relate obesity issues to other existing agendas • Identify congruent and conflicting policies and activities • Identify the stakeholders	• Observational studies • Experimental studies • Indirect evidence • Monitoring and surveillance data • Informed opinion (e.g., on what factors are modifiable)	• Evidence reviews of specific modifiable determinants of obesity and its pathways including levels of certainty and likely size of impact • Identified pathways and drivers of change
3. Define the range of opportunities for action (*How and where could we intervene?*)	• Create links and overlaps with existing plans, policies and programs • Outline the multi-dimensional nature of the action needed • Provide evidence of precedent	• Parallel evidence from other public health initiatives such as tobacco control • Pre-existing frameworks for action (e.g., Ottawa Charter, settings approaches) • Informed opinion (e.g., about other successful frameworks, modifiable and feasible strategies) • Program logic and theory	• Coherent obesity prevention strategic framework either as a stand-alone framework or part of a broader plan of action for nutrition and physical activity, and/or non-communicable diseases • Short and long term goals

4. Evaluate potential interventions (*What are the specific, potential interventions and their likely effectiveness?*)	• Estimate the likely effectiveness of concrete potential interventions in the target population • Progress obesity initiatives through the necessary processes • Identify resource implications	• Experimental studies • Observational studies • Effectiveness analyses, including modelling • Economic analyses • Program logic and theory • Program evaluation (e.g., from existing interventions)	• Specific descriptions of interventions and support actions • Estimates of impact, effectiveness, cost-effectiveness, or cost-utility, and related sensitivity and degree of uncertainty

5. Select a portfolio of policies, programs and actions (*What is a balanced portfolio of initiatives that is sufficient to prevent increases in obesity?*)	• Gain stakeholder input into judgements on policy and implementation implications
	• Gain stakeholder input into and support for priority interventions
	• Take action
		• Estimates of effectiveness and cost-effectiveness and their associated sensitivity and uncertainty
		• Informed opinion on specific interventions and actions about their:
		  • Feasibility and sustainability
		  • Other potential positive or negative effects
		  • Effects on equity
		  • Acceptability to stakeholders
			• Balanced portfolio of specific policies, programs and other actions to prevent obesity

Source: Adapted from Swinburn, Gill, & Kumanyika (2005).

Mullen Thompson, Woolf, Carande-Kulis, Anderson L, Hinman, McQueen, Teutsch, & Harris, 2000) and Harris and colleagues (Harris, Helfand, Woolf, Lohr, Mulrow, Teutsch, & Atkins, 2001) are other excellent resources for thinking through appropriate use of assimilating evidence to support public health based prevention strategies.

Challenges and Controversies

Shifting to a public health paradigm is quite challenging as it relates to obesity. The essence of the public health paradigm is one of societal responsibility to protect the health of the population at large. In countries such as the United States, we tend to expect the public health system to protect us in areas such as sanitation, food safety, clean water, air quality (which includes tobacco smoke), and communicable diseases, but personal behaviors such as eating and physical activity are more likely to be defined as the responsibility of individuals. Interventions on obesity are considered to be in the domain of medical and allied health professionals. Therefore, although it is in one sense quite obvious that people do not control many of the factors that influence eating and physical activity, there is a perception that people who really want to live a healthy life and control their weight can do this. This value orientation leads to a negative judgment about overweight or obese individuals or groups (see Chapter 6).

For example, the higher than average prevalence of obesity in some ethnic minority populations or in low income women, which was observed before the epidemic of obesity in the population overall, may be perceived as consistent with a presumed general pattern of social inadequacy in these groups. With increases in obesity in the population at large and especially in children—who are less socially autonomous and less likely to be blamed for their condition—attitudes have changed somewhat toward acknowledging the need for environmental and policy changes. The issue then becomes one of degree. How much and which changes are needed at the societal level compared to aspects where individuals should be held accountable? How much of what children do is the responsibility of their parents as opposed to school teachers, principals, or policy makers?

In any event, efforts to raise general public awareness of obesity and particularly any environmental or policy change approaches that are viewed as potentially discriminatory to overweight or obese people have been challenged by consumer groups and professionals. These arguments take on various forms. Some assert that any emphasis on obesity increases stigmatization and bias—making life more difficult for those who are already obese (see Chapter 6). One author sees a government conspiracy to stigmatize women in ethnic minority populations that have a high prevalence of obesity (Smith, 2004). These assertions are reminders of the need for sensitivity when formulating public campaigns and policy proposals. The other main type of argument attempts to demonstrate, with various statistics, that the health risks of obesity are being exaggerated (Campos, 2004). This argument is ultimately untenable given the amount of data available about the health risks of obesity, but may be used effectively by some whose interests are threatened by proposed interventions. The debate on interventions that touch the social fabric of society will be ongoing, as it exposes the contradiction of promising fullfledged individualism within a structured society.

The public health perspective on obesity prevention is also challenged on the grounds that it is impractical to try to make the types of broad changes that have been proposed. Gaining acceptance of and effecting changes in physical, economic, and policy environments—which reflect, interact with, and shape sociocultural environments—is certainly not something for which the process is straightforward and readily implemented by policy makers, program planners, or advocates or by any one sector or segment of society.

Nor are all consequences of societal changes easily identified and addressed. Many involve critical elements of the existing social structure and will, therefore, have ripple effects. Cultural, political, and commercial interests are threatened by various proposals for structural change. Currently observed eating and physical activity patterns and lifestyles relate to technological advancements that are viewed as essential, or are at least very popular, and they are also lucrative. Government interference with freedom of choice (to advertise food or to eat whatever foods one chooses to eat) is one accusation that arises. However, parallels have been drawn between obesity prevention and other health-related areas where individual freedoms have been influenced by government regulation: including tobacco control, seat belts, alcohol use, and family planning (Economos, Brownson, DeAngelis, Novelli, Foerster, Foreman, Gregson, Kumanyika, & Pate, 2001; Kersh & Morone, 2002a; Kersh & Morone, 2002b). Issues of individual freedom are always underlying considerations when public policies for the purpose of societal protection are made.

Obesity prevention is more controversial than related areas such as CVD prevention because it adds the element of the total *quantity* of food (calories) consumed. The issue of total calories triggers debate about the entire system of agricultural production and the availability of too many calories per capita in a society where levels of physical labor have declined to low levels (Nestle, 2002; Institute for Agriculture and Trade Policy, 2006). Debates about agricultural policies and food production as these pertain to obesity join other debates about agricultural policy, related to issues such as pesticide contamination and environmental sustainability (Lang & Heasman, 2004). Marketing of high calorie, low nutrition foods to children on television and through contracts with schools are also points of contention (Institute of Medicine, 2006).

Belief in the free market model implies that the interplay of supply and demand can correct any imbalance related to the food supply, while public health advocates point to current economic policies as favoring less healthful foods. The global situation with respect to both obesity and hunger challenges assumptions about the ability of market forces alone to protect the public's health with respect to food intake (Milio, 1990; World Health Organization, 2003). Incongruence between federal nutrition program guidelines or agricultural policies and federal dietary recommendations for weight control and chronic disease prevention have been likened to the federal government's providing agricultural subsidies for tobacco production while promoting smoking cessation. The dilemma that exists with obesity prevention is that, unlike tobacco, food and the systems that provide it are essential to human survival and fulfillment. Somehow, the solution to the obesity epidemic must involve a win-win scenario in which the food industry is involved (see Chapter 9). Figuring out how to create that scenario is proving to be very difficult. In this policy climate, the credibility of obesity prevention experts who work with the food industry may be questioned by public health

Table 5.3 Lessons learned from four social change models: key elements for success.

• Sense that there is a crisis
• Science base (research, data, and evidence)
• Economic benefits
• Charismatic leaders
• Coalition development
• Advocacy
• Government involvement
• Mass communication
• Environmental and policy change
• Overall plan for how the necessary elements can be synergistic

Source: Economos, C. et al. (2001). *Nutrition Reviews*, 59 (3), S40–S56.

advocates, and those who take positions that threaten food industry interests may find themselves or their work being attacked (Mooney, 2005).

Key Elements for Success

Recent successes in public health provide important insights for obesity prevention (Economos et al, 2001; Eriksen, 2005). For example, a set of retrospective case studies of how progress was made in the areas of automotive safety, breastfeeding, waste recycling, and tobacco control identified ten essential components needed, at minimum, to prevent obesity at the population level (see Table 5.3; Economos et al, 2001). The sense of crisis clearly exists and is accepted generally in spite of the aforementioned attempts to play down the importance of obesity. The sense of crisis with respect to children is critical from the perspective of cultural values because children are viewed as a vulnerable population needing societal protection.

As discussed previously, the nature of the science base required to support obesity prevention is still being differentiated from the evidence base that is appropriate for supporting obesity treatment initiatives (Swinburn et al, 2005). In addition, across many areas of public health and prevention science (including obesity prevention) much work remains in understanding how to effectively and efficiently translate scientific evidence into policy and practice (Swinburn et al, 2005; Kellam & Langevin, 2003; Brownson, Kreuter, Arrington, & True 2006). Some policy is made and some programs are mounted with little if any reference to evidence, while in other cases a lack of evidence may be used an excuse for not taking action.

As indicated (Table 5.3), other elements in the mix for success include: mass communication to increase public awareness; advocacy to shape public attitudes and facilitate policy changes; enabling legislation; and economic incentives, e.g., one or more industries whose potential profit will drive a favorable shift in market forces. In addition, an overall plan, a vision, is needed to see the potential for synergy and ultimate success (Economos et al, 2001). This plan may not emerge at the outset, but it is critical to show how various elements fit into a larger picture and the markers of success. The national action plan for childhood obesity prevention, developed by an Institute of Medicine Committee at the request of the U.S. Congress, provides an integrative vision for childhood obesity prevention (Institute of Medicine, 2005). No companion national plan for prevention of obesity in adults exists currently.

Some Guiding Frameworks

Developing effective solutions requires: (1) identifying factors that cause or perpetuate the problem and (2) reflecting on changing these factors to determine potentially useful actions. Which are the easiest or most difficult factors to change? What is the potential impact of changing them? What is involved in changing them? What are some pros and cons of changing them? That is, what are some potential ripple effects, and are they positive or negative? Curbing and ultimately reversing the obesity epidemic will reflect the culmination of many different types of solutions working together. Implementing obesity prevention approaches also requires being able to make the case for the types and intensity of actions that are needed. The review of various controversies associated with obesity prevention underscores the need for a clear articulation of the issues involved. The following frameworks provide some guidance in these respects.

These frameworks are congruent with approaches discussed in other chapters in the Handbook and some are used within other chapters. Many of these concepts are actively used to address other problems such as tobacco use, alcohol and drug use, automotive safety, HIV/AIDS prevention, injury prevention, and environmental health. As we move beyond treatment-oriented paradigms, obesity prevention can and should benefit from the knowledge base and experience within public health and health promotion practice in general (Brownson, Baker, & Novick, 1999; Brownson, Remington, & Davis, 1998; Bruce & McKane, 2000; Peterson & DiClemente, 2000; Raczynski & DiClemente, 1999; Smedley & Syme, 2000).

Disease Continuum

When chronic disease prevention is defined according to a continuum of disease emergence, the anchor points are the timing of disease diagnosis and of progression to increasingly greater levels of severity (see Figure 5.2). *Primary prevention* refers to intervention to prevent excess weight gain prior to the time of diagnosis of obesity, to reduce the incidence (new cases) of obesity. This can be contrasted with measures to reduce obesity prevalence (existing cases), which could include either prevention of excess weight gain among those not yet obese or weight loss to non-obese levels among those who are already obese). As discussed previously, reduction of obesity prevalence is also an important goal. *Primordial prevention* is sometimes used to depict the very earliest stage of the development of risk—akin to maintaining people in a healthy state. Interventions after the point of diagnosis are "treatments" but are also types of prevention in that they may prevent more serious consequences farther along the continuum. For example, *secondary prevention* refers to therapies applied when a disease process has become manifest but is still in the early

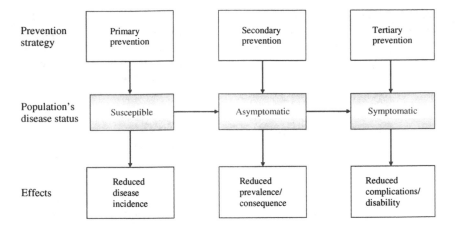

Figure 5.2. Primary, secondary, and tertiary prevention on disease continuum.

Source: Brownson, R. C., Remington, P., Davis, J.R., (1998). *Chronic Disease Epidemiology and Control*, 2nd Edition. Washington, D.C.: American Public Health Association.

stages, to arrest or retard progression and avoid serious complications. *Tertiary prevention* refers to treatment of advanced disease, to avoid death or disability.

The primary-secondary-tertiary prevention continuum can be confusing in that the designation of a particular strategy depends on what outcome is identified and where it falls on the continuum between good health and death or disability, as ultimate outcomes. For example, both obesity prevention and obesity treatment can be considered strategies for the primary prevention diabetes or hypertension. Diabetes and hypertension treatment are, in turn, strategies for the primary prevention of coronary heart disease. The term "*risk reduction*" also refers to actions undertaken to prevent or control the development or progression of risk factors or disease, e.g., primary or secondary prevention of high blood pressure, high cholesterol, or elevated fasting glucose levels to reduce the risk of developing CVD.

To apply the primary-secondary-tertiary prevention continuum to obesity, reference points for adults (ages 18 or 20 years and over) refer to the BMI ranges used to diagnose and indicate severity: BMI 25–29.9 (overweight), 30–34.9 (Class I obesity), 35–39.9 (Class II obesity), and 40 and over (Class III obesity) (National Heart, Lung, and Blood Institute, 1998) (see Chapter 2). Reference points for children up to age 18 or 20 years are the 85th–94.9th percentiles (overweight) and above the 95th percentile (obese) percentile of the relevant age-gender BMI reference[2] (Kuczmarski & Flegal, 2000) (see Chapter 2). For both adults and children, primary prevention would constitute interventions to prevent the overweight from becoming obese. Primary prevention of adult-onset obesity also includes prevention or treatment of obesity in children, since obese children are at significant risk of remaining obese in adulthood. Secondary prevention of obesity might be defined as weight stabilization or weight loss among those with Class I or Class II obesity, to prevent progression to Class III. Treatment of

---

[2]The CDC refers to these categories for children and youth as "as risk of overweight" and "overweight" respectively, rather than overweight and obesity. The terminology used here is consistent with the convention adopted by the Institute of Medicine Committee on Obesity Prevention in Children and Youth (Institute of Medicine, 2005).

Class III obesity, which is recognized as a severe condition with a high risk of complications, might be considered tertiary prevention.

The concept of a continuum, i.e., a gradual, progressive process of obesity development, does help to emphasize that one does not have to wait until people are obese before taking action to control weight and that the likelihood of adverse health consequences of obesity increases with increasing severity and duration. It identifies the population of interest for primary prevention of obesity as anyone who is not yet obese or perhaps overweight. The implied knowledge and behavioral targets relate to caloric intake, physical activity and voluntary weight control (e.g. weight monitoring with deliberate steps to maintain energy balance). This concept does not indicate how to intervene in order to influence these behavioral targets. The frameworks described below provide intervention guidance, which is then spelled out in great detail in subsequent chapters.

Population Focus

As noted in Chapter 1, The World Health Organization (WHO) Report on the Global Epidemic of Obesity (World Health Organization, 2000) proposed a three-level framework for classifying preventive interventions *according to the segment of the population to be reached* (Figure 5.3). This framework was adapted from one developed by the Institute of Medicine in relation to other aspects of public health (Institute of Medicine, 1994) and subsequently applied to obesity prevention as an alternative to the primary-tertiary-secondary continuum

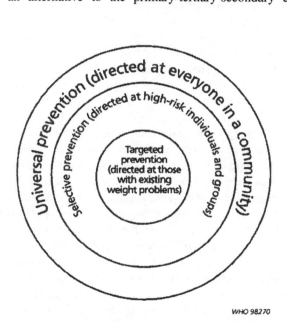

WHO 98270

The diagram shows the three different, but complementary, levels of preventive action for dealing with weight gain and obesity. The very specific targeted-prevention approach is represented by the central circle, the selective preventive approach directed at high-risk individuals and groups is represented by the middle ring, and the broader universal or populationwide prevention approach is represented by the outer ring.

Figure 5.3. Population levels of prevention measures.

Source: World Health Organization (2000). *Obesity, Preventing and Managing the Global Epidemic, Report of a WHO Consultation.* WHO Technical Report Series 894: Geneva, Figure 8.3 as adapted from Gill, T.P., 1997, Key issues in the prevention of obesity. *British Medical Bulletin, 53*, 359–388.

(Institute of Medicine,1995). As shown, in the WHO framework, *universal or public health prevention* is directed at everyone in a community without any selectivity on weight status or apparent risk of becoming obese. *Selective prevention* identifies population based strategies that focus on specific population subgroups and individuals in high risk categories, e.g., defined by race/ethnicity and socioeconomic status (see Chapter 1) or life stage (see Chapter 21). In the original IOM framework (Institute of Medicine, 1994) and also as adapted for obesity prevention (Institute of Medicine, 1995), "selective prevention" refers to high risk groups, and "indicated prevention" refers to high-risk individuals. The WHO framework (Figure 5.3) includes high-risk individuals in the selective prevention category and uses "targeted prevention" to refer to interventions for individuals with existing weight problems or at high risk of obesity related diseases.

The importance of a population approach to obesity prevention was described in Chapter 1. Such initiatives emphasize controlling the determinants of incidence (Rose, 1992) and involve social marketing campaigns, policy development, and programmatic initiatives to change aspects of the social structure related to food access and physical activity options. Our understanding of this approach to population health is often credited to Geoffrey Rose (Rose, 1992; McKinlay, 1992; McKinlay, 1998). This approach emphasizes the potential for influencing the behavior of individuals through altering the behavioral options that are presented and promoted within the environment.

Policy approaches that provide benefit to individuals without any deliberate action on their part are often called "passive" approaches, e.g., putting fluoride in drinking water, folic acid in grain products, or air bags in cars. "Active approaches" work by stimulating purposeful behavior change (e.g., educating people to stop smoking or to use seat belts. Passive and active strategies clearly work in concert at a general population level. Education and counseling to increase awareness of and motivation for more healthful eating and physical activity patterns increase the likelihood that individuals will respond to more healthful options as they become available (e.g., creating pedestrian only areas and also encouraging people to walk more). Much of the challenge in weight gain prevention relates to the difficulty of maintaining behaviors that are socially deviant and not supported in the environmental contexts in which people live and work. As the prevalence of more healthful options increases, so does the likelihood that these options will be viewed as normative, desirable, and accessible and chosen incidentally. In other words, more "passive", population wide approaches can change the landscape for weight control, consistent with the WHO tenet that the "healthy choice should be the easy choice" (Nutbeam, 1986).

Universal approaches aim to shift the entire population distribution. In cardiovascular epidemiology this has been explained using blood pressure as the case example (Rose, 1992), but the reasoning applies to any risk factor with a continuous distribution—where shifting the distribution, downward, re-centers the distribution of the risk factor around a lower mean. This also lowers the number of people crossing a high risk threshold at the upper end of the distribution. Rose demonstrated this principle for BMI using data from the cross-national Intersalt study (Rose, 1991) (see Figure 5.4). The BMI distributions of the diverse Intersalt study populations can be likened to changes in BMI distributions over time in populations such as the United States. As more people gain excess weight, the average BMI increases, the distribution widens, and the proportion of people above the cut off point of BMI 30 is higher.

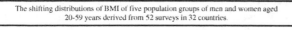

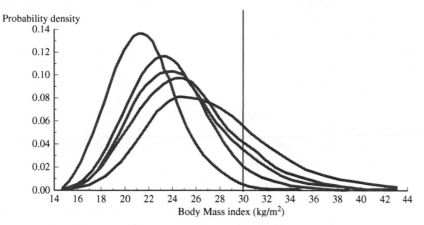

Figure 5.4. Concept of shifting distribution of body mass index.

Source: Adapted from Rose, G. (1991). Population distributions of risk and disease. *Nutr Metab Cardiovascular Dis, 1,* 37–40, Figure 1, page 38. Reprinted with permission of Springer Verlag.

Besides the need for policy and environmental changes to increase the ease of making more healthful choices, universal approaches are also more cost effective than individually-oriented approaches when applied to risk factors or conditions with a high prevalence (Rose, 1992). If almost everyone needs the intervention, there is no reason to screen and counsel each person individually. This is both labor intensive and costly. Furthermore, non-invasive interventions such as healthy eating and activity promotion can be applied universally without concern for harm.

Potential limitations to individually-oriented approaches are relevant here as well. Such approaches tend to de-contextualize risk behaviors, overlooking the influence of cultural and structural influences on individual options for choice—"blaming the victim" for an inability to overcome adverse forces that are clearly beyond individual control (Cockerham, Rütten, & Abel, 1997; McKinlay,1998). In addition, individually-oriented approaches may work best for those who are already health aware and in circumstances conducive to changing their eating and physical activity habits for the better. This is a lower risk segment of the population. Focusing on individuals may, therefore, inadvertently widen the gap between the "haves" and the "have-nots" and exacerbate health disparities.

Arguments against population wide approaches relate in part to concerns about the low benefit-to-risk ratio for individuals. To re-iterate the "prevention paradox" mentioned in Chapter 1, population-wide approaches designed to create population trends and promote modest changes in a large number of individuals are difficult to associate with the benefits for any given individual (Rose, 1992). According to this view, *"Why bother the entire population and take the chance of doing harm when not everyone is at risk?"* However, it is hard to exempt anyone from the need to avoid progressive gain of excess weight. Some people may not have to work as hard as others to accomplish this, but the need is applicable to the population at large.

Do universal prevention strategies threaten the ability of individuals to make free choices? Proponents of population-wide approaches point out that there are always limitations on choice within a social structure—it is central to understand what forces determine those limitations (Rose, 1992). For example, given the evidence that global market forces have shaped food choices in ways that promote the consumption of excess calories, often unintentionally (sometimes called passive overconsumption) (Blundell & Macdiarmid, 1997), is it not appropriate to take action to shift the range of options to one that is more balanced?

As noted previously, perhaps the harder question to answer is that of whose responsibility it is to effect universal strategies involving large societal forces underlying the obesity epidemic. Is this the domain of health care professionals or even public health workers? Even if convinced of the need for environmental changes to enable healthier behaviors in the population at large, many who are trained in health care or public health may be uncertain about how to promote such changes and also wary of the inherently political nature of challenging those who control and profit from the current scenario as it relates to eating and physical activity patterns. Health professionals who are used to being in control with respect to needed expertise in treatment settings may feel devalued or disempowered by approaches that relegate clinical or other technical health expertise to a lesser role in creating solutions. On the other hand, professionals in disciplines more directly related to the aspects of society that may need to be changed (e.g., city planners, economists, agricultural policy makers; sociologists; anthropologists) may not see themselves or be seen by others as having health-related mandates or jurisdictions. Problems like population-wide obesity actually re-define health to represent the net effects of a range of social processes. Obesity is then an adverse side effect of progress and development in a free market system where obesity-promoting eating and physical activity patterns were both socially desirable and good business.

Levels of Influence on the Problem

Ecological Models

The framing of obesity prevention issues from an ecological perspective was introduced in Chapter 1. Ecological models, or socio-ecological frameworks of health behavior are in the forefront of thinking about how to effect change at a population level because they emphasize the importance of the social and environmental contexts in which individuals live and make choices (Friedman, Hunter, & Parrish, 2002; Institute of Medicine, 2003; Stokols, 1992). These models generally depict circular or elliptical layers of influence extending from the individual to the societal, illustrating the principle that the layers are interdependent (See Figure 5.5 [also Figure 1.4 in Chapter 1] from Booth and colleagues (Booth, Sallis, Ritenbaugh, Hill, Birch, Frank, Glanz, Himmelgreen, Mudd, Popkin, Rickard, St. Jeor, & Hays, 2001)). Efforts to change behavior will be most effective when carried out at these multiple levels and including both individual and environmental and policy changes. Individually-oriented interventions are considered most effective when the social environment is in synchrony with the knowledge and behaviors addressed in these programs. Environmental and policy changes are considered most effective when they are combined with programs that motivate and educate individuals to want and respond to the types of change that are made.

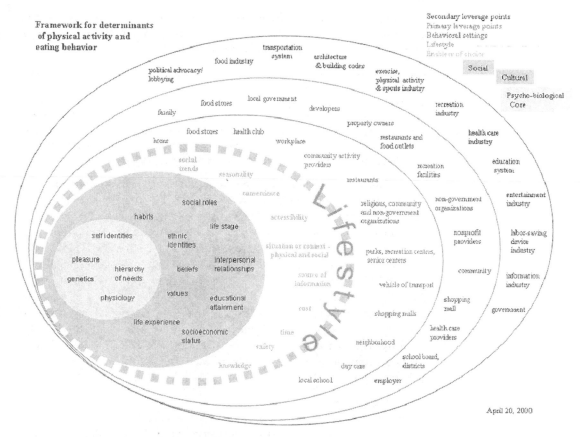

Figure 5.5. Framework for determinants of physical activity and eating behavior.

Source: Booth S.L. et al. (2001). Environmental and Societal Factors Affect Food Choice and Physical Activity: Rationale, Influences, and Leverage Points. *Nutrition Reviews 59 (3 Part 2),* S21–S29. Reprinted with permission of the International Life Sciences Institute (ILSI).

Ecological models are relevant to both treatment as well as prevention, in that the influences in the outer layers are in the background of treatment-oriented interventions. However, preventive interventions focusing on population-wide change actually attempt to address the outer layers to enable environments to support the targeted changes in individuals.

There is no one preferred version of an ecological model with respect to obesity prevention. Levels or layers can be labeled to fit the perspective in question with or without further detail. The ecological model in Figure 5.5 provides considerable detail on levels of influence on individual eating and physical activity behaviors to illustrate leverage points to intervene for change. Accompanying this framework are more detailed explanations about the factors within each level and rankings of specific factors based on the collective judgments of experts about which factors are potentially the most changeable and which, if changed, would have the most impact on eating and physical activity. There is an example of the use of this framework to identify potentially useful interventions to increase physical activity (Booth et al, 2001; Wetter, Goldberg, King, Sigman-Grant, Baer, Crayton, Devine, Drewnowski, Dunn, Johnson, Pronk, Saelens, Snyder, Novelli, Walsh, & Warland, 2001).

The Canadian Population Health Model, based on the principles set forth in the Ottawa Charter for Health Promotion (1986), is an alternative representation of an ecological model. Population health is characterized as:

"influenced by social, economic and physical environments, personal health practices, individual capacity and coping skills, human biology, early childhood development, and health services. As an approach, population health focuses on the interrelated conditions and factors that influence the health of populations over the life course, identifies systematic variations in their patterns of occurrence, and applies the resulting knowledge to develop and implement policies and actions to improve the health and well-being of those populations" (Health Canada, 2001, page 2)

This model posits that action must be taken at various levels within society for change to be accomplished (Evans & Stoddart, 2003). It is depicted as a cube showing areas for action, strategies for taking action, and settings, sectors, or stakeholders where or on whom actions would focus, on a platform that includes values, assumptions, experience, and evidence. The population health model serves as a planning and analysis tool for improving overall population health and for reducing inequities among population groups (Health Canada, 2001). It has been extensively developed with respect to key elements and pathways for effecting and assessing change, with accompanying tools to guide implementation of key elements. The Canadian Population Health Model has been adapted to provide a framework for a review of childhood obesity prevention interventions (Flynn, McNeil, Maloff, Mutasingwa, Wu, Ford, & Tough, 2006).

Obesity Causal Web
The International Obesity Task Force (IOTF) depicts the societal factors and processes contributing to obesity as a "causal web" (Kumanyika et al, 2002) (see Figure 5.6). At the right are the known determinants of weight status—energy intake and energy expenditure. Obesity in the general population results when there is a chronic excess of energy consumed in relation to that expended among a large number of individuals. Moving horizontally and working backward, the successive levels of influence extend from those that are proximal to the individual, i.e., work, school, and home, to those for which the control points are more remote and influences potentially less direct, although the pathways drawn show that many of the global factors operate both directly as well as through the other levels. Moving vertically, the different societal sectors, processes, and settings that influence individual and population eating and physical activity behaviors are represented.

The causal web emphasizes the structural organization of societal sectors, e.g., transportation, food, or education, and shows the interrelationships among sectors that converge on the individual's near environment. From this perspective, the role of the health sector as only one of several types of influences on the obesity epidemic is quite clear. Policies and initiatives in the other sectors are not necessarily "health conscious" although they create the physical, socio-cultural, and economic structures in which eating and physical activity occur. The health sector can take the lead but must work with these other sectors to prevent obesity. One, underutilized, intersectoral strategy is to identify and promote interventions that facilitate obesity prevention but are entirely driven and sustained by goals and methods that are unrelated to weight status or even to health. Robinson (2004) has referred to these

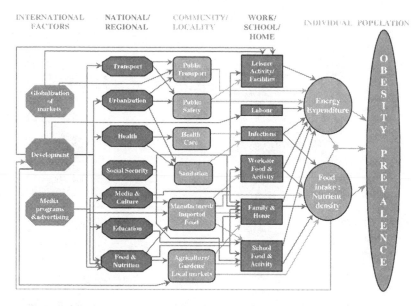

Figure 5.6. Causal web of societal processes influencing the population prevalence of obesity.

Source: International Obesity Task Force [www.iotf.org] see Kumanyika S et al *International Journal of Obesity* 2002; 26:425–36.

interventions as "stealth interventions" because they are not necessarily labeled as health-related. An example would be promoting physical activities such as dancing, games, or hikes for recreation, social interaction, social engagement, or environmental improvement. Activities can be supported by agencies and organizations devoted to these endeavors whether or not they take on the obesity prevention mission. These strategies, therefore, provide a basis for forming non-traditional alliances and for leveraging resources not controlled by health sector.

The causal web can be used for action planning and policy development (Kumanyika 2001; Kumanyika et al, 2002). For example, the Quebec Association for Public Health has developed a detailed plan for use of the causal web to mobilize community action on weight problems generally (ASPQ publication at http://www.aspq.org/view_publications.php?id = 17). The American Public Health Association has developed an on-line Tool Kit that uses the Causal Web to highlight possible actions to intervene on childhood and adolescent obesity (APHA Toolkit; http://www.apha.org/ppp/obesity_toolkit/index.htm).

Continuum of Action
As noted in Chapter 1, interventions involving policy or environmental changes at the levels distal to individuals are often termed "upstream" interventions, whereas those that address the problem by working with individuals one by one are termed "downstream". The upstream and downstream metaphor is often used to emphasize the importance of policy changes in enabling success with smoking cessation. McKinlay has cited Jette's application of this conceptualization to interventions on physical activity in older adults (McKinlay, 1998) and a similar adaptation was developed here, by Kumanyika applicable to

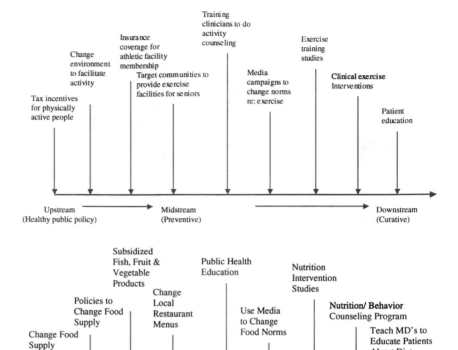

Figure 5.7. Illustration of health promotion and disease prevention interventions related to physical activity (top) and healthy eating (bottom) along a continuum from upstream to downstream.

Source: Top figure is from McKinlay, J.B. (1995). The New Public Health Approach to Improving Physical Activity and Autonomy in Older Populations", in Heikkinen, E., Kuusinen, J., Ruoppila, I., (eds). *Preparation for Aging,* New York, Kluwer/Plenum, reprinted with permission of Springer-Verlag. The bottom figure is S. Kumanyika's adaptation of the top figure.

healthy eating (see Figure 5.7). Upstream interventions target public policy related to economic and physical environment incentives or opportunities conducive to increased physical activity. Midstream interventions improve the service and media environments. Downstream interventions are individually-oriented and curative. This characterization of the spectrum of possible actions also illustrates solutions that are not based on a reversal of presumed causes. That is, regardless of the cause of insufficient activity in older adults, interventions to render activity more rewarding and feasible may foster an increase.

The Spectrum of Prevention, from Contra Costa County in California, is a related framework that is designed to be a tool for planning and coordination of initiatives undertaken by different groups working on the same issue (Rattray, Brunner, & Freestone, 2002). The seven levels of the spectrum are inclusive of the types of strategies needed in a comprehensive effort to address a public health issue: (1) influencing policy and legislation,

Environment size / Environment type	Micro-environment (settings)		Macro-environment (sectors)	
	Food	PA	Food	PA
Physical	What is/isn't available?			
Economic	What are the financial factors?			
Policy	What are the rules?			
Socio-cultural	What are the attitudes, beliefs, perceptions, values and practices?			

Figure 5.8. ANGELO framework: Analysis grid for environments linked to obesity.

Source: Egger, G., Swinburn, B., Rossner S. (2003). Dusting off the epidemiological triad: could it work with obesity? *Obes Rev. 4,* 115–9. Reprinted with permission of Blackwell Publishing.

(2) mobilizing neighborhoods and communities, (3) fostering coalitions and networks, (4) changing organizational practices, (5) educating providers, (6) promoting community education, and (7) strengthening individual knowledge and skills.

Analysis Grid for Environments Linked to Obesity (ANGELO)

The ANGELO framework was developed by obesity prevention researchers in Australia and New Zealand (Swinburn, Egger, & Raza, 1999). ANGELO is a conceptual model for thinking through the environmental influences on obesity. It is intended to be a practical tool for prioritizing strategies for intervention within a given setting. The ANGELO "grid" is shown in Figure 5.8. This grid can be used in a workshop format, e.g., with community coalition members representing diverse sectors as implied in the causal web in Figure 5.5. The approach uses familiar public health problem solving techniques. The first step is to generate potential areas for action—making a comprehensive list of potential elements looking at the environment through the four different lenses indicated on Figure 5.8: physical, economic, political, and sociocultural environments. Available data elements are then rated with respect to: (1) the evidence that this element has an important influence on food intake or level of physical activity (validity); (2) how important this issue is (relevance); (3) the potential for effecting change within this sphere (changeability).

Portfolio Approach

Use of a "portfolio approach has been suggested to help in determining which set of actions applies given evidence about the potential impact and effectiveness of specific interventions" (see Table 5.4) (Hawe & Shiell, 1995; Swinburn et al, 2005). The idea is similar to that for a financial investment portfolio—balancing risks by including a combination of low risk and high risk options—where the return on investment is small but relatively certain for the low risk options and large but uncertain for the high risk options. The portfolio approach helps to avoid having to exclude promising but untried strategies due to a lack of sufficient evidence. As shown in Table 5.4, various options are classified according to their potential benefits and their certainty of effect. An Australian report provides an example of the use of this approach in practice

Table 5.4 Promise table for categorizing potential interventions.

Certainty of effectiveness[*]	Potential population impact[†]		
	Low	**Moderate**	**High**
Quite high	**Promising**	**Very promising**	**Most promising**
Medium	Less promising	**Promising**	**Very promising**
Quite low	Least promising	Less promising	**Promising**

Source: Swinburn, Gill, & Kumanyika (2005).

[*] The certainty of effectiveness is judged by the quality of the evidence, the strength of the programmatic logic, and the sensitivity and uncertainty parameters in the modeling of the population impact.
[†] Potential population impact takes into account efficacy (impact under ideal conditions), reach, and uptake, and it can be measured in a number of ways such as effectiveness, cost-effectiveness, or cost utility.

(New South Wales Center for Public Health Nutrition & New South Wales Department of Health, 2005).

Evaluating Obesity Prevention

Methods for evaluating obesity prevention depend on the level of prevention, the type(s) of initiatives involved, the setting(s) and the time course over which outcomes are determined. Behavioral interventions directed to individuals are the easiest to evaluate in the sense of being able to infer directly cause and effect within a set time horizon. Besides the fact that these types of interventions cannot be the main approach in obesity prevention at the population level, they are also difficult to evaluate for the reasons outlined in the NIH obesity pilot studies workshops, e.g., the large sample sizes required to observe small BMI changes and the difficulty of measuring energy balance outside of laboratory settings (Kuczmarski, 2002; Kumanyika & Obarzanek, 2003).

Evaluation of population level interventions focuses on the particular outcome targeted by the intervention. The Institute of Medicine report on Progress in Childhood Obesity Prevention provides specific guidance on evaluation—with a detailed logic model for thinking through the presumed relationships between what resources and actions are applied and the types of outcomes observed, with attention to important aspects of the demographic and socio-political contexts (Institute of Medicine, 2007). Ecological models can be used to identify specific relationships to serve as focal points for evaluation. The action oriented frameworks help to differentiate the type of evaluation needed. Standard program evaluation techniques are only appropriate for conventional programs and conventional programs are only one type of approach. For example, if the strategy used relates to coalition building, then assessment of the characteristics and performance of the coalition would be appropriate.

Somewhat non-traditional approaches to evaluation are needed when policy change is the intervention. Schmid and colleagues have outlined a framework for policy evaluation and research that covers the span of relevant issues (Schmid, Pratt, & Witmner, 2006). That is, if policy is the target, then evaluations would focus on the quality or quantity of improved policy options. Establishing standards for minimally acceptable policies is an important component of policy evaluation and research. For example, this approach is now used with respect to improving the healthfulness of school environments (National Alliance for

Nutrition and Activity, 2006). Linking policy and changes in the environment to changes in individual behaviors adds a layer of complexity, but models and tools are available. For example, protocols for observing activity in recreational facilities and classrooms are available for assessing the impact of changes in these settings (McKenzie, Marshall, Sallis, & Conway, 2000; Rowe, Schuldheisz, & van der Mars, 1997) on individual or group behavior. Effects of changes in food prices or the mix of products offered can be assessed from sales receipts and use of exercise equipment or employee insurance benefits designed to promote increased physical activity can be tracked by keeping relevant records.

As a rule, the more distant the changes from the individual's point of choice, the harder it will be to interpret individual choices as attributable to the change. The influence of child or family level interventions involving "TV turnoffs" can be readily evaluated through assessment of individual behavior in a randomized trial format. Evaluating the effects of changes in television advertising or programming will be much more challenging. One issue is that experimentation with television programming and commercial advertising is not feasible. In addition, although it appears to be possible to link exposure to television advertising to children's food preferences and food consumption, it is much harder to make the connection to weight levels given the many other factors that influence weight (Institute of Medicine, 2006).

Conclusions

Some of the techniques used in obesity treatment are potentially relevant to prevention in clinical situations, but the main approaches needed to prevent obesity cannot be derived from therapeutic paradigms. Compared to obesity treatment, obesity prevention requires a less medically oriented or curative approach, one that is more oriented toward health promotion and population health, and one that focuses on system and policy change. Obesity prevention requires different types of expertise and involvement from health professionals than does treatment. Of crucial importance, effective obesity prevention strategies are likely to require involvement of professionals from a range of disciplines that are not identified with treatment. Obesity prevention requires a public health-oriented approach to obesity—a theme that is reflected throughout this Handbook.

Early on, when talk of "the obesity epidemic" might have been taken as hyperbole, the critical task was to foster recognition of the obesity problem among health professionals, policy makers, relevant private sector components, and the general public. Currently, although the ongoing dissemination of more evidence about the increasing prevalence of obesity and its consequences across the life span is still important, we are past the point of only describing the problem and well into the stage of developing, implementing and evaluating large scale solutions. Broad statements about the sweeping societal changes needed to curb the obesity epidemic must be followed by specifics. What can we actually do? Who should be doing it? How can it be done? Are we ready to do it? Indicated strategic directions include: (1) shifting emphasis from personal choice/individual control to environmental consequences/social context as the major driver; (2) redefining "ownership" of the problem to include non-health sectors, particularly the agricultural industry, food industry, travel, and urban planning sectors; (3) redefining the role of the health sector to one of involving and stimulating awareness and interest of other sectors in addressing the problem; (4) creating governmental mandates for action to initiate and achieve ameliorative policy shifts; (5) fostering cultural and economic changes as they relate to patterns of eating and physical activity. Obesity prevention can potentially contribute—better yet, must contribute to multiple objectives for improving society and its processes, objectives that go far beyond the seemingly narrow topic of weight control. This view of obesity prevention sets the stage for a much broader platform from which to take action.

References

Action for Healthy Kids (2007). http://www.actionforhealthykids.org/

Alliance for a Healthier Generation
http://www.healthiergeneration.org/engine/renderpage.asp

Antipatis, V. J., Kumanyika, S., Jeffery, R. W., Morabia, A., & Ritenbaugh, C. (1999). Confidence of health professionals in public health approaches to obesity prevention. *International Journal of Obesity and related metabolic disorders, 23*, 1004–1006.

Blundell, J. E., & Macdiarmid, J. I. (1997). Passive overconsumption. Fat intake and short-term energy balance. *Annals of the New York Academy of Science, 827*, 392–407.

Booth, S. L., Sallis, J. F., Ritenbaugh, C., Hill, J. O., Birch, L. L., & Frank, L. D. et al. (2001). Environmental and societal factors affect food choice and physical activity rationale, influences, and leverage points. *Nutrition Reviews, 59*(3 Pt 2), S21–S39.

Briss, P. A., Zaza, S., Pappaioanou, M., Fielding, J., Wright-De Aguero, L., & Truman, B. I. et al. (2000). Developing an evidence-based guide to community preventive services – methods. The task force on community preventive services. *American Journal of Preventive Medicine, 18*(1 Suppl.), 35–43.

Brownson, R. C., Baker, E. A., & Novick, L. E. (1999). *Community-based Prevention. Programs That Work*. Gaithersburg, MD: Aspen Publishers, Inc.

Brownson, R. C., Kreuter, M. W., Arrington, B. A., & True, W. R. (2006). Translating scientific discoveries into public health action: How can schools of public health move us forward? *Public Health Reports, 121*, 97–103.

Brownson, R. C., Remington, P., & Davis, J. R. (1998). *Chronic Disease Epidemiology and Control*, (2nd ed.). Washington, DC: American Public Health Association.

Brownson, R. C., Baker, E. A., Leet, T. L., & Gillespie, K. N. (2003). *Evidence-based Public Health*. New York: Oxford University Press.

Bruce, T. A., & McKane, S. U., (Eds.). (2000). *Community-based Public Health. A Partnership Model*. Washington, DC: American Public Health Association.

The California Endowment (2004). The California Endowment Commits $26 Million To Prevent Childhood Obesity. October 14.
http://www.calendow.org/news/press_releases/2004/10/101404.stm

Campos, P. (2004). *The Obesity Myth — Why America's Obsession with Weight is Hazardous to Your Health*. New York: Gotham Books.

Cockerham, W. C., Rütten, A., & Abel, T. (1997). Conceptualizing contemporary health lifestyles. Moving beyond Weber. *Sociological Quarterly, 38*, 321–341.

Economos, C. D., Brownson, R. C., DeAngelis, M. A., Novelli, P., Foerster, S. B., & Foreman, C. T. et al. (2001). What lessons have been learned from other attempts to guide social change? *Nutrition Reviews, 59*, S40–S56.

Eriksen, M. (2005). Lessons learned from public health efforts and their relevance to preventing childhood obesity, Appendix D, in Institute of Medicine. *Preventing Childhood Obesity. Health in the Balance*, (pp. 405–422). Washington, DC: National Academy Press.

Eriksson, C. (2000). Learning and knowledge-production for public health. A review of approaches to evidence-based public health. *Scandinavian Journal of Public Health, 28*, 298–308.

Evans, R. G., & Stoddart, G. L. (2003). Consuming research, producing policy? *American Journal of Public Health*, *93*, 371–379.

Flynn, M. A., McNeil, D. A., Maloff, B., Mutasingwa, D., Wu, M., Ford, C., & Tough, S. C. (2006). Reducing obesity and related chronic disease risk in children and youth: a synthesis of evidence with 'best practice' recommendations. *Obesity Review*, *7* (Suppl. 1), 7–66.

French, S. A., Story, M., & Jeffery, R. W. (2001). Environmental influences on eating and physical activity. *Annual Review of Public Health*, *22*, 309–335.

Friedman, D. J., Hunter, E. L., & Parrish, R. G. (2002). *Shaping a Vision of Health Statistics for the 21st Century*. Washington, DC: Department of Health and Human Services Data Council, Centers for Disease Control and Prevention, National Center for Health Statistics, and National Committee on Vital and Health Statistics. (Accessed on February 5, 2004 at: http://www.ncvhs.hhs.gov/21st%20final%20report.pdf).

Glenny, A. M., O'Meara, S., Melville, A., Sheldon, T. A., & Wilson, C. (1997). The treatment and prevention of obesity: A systematic review of the literature. *International Journal of Obesity and related metabolic disorders*, *21*, 715–737.

Green, L. W., & Glasgow, R. E. (2006). Evaluating the relevance, generalization, and applicability of research: issues in external validation and tranation methodology. *Evaluation & the Health Professions*, *29*, 126–153.

Hardeman, W., Griffin, S., Johnston, M., Kinmonth, A. L., & Wareham, N. J. (2000). Interventions to prevent weight gain. A systematic review of psychological models and behavior change methods. *International Journal of Obesity and related metabolic disorders*, *24*, 131–143.

Harris, R. P., Helfand, M., Woolf, S. H., Lohr, K. N., Mulrow, C. D., Teutsch, S. M., & Atkins, D.(2001). Methods Work Group, Third U.S. Preventive Services Task Force. Current methods of the U.S. Preventive Services Task Force. A review of the process. *American Journal of Preventive Medicine*, *20*(3 Suppl): 21–35.

Hawe, P., & Shiell, A. (1995). Preserving innovation under increasing accountability pressures: The health promotion investment portfolio approach. *Health Promotion Journal of Australia*, *5*(2), 4–9.

Health Canada (2001). The population health template: Key elements and actions that define a population health approach. Discussion paper. Available at: http://www.phac-aspc.gc.ca/ph-sp/phdd/pdf/discussion_paper.pdf

Institute for Agriculture and Trade Policy (2006). *Food without thought. How U.S. farm policy contributes to obesity*. Washington, DC www.iatp.org/iatp/publications.cfm?accountID=421&refID=80627

Institute of Medicine (1994). *Reducing risks for mental disorders. Frontiers for preventive intervention research*. Washington, DC: National Academy Press.

Institute of Medicine (2002). *Speaking of health. Assessing health communication strategies for diverse populations*. Committee on communication for behavior change in the 21st century. Washington, DC: National Academies Press.

Institute of Medicine (2003). *The future of the public's health in the 21st century*. Washington, DC: National Academies Press.

Kellam, S. G., & Langevin, D. J. (2003). A framework for understanding "evidence" in prevention research and programs. *Prev Sci*, *4*, 137–153.

Kersh, R. & Morone, J. (2002a). The politics of obesity: seven steps to government action. *Health Affairs (Millwood)*, *21*, 142–153.

Kersh, R. & Morone, J (2002b). How the personal becomes the political. Prohibitions, public health, and obesity. *Studies in American Political Development*, *16*, 162–175.

Koplan, J. P., Liverman, C. T., & Kraak, V. I. (Eds.). (2005). *Preventing childhood obesity, health in the balance*. Washington, DC: National Academies Press, Institute of Medicine.

Koplan, J. P., Liverman, C. T., Kraak, V. I., & Wisham, S. L. (Eds.). (2007). *Progress in preventing childhood obesity, How do we measure up?* Washington, DC: National Academy Press, Institute of Medicine.

Kuczmarski, R. (2002). *Second investigators workshop on innovative approaches to prevention of obesity. Workshop report.* National institute of diabetes and digestive and kidney diseases. National institutes of health. Available at: www.niddk.nih.gov/fund/other/archived-conferences/2002/obesity_report.pdf

Kuczmarski, R. (2004). *Summary Report of July 2004 Workshop on site specific approaches to prevention or management of childhood obesity.* National institute of diabetes and digestive and kidney diseases. National institutes of health. Available at: http://www.obesityresearch.nih.gov/news/meetings.htm

Kuczmarski, R. J. (1992). Prevalence of overweight and weight gain in the United States. *American Journal of Clinical Nutrition, 55,* 495S–502S.

Kuczmarski, R. J., Flegal, K. M., Campbell, S. M., & Johnson, C. L. (1994). Increasing prevalence of overweight among U.S. adults. The National Health and Nutrition Examination Surveys, 1960–1991. *Journal of the American Medical Association, 272,* 205–211.

Kuczmarski, R. J., & Flegal, K. M. (2000). Criteria for definition of overweight in transition: background and recommendations for the United States. *American Journal of Clinical Nutrition, 72,* 1074–1081.

Kumanyika, S., Jeffery, R. W., Morabia, A., Ritenbaugh, C., & Antipatis, V. J. (2002). Public Health Approaches to the Prevention of Obesity (PHAPO) Working Group of the International Obesity Task Force (IOTF). Obesity prevention: The case for action. *International Journal of Obesity and related metabolic disorders, 26,* 425–436.

Kumanyika, S. K. (1993). Special issues regarding obesity in minority populations. *Annals of Internal Medicine, 119,* 650–654.

Kumanyika, S. K. (2001). Minisymposium on obesity: overview and some strategic considerations. *Annual Review of Public Health, 22,* 293–308.

Kumanyika, S., Jeffrey, R. W., Morabia, A., Ritenbaugh, C., & Antipatis, V. J. (2002). Obesity prevention: the case for action. *International Journal of Obesity and related metabolic disorders, 26,* 425–436.

Kumanyika, S. K., & Obarzanek, E. (2003). Pathways to obesity prevention: report of a National institutes of health workshop. *Obesity Research, 11*(10), 1263–1274.

Lang, T., & Heasman, M. (2004). *Food wars. The global battle for mouths, minds, markets.* London: Earthscan.

League, C. A., & Dearry, A. (2004). *Summary report of May 2004 Workshop on obesity and the built environment. Improving public health through community design.* National institute of environmental health sciences. National institutes of health. Available at: www.niehs.nih.gov/drcpt/beoconf

McKenzie, T. L., Marshall, S. J., Sallis, J. F., & Conway, T. L. (2000 Jan). Leisure-time physical activity in school environments: an observational study using SOPLAY. *Preventive Medicine, 30*(1),70–77.

McKenzie, T. L., Sallis, J. F., Kolody, B., & Faucette, F. N. (1997). Long-term effects of a physical education curriculum and staff development program: SPARK. *Research Quarterly for Exercise and Sport, 68*(4), 280–291.

McKinlay, J. B. (1992). Health promotion through healthy public policy: The contribution of complementary research methods. *Canadian Journal of Public Health, 83*(Suppl. 1), S11–S19.

McKinlay, J. B. (1998). Paradigmatic obstacles to improving the health of populations. Implications for health policy. *Salud Publica De México, 40,* 369–379.

Mercer, S. L., Green, L.W, Rosenthal, A. C., Husten, C. G., Khan, L. K. & Dietz, W. H. (2003). Possible lessons from the tobacco experience for obesity control. *American Journal of Clinical Nutrition, 77*(Suppl. 4), 1073S–1082S.

Milio, N. (1990). Toward intersectoral health policy. In N Milio, (Ed.), *Nutrition Policy for Food Rich Countries. A Strategic Analysis* (pp. 155–172). Baltimore, MD: Johns Hopkins University Press.

Mooney, C. (2005). *The republican war on science, Chapter 9; Eating away at Science* (pp. 121–141). New York: Basic Books.

National Alliance for Nutrition and Activity. (2006 December 2). *Model school wellness policies.* Retrieved from http://www.Schoolwellnesspolicies.org/index.html

National Heart, Lung, and Blood Institute Obesity Education Initiative (1998). Clinical guidelines on the identification, evaluation, and treatment of overweight and obesity in adults. *Obesity Research, 6*(Suppl. 2).

National Obesity Task Force (2003). *Healthy weight 2008 – Australia's future.* Canberra: Department of Health & Aging.

The National Task Force on Prevention and Treatment of Obesity (1994). Towards prevention of obesity: research directions. *Obesity Research, 2,* 571–584.

Nestle, M. (2002). *Food politics: How the Food Industry Influences Nutrition and Health.* Berkeley CA: University of California Press.

New South Wales Center for Public Health Nutrition & New South Wales Department of Health (2005). *Best Options for Promoting Healthy Weight and Preventing Weight Gain in NSW.* http://www.cphn.biochem.usyd.edu.au/resources/index.html

Nutbeam, D. (1986). *Health promotion glossary. In Health promotion: An anthology* (pp. 343–358). Washington, DC: Pan American Health Organization.

Ottawa Charter for Health Promotion (1986). *Canadian Journal of Public Health, 77,* 425–430.

Persons, S. M. (1998). Prevention Conference Takes Topics From Headlines. *NIH Record,* December 15. Available at. http://obssr.od.nih.gov/Content/Publications/Articles/Prevartc.htm

Peterson, J. L., & DiClemente, R. J. (2000). *Handbook of HIV Prevention.* New York: Kluwer Academic.

Petticrew, M., & Roberts, H. (2003). Evidence, hierarchies, and typologies: Horses for courses. *Journal of Epidemiology and Community Health, 57,* 527–529.

Raczynski, J. M., & DiClemente, R. J., (Eds.). (1999). *Handbook of health promotion and disease prevention.* New York: Kluwer Academic.

Rattray, T., Brunner, W., & Freestone, J. (2002). *The new spectrum of prevention. A model for public health practice.* Martinez CA: Contra Costa Health Services.

Robert Wood Johnson Foundation (2006). *Childhood obesity.* www.rwjf.org/obesity

Robinson, T. (2004). *Behavior change interventions to prevent obesity.* Ancel keys symposium. University of Minnesota. Available at. http://www.epi.umn.edu/about/sem_robinson/robinson.shtm

Rose, G. (1991). Population distributions of risk and disease. *Nutr Metab Cardiovasc Dis, 1,* 37–40.

Rose, G. (1992). *The strategy of preventive medicine.* New York: Oxford University Press.

Rothman, A. J. (2000). Toward a theory-based analysis of behavioral maintenance. *Health Psychology, 19*(Suppl. 1), 64–69.

Rowe, P. J., Schuldheisz, J. M., & van der Mars, H. (1997). Measuring physical activity in physical education: Validation of the SOFIT direct observation instrument for use with first to eighth grade students. *Pediatric Exercise Science, 9,* 136–149.

Ryan, K. W., Card-Higginson, P., McCarthy, S. G., Justus, M. B., & Thompson, J. W. (2006). Arkansas fights fat: translating research into policy to combat childhood and adolescent obesity. *Health Affairs (Millwood), 25,* 992–1004.

Rychetnik, L., Frommer, M., Hawe, P., & Shiell, A. (2002). Criteria for evaluating evidence on public health interventions. *Journal of Epidemiology and Community Health, 56,* 119–127.

Rychetnik, L., Hawe, P., Waters, E., Barratt, A., Frommer, M. (2004). A glossary for evidence based public health. *Journal of Epidemiology and Community Health, 58*(7), 538–545.

Sallis, J. F., Moudon, A. V., Linton, L. S., & Powell K. E. (Eds.). (2005) Active living research. *American Journal of Preventive Medicine, 28*(Suppl. 2), entire issue.

Sallis, J. F., Cervero, R. B., Ascher, W., Henderson, K. A., Kraft, M. K., & Kerr, J. (2006). An ecological approach to creating active living communities. *Annual Review of Public Health, 27,* 297–322.

Schmid, T. L., Pratt, M., & Witmer, L. (2006). A framework for physical activity policy research. *Journal of Physical Activity and Health, 3*(Suppl.1).

Schmitz, M. K., & Jeffery, R. W. (2000). Public health interventions for the prevention and treatment of obesity. *Medical Clinics of North America, 84,* 491–512.

Serdula, M. K., Mokdad, A. H., Williamson, D. F., Galuska, D. A., Mendlein, J. M., & Heath, G. W. (1999). Prevalence of attempting weight loss and strategies for controlling weight. *Journal of the American Medical Association, 13,* 1353–1358.

Smedley, B. D., & Syme, S. L. (Eds.). (2000). *Promoting health. Intervention strategies from social and behavioral research.* Washington, DC: National Academy Press.

Smith, D. (2004 May 1). Demonizing fat in the war on weight. *New York Times.*

Stokols, D. (1992). Establishing and maintaining healthy environments. Toward a social ecology of health promotion. *American Psychologist, 47,* 6–22.

Story, M., & Orleans, C. T. (2006). Building evidence for environmental and policy solutions to prevent childhood obesity: The healthy eating research program. *American Journal of Preventive Medicine, 30,* 96–97.

Stoto, M. A., Green, L. W., & Bailey, L. A. (Eds.). (1997). Linking research to public health practice. A Review of the CDC's Program of Centers for Research and Demonstration of Health Promotion and Disease Prevention. Washington, DC: National Academy.

Swinburn, B., Egger, G., & Raza, F. (1999). Dissecting obesogenic environments. The development and application of a framework for identifying and prioritizing environmental interventions for obesity. *Preventive Medicine, 29,* 563–570.

Swinburn, B, Gill, T, Kumanyika S. (2005). Obesity prevention: a proposed framework for translating evidence into action. *Obesity Review, 6,* 23–33.

Thomas, P. R. (Ed.). (1995). *Weighing the options: Criteria for evaluating weight-management programs.* Washington, DC: National Academy of Sciences, Institute of Medicine.

U.S. Department of Health and Human Services (2001). *The Surgeon General's Call to Action to Prevent and Decrease Overweight and Obesity, 2001.* Washington, DC: U.S. Department of Health and Human Services, Public Health Service.

Waxman, A. (2003). Prevention of chronic diseases: WHO global strategy on diet, physical activity and health. *Food and Nutrition Bulletin, 24,* 281–284.

Wetter, A. C., Goldberg, J. P., King, A. C., Sigman-Grant, M., Baer, R., & Crayton, E., et al. (2001). How and why do individuals make food and physical activity choices? *Nutrition Reviews, 59*(3 Pt 2), S11–S20.

Winkleby, M. A., Feldman, H. A., & Murray, D. M. (1997). Joint analysis of the three U.S. community intervention trials for reduction of cardiovascular risk. *Journal of Clinical Epidemiology, 50,* 645–658.

World Health Organization (2000). *Obesity: Preventing and managing the global epidemic.* Report of a WHO Consultation. WHO Technical Report Series 894: Geneva.

World Health Organization (2003). *WHO Technical report series 916. Diet, nutrition and the prevention of chronic diseases.* Geneva: Joint FAO/WHO expert consultation.

Youth, J., McGinnis, M., Gootman, J. A., & Kraak V. I. (Eds.). (2006). *Committee on food marketing and the diets of children and food marketing to children and youth. Threat or opportunity?* Washington, DC: National Academies Press, Institute of Medicine.

Chapter 6

Consumer Perspectives and Consumer Action

Kelly D. Brownell

It is appropriate to begin considerations of how one might approach obesity prevention with a view of the relevant landscape, at the center of which are those individuals who are overweight and obese as well as others at risk for becoming overweight and who may experience constant worry about weight. The statistics are alarming as indicated by figures from the National Center for Health Statistics: only a third of adults have body weights in the range considered healthy while 65% are overweight or obese; 16% of children are overweight (the category that is equivalent to obesity in adults), and another 14% of children are at risk of overweight (Hedley et al., 2004). These percentages are even higher in African American and Mexican Americans. If weight concern is assessed by asking people if they are actively trying to lose or maintain their weight, then even larger proportions are affected. For example, Behavioral Risk Factor Survey data for 2000 indicate that 76% of adults are trying to lose or maintain weight, and this does not include all of those in the obese categories who could, presumably, obtain health benefits from losing some weight (Bish et al., 2005).

In an ideal society, this large group of consumers would be understood, served, protected, and empowered by their government(s) and by those in a position to affect their well-being. Unfortunately, however, the consumer experience with food, physical activity and obesity is fraught with mixed messages and with powerful influences pulling in opposite directions. The net impact is a major public health problem, widespread personal distress and societal concern about chaotic eating, unprecedented sedentary behavior, and body weight rising around the world in what appears to be an inexorable triumph of a toxic or obesigenic environment over self-regulation.

The purpose of this chapter is to examine the factors that shape individual's experience with food, activity, and obesity from a consumer perspective and to discuss how this experience can inform the changes necessary to reverse the rising prevalence of obesity and therefore prevent the consequent diseases.

A Consumer Perspective Should be Worldwide

This text focuses on obesity in the United States, but it is critical to avoid a U.S.-centered view of public health issues, including obesity. Obesity is very much a global problem (Brownell & Yach, 2005; Lobstein et al., 2004; Rigby,

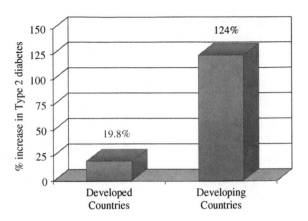

Figure 6.1 Projected percentage increases in the number of cases of Type 2 diabetes in developed and developing countries. Data taken from Yach, Stuckler, & Brownell (2006).

Kumanyika & James, 2004; Yach, Stuckler, & Brownell, 2006; World Health Organization, 2000; 2005). What happens in the United States affects consumers elsewhere, and vice versa. The global context of obesity is covered in detail in Chapter 11, but a few points merit discussion here.

The tobacco experience provides a compelling case to warn against viewing the problem or solutions to obesity as only a national problem. Much of the world has been complacent on tobacco issues. While American authorities celebrated reductions in the number of U.S. smokers, the tobacco industry expanded their business elsewhere so there are now more smokers worldwide than ever. It is important to avoid this trap with obesity (Yach, Hawkes, Gould, & Hofman, 2004; Yach, Leeder, Bell, & Kistnasamy, 2005). As a sign of how the obesity problem will hit developing countries hard, Figure 6.1 shows the projected increase in diabetes in these compared to developed countries.

Many of the factors that contribute to obesity and to the consumer experience are global in nature (Chopra, Galbraith, & Darnton-Hill, 2002; Yach, Stuckler, & Brownell et al., 2006). The price of food is affected by international trade policy, agriculture subsidies that affect the cost of food internationally, expansion of global markets by multinational food companies, technology that decreases the need for physical labor, and more. Perceptions of obesity affect national and international policies on prevention. And finally, much of the creative thinking on the obesity problem, especially among government officials, is occurring outside the U.S., particularly in countries from the European Union (European Union, 2005). It is important, therefore, to consider what occurs outside the United States.

Personal Responsibility: The Politics, Scientific Evidence, and a Possible Balance

At the heart of the consumer experience is a dominating paradox, one that strikes to the heart of what causes obesity and who is responsible for the solution (Brownell & Horgen, 2004). At the same time individuals face a "toxic" or "obesogenic" environment that undermines personal responsibility and guarantees rising prevalence, people are blamed for their weight, face discrimination by virtue of being stigmatized, and are expected to prevail over the environment no matter how unhealthy it becomes.

Personal responsibility may be the two most important words pertaining to the obesity issue, partly because it assigns blame for the problem. Positions that people, institutions, and governments take on obesity are influenced to a great extent by assumptions of cause. There is a massive, heavily funded campaign designed to frame obesity as a deficit in personal behavior and hence to steer solutions away from government of corporate responsibility to the individual (Brownell & Horgen, 2004). Inherent in this stance are assumptions that the body can be shaped as desired, that willpower is what separates obese people from others, that an imperfect body reflects an imperfect person, and that rising prevalence is due to personal irresponsibility. Education is the default recommendation by those embracing this stance, and because this approach is likely to be weak and ineffective, one unspoken message is "suck it up and behave better." Another, perhaps more harmful message over the long term is to reinforce the stereotypes that obese individuals are not competent.

The U.S. food industry, its trade associations and "scientific" advocacy groups, conservative political groups, shadow organizations masquerading as consumer groups, and political allies of these organizations are aggressive in pushing this responsibility position. The administrative branch of the U.S. government also issues forth a consistent message with personal responsibility as the central theme. People are responsible for their weight and parents are responsible when their children are overweight, so the position claims. Often evoked in this discussion are allusions to core American values of freedom and liberty. Public health advocates suggesting changes in the food environment are sometimes labeled as the "food police" and the "food Nazis." The food industry funds this campaign in part through groups with names the opposite of what is warranted, with the Center for Consumer Freedom as the prime example.

It is to be expected that the food industry, more so than other industries that are potentially affected by efforts to curb the obesity epidemic, will behave in this way because their financial and legal exposure is considerable. Some of the highest profits are on processed foods such as soft drinks, fast foods, and snack foods, the very food most heavily marketed, particularly to children. Most discouraging is that government officials carry forth the same message, as if their script is written by industry. One of many examples is comments made by Surgeon General Richard Carmona in a visit to South Carolina:

"Surgeon General Richard Carmona says regulation isn't the answer to stemming that epidemic. 'It has to start with the individual," said Dr. Carmona . . . Do you really want the government to tell you what to eat?' 'I would hope that the average person, armed with the right information, would make the right decision . . .'" (Reid, 2006).

The irony is that the government *does* tell you what to eat. With a trivial amount of funding it creates dietary guidelines and educates the public, but with massive subsidies and legislation favorable to the food industry, it establishes policies that favor some foods over others. A consumer may wonder why a salad and drink at McDonald's costs more than a Quarter Pounder with Cheese Value Meal. The answer can be found in the subsidies. The government subsidizes corn used to feed cattle (driving down the cost of the hamburger and cheese) and high fructose corn syrup (lowering the cost of soft drinks), but offers little subsidy for fruit and vegetable farmers. As another example, Nestle (2002) estimated that the entire U.S. government budget for nutrition education came to one fifth the annual advertising budget for Altoids Mints!

The personal responsibility argument applied to obesity is startlingly reminiscent of tobacco industry positions which emphasized the right of adults to use the product and claims the industry only encouraged "responsible" use, while in fact the industry distorted scientific evidence on the dangers of smoking, the addictive nature of nicotine, and advertising to children, and decried government intervention as intrusions on freedom. David Kessler, former FDA Commissioner, described the industry playbook:

"Devised in the 1950s and '60s, the tobacco industry's strategy was embodied in a script written by the lawyers. Every tobacco company executive in the public eye was told to learn the script backwards and forwards, no deviation was allowed. The basic premise was simple – smoking had not been proved to cause cancer. Not proven, not proven, not proven – this would be stated insistently and repeatedly. Inject a thin wedge of doubt, create controversy, never deviate from the prepared line. It was a simple plan and it worked." (Kessler, 2002).

A clear playbook exists for much of the food industry. The distortion of scientific evidence, the undermining of public health recommendations (Brownell & Nestle, 2004; Nestle, 2002), cries of freedom being usurped, and policy recommendations that guarantee the status quo, with enough repetition, will ring true to many consumers.

It is important that we "get it right" on this issue of responsibility. How one balances the personal responsibility and public health positions helps determine public policy and affects key issues such as price and availability of different foods, how obesity is addressed in the media, and the way in which consumers experience their environment and deal with understanding their own weight issues. Movement forward is possible only if these positions can be reconciled and placed in the proper context.

I believe these positions can and should be reconciled, but doing so finds the personal responsibility position as stated difficult to defend. Consider that:

- High fat diets cause overeating (and increased fatness) even in animal species that may otherwise have effective appetite regulatory mechanisms (West & York, 1998; Bray, Paeratakul & Popkin, 2004).
- People moving to the U.S. from other countries typically gain weight (Lauderdale & Rathouz, 2002; Goel, McCarthy, Phillips & Wee, 2004).
- The prevalence of obesity is increasing in nearly every country in the world, in both adults and children (World Health Organization, 2000; Ebbeling et al, 2002); it seems unlikely to posit a global epidemic of personal irresponsibility.
- There is scientific evidence showing that classes of foods most heavily marketed such as soft drinks and fast food are linked to risk for obesity (Ebbeling et al., 2006; Pereira et al., 2005; Vartanian, Schwartz, & Brownell, 2007).
- The personal responsibility approach has prevailed for years and must be considered a failed experiment given that the prevalence of obesity has only increased.

A key question, therefore, is where the principle and practice of personal responsibility fit as we decide how to reduce the prevalence and impact of obesity across large populations. One point of reconciliation in this debate is to appreciate that personal responsibility *is* beneficial and should be enhanced. People taking successful action "own" the behavior and make government intervention less necessary. A related question then, is what set of conditions have so undermined the ability of individuals to be "responsible." It is the answer to this question that points to the responsibility of governments. The role of government policies, at federal, state, local, and global levels in contributing to the obesigenic environment is well documented (Brownell & Horgen 2004; Nestle, 2002), even though some of the factors are unintended side effects of policies and programs from which individuals and the society at large derive some benefits.

Nevertheless, governments owe their citizens a safe and healthy environment, so officials who hold dear the concept of personal responsibility should improve conditions such that people find it easier to meet expectations about responsible behavior with respect to eating, physical activity, and weight control. We readily accept that we should have clean air and water and that government must undertake the necessary regulation. With smoking, policy level interventions to protect those who do not voluntarily choose to inhale cigarette smoke are now part of the legislative culture. With food and physical activity, the extent to which individual choices are influenced, i.e., limited, or shaped in specific directions, by market forces—although well documented—is variably acknowledged by both the general public and by policy makers.

Promotion of personal responsibility and health education will be more appropriate once policy makers acknowledge their role in helping to create or maintain environments conducive to a more healthful set of food and physical activity choices for consumers. As this evolves, it is nonsensical to think that modestly funded health education efforts could complete with the billions spent by the food industry (see Chapter 10) or that consumers can be expected to fend for themselves in a well-funded marketing environment that has commercial interests rather than public health as the primary driver. Much has been written about the specific policies and programs that might follow from this perspective on government responsibility (Brownell & Horgen, 2004; Dietz & Gortmaker, 2001; Ebbeling, Pawlak, & Ludwig, 2002; Koplan, Liverman, & Kraak, 2005; McGinnis, Gootman, & Kraak, 2006; Nestle, 2002; Nestle & Jacobson, 2000; Wang & Brownell, 2005).

A heavy focus on personal responsibility, without full appreciation of the environmental factors that compromise it, leads to assumptions of blame that can affect how obese people are viewed and treated by the culture. The consequence can be an intensification of bias and stigma directed at overweight individuals. This may even be true when well intended public health advocates cite the increasing financial costs to society associated with an increasing number of obese and, particularly, severely obese individuals (costs of obesity are discussed in Chapter 4). Some may use this as further justification for hostility toward the obese themselves rather than as an argument for urgent, high level policy solutions. The question is how to attack obesity with creative public policy solutions while not attacking the individuals with the problem.

The Experience of Being Obese: Bias and Discrimination

Opinions about body weight are very much a function of culture. In varying times and places, excess weight has been revered as beautiful and as a sign of wealth (only the wealthy could afford the food and be exempt from physical labor). There is some variation even within a country, such as the often cited attitudes about obesity in African Americans that are more mixed and less negative than in the general population (Baturka, Hornsby, & Schorling, 2000; Kumanyika, Morssink, & Agurs, 1992). Overall, however, obesity is a highly stigmatized condition (Brownell, Puhl, Schwartz, & Rudd, 2005).

The consequences of weight bias can be severe. There are numerous anecdotal reports of psychological and social distress caused by stigmatizing experiences. A few examples are:

When I was a child, I was sick and absent from school one day. The teacher taking attendance came across my name and said "She must have stayed home to eat". The other kids told me about this the next day. (from Brownell (2005a))

I remember one incident when I was in the 6th grade and my teacher was looking at my latest handwriting assignment and she announced to the whole class that my handwriting was just like me – "fat and squatty" . . . The pain and humiliation aimed at you as an innocent child never leaves you! (from Brownell (2005a))

"Gina Score, a 14-year-old girl in South Dakota, was sent in the summer of 1999 to a state juvenile detention camp. Gina was characterized as sensitive and intelligent, wrote poetry, and was planning to skip a grade when she returned to school. She was sent to the facility for petty theft – stealing money from her parents and from lockers at school "to buy food". She was said to have stolen "a few dollars here, a few dollars there" and paid most of the money back. The camp, run by a former Marine and modeled on the military, aimed, in the words of an instruction manual, to "overwhelm them with fear and anxiety." On July 21, a hot humid day, Gina was forced to begin a 2.7 mile run/walk. Gina was 5'4" tall, weighed 224 pounds, and was unable to complete even simple physical exercises such as leg lifts. She fell behind early but was prodded and cajoled by instructors. A short time later, she collapsed, lay on the ground panting, with pale skin and purple lips. She was babbling incoherently and frothing from the mouth, with her eyes rolled back in her head. The drill instructors sat nearby drinking sodas, laughing and chatting, accusing Gina of faking, within 100 feet of an air-conditioned building. After four hours with Gina lying prostrate in the sun, a doctor came by and summoned an ambulance immediately. Gina's organs had failed and she died." (from Puhl & Brownell (2001))

Anecdote does not prove a problem is widespread, but can help offer a human context for what people face. Turning to available scientific evidence, it is clear that weight bias is indeed widespread, is powerful, and is very resistant to change (Brownell et al., 2005; Puhl & Brownell, 2001). Some have labeled obesity as the last acceptable form of discrimination (Falkner et al., 1999; O'Hara, 1996; Puhl & Brownell, 2001).

Dating back to the classic study by Richardson et al. (1961), deep seated bias has been shown in study after study. The Richardson et al. study involved 640 children ages 10–11 who were shown six drawings of other children; four drawings were of children with disabilities and one each was a normal weight or overweight child. The overweight child was rated as least likeable by a considerable extent.

One might speculate that in today's world, with obesity much more the statistical norm, bias might have decreased. Latner and Stunkard (2003) replicated the Richardson study with 458 fifth- and sixth-grade children and found the overweight child was still ranked as least likeable and was ranked significantly lower than in 1961.

Early studies of bias toward obese adults consisted of a combination of clinical observations (Stunkard, 1976), some empirical work (Allon, 1979), and writings about fat and feminism as political and social issues (Orbach, 1978).

More recent empirical and theoretical work has advanced the field considerably. Some of the advance is due to progress in measuring implicit bias for work done initially on race and gender bias (Greenwald & Banaji, 1995; Greenwald, McGhee, & Schwartz, 1998). The primary implicit measure has been the Implicit Associations Test (IAT) developed by Greenwald and colleagues (1998). The IAT measures implicit memory-based associations using an assessment of reaction time to pairs of words such as fat-bad or fat-good. The assumption is that processing speed is an indirect measure of association between two concepts, and that the implicit association reflects unconscious or implicit attitude. The measure evaluates associations outside conscious control. It can be compared to explicit attitude measures to evaluate how a person's conscious or public attitudes compare to implicit attitudes. This is important because most people consider themselves fair-minded or least wish to appear so and are reluctant to report explicit bias.

The IAT has now been used in a number of studies on attitudes about obesity. Teachman and Brownell (2001) compared weight attitudes in the general population to those in health care professionals specializing in the treatment of obesity. Bias in the general population was very strong, while in health professionals was strong but attenuated somewhat. A subsequent study found similarly strong bias in the general population, but even more discouraging was that interventions designed to provoke empathy or to offer information about causes of obesity did not lower the bias (Teachman et al., 2003). Subsequent studies have demonstrated bias in other populations (Brownell et al., 2005; Chambliss, Finley, & Blair, 2004) and in obese people themselves (Wang, Brownell, & Wadden, 2004).

Many studies also use explicit measures of bias. People sometimes report explicit bias, as in the case of studies on attitudes of health care professionals about obese patients, but explicit measures often show no bias. When implicit and explicit measures differ, one can look to the way a stigmatized group is treated as an indication of which attitudes are acted out. For instance, overweight people are portrayed in negative ways in entertainment television (Greenberg et al., 2003) suggesting that explicit measures showing no bias ring less true than implicit measures showing strong bias.

Being subject to bias and stigma brings many practical consequences in everyday life. There is evidence that obese people face discrimination in employment, earn lower wages, fare less well in education settings (after controlling for performance), and face negative attitudes and behaviors in the health care system (see Brownell et al., 2005; Puhl & Brownell, 2001). The bias and its manifestation in discriminatory attitudes and actions cross many key areas of living and can affect overweight individuals in profound ways. People cope with these threats in different ways, ranging from internalization of distress leading to depression to social action such as filing anti-discrimination lawsuits and forming size acceptance groups (Puhl, 2005). Little is known about the impact of these varying approaches either on individuals or the culture.

The unexplored but important area of study is the extent to which living in a biased culture and experiencing acts of discrimination can affect health. This relationship might explain at least some of the association of obesity with health outcomes (Figure 6.2). Being overweight changes social, psychological, financial, and other relationships one has in the society at large; hence,

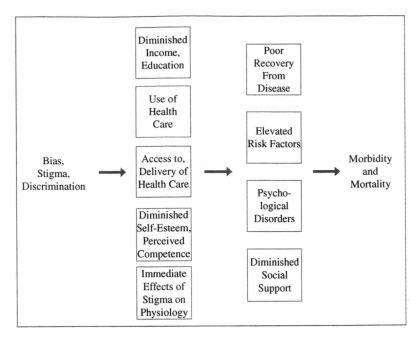

Figure 6.2 A hypothetical scheme representing possible ways that the experience of bias and discrimination may be linked to important health outcomes. From Brownell (2005).

acts of bias might affect physiology directly (e.g., through blood pressure), could make a person reluctant to receive preventive care, could drive down income which in turn is disadvantageous for health, and more. When factoring in the groups with especially high prevalence of obesity, say in the case of African American women, biases related to weight may interact with those related to race and gender to create especially damaging effects.

Being overweight carries the double burden of impaired health and quality of life combined with exposure to negative attitudes and overt acts of bias and discrimination. There is no sign that the bias is easing, and in fact the Latner and Stunkard (2003) study suggested the bias grows worse. People are blamed for being overweight and in some quarters are expected to solve the problem with no outside help from institutions such as government and the food industry (the personal responsibility argument). This is another stance that is difficult to defend with scientific evidence, given the strong role of biological and environmental factors in etiology.

Progress is being made on countering weight stigma in health care settings (Chambliss & Blair, 2005; Early & Johnston, 2005; Wee & Yanovski, 2005), through legal means (Solovey, 2005; Theran, 2005), and through other means (see Brownell et al., 2005). This work is in its beginning stages, so much more will be necessary to prevent bias, stigma, and discrimination based on weight.

Consumer Action: Power from the Grassroots

Consumer attitudes about the obesity issue are fascinating and point to clear change on the horizon. Polls indicate that the percentage of consumers who believe obesity is a major problem ranges from 70 to 95% (Brownell, 2005b).

Table 6.1 Trends in public opinion based on poll data.

	2001	2003	2004
Favor taxing foods	33%	40%	54%
Favor restricting children's food advertising	57%	56%	73%
Favor soft drink/snack food bans in schools	47%	59%	69%
Favor required calorie labeling in restaurants		74%	80%

From Brownell (2005b)

When asked who is responsible for obesity, consumers will often point to the individuals as the responsible agent but at the same time look to institutional change for solutions.

Table 6.1 shows trends in public opinion from polls discussed in an article by Brownell (2005b). Even the most controversial proposal, to tax foods, is now supported by over 50% of the population. Policies such as mandatory calorie labeling on restaurant menus and ridding schools of soft drinks are supported by strong majorities. These results indicate consumer recognition of the environmental contributions to obesity, consensus about the emergency nature of the problem, and awareness that institutions such as government, schools, and the food industry must better protect the population, particularly children. These beliefs signal what will probably be a rising tide of consumer action to promote systemic change, including advocacy for policy change as well as legal actions.

Consumers can become powerful change agents in the fight to prevent obesity. This speaks to a fundamental issue in provoking change – whether the emphasis should be on top-down change (actions of central governments) or change originating in the grass roots. Ideally, change would occur from both the top down and bottom up. This may be happening in relation to the obesity epidemic. However, consumer action cannot, and should not, wait for those in government and industry to take the lead. In fact, one of the arguments used by both governments and industries is that they cannot make changes without infringing upon what consumers want. Consumer action can motivate and, in some cases, compel action from the top.

As noted in Chapter 13, much consumer action occurs at state and local levels where there are readily identifiable and accessible targets for action. Consumers are exerting their influence by working with local and state legislators. A number of states have considered obesity and nutrition legislation. The likelihood that these efforts will be successful increases when health and advocacy groups combine into coalitions and when citizens work closely with local legislators.

Consumers-stimulated action at the federal level is much more complex (see Chapter 7). While it is true that some federal legislators have proposed progressive action, these individuals are in the minority. Overall, federal officials may be doing more harm than good by giving the appearance of action and overemphasizing what can be accomplished by educational strategies alone while supporting practices, e.g., food subsidy programs, that contribute to the problem. It is important to work for change at the federal level, but this might occur only when there is enough state and local change to force the central government to act.

Several chapters in this book relate to aspects of consumer action through various settings. Examples of where consumer attitudes and actions have fit into other successful or partly successful public health efforts may provide guidance (Economos et al., 2001; Kersh & Morone, 2002). Encouraging consumers to express their voice, to organize, to be creative, to evaluate the impact of local programs, and to share their results with others may be an effective means of facilitating broad changes. In local communities, consumers are focusing their awareness and in some cases outrage at current conditions by creating farm to school programs, initiating community supported agriculture through local farms, opening farmer's markets in inner cities, working with schools to limit or expel soft drinks and snack foods, pressuring schools to add back physical education, forming walking school buses, lobbying for walking and biking trails, and more (Brownell & Horgen, 2004). Each victory gets noted locally and regionally, encouraging others to do the same. An ongoing problem with leveraging these successes to motivate institutional change is the typical lack of evaluation for these efforts. However, clever use of funds from agencies such as the NIH and CDC as well as from local and national foundations could help in the evaluation of such efforts and insure that progress is maximally contagious.

Summary

Beliefs about the causes of obesity have a significant impact on consumers. Such beliefs, often couched in terms of personal vs. social responsibility, help shape cultural attitudes about obesity and obese people as well as actions people are or are not willing to have taken to prevent the problem. Ideally these attitudes would be based on some truth (scientific evidence) but such is not typically the case. More often political and moral views shaped in part by industry financing, prevail in establishing public policies.

Consumer protection, particularly of children, is a value that must be embraced before progress can be made on obesity. Current conditions so undermine personal resources that pleas from officials and industry for people to be more responsible will have little or no impact and are not credible given all that these institutions do to encourage overeating and sedentary behavior.

In the United States, the ingenuity in addressing obesity is occurring at the grass roots. Changes beginning at the grass roots can grow into a powerful social movement, one that builds in size and momentum and then forces the systemic change necessary for national action. The relatively limited and weak—in a structural sense—actions of the U.S. government cause America—a major contributor the problem on a global scale—to lag behind many other nations or regions in progress on the obesity epidemic. While it would be best to see change emanating from both the bottom up and the top down, the fact that consumers are mobilizing to create or at least demand change is a positive sign and should be expected, within a short time, to generate a much needed social movement that will change the food and activity landscape as profoundly as needed.

References

Allon, N. (1979). Self-perceptions of the stigma of overweight in relationship to weight-losing patterns. *American Journal of Clinical Nutrition, 32*, 470–480.

Baturka, N., Hornsby, P. P., & Schorling, J. B. (2000). Clinical implications of body image among rural African-American women. *Journal of General Internal Medicine, 15*, 235–241.

Bish, C. L., Blanck, H. M., Serdula, M. K., Marcus, M., Kohl III, H. W., & Khan, L. K. (2005). Diet and physical activity behaviors among Americans trying to lose weight: 2000 Behavioral risk factor surveillance system. *Obesity Research, 13*, 596–607.

Bray, G. A., Paeratakul, S., & Popkin, B. M. (2004). Dietary fat and obesity: A review of animal, clinical and epidemiological studies. *Physiology and Behavior, 83*, 549–555.

Brownell, K. D. (2005a). The social, scientific, and human context of prejudice and discrimination based on weight. In K. D. Brownell, R. B. Puhl, M. B. Schwartz, & L. C. Rudd (Eds.), *Weight bias: Nature, consequences, and remedies* (pp. 1–11). New York: Guilford.

Brownell, K. D. (2005b). The chronicling obesity: Growing awareness of its social, economic, and political contexts. *Journal of Health Politics, Policy and Law, 30*, 955–964.

Brownell, K. D., & Horgen, K. B. (2004). *Food fight: The inside story of the food industry, America's obesity crisis, and what we can do about it.* New York: McGraw-Hill/Contemporary Books.

Brownell, K. D., & Nestle, M. (2004 January). The sweet and lowdown on sugar (OpEd). *New York Times, 23*, A23.

Brownell, K. D., Puhl, R. B., & Schwartz, M. B., & Rudd, L. C. (Eds.). (2005). *Weight bias: Nature, consequences, and remedies.* New York: Guilford.

Brownell, K. D., & Yach, D. (2005 Nov–Dec). The battle of the bulge. *Foreign Policy*, 26–27.

Chambliss, H. O., & Blair, S. N. (2005). Improving the fitness landscape. In K. D. Brownell, R. B. Puhl, M. B. Schwartz, & L. C. Rudd (Eds.), *Weight bias: Nature, consequences, and remedies* (pp. 248–264). New York: Guilford.

Chambliss, H. O., Finley, C. E., & Blair, S. N. (2004). Attitudes toward obese individuals among exercise science students. *Medicine and Science in Sports and Exercise, 36*, 468–474.

Chopra, M., Galbraith, S., & Darnton-Hill, I. (2002). A global response to a global problem: The epidemic of overnutrition. *Bulletin of the World Health Organization, 80*, 952–958.

Dietz, W. H., & Gortmaker, S. L. (2001). Preventing obesity in children and adolescents. *Annual Review of Public Health, 22*, 337–353.

Early, J. L., & Johnston, J. A. (2005). Improving medical practice. In K. D. Brownell, R. B. Puhl, M. B. Schwartz, & L. C. Rudd (Eds.), *Weight bias: Nature, consequences, and remedies* (pp. 223–233). New York: Guilford.

Ebbeling, C. B., Feldman, H. A., Osganian, S. K., Chomitz, V. R., Ellenbogen, S. J., & Ludwig, D. S. (2006). Effects of decreasing sugar-sweetened beverage consumption on body weight in adolescents: A randomized, controlled pilot study. *Pediatrics, 117*, 673–680.

Ebbeling, C. B., Pawlak, D. B., & Ludwig, D. S. (2002). Childhood obesity: Public health crisis, common sense cure. *Lancet, 360*, 473–482.

Economos, C. D., Brownson, R. C., DeAngelis, M. A., Novelli, P., Foerster, S. B., & Foreman, C. T. et al. (2001). What lessons have been learned from other attempts to guide social change? *Nutrition Reviews, 59*, S40–S56.

European Union (2005). EU platform on diet, physical activity, and health. Retrieved on March 27, 2006, from http://europa.eu.int/comm/health/ph_determinants/life_style/nutrtion/platform/docs/platform_members.pdf.

Falkner, N. H, French, S. A., Jeffery, R. W., Neumark-Sztainer, D., Sherwood, N. E., & Morton, N. (1999). Mistreatment due to weight: Prevalence and sources of perceived mistreatment in women and men. *Obesity Research, 7*, 572–576.

Goel, M. S., McCarthy, E. P., Phillips, R. S., & Wee, C. C. (2004). Obesity among U.S. immigrant subgroups by duration of residence. *Journal of the American Medical Association, 292*(23), 2860–2867.

Greenberg, B. S., Eastin, M., Hofschire, L., Lachlan, K., & Brownell, K. D. (2003). Portrayals of overweight and obese individuals on commercial television. *American Journal of Public Health, 93*, 1342–1348.

Greenwald, A. G., & Banaji, M. (1995). Implicit social cognition: Attitudes, self-esteem, and stereotypes. *Psychological Review, 105*, 4–27.

Greenwald, A. G., McGhee, D. E., & Schwartz, J. L. K. (1998). Measuring individual differences in implicit cognition: The implicit association test. *Journal of Personality and Social Psychology, 74*, 1464–1480.

Hedley, A. A., Ogden, C. L., Johnson, C. L., Carroll, M. D., Curtin, L. R., & Flegal, K. M. (2004). Prevalence of overweight and obesity among U.S. children, adolescents, and adults, 1999–2002. *JAMA, 291*, 2847–2850.

Kersh, R., & Morone, J. (2002). The politics of obesity: Seven steps to government action. *Health Affairs, 21*,142–153.

Kessler, D. A. (2002). *A question of intent: A great American battle with a deadly industry*. New York: Public Affairs.

Koplan, J. P., Liverman, C. T., & Kraak, V. I. (2005). *Preventing childhood obesity: Health in the balance*. Washington, DC: Institute of Medicine of the National Academies, National Academies Press.

Kumanyika, S. K., Morssink, C., & Agurs, T. (1992). Models for dietary and weight change in African-American women: identifying cultural components. *Ethnicity and Disease, 2*, 166–175.

Latner, J. D., & Stunkard, A. J. (2003). Getting worse: The stigmatization of obese children. *Obesity Research, 11*, 452–456.

Lauderdale, D. S., & Rathouz, P. J. (2002). Body mass index in a U.S. national sample of Asian Americans: effects of nativity, years since immigration and socioeconomic status. *International Journal of Obesity, 24*, 1188–1194.

Lobstein, T., Baur, L., Uauy, R., & IASO International Obesity Task Force. (2004). Obesity in children and young people: A crisis in public health. *Obesity Reviews, 5*(Suppl. 1), 4–104.

McGinniss, J. M., Gootman, J. A., & Kraak, V. I. (2006). Food marketing to children and youth: Threat or opportunity? Washington, DC: Institute of Medicine of the National Academies, National Academies Press.

Nestle, M. (2002). *Food politics: How the food industry influences nutrition and health*. Berkeley, CA: University of California Press.

Nestle, M., & Jacobson, M. F. (2000). Halting the obesity epidemic: A public health policy approach. *Public Health Reports, 115*, 12–24.

O'Hara, M. D. (1996). Please weight to be seated: Recognizing obesity as a disability to prevent discrimination in public accommodations. *Whittier Law Review, 17*, 895–954.

Orbach, S. (1978). *Fat is a feminist issue: The anti-diet guide to permanent weight loss*. New York: Paddington.

Pereira, M. A., Kartashov, A. I., Ebbeling, C. B., Van Horn, L., Slattery, M. L., Jacobs, D. R. Jr., & Ludwig, D. S. (2005). Fast-food habits, weight gain, and insulin resistance (the CARDIA study): 15-year prospective analysis. *Lancet, 365*, 36–42.

Puhl, R. M. (2005). Coping with weight stigma. In K. D. Brownell, R. B. Puhl, M. B. Schwartz, & L. C. Rudd (Eds.), *Weight bias: Nature, consequences, and remedies* (pp. 275–284). New York: Guilford.

Puhl, R., & Brownell, K. D. (2001). Bias, discrimination, and obesity. *Obesity Research, 9*, 788–805.

Reid, C. M. (2006). Should obesity be regulated? Surgeon general to tackle the issue at USC forum. *The State*, Feb. 27.

Richardson, S. A., Goodman, N., Hastorf, A. H., & Dornbusch, S. M. (1961). Cultural uniformity in reaction to physical disabilities. *American Sociological Review, 26,* 241–247.

Rigby, N. J., Kumanyika, S., & James, W. P. (2004). Confronting the epidemic: The need for global solutions. *Journal of Public Health Policy, 25,* 418–434.

Solovay, S. (2005). Remedies for weight-based discrimination. In K. D. Brownell, R. B. Puhl, M. B. Schwartz, & L. C. Rudd (Eds.), *Weight bias: Nature, consequences, and remedies* (pp. 212–222). New York: Guilford.

Stunkard, A. J. (1976). *The pain of obesity*. Palo Alto, CA: Bull Publishing.

Teachman, B. A., & Brownell, K. D. (2001). Implicit anti-fat bias among health professionals: Is anyone immune? *International Journal of Obesity, 25,* 1525–1531.

Teachman, B. A., Gapinski, K. D., Brownell, K. D., Rawlins, M., & Jeyaram, S. (2003). Demonstrations of anti-fat bias: The impact of providing causal information and evoking empathy. *Health Psychology, 22,* 68–78.

Theran, E. E. (2005). Legal theory on weight discrimination. In K. D. Brownell, R. B. Puhl, M. B. Schwartz, & L. C. Rudd (Eds.), *Weight bias: Nature, consequences, and remedies* (pp. 195–211). New York: Guilford.

Vartanian, L. R., Schwartz, M. B., & Brownell, K. D. (2007). Effects of soft drink consumption on nutrition and health: A systematic review and meta-analysis. *American Journal of Public Health, 97*(4): 667–75. [Epub 2007 Feb 28].

Wang, S. S., & Brownell, K. D. (2005). Public policy and obesity: The need to marry science with advocacy. *Psychiatric Clinics of North America, 28,* 235–252.

Wang, S. S., Brownell, K. D., & Wadden, T. A. (2004). The influence of the stigma of obesity on overweight individuals. *International Journal of Obesity, 28,* 1333–1337.

Wee, C. C., & Yanovski, S. Z. (2005). Improving the health care system. In K. D. Brownell, R. B. Puhl, M. B. Schwartz, & L. C. Rudd (Eds.), *Weight bias: Nature, consequences, and remedies* (pp. 234–247). New York: Guilford.

West, D. B. & York, B. (1998). Dietary fat, genetic predisposition, and obesity: Lessons from animal models. *American Journal of Clinical Nutrition, 67*(3 Suppl), 505S–512S.

World Health Organization (2000). *Obesity: Preventing and managing the global epidemic*. Geneva, Switzerland: World Health Organization. Technical Report Series 894.

World Health Organization (2005). *Preventing chronic disease: A vital investment*. Geneva, Switzerland: World Health Organization.

Yach, D., Hawkes, C., Gould, C. L., & Hofman, K. J. (2004). The global burden of chronic diseases: Overcoming impediments to prevention and control. *JAMA, 291,* 2616–2622.

Yach, D., Leeder, S. R., Bell, J., & Kistnasamy, B. (2005). Global chronic diseases (editorial). *Science, 307,* 317.

Yach, D., Stuckler, D., & Brownell, K. D. (2006). Epidemiologic and economic consequences of the global epidemics of obesity and diabetes. *Nature Medicine, 12,* 62–66.

Chapter 7

The Role of Government in Preventing Obesity

Debra Haire-Joshu, Christopher Fleming and Rebecca Schermbeck

Introduction

The traditional role of government is to promote the health and well being of its population (Blackburn & Walker, 2005). Today obesity is occurring in epidemic proportions, threatening the immediate and long-term health of citizens in the U.S. and abroad (see Chapters 3 and 11) and requiring government to act in order to meet its basic mission. However, unlike specific diseases (e.g. polio, smallpox), the causes of the obesity epidemic are not singular but rather are immensely complex; the result of changes in an individual's diet and physical activity patterns as influenced by broader factors such as industrialization, urbanization, economic development and increasing food market globalization.

To date, several countries have worked to systematically develop model plans to combat obesity (including Australia and Denmark) (Australian Government National Health and Medical Research Council, 1997; Popkin & Gordon-Larsen, 2004; Sweden National Board of Health, 2001). This is in contrast to the United States government—the focus of this chapter–which does not have a singular national plan designed to combat obesity but rather has addressed the public health burden of obesity through multiple government actions across federal, state, and local levels without deliberate coordination (Oliver, 2006). It is within this context that public health advocates pursue governmental action to influence policy and produce outcomes that individuals may be unlikely to achieve by themselves (Blackburn & Walker, 2005; Brownson, Haire-Joshu, & Luke, 2006; Oliver, 2006).

In 2001 the U.S. Surgeon General's Office produced the report entitled "Call to Action to Prevent and Decrease Overweight and Obesity" (U.S. Department of Health and Human Services, Public Health Service, & Office of the Surgeon General, 2001). The report offered a review of key evidence and offered recommendations for obesity prevention, providing a foundation for policies promoting improvement in food and activity environments, but without a specific plan for how these recommendations could be achieved. The need for a prevention-focused action plan to decrease obesity among the youth in the United States (Koplan, Liverman, & Kraak, 2004) was addressed in 2002, when the U.S. Congress charged the Institute of Medicine (IOM) to develop such a plan. The primary emphasis was to examine the behavioral, social, cultural, and other broad environmental factors involved in childhood obesity and make recommendations

Box 7.1. Institute of Medicine, Preventing Childhood Obesity: Health in the Balance (Koplan et al., 2004)

Recommendations: Role of the Federal Government

The President should request that the Secretary of the Department of Health and Human Services convene a high-level task force to ensure coordinated budgets, policies, and program requirements and to establish effective interdepartmental collaboration and priorities for action. An increased level and sustained commitment of federal and state funds and resources are needed.

The Federal Government should:

- Strengthen research and program efforts addressing obesity prevention, with a focus on experimental behavioral research and community-based intervention research and on the rigorous evaluation of the effectiveness, sustainability, and scaling up of prevention interventions.
- Support extensive program and research efforts to prevent childhood obesity in high-risk populations with health disparities, with a focus both on behavioral and environmental approaches.
- Support nutrition and physical activity grant programs, particularly in states with the highest prevalence of childhood obesity.
- Strengthen support for relevant surveillance and monitoring efforts, particularly the National Health and Nutrition Examination Survey (NHANES).
- Undertake an independent assessment of federal nutrition assistance programs and agricultural policies.
- Ensure that they promote healthful dietary intake and physical activity levels for all children and youth.
- Develop and evaluate pilot projects within the nutrition assistance programs that would promote healthful dietary intake and physical activity and scale up those found to be successful.

Recommendations: Role of the State and Local Governments

State and local governments should:

- Provide coordinated leadership and support for childhood obesity prevention efforts, particularly those focused on high-risk populations, by increasing resources and strengthening policies that promote opportunities for physical activity and healthful eating in communities, neighborhoods, and schools.
- Support public health agencies and community coalitions in their collaborative efforts to promote and evaluate obesity prevention interventions.

Box 7.2. Case Study: Arkansas and the Case of Governor Mike Huckabee

In June of 2003, Arkansas Governor Mike Huckabee's doctor diagnosed him with diabetes. Wishing to halt the progression of a disease with which both of his parents had suffered, Gov. Huckabee underwent a dramatic change in lifestyle – he began to eat the right foods and regularly exercise. Twelve months later, Gov. Huckabee had lost 105 pounds, and his doctor informed him that he exhibited no signs of diabetes.

In March of 2003, the Arkansas state legislature signed into law House Bill 1583, which:

• created a "Child Health Advisory Committee";
• earmarked up to 5% of Health Master Settlement Agreement funds for model or pilot programs created under the Act (1220);
• prohibited food and beverage vending machine access for elementary students; and
• required schools "to include as part of the student report card to parents an annual body mass index by age for each student."

The legislature's activities, coupled with Gov. Huckabee's very public campaign to promote his personal success story while emphasizing the importance of a healthy lifestyle, have been very effective in shaping a 'model' state plan to combat obesity. In fact, in the Child Nutrition and Reauthorization Act of 2004 (P.L. 108–265), Congress acknowledges the state of Arkansas as the "first state in the United States to have a comprehensive statewide initiative to combat and prevent childhood obesity" and promotes Arkansas' program as a "model for States across the United States."

The legislature has since taken more progressive actions, and Governor Huckabee, with the input of many interests, has instituted "Healthy Arkansas", which is highlighted in Table 7.4.

---

for prevention efforts. As a result of this report, the IOM made recommendations for various sectors of society to take action in preventing obesity among children. The boxes above highlight the IOM recommendations made for federal, state, and local government. These recommendations call for high level federal government leadership and coordination as well as focused research, surveillance, policy and programs and also for coordination and programmatic support in states and localities. Given that the epidemic of childhood obesity is embedded within the overall societal context that has led to the epidemic in adults, these recommendations provide a useful reference point for considering the role of government in the U.S. population at large.

The purpose of this chapter is to review key elements of the U.S. federal, state, and local infrastructures for taking the types of actions recommended by the IOM and to identify potential ways to enhance the impact of current or future initiatives. The guiding question is: Which agencies or types of agencies, which policies or types of policies, and which programs or types of programs do or could governments have that influence obesity determinants? Are the influences of these agencies, policies, and programs—regardless of their primary intent—generally favorable or adverse for obesity prevention? How can available funding and programs be better leveraged to improve the potential for short and long term obesity prevention? After briefly highlighting relevant frameworks from a global perspective, we then provide a detailed review of the U.S. situation.

Global Frameworks

Concepts and actions related to the role of government have been well articulated in international settings motivated in part by the role of global marketing in obesity determinants such as food availability within specific countries and by the commonalities among countries with respect to the influence of economic development and urbanization of eating and activity lifestyles. For example, the International Obesity Task Force (IOTF) developed a "causal web", shown in Figure 7.1, to depict the interplay of various sectors that influence energy intake and expenditure (i.e. food marketing, media, national and state level nutrition policies, education, and transportation) at international, national/regional/state, community, and work/school/home levels (Kumanyika, Jeffery RW, Morabia A, Ritenbaugh C, & Antipatis VJ, 2002). Many of the processes shown are controlled or shaped by government regulatory actions or funding patterns.

The World Health Organization (WHO) recently adopted a "Global Strategy on Diet, Physical Activity and Health" which also addresses the role of poor diet and inactivity as impacted by multiple factors including food and agriculture policies; fiscal policies; regulatory policies; consumer marketing, and school food and activity policies (World Health Organization, 2002). The WHO strategy provides a platform for addressing certain global influences that can only be addressed by international agencies (Chopra M, Galbraith S, & Damton-Hill I, 2002; Report of a World Health Organzation consultation, 2000) and also emphasizes the need for countries to develop national long-term strategies with broad impact across individual and community levels. The above-cited IOM recommendations for governmental action on childhood obesity (see Boxes 7.1 and 7.2) address the need for national level planning within the United States.

Causal Web of Societal Processes influencing the **population prevalence** *of obesity*

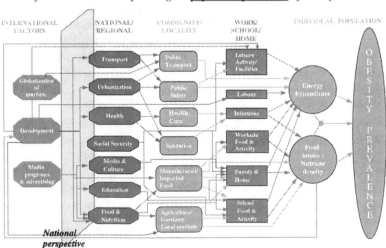

Figure 7.1 International Obesity Task Force Framework for Obesity Prevention (Kumanyika et al., 2002).

The U.S. Federal Government

The many branches and other components of the federal government and the major organizational relationships are shown in Figure 7.2. Given the breadth of influences on food intake and physical activity as depicted in Figure 7.1, policies and programs that directly or indirectly affect obesity or obesity prevention may be housed in a diverse array of these entities. In the current context, the federal government is limited in its ability to regulate behavior that directly affects the prevalence of overweight and obesity (namely, the physical activity and dietary behaviors of individuals). As a result, relatively little federal legislation has been passed that directly addresses obesity prevention. Instead, through sometimes complex and obscure legislative processes, Congress designates and oversees funding of federal programs addressing some aspect of obesity through the authorization and appropriation processes of the federal budget.

Given this governmental structure, we first review executive agency programs, as this is where the federal government is most visible in obesity prevention efforts. These programs include both longstanding federally-sponsored food and nutrition programs, for which alignment with obesity prevention goals is a relatively recent development, as well as newer programs specifically designed to address the epidemic. Here and throughout the chapter, the descriptions are not intended to be an exhaustive or comprehensive listing, but rather to provide examples of the diversity and nature of what the federal government is doing to address obesity prevention needs as well as indicating where one might look to identify modified or newly initiated programs and policies that continue to emerge. We then provide an overview of the legislative processes that govern agency funding and program and policy initiatives related to obesity prevention.

Current Federal Obesity Initiatives – Executive Departments and Agencies

Department of Health and Human Services (DHHS)
The DHHS is the second largest department in the United States government and is charged with protecting the health and safety of all Americans and for providing essential human services (U.S. Department of Health and Human Services). Hence, obesity prevention is part of the primary mission of this department. DHHS' interest in preventing obesity includes not only the fulfillment of the health protection function but also the health care burden and costs that are associated with obesity (see Chapter 4). An overview of DHHS agencies is provided in Figure 7.3. As discussed below and summarized in Table 7.1, several of these agencies cite some aspect of obesity prevention and/or treatment as an activity.

Centers for Disease Control and Prevention (CDC)
The CDC is the lead agency for a large number of federal government programs aimed at combating obesity within the population at large (Centers for Disease Control and Prevention). CDC focuses on public health efforts to prevent and control infectious and chronic diseases, injuries, workplace hazards, disabilities, and environmental health threats in a variety of community settings. Activities within the CDC, as opposed to other agencies in DHHS, focus on intervention or applied research designed to improve the general health of the public or respond to health emergencies, described as follows. The CDC has played a key role in catalyzing change around obesity prevention by raising

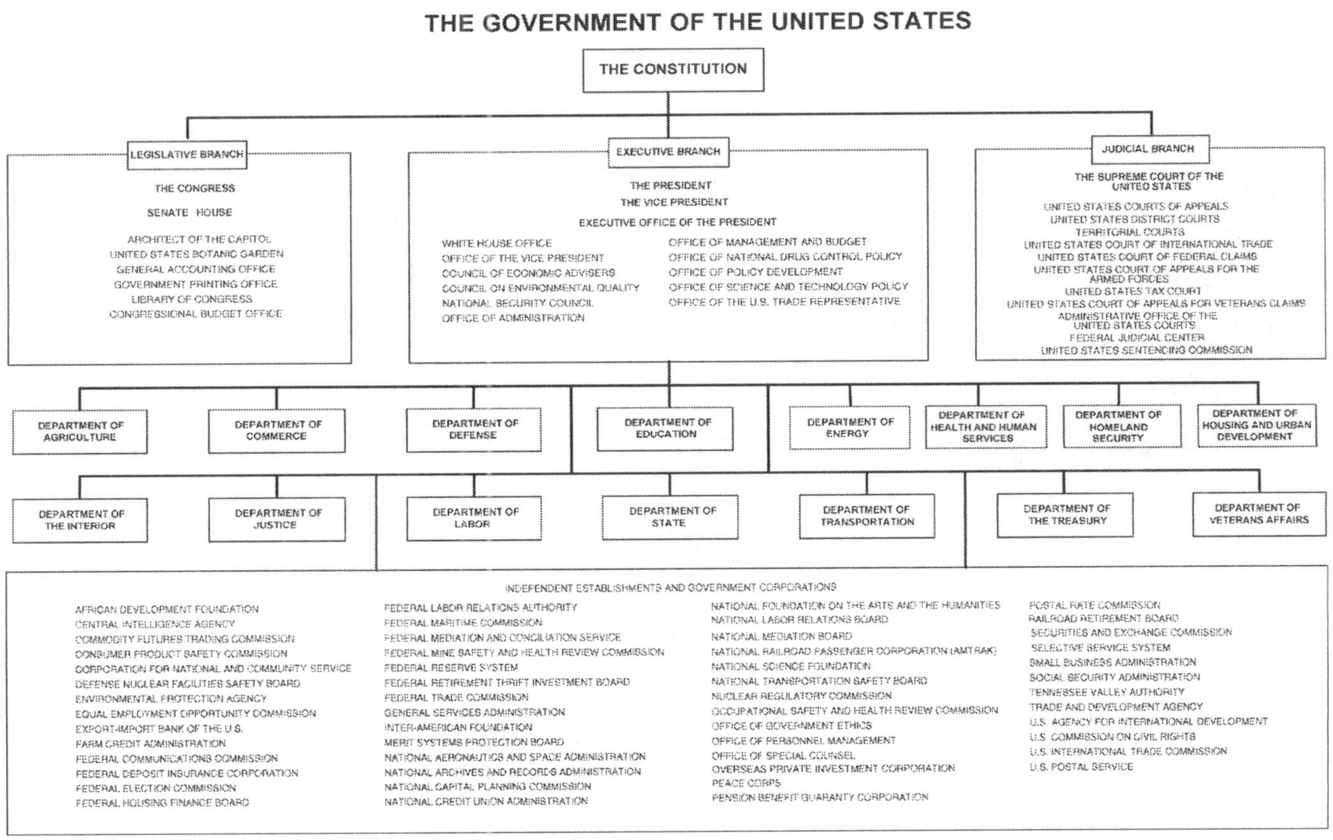

THE GOVERNMENT OF THE UNITED STATES

THE CONSTITUTION

LEGISLATIVE BRANCH

THE CONGRESS
SENATE HOUSE

ARCHITECT OF THE CAPITOL
UNITED STATES BOTANIC GARDEN
GENERAL ACCOUNTING OFFICE
GOVERNMENT PRINTING OFFICE
LIBRARY OF CONGRESS
CONGRESSIONAL BUDGET OFFICE

EXECUTIVE BRANCH

THE PRESIDENT
THE VICE PRESIDENT
EXECUTIVE OFFICE OF THE PRESIDENT

WHITE HOUSE OFFICE
OFFICE OF THE VICE PRESIDENT
COUNCIL OF ECONOMIC ADVISERS
COUNCIL ON ENVIRONMENTAL QUALITY
NATIONAL SECURITY COUNCIL
OFFICE OF ADMINISTRATION
OFFICE OF MANAGEMENT AND BUDGET
OFFICE OF NATIONAL DRUG CONTROL POLICY
OFFICE OF POLICY DEVELOPMENT
OFFICE OF SCIENCE AND TECHNOLOGY POLICY
OFFICE OF THE U.S. TRADE REPRESENTATIVE

JUDICIAL BRANCH

THE SUPREME COURT OF THE UNITED STATES

UNITED STATES COURTS OF APPEALS
UNITED STATES DISTRICT COURTS
TERRITORIAL COURTS
UNITED STATES COURT OF INTERNATIONAL TRADE
UNITED STATES COURT OF FEDERAL CLAIMS
UNITED STATES COURT OF APPEALS FOR THE ARMED FORCES
UNITED STATES TAX COURT
UNITED STATES COURT OF APPEALS FOR VETERANS CLAIMS
ADMINISTRATIVE OFFICE OF THE UNITED STATES COURTS
FEDERAL JUDICIAL CENTER
UNITED STATES SENTENCING COMMISSION

DEPARTMENT OF AGRICULTURE
DEPARTMENT OF COMMERCE
DEPARTMENT OF DEFENSE
DEPARTMENT OF EDUCATION
DEPARTMENT OF ENERGY
DEPARTMENT OF HEALTH AND HUMAN SERVICES
DEPARTMENT OF HOMELAND SECURITY
DEPARTMENT OF HOUSING AND URBAN DEVELOPMENT
DEPARTMENT OF THE INTERIOR
DEPARTMENT OF JUSTICE
DEPARTMENT OF LABOR
DEPARTMENT OF STATE
DEPARTMENT OF TRANSPORTATION
DEPARTMENT OF THE TREASURY
DEPARTMENT OF VETERANS AFFAIRS

INDEPENDENT ESTABLISHMENTS AND GOVERNMENT CORPORATIONS

AFRICAN DEVELOPMENT FOUNDATION
CENTRAL INTELLIGENCE AGENCY
COMMODITY FUTURES TRADING COMMISSION
CONSUMER PRODUCT SAFETY COMMISSION
CORPORATION FOR NATIONAL AND COMMUNITY SERVICE
DEFENSE NUCLEAR FACILITIES SAFETY BOARD
ENVIRONMENTAL PROTECTION AGENCY
EQUAL EMPLOYMENT OPPORTUNITY COMMISSION
EXPORT-IMPORT BANK OF THE U.S.
FARM CREDIT ADMINISTRATION
FEDERAL COMMUNICATIONS COMMISSION
FEDERAL DEPOSIT INSURANCE CORPORATION
FEDERAL ELECTION COMMISSION
FEDERAL HOUSING FINANCE BOARD
FEDERAL LABOR RELATIONS AUTHORITY
FEDERAL MARITIME COMMISSION
FEDERAL MEDIATION AND CONCILIATION SERVICE
FEDERAL MINE SAFETY AND HEALTH REVIEW COMMISSION
FEDERAL RESERVE SYSTEM
FEDERAL RETIREMENT THRIFT INVESTMENT BOARD
FEDERAL TRADE COMMISSION
GENERAL SERVICES ADMINISTRATION
INTER-AMERICAN FOUNDATION
MERIT SYSTEMS PROTECTION BOARD
NATIONAL AERONAUTICS AND SPACE ADMINISTRATION
NATIONAL ARCHIVES AND RECORDS ADMINISTRATION
NATIONAL CAPITAL PLANNING COMMISSION
NATIONAL CREDIT UNION ADMINISTRATION
NATIONAL FOUNDATION ON THE ARTS AND THE HUMANITIES
NATIONAL LABOR RELATIONS BOARD
NATIONAL MEDIATION BOARD
NATIONAL RAILROAD PASSENGER CORPORATION (AMTRAK)
NATIONAL SCIENCE FOUNDATION
NATIONAL TRANSPORTATION SAFETY BOARD
NUCLEAR REGULATORY COMMISSION
OCCUPATIONAL SAFETY AND HEALTH REVIEW COMMISSION
OFFICE OF GOVERNMENT ETHICS
OFFICE OF PERSONNEL MANAGEMENT
OFFICE OF SPECIAL COUNSEL
OVERSEAS PRIVATE INVESTMENT CORPORATION
PEACE CORPS
PENSION BENEFIT GUARANTY CORPORATION
POSTAL RATE COMMISSION
RAILROAD RETIREMENT BOARD
SECURITIES AND EXCHANGE COMMISSION
SELECTIVE SERVICE SYSTEM
SMALL BUSINESS ADMINISTRATION
SOCIAL SECURITY ADMINISTRATION
TENNESSEE VALLEY AUTHORITY
TRADE AND DEVELOPMENT AGENCY
U.S. AGENCY FOR INTERNATIONAL DEVELOPMENT
U.S. COMMISSION ON CIVIL RIGHTS
U.S. INTERNATIONAL TRADE COMMISSION
U.S. POSTAL SERVICE

Figure 7.2 Federal Government Organizational Chart Federal government organization.pdf.

(Available from The U.S. Government Official Web Portal, 2006. http://www.firstgov.gov/Agencies.shtml.)

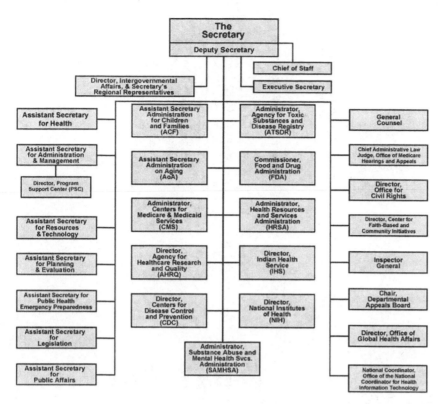

Figure 7.3 U.S. Department of Health and Human Services Organizational Chart
HHS – Department of Health & Human Services Organizational Chart.pdf.

(Available from http://www.hhs.gov/about/orgchart.html.)

awareness of obesity as a public health issue, documenting the disease burden
it presents, particularly for children, and promoting the development and implementation of comprehensive, evidence-based interventions, including those
addressing environmental and policy change (*Statement by William H. Dietz:
CDC's Role in Combating the Obesity Epidemic,* 2002). See Figure 7.4 for the
current CDC organizational chart.

CDC obesity prevention efforts are primarily coordinated through the
National Center for Chronic Disease Prevention and Health Promotion (NCCD-
PHP), which oversees the work of multiple divisions engaged in programming.

The Division of Nutrition and Physical Activity (DNPA) offers public health
approaches to address the role of nutrition and physical activity in improving
the public's health and preventing and controlling chronic diseases (Centers for
Disease Control and Prevention). The scope of DNPA activities includes epidemiological and behavioral research, surveillance, training and education, intervention development, health promotion and leadership, policy and environmental
change, communication and social marketing, and partnership development.
Activities potentially relevant to obesity prevention include promotion of fruit and
vegetable intake through the 5-A-Day program (which received 4 million dollars
FY2004) (Foerster et al., 1995; Havas et al., 1994; National Cancer Institute,
2006), and the promotion of physical activity in youth through the VERB
campaign. The VERB campaign has been very successful but, despite evidence

Table 7.1 Department of Health and Human Services—obesity related initiatives (Current and recent).

Dept. of Health and Human Services (DHHS)	Center for Disease Control (CDC) –	Obesity related programs	Target population	Type/Format of program
	Control (CDC) – National Center for Chronic Disease and Prevention and Health Promotion (NCCD-PCP)			
	Division of Nutrition and Physical Activity (DNPA)	5 a Day	U.S. population	Funding to states, Media campaign, Website, Partnerships, Print materials
		VERB! (inactive as of FY2006)	Ages 9–13	Social marketing, Media campaign, Partnerships Website, Teacher's website
		BAM! Body and Mind	Ages 9–13	
		Nutrition and Physical Activity Program to Prevent Obesity and other Chronic Disease	U.S. population	Funding delivered to states to promote nutrition and physical activity
	Division of Adolescent and School Health (DASH)	Coordinated School Health Program	School Age Children (K-12th grade)	Eight component model for school health education
	Health Protection Research Initiative (HPRI)	Workplace Prevention Programs	U.S. population	Research and Evaluation
	Prevention Research Centers (PRCs)	Planet Health, CATCH, PRCs at Universities	U.S. population	Research, Toolkit development
	Healthier U.S.	STEPS	U.S. population	Funding to states, Website, Media campaign
National Institutes of Health (NIH)	National Heart Lung and Blood Institute	We Can! Program (a collaboration of all NIH departments)	Children ages 8–13	Research, Tool kit, Website
		Portion Distortion Quiz	U.S. population	Website
		Aim for a Healthy Weight	Adults	Toolkit
	National Institute of Diabetes and	WIN Weight Control	Adults	Research

Agency	Program	Target Audience	Product/Format
	Digestive and Kidney Diseases (NIDDK) Information Network	Public Health Professionals	Resource website
National Cancer Institute	Cancer Control Planet Body and Soul	African American Church members	Toolkit, Website, DVD
National Institute of Environmental Health Sciences	Fitness Fighters	Children	Television show
Food and Drug Administration (FDA) Obesity Working Group	Labeling Initiative	U.S. population	A group of obesity specialists informing the FDA on what types of programs to initiate regarding obesity, food labeling construction and modification
Health and Resources and Services Administration (HRSA) Maternal Child Health Bureau Bureau of Primary Care		U.S. Population focus on women, minorities, child/maternal health	Toolkits, Personnel training, Partnerships
Office of Public Health and Science (OPHS) Office of Disease Prevention and Health Promotion	Healthy People 2010	U.S. population	Health objectives in print and internet format
The President's Council on Physical Fitness and Sports (PCPFS)	www.fitness.org (The website for PCPFS)	U.S. population	Website
	The President's Challenge	With Presidential Active Lifestyle Awards (PALA) for participants as well as State Champion Awards and National School Demonstrations	Website
	May Month (National	U.S. population	Website, National media campaign, Print material

(Continued)

Table 7.1 (Continued)

	Obesity related programs	Target population	Type/Format of program
	Physical Fitness and Sports Month)		
	PCPFS Research Digest	Fitness professionals and interested citizens	Quarterly publication, Website
Office of Women's Health	Pick Your Path to Health	Women of color	Toolkit, Listserv, Media campaign, Partnerships, Community groups
	Powerful Bones. Powerful Girls.	9–12 year old girls	Website
Office of Minority Health	African American Anti-Obesity Initiative	Minority population	Health policy development and programs
Indian Health Services		American Indian and Alaska Native Population	Culturally acceptable health services and programs
The Surgeon Generals Office	Call to Action to Prevent and Decrease Overweight and Obesity	U.S. population, policymakers	Reports
Administration on Aging	You Can!	Older U.S. population	Print materials, Toolkit
Medicare/Medicaid Services	Obesity related reimbursement	U.S. population	Reimbursement program
Administration for Children and Families	Head Start, Early Head Start	Low income pregnant women, infants, and children up to age 5, families receiving TNAF, foster care children, handicapped children, families at 100% of poverty	Nutrition education, nutritious meals and snacks

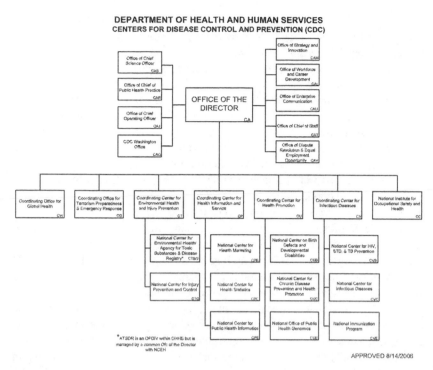

Figure 7.4 Centers for Disease Control Organizational Chart CDC organizational chart.pdf).

(Available from http://www.cdc.gov/maso/pdf/CDC.pdf.)

of its effectiveness (Centers for Disease Control and Prevention, 2005g) was not refunded for fiscal year 2006.

The DNPA also provides grants to states to develop plans and comprehensive programs to prevent obesity and chronic disease. States are provided capacity building grants to develop state plans and build coalitions for change, with implementation grants providing support for environmental and community interventions. As of 2005, 18.6 million dollars was available to 28 states for obesity programs through DNPA. The agency received almost double that number of applications but had insufficient funds to support the high demand from states (Glendening, Hearne, Segal, Juliano, & Earls, 2005).

The Division of Adolescent and School Health (DASH) addresses health needs of adolescents through (1) surveillance of health risk behaviors and school health policies (including the Youth Risk Behavior Surveillance System and School Health Profiles); (2) practitioner-focused application tools to aid in synthesis of research; (3) implementation of comprehensive adolescent and school and health programs; and (4) technical evaluation assistance to state and local education agencies. DASH oversees the Coordinated School Health Program (CSHP) which encourages cooperation of state health and education departments with schools in promoting policies and programs that address obesity and chronic disease. In FY2005, $56.7 million was available to fund 23 of 39 state applicants (Centers for Disease Control and Prevention, 2005a; 2005e).

Health Protection Research Initiative (HRPI) was developed in 2004 as a multiyear initiative in which CDC provided $21.7 million in funding 57 research grants to develop health promotion and prevention workplace programs (31 awards), encourage career development in public health research (24 awards), and create health promotion economic centers (two awards). Of the workplace-focused grants, 21 involve projects designed to increase physical activity, improve nutrition, and reduce obesity (Centers for Disease Control and Prevention, 2005d).

Prevention Research Centers (PRCs) conduct applied research targeting chronic disease prevention and control. The 33 PRCs partner academic researchers, public health agencies, and community members for the purpose of conducting research projects on health- or population-specific issues. Several centers conduct projects that address some aspect of energy balance (Centers for Disease Control and Prevention, 2005f).

Steps to a Healthier U.S. (STEPS) is a national initiative which is a component of the President's Healthier U.S. initiative, and is coordinated through NCCD-PHP (U.S. Department of Health and Human Services, 2005g). It began in 2003 as a cooperative agreement program that identifies, promotes, and strengthens evidence-based school and community programs focused on decreasing three related risk factors – physical inactivity, poor nutrition, and tobacco use. Interventions encourage cooperative initiatives among policy makers, education and health agencies, schools and communities. In FY2004, $35.8 million was available to fund 40 STEPs communities nationwide (U.S. Department of Health and Human Services, 2005g).

National Institutes of Health (NIH)

The NIH is home to 27 institutes and centers charged with the conduct of "science in pursuit of fundamental knowledge about the nature and behavior of living systems." (National Institutes of Health, 2005). The focus of NIH activities is on scientific discovery, designed to be complementary to the public health research focus of the CDC. The escalating obesity epidemic, and its association with specific diseases such as diabetes, heart disease, and cancer, has led to relevant research efforts at multiple institutes within NIH (see Table 7.1).

NIH has a long history of conducting obesity related research at fundamental, clinical, and epidemiologic levels (National Institutes of Health, 2005). For example, research in fundamental sciences led to the discovery of the hormone leptin, which drastically alters the fat tissue as a storehouse for energy, and ghrelin which stimulates appetite just before meals. The Diabetes Prevention Program, funded by the National Institute of Digestive, Diabetes, and Kidney Disorders (NIDDK), provided evidence for lifestyle behavioral modification and limited weight loss in the prevention and treatment of type 2 diabetes. The National Heart, Lung, and Blood Institute (NHLBI) funded The Coronary Artery Risk Development in Young Adults (CARDIA), a long-term epidemiologic study examining the distribution and evolution of coronary heart disease risk factors and the development of obesity during transition years to adulthood in 5,115 African American and white men and women. The Framingham Heart Study is a longitudinal investigation of constitutional, environmental, and genetic factors influencing the development of cardiovascular disease in over 14,000 men and women in three generations. And finally, beginning in 1990, the CHIC Study (Cardiovascular Health in Children and Youth Study) has collected data on almost 4,000 school children and adolescents in North Carolina—from ages 8 through 16, monitoring obesity, eating habits and physical activity, and related risk factors.

Most recently, as noted in Table 1, NIH has funded We Can!, a new initiative of four agencies within NIH (NIDDK, NHLBI, the National Cancer Institute [NCI], and the National Institute of Child Health and Human Development [NICHD]). *Ways to Enhance Children's Activity and Nutrition* was launched in June 2005 as a collaborative effort with the National Recreation and Parks Association. This program is targeted to children 8–13 years of age with objectives of improving nutritional choices, increasing physical activity, and decreasing screen time for this population. This program is unique among government obesity initiatives because it focuses on family activities, community outreach, national media, and relationship development with corporations to ensure acceptance and utilization of the program (National Heart Lung and Blood Institute, National Institute of Diabetes and Digestive and Kidney Disease, National Institute of Child Health and Human Development, & National Cancer Institute, 2006).

Finally, to avoid duplication and enhance efforts, the NIH Director, Dr. Elias Zerhouni, established the NIH Obesity Research Task Force in April 2003, as a new effort to accelerate progress in obesity research across the NIH. The task force is co-chaired by the Directors of NIDDK and NHLBI and includes as members representatives from 24 other NIH Institutes and Centers with relevant expertise (see www.obesityresearch.nih.gov). A key task force activity was the development of a Strategic Plan for NIH Obesity Research as a guide for coordinating obesity research activities (National Institutes of Health, 2005; National Institutes of Health Obesity Research Task Force, 2004). The plan development addressed four themes: lifestyle modification; pharmacologic, surgical, or other medical approaches; breaking the link with chronic diseases; and, cross-cutting research topics including health disparities, technology, interdisciplinary research, training, translational research, education, and outreach. This plan will guide NIH research to address obesity prevention and control.

Food and Drug Administration (FDA)
The FDA began in 1906 with the passage of the Federal Food and Drug Act, and is a "scientific, regulatory, and public health agency charged with monitoring the manufacture, import, transport, storage, and sale of food products (other than meat and poultry) . . ." (U.S. Department of Health and Human Services, 2005c). In 1990, Congress passed the Nutrition Labeling and Education Act which gave the FDA authority to initiate a uniform and science-based food label. Estimates are that two-thirds of shoppers read food labels before buying new items, while one-third cite labels as influencing purchases, making this a powerful nutrition education initiative (French, Story, & Jeffery, 2001). In 2003, the FDA formed an Obesity Working Group, which outlined an action plan to cover critical dimensions of the obesity problem from the FDA's perspective. The working group recommended: better defining of labeling terms relative to calories; more accurate information from manufacturers concerning portion size; an educational campaign focusing on calories; expansion of nutritional information provided to consumers at restaurants; review of obesity-related drug therapies; and research (U.S. Food and Drug Administration, 2005).

Health Resources and Services Administration (HRSA)
HRSA provides "national leadership, program resources and services needed to improve access to culturally competent, quality health care." Obesity information is provided through the Maternal Child Health Bureau, which offers programs, materials, and online resources encouraging positive nutrition and exercise, as well

as the Bureau of Primary Care, which informs regarding treatment of overweight students in schools through screening and intervention (U.S. Department of Health and Human Services Health Resources and Services Administration, 2005d).

Office of Public Health and Science (OPHS)

The OPHS houses several offices that address some aspect of obesity.

The Office of Disease Prevention and Health Promotion (ODPHP) is home to the Healthy People 2010 program, which designates national health objectives and establishes national goals to reduce these threats. This office coordinates the efforts of numerous partners from the federal government and the public at large in developing and reporting on these objectives (Office of Disease Prevention and Health Promotion, 2007).

The President's Council on Physical Fitness and Sports, which began in 1956, is a committee of 20 volunteers appointed by the President to advise on means of promoting physical activity in America. The Council does not specifically target obesity but rather addresses physical activity as a key component of the energy balance equation. The Council is designed to be a catalyst for recommendations and actions that support health initiatives of the President, DHHS, and Healthy People 2010 (U.S. Department of Health and Human Services, 2005h).

The Office of Women's Health, The Office of Minority Health (U.S. Department of Health and Human Services, 2005f) and the *Indian Health Service* (U.S. Department of Health and Human Services, 2005e) partner with other federal agencies in obesity-related research and offer linkages to information and research relevant to the target populations, or access to model educational programs addressing obesity via the website (see Table 7.1).

The Surgeon General's Office provides leadership and advocates for evidence-based health education and behaviors. As noted in the Introduction to this chapter, the Surgeon General's Office issued a "Call to Action to Prevent and Decrease Overweight and Obesity" (U.S. Department of Health and Human Services et al., 2001). The office does not financially support activities but, rather, serves as a 'bully pulpit' for calling attention to key public health issues.

Other DHHS Initiatives

The *Administration on Aging* supports the 'You Can! Campaign,' designed to increase the number of older adults who stay active and healthy (U.S. Department of Health and Human Services, 2005a). And the *Centers for Medicare and Medicaid Services*, which designated obesity a disease in 2005, began providing reimbursement for specified treatments (U.S. Department of Health and Human Services, 2005b).

United States Department of Agriculture (USDA)

The USDA also plays a major role in federal obesity policy and initiatives. The USDA was formed in 1862 with policies historically rooted in supplying the nation with adequate and safe food by increasing agricultural productivity, efficiency, and commodity production. These goals have been successfully accomplished with the threat of famine virtually eliminated by abundant availability and reduced cost of foods (Tillotson, 2003; 2004). The USDA now has assumed a major role in a range of food and nutrition programs for the population at large, and provides not only oversight of food safety but also nutrition education and information, labeling regulations, and food distribution. However, compared to the objectives of reducing hunger and under-nutrition, objectives related to obesity prevention are much less inherently compatible with and sometimes appear counter to the push for high levels of food production, at least if that food is channeled into the domestic market. A related issue is one of agricultural subsidies. For example, the IOM report recommended "an independent assessment of federal nutrition assistance programs and agricultural policies" to determine the extent to which they are or can be harmonious with childhood obesity prevention. High levels of food production may lead to over-consumption, i.e., the calories available per capita are currently in excess of the energy intake needs of most individuals in the population. Commodity-based programs that emphasize high calorie or high fat foods may render it more difficult for program participants to achieve healthy weights. To provide nutrition assistance, dietary guidance and other educational programs which are conducive to obesity prevention while also fully supporting agricultural productivity *within the same agency* is ever present under the current circumstances.

Figure 7.5 shows the USDA organizational structure and components. Of its seven agencies, the *Food, Nutrition and Consumer Service Agency* (FNCSA) is most associated with obesity prevention activities (see Table 7.2). The FNCSA is home to two centers that oversee nutrition assistance programs for underserved populations: The Food and Nutrition Service and the Center for Nutrition Policy and Promotion.

Food and Nutrition Service (FNS)

The FNS is responsible for food distribution through the Food Stamp Program, the Special Supplemental Nutrition Program for Women, Infants, and Children (WIC), and the National School Lunch Program (NSLP). The FY2004 budget included $42.9 billion for domestic food assistance programs (Institute of Medicine, 2005; U.S. Department of Agriculture, 2002; 2005a).

• The Food Stamp Program is administered through the states and serves an estimated 23.9 million participants each day (U.S. Department of Agriculture, 2005a). It is the largest food assistance program in the country ($30.5 million in FY2004) and is designed to increase the food purchasing power of eligible low-income households. One outcome of the program is that food stamp recipients have a higher caloric intake on average than non-recipients (Institute of Medicine, 2005; U.S. Department of Agriculture, 2002). WIC was established in 1974 and provides federal grants to states for supplemental foods, health care referrals, and nutrition education for low-income pregnant, breastfeeding, and non-breastfeeding postpartum women, and to infants who are found to be at nutritional risk. In 2000, WIC served 54% of all U.S. infants and 25% of children between the ages of 1 and 4 (Institute of Medicine, 2005; U.S. Department of Agriculture, 2002). In 2005, WIC distributed to states over $5 billion dollars for the program. WIC offers information and modules on obesity prevention programs, including FIT-WIC for children. Concerns have been raised suggesting that WIC food packages include and encourage high calorie and high cholesterol items. In addition, breast feeding is also reduced among WIC mothers (13% WIC mothers versus 30% non-WIC mothers) (U.S. Department of Agriculture, 2002). In response, the Institute of Medicine (IOM) evaluated dietary needs and intake of WIC participants and recommended strategies for program improvement (Institute of Medicine, 2005).

• The National School Lunch Program (NSLP) was established in 1946 as a federally assisted meal program operating in public and nonprofit private schools and child care institutions. It is designed to provide nutritionally

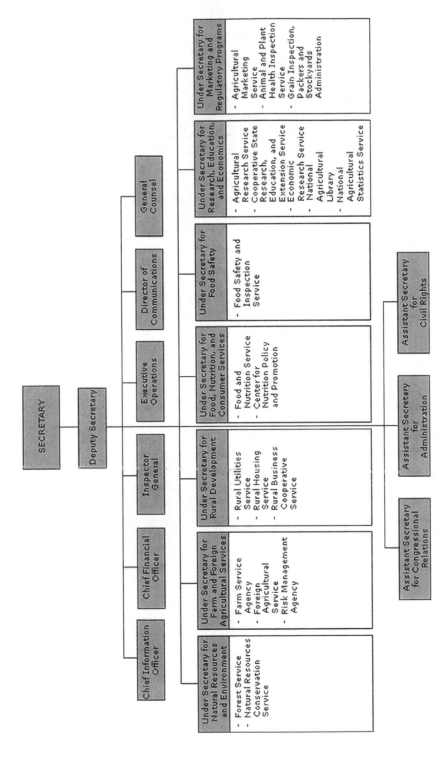

Figure 7.5 U.S. Department of Agriculture. Organization chart. 2006 USDA Organizational Chart.pdf. (Available from http://www.usda.gov/img/content/org_chart_enlarged.jpg.)

Table 7.2 U.S. Department of Agriculture – Agencies and programs relevant to obesity prevention.

Dept. of Agric. (USDA)	Food and Nutrition Services (FNS)	Programs	Target population	Type of program
		Food Stamp Program	Low-income, working families with dependents. Those without dependents are eligible for a shorter time period.	EBT (Electronic Bank Transfer), print material
		Women, Infant, and Children (WIC)	Low-income women, infants, and children up to age 5 who are at nutritional risk.	Individual and group nutrition counseling, Distribution at the federal, state, and county level
		School Meals — National School Lunch (NSLP) School Breakfast	High school students and younger at public or non-profit private schools and in residential care.	Food distribution
		Special School Milk Program	Children in schools, child care institutions and eligible camps that do not participate in other Federal child nutrition programs.	Milk distribution
		Team Nutrition	Kindergarten through 12th grade	Toolkit, Nutrition education food service training
		Food Distribution — School/Child Nutrition Commodity Program	Groups listed for NSLP, CACFP, and SFSP	Commodity foods distribution
		Food Distribution Program on Indian Reservations	Low income elderly living on an Indian Reservation or Native Americans	Commodity foods distribution

(*Continued*)

Table 7.2 (Continued)

	Programs	Target population	Type of program
	Nutrition Services Incentive Program	Older adults	Commodity foods and monetary funds distribution
	Commodity Supplemental Food Program	WIC and the elderly	Commodity foods and funds allocated to states for distribution
	The Emergency Food Assistance Program	Low-income Americans, including the elderly	Commodity foods distribution
	Child and Adult Care Food Program (CACFP)	Children and adults in non-residential or licensed residential day care centers, children in homeless shelters and youth in after school programs.	Food and funds allocated to states for distribution
	Summer Food Service Programs (SFSP)	Children (18 years or younger) in low-income communities.	Food distribution to state and county agencies
	Farmer's Market Nutrition Programs (WIC & Senior)	WIC target population and low-income (<185% below poverty line) seniors (>60y/o).	Local farmers' produce distribution
Center for Nutrition Policy and Promotion (CNPP)	Dietary Guidelines for Americans (collaboration with Department of Health and Human Services)	U.S. population	Print materials, Website
	Food Pyramid	Adults	Website, Print materials
	Food Pyramid for Kids	Young children	PDF files, Print material
	Healthy Eating Index	U.S. population	PDF files, Print materials
	Nutrition Insight	U.S. population	PDF files

balanced, low-cost or free lunches to children each school day and is administered by the states through state school food authorities (SFAs). Foods for the NSLP are also dependent upon a varying agricultural surplus. The school-lunch reauthorization bill enacted by Congress in 2004 contained measures to improve the nutritional content of school lunches, creating initiatives to encourage partnerships between schools and local produce farms and increase the availability of whole grains in school meals. Additionally, Public Law 108–265 (described in detail later in this chapter) requires that schools have a local wellness policy in place and set goals for nutrition education, physical activity, and school-based activities to promote wellness (U.S. Department of Agriculture, 2005b).

- The FNS coordinates Team Nutrition, which provides educational materials for children, oversees after-school initiatives promoting appropriate nutrition, and teaches food service members how to prepare healthy school foods. Team Nutrition provides training and technical assistance for food service, nutrition education for children and caregivers, and school and community support for healthy eating and physical activity. Team Nutrition also sponsors the Power to Choice program, intended for after-school program leaders working with adolescents (USDA Food and Nutrition Service, 2006).

Center for Nutrition Policy and Promotion (CNPP)

The CNPP is an agency of the FNS that conducts applied research and analysis in nutrition knowledge and attitudes, dietary survey methodology, and dietary guidance and nutrition education techniques. CNPP coordinates the review and publication of the *Dietary Guidelines for Americans*, which have been published jointly every 5 years since 1980 by the Department of Health and Human Services (HHS) and the Department of Agriculture (USDA) (U.S. Department of Agriculture, 2005). They provide "authoritative advice for people two years and older about how good dietary habits can promote health and reduce risk for major chronic diseases" (U. S. Department of Health and Human Services & U. S. Department of Agriculture, 2005). These guidelines are the basis for U.S. government food and nutrition education programs, and nutrition policy initiatives. The CNPP also coordinates the production of MyPyramid, the Healthy Eating Index, and materials on nutrient content of foods and food expenditures. Educational and interactive information designed to promote energy balance is made available to the population at large and nutrition educators per the FY2006 budget of $2.9 million.

Other Executive Branch Activities

Department of Defense (DOD) The DOD identifies obesity as a health and fitness concern for incoming recruits and current personnel as well as a condition of continued employment. DOD pays an estimated $15 million per year in bariatric surgery for military personnel and dependents (see Table 7.3) (U.S. Department of Defense, 2006a). In addition, many service branches have developed obesity treatment and prevention programs for members. The Navy offers ShipShape, an 8-week program designed to provide active-duty personnel with basic information on nutrition, stress management, physical activity, and behavior modification techniques (U.S. Department of Defense, 2006a). The Army offers Weigh to Stay, an intensive, standardized three part weight management and education program with designated follow-ups (U.S. Department of

Table 7.3 Other federal agencies and programs relevant to obesity prevention.

Government agency	Obesity related programs	Target population	Type of program
Dept. of Defense	ShipShape	Military personnel and incoming recruits	Physical fitness, Weight management and education programs, Obesity related medical treatment and prescriptions
	Weigh to Stay		
Dept. of Education	Carol M White Physical Education Program (PEP)	Students in school and at after school programs grades kindergarten through 12th	Grants to educational agencies and community based organizations to initiate, expand or improve physical education programs and equipment, including after school programming
Dept. of the Interior	National Park Service: National Trails System — Pathways to Walk program	U.S. population	Maintaining national trails for recreational use
Dept. of Transportation	Bicycle and Pedestrian Programs	Non-motorized street users	Federal funding to states for the promotion of non-motorized transportation, education, and safety
Federal Highway Administration	Recreational Trails Program (RTP)	U.S. population	Federal funding to states to provide and tend to recreational trails
	Safe Routes to School (Collaboration with the National Highway Traffic Safety Administration)	Kindergarten through 8th grade children	Federal funding to states to encourage, develop, and implement safe walking and biking to school programs
Dept. of Veteran Affairs	MOVE!	Veterans	Individual and group counseling, PSA, website based questionnaire to assess needs for tailoring counseling
VA National Center for Health Promotion and Disease Prevention (NCP)			
Federal Trade Commission (FTC)	Division of Advertising Practices	U.S. population	Guidelines for advertising workshops, literature and workshops and advertising to children
	For the Consumer: Diet, Health and Fitness	Literate U.S. population	Internet based text and PDF, workshops, Internet marketing campaigns
Office of Personnel Management	Healthier Feds Campaign	Federal Employees and retires	Workplace initiative, website

Defense, 2006). In 2003, the IOM published a report that made recommendations to DOD on strategies for preventing weight gain in military personnel, and noted the necessary components for weight loss programs in the military (Institute of Medicine, 2003). This report recommended standardization of programs across the different Service branches.

Department of Education (DOE) The DOE coordinates the Carol M. White Physical Education Program, which awards grants to local educational agencies (LEA) and community-based organizations to initiate, expand, or improve physical education programs (U.S. Department of Education, 2005). This includes after-school programs for students in one or more grades from kindergarten through 12th grade, in order to help students make progress toward meeting state standards for physical education. In 2005, $73,408,000 was appropriated for this program.

The Department of the Interior developed a "Pathways to Health" program encouraging trail use (U.S. Department of the Interior, 2005).

Department of Transportation (DOT) The DOT is home to the federally funded, "Safe Routes to School" program, initiated in 2005 as a collaborative effort of the Federal Highway Administration and National Highway Traffic Safety Administration. This joint effort is based on the premise that a comprehensive approach to encourage child activity must include infrastructure-related projects, such as sidewalks and bicycle paths, and other projects stressing awareness and education (U.S. Department of Transportation-Federal Highway Administration, 2005).

Department of Veterans Affairs (VA) The VA is testing MOVE!, a program designed by the VA National Center for Health Promotion and Disease Prevention (NCP) to help veterans lose weight, keep it off, and improve their health. It includes materials and support via individual and group weight loss counseling (U.S. Department of Veterans Affairs, 2005).

Obesity Prevention Activities of Independent Federal Organizations

Federal Trade Commission (FTC) The FTC is an independent agency headed by five Commissioners, with a goal to protect consumers against unfair, deceptive, or fraudulent practices. The FTC houses the Division of Advertising Practices, which is charged with protecting consumers from deceptive and unsubstantiated advertising. This agency has a critical role to play with regard to recent calls to limit the advertising of unhealthy foods to children or balance the efforts with healthy claims (Federal Trade Commission, 2007). The FTC has worked collaboratively in sponsoring workshops to examine various perspectives on marketing and childhood obesity.

Office of Personnel Management (OPM) is within the executive branch of government and coordinates the 2004 *HealthierFeds* campaign (Office of Personnel Management, 2005). The *HealthierFeds* initiative educates Federal employees and retirees on healthy living and best-treatment strategies via website information and promotes individual responsibility for personal health.

Monitoring and Surveillance Activities

Monitoring and surveillance of nutritional status and other health status data are key functions of the U.S. government. These surveillance systems were mandated by the National Nutrition Monitoring and Related Research Act of 1990, which includes a plan for: collecting continuous, coordinated, timely, and reliable data; using comparable methods for data collection and reporting of results; conducting research; and disseminating information (Moshfegh, 1994). These types of activities are funded by Congress via annual appropriations, and the majority of surveillance activities are coordinated by the National Center for Health Statistics (NCHS), located within CDC and home to the Interagency Board for Nutrition Monitoring and Related Research (a group comprised of most departments of the federal government involved in any aspect of nutrition) (Centers for Disease Control and Prevention, 2006a). Some of the data are sample surveys, while others are compilations of data from local health programs. Select highlights of nutrition-related monitoring and surveillance activities conducted by the NCHS are described below.

National Health and Nutrition Examination Survey (NHANES I, II, III, 1999–2004)

This is a series of periodic surveys given to the public to self-report information on height, weight, and a variety of health information. The NHANES surveys are based on national probability samples that do not yield state or local level data, although some data have been reported for major U.S. regions. Over-sampling of high risk groups or, more recently, of black Americans and Mexican Americans helps to support analyses by important subgroups. Beginning in 1999, the NHANES is ongoing rather than periodic-data is reported for each 2 year interval. The information collected from these surveys has enabled the government to produce the height-for-weight charts, monitor the relationship between nutrition, diet, and health, as well as monitor disease. NHANES is unique in that it is the only survey collecting a representative sample of biological specimens from the U.S. population (Centers for Disease Control and Prevention, 2006a).

Hispanic Health and Nutrition Examination Survey (HHANES)

This survey was implemented between 1982 and 1984. Hispanic Americans had been included in the NHANES up to that time, but in too few numbers to draw conclusions about their health. This survey offers specific health related information for Puerto Ricans, Mexican Americans, and Cuban Americans (Centers for Disease Control and Prevention, 2006a). Hispanic HANES has not been repeated; however, Mexican Americans are now over-sampled in the NHANES.

The Pediatric Nutrition Surveillance Survey (PedNSS)

This survey provides nutrition surveillance of infants and children in federally funded child health programs (Centers for Disease Control and Prevention, 2006b).

The Pregnancy Nutrition Surveillance Survey (PNSS)

This survey offers nutrition surveillance of women in federally funded maternal health programs (Centers for Disease Control and Prevention, 2006b).

Behavioral Risk Factor Surveillance System (BRFSS)

This is sponsored by the National Center for Chronic Disease Prevention and Health Promotion. This is a state based assessment of the prevalence of personal health practices that are related to the leading causes of death. Data are collected by telephone. BRFSS has been used by state health departments to plan, initiate and guide health promotion and disease prevention programs, and to monitor their progress over time. The BRFSS has been conducted continuously since 1984 (Centers for Disease Control and Prevention & National Center for Chronic Disease Prevention and Health Promotion, 2006).

Youth Risk Behavior Surveillance Survey (YRBSS)
This national probability sample survey is designed to evaluate the major health risk behaviors among American youth and young adults that lead to death, disability, and social problems (Centers for Disease Control and Prevention, 2006). Data results for the YRBSS are available at state and local levels for those states and localities that participate in the survey.

School Health Policies and Programs Survey (SHPPS)
The SHPPS is a different type of surveillance activity than those previously mentioned, as it assesses health policies and programs at the state, district, school, and classroom levels nationwide (Centers for Disease Control and Prevention, 2006c). The survey was conducted in 1994 and 2000, and data collection for the 2006 survey began in January 2006.

Funding of Federal Obesity Prevention Activities

Funding Mechanisms
At the federal level, Congress has a primary effect on obesity prevention efforts through its use of Constitutional authority to authorize and appropriate funds to the various departments of the federal government. These "powers of the purse" (to tax and spend) are found in Article I, Section 8 of the Constitution – "the spending power provides Congress with independent authority to allocate resources for the public good; Congress need not justify its spending by reference to a specific enumerated power" (Gostin, 2000).

Funding for obesity related programs implemented by executive agencies generally takes place via two avenues: authorization – a statutory provision that obligates funding for a program or agency; and appropriations, which assures the provision of funds through an annual appropriations act or a permanent law for specified purposes. Authorization acts establish, continue, or modify agencies or programs. The authorization act also authorizes appropriations for specific agencies and programs, frequently setting spending ceilings, or it may provide permanent, annual, or multi-year authorizations. Authorizing legislation pertaining to a certain department of the federal government emanates from the committee responsible for the oversight of that department (e.g. the committee on Health, Education, Labor and Pensions is responsible for authorizations relating to the Department of Health and Human Services) (Fisher, Kaiser, Oleszek, & Rosenberg, 2004). The Congressional committees provide information to the Budget Committees of the House and Senate, which are responsible for drawing up the budget resolutions that are adopted each year to establish aggregate spending and revenue levels of the government for at least five fiscal years (Fisher et al., 2004; Sachs, 2000, 2003). Congress is not required to provide appropriations for an authorized program (Streeter, 2004).

Appropriations measures provide new budget authority for the program, activity, or agency previously authorized. Members of Congress who sit on the Budget or Appropriations committees are responsible for writing the twelve annual appropriations acts that fund the departments and agencies of the federal government (United States Government Accountability Office (Office of the General Counsel), January 2004). These annual appropriations bills fund multiple nutrition or obesity-related programs within the Department of

Health and Human Services and the Department of Agriculture (e.g. food stamp and child nutrition programs) (Womach, 2005).

Organizations that Influence the Legislative Processes

Throughout the budgetary process congressional committees frequently seek information from relevant governmental agencies and experts external to the government, located in independent research groups, universities, and think tanks or advocacy groups. These organizations serve critical roles in informing the agenda and debate over policy initiatives and outcomes when Congress considers adopting measures to reauthorize or re-appropriate funds for agencies or programs (Sachs, 2000; 2003).

Within the government, there are several authoritative and nonpartisan agencies charged with providing information and evidence to inform the crafting of policy. These agencies include the Congressional Budget Office (CBO), the Congressional Research Service (CRS), and the Government Accountability Office (GAO), which are dependable sources of information pertaining to authorizations, appropriations, budget or other legislative measures being considered by Congress.

Outside of the government, numerous other organizations, including academic, advocacy, or think tank groups, offer advice and resources to congressional staff. These organizations are diverse in composition and philosophy but fill an important role in identifying gaps in policy initiatives. A comprehensive listing of many of these groups is available elsewhere (Carlisle Fountain, 2005). Following are select examples of several of these groups.

Most notably, The Institute of Medicine (IOM) fills an invaluable role to Congress through its service as "adviser to the nation to improve health." Since 1970, as a charter of the National Academy of Sciences, the Institute of Medicine has provided independent, unbiased, evidence-based advice to policymakers, health professionals, industry, and the public. In relation to obesity, the IOM has conducted numerous studies requested by Congress and provided evidence and recommendations for prevention of childhood obesity (Koplan et al., 2004), prevention of obesity in military and other settings (Institute of Medicine, 2003), guidance for food and nutrition in schools and WIC programs, (Institute of Medicine, 2005; Institutes of Medicine, 2006), and physical activity and the built environment (Institute of Medicine & Transportation Research Board, 2005).

Other groups that inform the national debate on obesity include The Henry J. Kaiser Family Foundation, a non-profit, private operating foundation which provides information to policymakers through the conduct of studies on media and other factors influencing obesity in children (The Henry J. Kaiser Family Foundation, 2006). The Center for Science in the Public Interest (CSPI) is a high profile consumer advocacy organization which conducts research and advocacy programs in health and nutrition with a strong focus on obesity prevention (Center for Science in the Public Interest, 2006). The American Obesity Association works to secure funds in support of research and treatment for obesity from government, the health care profession and the insurance industry, and is focused on ending obesity discrimination (American Obesity Association, 2006). And finally, The University of Baltimore Obesity Initiative is an example of an academic center that provides information on status of state initiatives by providing a "report card" for each state, based on efforts to pass obesity control measures (University of Baltimore Obesity Initiative, 2006).

Overview of Pertinent Legislation

Several key pieces of legislation play a primary role in influencing the nutrition and activity environment of our country. These bills are the focus of discussion and debate within the federal government, and among watchdog and advocacy groups, all of which strive to influence or inform the bill in a way that is consistent with their understanding of the evidence for obesity prevention. Highlights of these key pieces of legislation are as follows:

Labor, Health & Human Services, and Education (HHS): Annual Appropriations

The HHS appropriations bill is typically the second largest source of discretionary fund expenditures – the FY2005 bill accounted for 17.3% of all federal discretionary budget authority in FY2005 (the Defense appropriations bill accounted for 47.5% of FY2005 discretionary budget authority) (Irwin, 2005). Included in this annual bill is funding for federal agencies that, as previously discussed, play major roles in obesity prevention and reduction efforts. It also includes provisions for two block grant programs administered by the CDC that fund certain state and local initiatives addressing the obesity epidemic.

The Preventive Health and Health Services Block grants (PHHS) (authorized under P.L. 103–0183 "Preventive Health Amendments of 1993") received $100 million in unauthorized appropriations for FY2006 (Congressional Budget Office, January 13, 2006). Local public health departments reportedly receive about 40% of PHHS grants that allow departments to carry out programs promoting healthy nutrition and physical activity (Congressional Budget Office, January 13, 2006). The PHHS grants are in danger of being eliminated in FY2007, as new authorizing language has not passed Congress, and the grants again are not present in President Bush's FY2007 Budget Request to Congress.

The Community Services Block Grant (CSBG) program provides grants to state agencies responsible for distributing the funds to local eligible entities generally dedicated to "reducing poverty" (Spar & Laney, 2005). Within the CSBG program is a *Community Food and Nutrition Program* that provides grants to public and private nonprofit organizations "to coordinate food assistance resources, to help identify potential sponsors of child nutrition programs . . . and to develop innovative approaches at the state and local level to meet the nutritional needs of low-income people" (Spar & Laney, 2005).

Agriculture and Related Agencies: Annual Appropriations

Approximately 80% of the USDA's spending is classified as mandatory, which by definition occurs outside of annual appropriations; however, programs such as the food stamp program, most child nutrition programs, and the farm commodity price and income support programs ultimately receive funds in the annual appropriations acts (Monke, 2005). These are described briefly below.

Child Nutrition and WIC Reauthorization Act of 2004 (P.L. 108–265) reauthorizes the School Lunch Program, School Breakfast Program, Summer Food Service Program, Child and Adult Care Food Program, and WIC (Special Nutrition Program for Women, Infants, and Children) for five years, through

2009. It contains provisions for nutrition education and promotion including funding that: promotes nutrition in child nutrition programs; expands the types of milk that can be served under the Child Nutrition Act; requires the USDA to issue regulations for increased consumption of foods and food ingredients in accordance with the most recent Dietary Guidelines for Americans; establishes fresh fruit and vegetable programs for children; authorizes grants to support farm-to-cafeteria activities such as school gardens; and directs LEAs to establish a local school wellness policy for schools, and allows for an independent evaluation of the Team Nutrition program. This bill leaves appropriations of funds for several programs (e.g. demonstration projects of fruit and vegetables in schools) up to Congress, meaning these activities may not get funded. Second, the bill directs LEAs to establish, but not implement, wellness policies (House Education and the Workforce Committee, 2004).

The Farm Security and Rural Investment Act of 2002 (Pub. L 107–171) or "Farm Bill". Congress periodically adopts major farm and food legislation in an "omnibus multi-year authorizing law," commonly referred to as the "farm bill" that covers federal farm support, food assistance, agricultural trade, marketing, and rural development policies (Womach, 2005). Farm bills are massive in scope and determine the methods and levels of support that the government provides to agricultural producers. Farm subsidies were originally developed to help small farmers. However, farm subsidy payments are distributed in proportion to past or present sales of the "program commodities," so the largest producers of those commodities reap the largest benefits (International Food and Agricultural Trade Policy Council, September 2005). In 2002, farms in the highest quintile of annual sales ($500,000 dollars or more, in 2002 dollars) received the largest proportion of commodity program payments (MacDonald, Hoppe, & Banker, 2005). One-half of commodity program payments went to farm households with an income higher than $60,580 – the median household income for all U.S. households in 2002 was $42,409.

The evolution of farmer subsidies in America has made corn and other grains abundant and cheap, encouraging the manufacture of mal-nutritious items such as corn sweeteners, corn-fed meat and chicken, and all types of highly processed foods (International Food and Agricultural Trade Policy Council, September 2005; Pollan, 2003; Tillotson, 2004; Womach, 2005). Farm policies instituted in the 1930s had effectively used government price supports in the form of loans to keep cheap grain out of the market (Pollan, 2003; Tillotson, 2004). In the early 1970s, however, the federal government replaced loans with direct payments to farmers, which encouraged farmers to grow as much as possible (Pollan, 2003). The 1996 Farm Bill actually pushed U.S. farm policy closer to "market-orientation," but the 2002 Farm Bill reversed the course, increasing government spending on farm subsidies and alienating the United States from other countries participating in the World Trade Organization (WTO) negotiations (International Food and Agricultural Trade Policy Council, September 2005). The 2007 farm bill will be written within the context of the WTO Doha Development Round of Negotiations, which encourages more open international agricultural markets (International Food and Agricultural Trade Policy Council, September 2005).

The Food Security and Rural Investment Act of 2002 amended the Farm Bill of 2002 and reauthorized the Food Stamp Program (described previously), which has been in existence since 1939. The program reached an estimated

25.8 million persons per month in May of 2005 and expenditures reached an estimated $32 billion for FY2005 (Womach, 2005). Additionally, the *Food Stamp Program* provides matching funding for nutrition education and outreach activities by states.

Department of Transportation Appropriations

The passage in 2005 of the Safe, Accountable, Flexible, Efficient Transportation Equity Act – A Legacy for Users (SAFETEA-LU) (P.L. 109–59) reauthorized federal surface transportation programs through FY 2009, and it also established the Safe Routes to School Program (Fischer, 2005). This program provides grants to state, local, and regional agencies, including nonprofit organizations, that demonstrate an ability to: carry out programs designed to encourage children to walk and bicycle to school; make bicycling and walking a safer and more appealing alternative; and facilitate the planning, development, and implementation of projects and activities. Earlier versions of this transportation appropriation (e.g., The Transportation Equity Act for the 21st Century (TEA-21)) have been useful in initiating local effort through grant programs.

State and Local Governments

The states possess considerable regulatory authority in protecting the "health, safety, morals, and general welfare" of citizens. In fact, courts have upheld the delegation of this regulatory authority (commonly known as "police powers") to state and local governments on the basis of, "first, the Tenth Amendment to the U.S. Constitution, which delegates police power to the states, and, second, state constitutions, which typically delegate police powers to local governments." (Gostin, 2000) The states' police powers to protect the health and welfare of its inhabitants are "inherent aspects of sovereignty," and it is from this authority that, following the Civil War, states began forming boards of health and creating administrative agencies devoted to safeguarding citizens' health (Gostin, 2000).

The nexus of actual programs and activities concerned with combating the obesity epidemic lies loosely within the sometimes interconnected, sometimes disparate network of governmental executive agencies and programs operating and coordinating at state and local levels. Complicating the picture is a relative lack of funds available for direct state- and local-level agency intervention, so it is often federal funds and grant programs that provide the financial resources necessary for various entities involved in obesity prevention (state agencies, local boards of health, nonprofit community organizations, for instance) to "fill the gaps." (Glendening et al., 2005; Health Policy Tracking Service: A Thomson West Business, 2005; *Statement submitted by the National Association of County and City Health Officials: FY2006 Appropriations for the Centers for Disease Control and Prevention*) Regulatory authority is available to state agencies (departments of education, health agencies, LEAs, and School food Authorities (SFAs), in particular) that wish to affect changes in certain environments, so as to induce healthy dietary and physical activity behaviors (Gostin, 2000). The willingness to use such authority often relies on availability of resources and political viability (whether the public and/or legislators back a given initiative). In general, obesity prevention efforts at the state level inevitably involve some combination of legislative and state agency actions, federal assistance, and participation among active and capable local entities.

State Health Costs and State Health Spending

It is important to reiterate the economic consequences that increases in the prevalence of overweight and obesity are having on health care spending. It has been estimated that direct medical costs attributable to adult overweight and obesity have reached $75 billion (in 2003 inflation-adjusted dollars) per year, and state-level expenditures were estimated to range from $87 million per year in Wyoming to $7.7 billion per year in California (Finkelstein, Fiebelkorn, & Wang, 2004; Milbank Memorial Fund, 2005). Further, the public sector finances approximately one-half of obesity-attributable direct medical costs via Medicare and Medicaid (Finkelstein, Fiebelkorn, & Wang, 2003; Finkelstein et al., 2004; Finkelstein, Ruhm, & Kosa, 2005). An independent report analyzing 2002–2003 state health expenditures examined state and federal funds spent on such programs and categories as Medicaid, the State Children's Health Insurance Program (SCHIP), state employees' health benefits, direct public health care, state facility-based services, and population health (Milbank Memorial Fund, 2005). The report concluded that state governments in fiscal year 2003 spent $357.8 billion on health, yet only 5.4 percent of health expenditures was expended on "population health" (e.g. nutrition education, preventive health, food stamps); similarly, "direct public health care" (e.g. health clinics, grants, WIC) accounted for a mere 0.9% of spending, while spending on "infrastructure" (including data analysis and surveillance activities) totaled only $2.5 billion of total state health expenditures (Milbank Memorial Fund, 2005).

A survey examining state and territorial health agencies' expenditures for chronic disease control activities speaks to the need for greater allocation and coordination of both resources and efforts aimed at obesity prevention activities (Chronic Disease Directors, November 2004). The results show that the adjusted per capita expenditures by state health agencies (SHAs) on prevention were $4.18; for every $1 spent on chronic disease prevention, $445 is spent on medical care for chronic diseases, with more than half of chronic disease expenditures by SHAs going to tobacco prevention and control (Chronic Disease Directors, November 2004). While many state budgets are strained, there remains a need for greater resource allocation devoted to obesity prevention efforts (Dunet, Butterfoss, Hamre, & Kuester, 2005).

State Level Authority and Actions

Several states have developed comprehensive and well-coordinated plans in an effort to promote healthy lifestyles and prevent and control the prevalence of overweight and obesity. The obesity prevention strategies that appear to most effectively promote healthy behaviors are those that are informed by a number of governmental entities and community-level interests and organizations (Dunet et al., 2005). Table 7.4 highlights ongoing efforts, at various stages, which have been initiated in several states and may be considered "model" obesity prevention plans. Often, these plans are led by executive agencies or offices that, sometimes in coordination with the legislature, institute obesity prevention

Table 7.4 Examples of coordinated state programs which focus on obesity-related outcomes.

State program	Who's involved?	Actions	Goals
Arkansas, Healthy Arkansas	• Governor's Office • Dept. of Health and Human Services • Dept. of Education • Stamp Out Smoking Program • Eli Lily, Gerber Foods Company	• State employee health promotion programs • Buy-in from worksites and insurance programs • Public health education campaigns • Fiscal and other incentives to be healthier	• Targets for state rates of obesity • Targets for state physical activity levels • Provision of preventive care health services • Healthier state employees
Maine, Healthy Maine Partnerships	• Bureau of Health (BOH) • 3 BOH programs: Partnership For A Tobacco-Free Maine; Maine Cardiovascular Health Program; Community Health Promotion Program • Dept. of Education • 31 local Healthy Maine Partnerships	• Assist schools in developing coordinated school health programs • Training and technical assistance to local Partnerships • Monitor and evaluate all activities of Healthy Maine Partnerships	• Decrease tobacco use • Reduce death, disability, and health care costs due to cardiovascular disease • Empower communities to plan, implement, and evaluate health initiatives on a local basis • Improve nutrition standards & increase physical activity at Maine schools
Missouri, Healthy Missourians Initiative	• Dept. of Health and Senior Services • Schools • Communities • Colleges, universities • Healthcare systems	• Assist schools and child care facilities in improving food choices and access to physical activity • Foster changes in the workplace • Provide incentives for health care systems to promote healthful habits • Develop and support state-level public policies promoting healthy lifestyles	• Increase intake of fruits and vegetables • Increase intake of dairy products • Increase physical activity • Increase breastfeeding • Decrease TV viewing
Texas, AIM for a healthy weight	• Dept. of State Health Services • Colleges, Universities • Community Groups • Schools/School Organizations • Dept. of Agriculture	• Social marketing campaigns • Identify and evaluate existing plans and activities • Increase advocacy for policies supporting healthy lifestyles • Create and implement effective data collection and data management systems	• Increase prevalence of healthy weight Texans • Obtain high levels of physical activity participation and healthful eating • Reduce the burden of weight related disease

initiatives. What follows is a discussion of the agencies, offices, and legislative efforts that are often at the center of or instigators of such initiatives.

State governors often use their positions to alert the public (and, in turn, the legislature) to the importance of adopting healthy lifestyles and assemble (sometimes through legislation) task forces and coalitions charged with adopting and coordinating statewide obesity prevention and control plans. In 2005, five governors talked about nutrition and obesity in their "State of the State" addresses (Health Policy Tracking Service: A Thomson West Business, 2005). Governors also often support their "Councils on Physical Fitness", "Food Policy Councils", and "5-a-Day" Coalitions (or other state groups similar in function) in promoting healthy lifestyles (Fierro, 2005). In short, offices of the Governor may serve as powerful instigating and coordinating agents of statewide obesity prevention plans. An example of this can be seen in the case study previously discussed in Box 7.2.

State Health Agencies (SHAs) are often the lead agency in statewide obesity prevention plans and are crucial entities in efforts aimed at curbing the prevalence of overweight and obesity. In partnership with the CDC, state health departments oversee the federally funded obesity prevention and control programs. SHAs may be a freestanding, independent department or a component of a larger state agency; the trend since the 1960s has been to merge state health departments with other departments, usually social services, mental health, or substance abuse agencies (Gostin, 2000). The head of the SHA is often politically appointed; changing leadership at SHAs coupled with shifting political landscapes may preclude sustained obesity prevention efforts.

SHAs rely on strong surveillance and epidemiological systems to guide intervention development and implementation (Association of State and Territorial Health Officials, 2004). However many SHAs do not have adequate surveillance systems in place. A review conducted by the independent Trust for America's Health in 2005 found that 13 states failed to report adequate surveillance data for childhood overweight rates in federally funded maternal and child health programs while 18 states and the District of Columbia failed to report rates of overweight high school students (Glendening et al., 2005). Nevertheless, SHAs are undertaking substantive efforts in building and implementing obesity prevention programs and activities. The following highlights some relevant SHA activities.

Michigan's Department of Community Health, in partnership with the country's first and only state-level Surgeon General in April 2004 issued "Healthy Michigan 2010: A Health Status Report." As a product of useful surveillance and analysis, the report called on Michigan leaders and residents to focus on prevention in health care, and it served as an effective tool in publicizing increases in the cost of health care resulting from "higher obesity, diabetes, heart disease, and other chronic disease rates" (Michigan Department of Community Health, 2005).

Utah's Department of Health, utilizing funds received from the CDC's Block Grant, and in partnership with the State Office of Education and local health departments, crafted the Gold Medal Initiative (Centers for Disease Control and Prevention, 2005c). The Initiative aims to make policy and environmental changes to encourage elementary schools to adopt a healthy culture by providing more physical activity, and better nutrition and healthier food choices.

Pennsylvania's Department of Health in 2003 began a pilot that has since been expanded state-wide, which requires schools to track Body Mass Index (BMI) measurements of its students (Centers for Disease Control and Prevention, 2005c). This is a practice that has been implemented in Arkansas schools, and it may serve as an invaluable surveillance technique that alerts the public to the magnitude of the obesity epidemic while serving as a performance measurement for other obesity prevention programs and activities.

State Departments of Education are important agents for informing and implementing policies that focus on promoting healthy school environments. Departments of Education often possess regulatory authority over the nutritional content of school meals as well as the authority to mandate certain levels of daily physical activity via physical education classes. Local SFAs that administer federal meals programs to schools by law must adhere to USDA nutritional standards. These standards include requirements for nutrients, and no more than 30% of calories may come from fat. Yet, a 2003 Government Accountability Office (GAO) report demonstrated that fat still accounted for 34% of calories in lunches served under the program in the 1998–1999 school year (United States Government Accountability Office, 2003).

SFAs also have wide discretion in adopting regulations around the competitive school foods. This is due to a 1983 ruling by the District of Columbia Federal Court of Appeals, *National Soft Drink Association v. Block*, which struck down USDA regulations prohibiting the sale of foods of minimal nutritional value anywhere on school grounds until the last lunch period had ended (United States Government Accountability Office, 2005). In a survey of school districts across the country, the GAO reported that 9 out 10 schools offered competitive foods through "one or more of the following venues in 2003–2004: a la carte cafeteria lines, vending machines, and school stores," and that the sale of competitive foods provides schools and school districts with substantial sources of revenue (United States Government Accountability Office, 2005).

In 2005, approximately 200 bills were introduced in 40 states providing some form of nutritional guidance; 24 states introduced 48 bills advocating health education; and 43 states introduced measures that would enhance physical education or activity standards, and 18 of these states adopted such legislation (Health Policy Tracking Service: A Thomson West Business, 2005). There has been state legislation that has either mandated nutritional requirements for or instituted restrictions on competitive foods, or creatively directed state departments of education to phase in nutritional guidelines for competitive foods. Several examples are listed below.

- In 2004, Colorado Senate Bill 04–103 encouraged "school districts work with contractors to increase over time the nutritional value of foods offered to students in school vending machines and to phase in higher nutritional standards as vendor contracts are renewed." The bill sets forth the nutritional guidelines and goes on to direct school districts to adopt a policy providing "that, by the 2006–2007 school year, at least fifty percent of all items offered in each vending machine or adjoining set of vending machines located in each school of the school district shall meet the criteria set forth" in the bill (Health Policy Tracking Service: A Thomson West Business, 2005).
- In 2003, California enacted Senate Bill 677, which stipulates that "the sale of all foods on school grounds shall be approved for compliance with the nutrition standards" set forth within the bill. The bill stipulates rather precise standards (Health Policy Tracking Service: A Thomson West Business, 2005).
- Kentucky's 2005 Senate Bill 172 designates the Kentucky Board of Education as the agency responsible for promulgating "an administrative regulation . . . to specify the minimum nutritional standards for all foods and beverages that are sold outside the National School Lunch programs, whether in vending machines, school stores, canteens, or a la carte sales" (Health Policy Tracking Service: A Thomson West Business, 2005).

Due to increased testing requirements required by the federal No Child Left Behind Law and the penalties imposed for not meeting certain test score standards, many school districts and LEAs have diverted resources away from physical education courses (Jurist: Legal News and Research, 2005). This is despite evidence that demonstrates positive effects of physical activity on academic performance (Department of Education-State of California, 2005; Sibley & Etnier, 2003). More recently, states have considered bills to "recommend" or "allow" a certain number of minutes per day or per week in which school children are to participate in physical activity or physical education, while other bills "require" or "direct" departments of education, LEAs, or school districts to provide a set amount of daily or weekly physical education instruction.

There have been a growing number of state-level legislative initiatives (such as those previously mentioned) aimed at addressing the obesity epidemic. States have introduced many such bills and resolutions: one study estimated that, between 2003 and 2005, over 800 relevant bills and resolutions pertinent to obesity prevention had been introduced, with 17% of bills being passed and 53% of resolutions being passed (Boehmer, Brownson, Haire-Joshu, & Dreisinger, 2007). Initial inquiries on policy development and implementation as it relates to obesity prevention suggest further assessment is needed to determine whether various socio-cultural, economic, and political conditions may facilitate or impede successful introduction and implementation of effective obesity prevention policies (Boehmer et al., 2007; Dietz, Bland, Gormaker, Molloy, & Schmid, 2002). Further, it is becoming clear that more comprehensive policy surveillance is needed to assess the effectiveness of implemented obesity prevention health policies; and such surveillance may also aid in the development of more effective and applicable policies.

State Departments of Transportation or departments engaged in areas of *conservation and natural resources* often possess the authority to develop policies and plans for neighborhoods and communities to support pedestrian-oriented transportation facilities, or preserve parks, trails, and other "open spaces" conducive to physical activity (Active Living National Office). Similarly, state planning agencies or state departments involved in areas of *economic development or commerce* may provide incentives for businesses, civic groups, and other interested entities to develop in communities that support healthy lifestyles among residents (Emerine & Feldman, 2003).

Federal funds are available to state departments of transportation (and any other state, local, or regional agency, including nonprofit organizations) due to the 2005 passage of the SAFETEA-LU reauthorization bill for federal surface transportation programs (Fischer, 2005). The reauthorization bill funded the "Safe Routes to School" program at $612 million for FY2004-FY2009 (see also Chapter 8). Under the program, state agencies and other eligible entities that display an ability to meet the requirements of the program may be apportioned funds. The funds "may be used for planning, design, and construction of infrastructure-related projects that will substantially improve the ability of students to walk and bike to school." Funds may also be used by eligible entities for behavioral activities that promote walking and bicycling to school (Fischer, 2005).

Social Service Agencies, including those administering Medicaid, SCHIP, WIC, and food stamp programs, can implement public health education campaigns and policies that aim to promote healthy lifestyles among beneficiaries.

For instance, Arkansas Medicaid recipients are receiving more preventive care, including reimbursement for sessions with a nutritionist (Bayard, 2005).

State governments are employers and have promoted healthy lifestyles among state employees by providing health benefit plans favorable to healthy lifestyles. For example, preventive care co-payments are being phased-out for Arkansas state employees, and state employee insurance now covers a more expansive range of preventive care. Further, 18,000 Arkansas state employees and 4,000 of their spouses in 2005 received $20 monthly discounts on their 2005 health premiums because they underwent a voluntary health risk assessment (Glendening et al., 2005).

Taxation. Given that dietary and physical activity behaviors cannot be directly regulated by the government, the states' power to tax also has the ability to regulate risk behavior and influence health-promoting activities. Small taxes on various food and beverage products have been found to have little effect on overall consumption. Researchers with the USDA's Food and Rural Economics Division, Economic Research Service, estimated that a nationwide 1% tax on potato chips alone would reduce annual household purchases (average of 156.28 ounces) by 0.71 ounces, equivalent to 0.28 ounces per person per year, or 42 calories per person (Kuchler, Tegene, & Harris, 2004). The revenue-raising potential of even a minimal tax, however, is impressive: the USDA researchers found that national taxes between 1% and 20% on potato chips alone could generate revenue in the range of $27 million to $501 million. The revenue created from such a tax could be directed to programs at federal, state, and local levels aimed at reducing obesity.

There are currently taxes on such products as soft drinks and snack foods in place in many states and municipalities, yet most of these tax revenues are earmarked for general funds, meaning that the funds are not designated for a specific program (Jacobson & Brownell, 2000). Several states currently have taxes on the books that raise substantial revenues. Arkansas taxes $0.21 per gallon of liquid soft drink and $2 per gallon of soft drink syrups, generating about $40.4 million dollars in annual income. There are some other states that have sales taxes on soft drinks and snack foods. California has a 7.25% sales tax on soft drinks that produces an estimated $218 million in annual income for the state, deposited into general funds. Indiana taxes candy, gum, soft drinks, bottled water, and dietary supplements at a rate of 5%; this tax has been estimated to raise $43 million in annual revenue, and this money, too, is designated for general funds (Jacobson & Brownell, 2000). Although not yet documented, it is likely that the most effective approaches will involve taxation with an earmark of funds for obesity prevention efforts, as has been successful in tobacco control (Siegel, 2002).

Local Initiatives

Like state government agencies and legislatures, city councils, local school boards, and county and city health departments often have the ability to initiate, coordinate, and implement obesity prevention plans at the local level. Local entities may also act as implementation agents of state (and federal) policies and programs.

At the level of the school, many local school boards have been active in banning soft drinks. The school systems of New York City, Los Angeles, Philadelphia, and Chicago have banned the sale of soft drinks in all schools within their jurisdictions (Glendening et al., 2005). The ban initiated by Chicago Public Schools also includes certain "junk foods" (defined by fat content) and gum.

The New York City Department of Health and Mental Hygiene has taken proactive steps in combating the obesity epidemic. The health department is partnering with local "convenience" stores in certain areas of the city and promoting the availability of 1% milk (New York City Department of Health and Mental Hygiene, 2006b). "Bodega" owners that have agreed to participate are stocking 1% milk, offering discounts, and distributing health information to customers.

New York City's health department is also initiating educational campaigns and innovative physical activity training (which involves training of close to 500 pre-Kindergarten teachers in the SPARK program (Sport, Play, and Active Recreation for Kids), in an effort to prevent childhood overweight and obesity (Dowda et al., 2005; McKenzie, Sallis, Kolody, & Faucette, 1997; New York City Department of Health and Mental Hygiene, 2006a; Sallis et al., 1997; Sallis et al., 1999). The New York City Department of Health and Mental Hygiene asked city restaurateurs and food suppliers to "voluntarily make an oil change by eliminating partially hydrogenated vegetable oils from the kitchen" (New York City Department of Health and Mental Hygiene, 2006).

Some local health agencies leverage federal funds or become involved in state-led programs. The federal STEPS grant program provides insight into the collaborative efforts taking place at the state and local level. Examples from two *STEPS* programs are noted in Box 7.3.

Box 7.3 Example of STEPS Programs

STEPS to a Healthier Austin Program *Austin, TX,* involves the Austin/Travis County Health and Human Services Department with chambers of commerce, universities, a local housing authority, faith-based organizations and many other parties in an effort to initiate interventions affecting school children, low-income individuals, employers and employees at work sites, among other environments (Steps to a Healthier U.S.). Program actions include:

• removing foods with low-nutritional value from school campuses;
• advocating for daily physical education classes at local schools;
• promoting healthy nutritional choices and physical activity among Austin's city and school district employees;
• implementing a diabetes disease management model at a local community health center (Steps to a Healthier U.S.).

STEPS to a Healthier Philadelphia led by the *Philadelphia Department of Health,* aims to reach racial and ethnic minorities, low-income families, people without health insurance, disabled individuals, and people with limited English proficiency (Steps to a Healthier U.S.). A social marketing campaign is delivered via radio, television, town meetings, and digital broadcasts. Actions include encouraging healthy lifestyles, efforts to implement consistent standards of care for providers in managed care plans treating obesity, diabetes, and asthma, and influencing local restaurants to carry healthy food options (Steps to a Healthier U.S.).

Other interesting activities on the local level include efforts by local governments and city and regional planners that have sought to utilize zoning laws and other legal instruments in encouraging development of "mixed use" communities and neighborhoods facilitating physical activity and community access to healthy foods (Ashe, Jernigan, Kline, & Galaz, 2003; Glendening et al., 2005; Mair, Pierce, & Teret, 2005; Schilling & Linton, 2005).

Local boards of health and health departments can certainly be effective agents in state obesity prevention and control efforts, but, as is the case with all public health officials working in government, there is a need to intensify work with elected officials, especially given the fact that some politically appointed public health officials have a relatively short term in their position. Additionally, past surveys of local boards of health have revealed that most board members are appointed, and a recent survey noted a lack of training, information, or technical assistance available to local boards of health (National Association of Local Boards of Health, 2005).

Summary and Conclusions

Obesity is a health priority requiring broad governmental action. The multiple efforts which have been instituted across all levels of government are positive and an important step forward in addressing this epidemic. However, additional steps now need to be taken to assure government efforts and policies are appropriate, systematically evaluated, and achieve optimal impact. As noted by the Institute of Medicine Report on Prevention of Childhood Obesity, a more coordinated approach is needed which ensures the use of evidence-based methods, requires systematic and rigorous evaluation of initiatives, and ongoing surveillance of impact (Koplan et al., 2004).

Over 300 initiatives sponsored by the federal government address some aspect of obesity (Glendening et al., 2005). This number reflects the recognition of obesity as a high health priority for our population and is an important finding. However, the current structure results in obesity being addressed by policymakers located across numerous departments and agencies within the federal government. As a result, obesity-related interventions can have conflicting missions, objectives, and mandates. These multiple interventions often reflect reactions to pressures brought to bear by the public response to the obesity epidemic, the impact on the population at large, and the federal workforce in particular. While these many initiatives offer some level of incremental change, they do not address obesity from a coordinated or comprehensive approach. In addition, it is unclear that the current initiatives reflect the current evidence base, or undergo systematic evaluation of impact to assure the most effective outcomes.

Coordinated leadership by the federal government is a critical step in prevention of obesity. Evidence-based approaches are needed to guarantee that available funds are used in the most effective and appropriate ways and such approaches are essential in assuring that federal policies impacting food production and distribution, or transportation and activity, are optimal in promoting energy balance behaviors and outcomes. The federal government has an increasing interest in preventing obesity given the rise in obesity-related medical expenditures that impact the health care system, in addition to the effects of widespread obesity on the health status and quality of life of the population. However, there are differing perspectives as to the appropriate federal role in establishing policies that address obesity. One view is that the federal government should have a very limited role since obesity is the ultimate result of lifestyle choices falling within the purview of individual and personal responsibility. This perspective encourages federal policies and programs designed to improve individual awareness and knowledge through education. In contrast, proponents of a more active governmental role point to evidence that obesity causes harm not only to the individual but to the public at large, and is the result of negative health influences across multiple behavioral, environmental, and genetic factors (Brownson et al., 2006; Haire-Joshu & Nanney, 2002; Institute of Medicine & Transportation Research Board, 2005; Koplan et al., 2004; Kumanyika et al., 2002; World Health Organization, 2002). As such, broader actions impacting institutions or environments are needed to prevent risk to the individual. This perspective advocates for comprehensive federal initiatives that regulate food and physical activity environments in schools and communities and also fund state and local programs to combat obesity. Clearly both policy changes and individually-oriented interventions are complementary, especially to enable individual change in low resource communities where environments related to the targeted changes may be particularly adverse or unsupportive. In addition, there is ample precedent for government intervention to facilitate individual behavior change (Gostin, 2000).

States and local governments will also continue to have a major role to play in reducing obesity. States have already attempted to regulate several environments through various legislative, regulatory, and organic efforts that receive funding through varied channels, which speaks to a need for additional and coordinated resources for comprehensive obesity prevention plans. Coordinated efforts are needed to assure evidence based practices are readily shared across state and local communities. Systematic communication guiding state and local governments in implementing the most effective evidence-based intervention and technical assistance needs to be available to facilitate the most effective obesity prevention and control initiatives.

References

Active Living National Office. *Working with government leaders to create and promote active living.* Retrieved December 15, 2005, from http://www.leadershipforactiveliving.org/tools.htm

American Obesity Association. (2006). Retrieved December 21, 2005, from http://www.obesity.org/

Ashe, M., Jernigan, D., Kline, R., & Galaz, R. (2003). Land Use Planning and the Control of Alcohol, Tobacco, Firearms, and Fast Food Restaurants. *American Journal of Public Health, 93*(9), 1404–1408.

Association of State and Territorial Health Officials. (2004). *Issue Report: Increasing Physical Activity Among Youth.* Washington, DC: Association of State and Territorial Health Officials.

Australian Government National Health and Medical Research Council. (1997). Acting on Australia's weight: a strategic plan for the prevention of overweight and obesity.

Bayard, M. (2005). *Issue Brief: State Employee Wellness Initiatives*. Washington, DC: NGA Center for Best Practices.

Blackburn, G., & Walker, W. (2005). Science-based Solutions to Obesity: What are the Roles of Academia, Government, Industry, and Health care? *American Journal of Clinical Nutrition, 82*(1), 207S–210.

Boehmer, T., Brownson, R., Haire-Joshu, D., & Dreisinger, M. (2007). Patterns of childhood obesity prevention legislation in the United States. *Preventing Chronic Disease, 4*(3). [serial online]. Retrieved from http://www.cdc.gov/pcd/issues/2007/jul/06_0082.htm.

Brownson, R., Haire-Joshu, D., & Luke, D. (2006). Shaping the Context of Health: A Review of Environment and Policy Approaches in the Prevention of Chronic Diseases. *Annual Review of Public Health, 27*, 341–370.

Carlisle Fountain, K. (2005). *Political advocacy groups, alphabetic list*. Retrieved December 21, 2005, from http://www.csuchico.edu/~kcfount/about.html

Center for Science in the Public Interest. (2006). Retrieved December 22, 2005, from http://www.cspinet.org/

Centers for Disease Control and Prevention. (2005) *About CDC: Mission*. Retrieved December 21, 2005, from http://www.cdc.gov/about/mission.htm

Centers for Disease Control and Prevention. (2005a) *Coordinated School Health Program*. Retrieved December 21, 2005, from http://www.cdc.gov/HealthyYouth/CSHP/

Centers for Disease Control and Prevention. (2005b) *Division of Nutrition and Physical Activity: Home*. Retrieved December 21, 2005, from http://www.cdc.gov/nccdphp/dnpa

Centers for Disease Control and Prevention. (2005c) *Exemplary State Programs*. Retrieved December 21, 2005, from http://www.cdc.gov/nccdphp/publications/exemplary/

Centers for Disease Control and Prevention. (2005d) *Health Protection Research Initiative*. Retrieved December 21, 2005, from http://www.cdc.gov/about/hpri.htm

Centers for Disease Control and Prevention. (2005e) *Healthy Schools and Healthy Youth*. Retrieved December 21, 2005, from http://www.cdc.gov/HealthyYouth/

Centers for Disease Control and Prevention. (2006) *National Center for Chronic Disease Prevention and Health Promotion: YRBSS: Youth Risk Behavioral Surveillance System*. Retrieved April 24, 2006, from http://www.cdc.gov/HealthyYouth/yrbs/index.htm

Centers for Disease Control and Prevention. (2006a) *National Center for Health Statistics: National Health and Nutrition Examination Survey*. Retrieved April 24, 2006, from http://www.cdc.gov/nchs/nhanes.htm

Centers for Disease Control and Prevention. (2006b) *Pediatric and Pregnancy Nutrition Surveillance System*. Retrieved April 24, 2006, from http://www.cdc.gov/pednss/

Centers for Disease Control and Prevention. (2005f) *Prevention Research Centers: Center Profiles*. Retrieved December 21, 2005, from http://www.cdc.gov/prc/centers/index.htm

Centers for Disease Control and Prevention. (2006c) *SHPPS: School Health Policies and Programs Study*. Retrieved July 24, 2006, from http://www.cdc.gov/HealthyYouth/shpps/index.htm

Centers for Disease Control and Prevention. (2005g). *VERB Youth Campaign*. Retrieved December 21, 2005, from http://www.cdc.gov/youthcampaign/index.htm

Centers for Disease Control and Prevention, & National Center for Chronic Disease Prevention and Health Promotion. (2006). *Behavioral risk factor surveillance system*, from http://www.cdc.gov/brfss/

Chopra M, Galbraith S, & Damton-Hill I. (2002). A global response to a global problem: the epidemic of overnutrition. *Bulletin of the World Health Organization, 80*(12), 952–958.

Chronic Disease Directors. (November 2004). *Chronic Disease Burden and Expenditures in the United States: A Report from State and Territorial Health Agencies*. McLean, VA: Chronic Disease Directors.

Congressional Budget Office. (January 13, 2006). *CBO Report: Unauthorized Appropriations and Expiring Authorizations*. Washington, DC.

Department of Education-State of California. (2005). *A Study of the Relationship between Physical Fitness and Academic Achievement in California Using 2004 Test Results*.

Dietz, W., Bland, M., Gormaker, S., Molloy, M., & Schmid, T. (2002). Policy tools for the childhood obesity epidemic. *J Law Med Ethics, 30*(3 Suppl), 83–87.

Dowda, M., James, F., Sallis, J. F., McKenzie, T. L., Rosengard, P., & Kohl, H. W., 3rd. (2005). Evaluating the sustainability of SPARK physical education: a case study of translating research into practice. *Res Q Exerc Sport, 76*(1), 11–19.

Dunet, D., Butterfoss, F., Hamre, R., & Kuester, S. (2005). Using the state plan index to evaluate the quality of state plans to prevent obesity and other chronic diseases. *Preventing Chronic Disease: Public Health Research, Practice, and Policy, 2*(2), 1–10.

Emerine, D., & Feldman, E. (2003). *Active Living and Social Equity: Creating Healthy Communities for All Residents*. Retrieved December 15, 2005, from http://icma.org/main/topic.asp?tpid=31&hsid=1&t=0

Federal Trade Commission. (July 25, 2007). *Home Page*. Retrieved July 27, 2007, from http://www.ftc.gov/ftc/about.shtm

Fierro, M. (2005). *The Obesity Epidemic - How States Can Trim the "Fat"*. Washington, DC: NGA Center for Best Practices.

Finkelstein, E., Fiebelkorn, I., & Wang, G. (2003). National Medical Spending Attributable to Overweight and Obesity: How Much, And Who's Paying? *Health Affairs*, W3-219.

Finkelstein, E., Fiebelkorn, I., & Wang, G. (2004). State-Level Estimates of Annual Medical Expenditures Attributable to Obesity. *Obesity Research, 12*(1), 18–24.

Finkelstein, E., Ruhm, C., & Kosa, K. (2005). Economic Causes and Consequences of Obesity. *Annual Review of Public Health, 26*(1), 239–257.

Fischer, J. (2005). *Safe, Accountable, Flexible, Efficient Transportation Equity Act: A Legacy for Users (SAFETEA-LU or SAFETEA): Selected Major Provisions*. Retrieved December 21, 2005, from http://digital.library.unt.edu/govdocs/crs/

Fisher, L., Kaiser, F., Oleszek, W., & Rosenberg, M. (2004). *Congressional Oversight Manual*. Retrieved December 13, 2005, from http://digital.library.unt.edu/govdocs/crs/

Foerster, S., Kizer, K., DiSogra, L., Bal, D., Krieg, B., & Bunch, K. (1995). California's 5 a Day-for Better Health! Campaign: An Innovative Population-based Effort to Effect Large-Scale Dietary Change. *American Journal of Preventive Medicine, 2*, 124–131.

French, S., Story, M., & Jeffery, R. (2001). Environmental Influences on Eating and Physical Activity. *Annual Review of Public Health, 22*(1), 309–335.

Glendening, P., Hearne, S., Segal, L., Juliano, C., & Earls, M. (2005). F as In Fat: How Obesity Policies are Failing in America, Trust for America's Health.

Gostin, L. (2000). *Public Health Law: Power, Duty, Restraint*. Berkely, CA: University of California Press.

Haire-Joshu, D., & Nanney, M. (2002). Prevention of Overweight and Obesity in Children: Influences on the Food Environment. *Diabetes Educator, 28*, 415–423.

Havas, S., Heimendinger, J., Reynolds, K., Baranowski, T., Nicklas, T., Bishop, D., et al. (1994). 5 A Day for Better Health: A New Research Initiative. *Journal of American Dietetics Association, 94*(1), 32–36.

Health Policy Tracking Service: A Thomson West Business. (2005). *State Actions to Promote Nutrition, Increase Physical Activity and Prevent Obesity: A Legislative Overview*. Falls Church, VA: NETSCAN iPublishing, Inc.

House Education and the Workforce Committee. (2004). *Child Nutrition and WIC Reauthorization Act*. Retrieved December 17, 2005, from http://www.house.gov/ed_workforce/issues/108th/education/childnutrition/billsummaryfinal.htm

Institute of Medicine. (2003). *Weight management: state of the science and opportunities for military programs*. Retrieved January 11, 2006, from http://www.iom.edu/CMS/3788/6901/14425.aspx

Institute of Medicine. (2005). *WIC Food Packages. Time for A Change*. Washington DC: National Academies Press.

Institute of Medicine, & Transportation Research Board. (2005). *Does the built environment influence physical activity? Examining the evidence*. Retrieved January 7, 2006

Institutes of Medicine. (2006, January 13, 2006). *Nutrition Statndards for Foods in Schools*. Retrieved January 25, 2006, from http://www.iom.edu/CMS/3788/30181.aspx

International Food and Agricultural Trade Policy Council. (September 2005). The U.S. Farm Bill and the Doha Negotiations: On Parallel Tracks or a Collision Course? Issue Brief.

Irwin, P. (2005). *Labor, Health and Human Services, and Education: FY2006 Appropriations*. Retrieved December 16, 2005, from http://digital.library.unt.edu/govdocs/crs/

Jacobson, M., & Brownell, K. (2000). Small taxes on soft drinks and snack foods to promote health. *American Journal of Public Health, 90*, 854–857.

Jurist: Legal News and Research. *NEA, school districts file No Child Left Behind lawsuit*. Retrieved December 15, 2005, from http://jurist.law.pitt.edu/paperchase/2005/04/nea-school-districts-file-no-child.php

Koplan, J., Liverman, C., & Kraak, V. (2004). *Preventing Childhood Obesity: Health in the Balance*: National Academies Press.

Kuchler, F., Tegene, A., & Harris, J. (2004). Taxing snack foods: manipulating diet quality or financing information programs? *Review of Agricultural Economics, 27*(1), 4–20.

Kumanyika, S., Jeffery RW, Morabia A, Ritenbaugh C, & Antipatis VJ. (2002). Obesity prevention: the case for action. *Int J Obes Relat Metab Disord, 3*, 425–436.

MacDonald, J., Hoppe, R., & Banker, D. (2005). Growing Farm Size and the Distribution of Commodity Program Payments. *Amber Waves, 2*, 10–11.

Mair, J., Pierce, M., & Teret, S. (2005). *The City Planner's Guide To The Obesity Epidemic: Zoning and Fast Food*: The Center for Law and the Public's Health at Johns Hopkins & Georgetown Universities.

McKenzie, T. L., Sallis, J. F., Kolody, B., & Faucette, F. N. (1997). Long-term effects of a physical education curriculum and staff development program: SPARK. *Res Q Exerc Sport, 68*(4), 280–291.

Michigan Department of Community Health. *Michigan Surgeon General's Health Status Report: Healthy Michigan 2010*. Retrieved January 4, 2006, from http://www.michigan.gov/mdch/0,1607,7-132—90327—,00.html

Milbank Memorial Fund. (2005). *2002-2003 State Health Expenditure Report*. New York: Milbank Memorial Fund, National Association of State Budget Officers, Reforming States Group.

Monke, J. (2005). *Agriculture and Related Agencies: FY2006 Appropriations*. Retrieved December 22, 2005, from http://digital.library.unt.edu/govdocs/crs/

Moshfegh, A. J. (1994). The National Nutrition Monitoring and Related Research Program: progress and activities. *J Nutr, 124*(9 Suppl), 1843S-1845S.

National Association of Local Boards of Health. *About Local Boards of Health*. Retrieved December 15, 2005, from http://www.nalboh.org/publications

National Cancer Institute. (March 1, 2006). *5 A Day to Better Health Program Evaluation Report*. Retrieved July 27, 2007, from http://www.cancercontrol.cancer.gov/5ad_1_intro.html

National Heart Lung and Blood Institute, National Institute of Diabetes and Digestive and Kidney Disease, National Institute of Child Health and Human Development, & National Cancer Institute. (2006). *Ways to enhance children's activity and nutrition*. Retrieved December 20, 2005, from http://www.nhlbi.nih.gov/health/public/heart/obesity/wecan/

National Institutes of Health. (2005). *Home Page for NIH Institutes*. Retrieved December 15, 2005, from http://www.nih.gov/

National Institutes of Health Obesity Research Task Force. (2004). *Strategic Plan for NIH Obesity Research*. Retrieved December 15, 2005, from http://www.obesityresearch.nih.gov/About/strategic-plan.htm

New York City Department of Health and Mental Hygiene. (2006) *Health Department Asks Restaurateurs and Food Suppliers to Voluntarily Make an Oil Change and Eliminate Artificial Trans Fat*. Retrieved January 25, 2006, from http://www.nyc.gov/html/doh/html/home/home.shtml

New York City Department of Health and Mental Hygiene. (2006a) *Health Department Launches New Initiatives to Prevent Childhood Obesity*. Retrieved January 17, 2006, from http://www.nyc.gov/html/doh/html/home/home.shtml

New York City Department of Health and Mental Hygiene. (2006b). *Mooove to 1% milk project*. Retrieved January 17, 2006, from http://www.nyc.gov/html/doh/html/home/home.shtml

Office of Disease Prevention and Health Promotion. (March 28, 2007). *In the Office of Public Health and Science*. Retrieved July 27, 2007, from http://odphp.osophs.dhhs.gov

Office of Personnel Management. *Healthier Feds Campaign*. Retrieved December 15, 2005, from http://www.opm.gov/healthierfeds/

Oliver, T. (2006). The Politics of Public Health Policy. *Annual Review of Public Health, 27*(21), 1–21.39.

Pollan, M. (2003, October 12). The (Agri)Cultural Contradictions of Obesity. *The New York Times Magazine*.

Popkin, B. M., & Gordon-Larsen, P. (2004). The nutrition transition: worldwide obesity dynamics and their determinants. *Int J Obes Relat Metab Disord, 28 Suppl 3*, S2-9.

Report of a World Health Organzation consultation. (2000). *Obesity: preventing and managing the global epidemic*.

Sachs, R. (2000). *Hearings in the House of Representatives: A Guide for Preparation and Procedure*. Retrieved December 15, 2005, from http://digital.library.unt.edu/govdocs/crs/

Sachs, R. (2003). *Hearings in the U.S. Senate: A Guide for Preparation and Procedure*. Retrieved December 16, 2005, from http://digital.library.unt.edu/govdocs/crs/

Sallis, J. F., McKenzie, T. L., Alcaraz, J. E., Kolody, B., Faucette, N., & Hovell, M. F. (1997). The effects of a 2-year physical education program (SPARK) on physical activity and fitness in elementary school students. Sports, Play and Active Recreation for Kids. *Am J Public Health, 87*(8), 1328–1334.

Sallis, J. F., McKenzie, T. L., Kolody, B., Lewis, M., Marshall, S., & Rosengard, P. (1999). Effects of health-related physical education on academic achievement: project SPARK. *Res Q Exerc Sport, 70*(2), 127–134.

Schilling, J., & Linton, L. (2005). The Public Health Roots of Zoning: In Search of Active Living's Legal Genealogy. *American Journal of Preventive Medicine, 28*(2, Supplement 2), 96.

Sibley, B., & Etnier, J. (2003). The relationship between physical activity and cognition in children: a meta-analysis. *Pediatric Exercise Science, 15*, 243–256.

Siegel, M. (2002). The effectiveness of state-level tobacco control interventions: a review of program implementation and behavioral outcomes. *Annual Review of Public Health, 23,* 45–71.

Spar, K., & Laney, G. (2005). *Community Services Block Grants (CSBG): Funding and Reauthorization.* Retrieved December 21, 2005, from http://digital.library.unt.edu/govdocs/crs/

Statement by William H. Dietz: CDC's Role in Combating the Obesity Epidemic, United States Senate, 107 Sess. (2002).

Statement submitted by the National Association of County and City Health Officials: FY2006 Appropriations for the Centers for Disease Control and Prevention, United States Senate.

Steps to a Healthier US. (2004). *Steps to a Healthier Philadelphia.* Retrieved January 22, 2006, from http://www.healthierus.gov/steps/grantees/2004/philadelphia.html

Steps to a Healthier U.S.. *Steps to a Healthier Austin.* Retrieved January 22, 2006, from http://www.healthierus.gov/steps/grantees/austin.html

Streeter, S. (2004). *The congressional appropriations process: an introduction.* Retrieved January 9, 2006, from http://digital.library.unt.edu/govdocs/crs/

Sweden National Board of Health. (2001). National action plan against obesity, recommendations and perspectives.

The Henry J. Kaiser Family Foundation. (2006). Retrieved January 5, 2006, from http://www.kff.org/

Tillotson, J. (2003). Pandemic Obesity: Conflicted Policy Consequences. *Nutrition Today, 38,* 116–119.

Tillotson, J. (2004). America's Obesity: Conflicting Public Policies, Industrial Economic Development, and Unintended Human Consequences. *Annual Review of Nutrition, 24*(1), 617–643.

U. S. Department of Health and Human Services, & U. S. Department of Agriculture. (May 25, 2005). *Dietary Guidelines for Americans 2005.* Retrieved April 24, 2006, from http://www.health.gov/dietaryguidelines/dga2005/document/html/chapter1.htm

U.S. Department of Agriculture. (2005) *Center for Nutrition Policy and Promotion Home Page.* Retrieved December 16, 2005, from http://www.usda.gov/cnpp/index.html

U.S. Department of Agriculture. (2005a) *Food and Nutrition Service Food Stamp Program.* Retrieved December 10, 2005, from http://www.fns.usda.gov/fsp/faqs.htm#1

U.S. Department of Agriculture. (2005b) *National School Lunch Program Fact Sheet.* Retrieved December 20, 2005, from http://www.fns.usda.gov/cnd/lunch/

U.S. Department of Agriculture. (2002). *Food and Nutrition Service, WIC Participants and Program Characteristics 2000* (No. WIC 02-PC). Alexandria, VA: U.S. Department of Agriculture.

U.S. Department of Defense. (2006) *Department of the Army.* Retrieved January 11, 2006, from http://web.usf.edu/~usfarotc/docs/links/AR600-9.pdf.

U.S. Department of Defense. (2006a) *Navy Environmental Health Center.* Retrieved January 11, 2006, from http://www-nehc.med.navy.mil/hp/shipshape/About_WM/Weight_Management.htm

U.S. Department of Education. *Carol M. White Physical Education Program.* Retrieved December 15, 2005, from http://www.ed.gov/programs/whitephysed/index.html

U.S. Department of Health and Human Services. (2005) Retrieved December 21, 2005, from http://www.hhs.gov/

U.S. Department of Health and Human Services. (2005a) *Administration on Aging.* Retrieved December 12, 2005, from http://www.aoa.gov/youcan/youcan.asp

U.S. Department of Health and Human Services. (2005b) *Centers for Medicare and Medicaid Services.* Retrieved December 12, 2005, from http://www.cms.hhs.gov/

U.S. Department of Health and Human Services. (2005c) *Food and Drug Administration.* Retrieved December 21, 2005, from http://www.fda.gov/

U.S. Department of Health and Human Services. (2005d). *Health Resources and Services Administration.* Retrieved December 18, 2005, from http://www.hrsa.gov

U.S. Department of Health and Human Services. (2005e) *Indian Health Service.* Retrieved December 18, 2005, from http://www.ihs.gov/

U.S. Department of Health and Human Services. (2005f). *Office of Minority Health Resource Center.* Retrieved December 20, 2005, from http://www.omhrc.gov/omhrc

U.S. Department of Health and Human Services. (2005g). *Steps to a healthier U.S. initiative.* Retrieved December 20, 2005, from http://www.healthierus.gov/steps/index.html

U.S. Department of Health and Human Services. (2005h). *The President's council on physical fitness and sports.* Retrieved December 20, 2005, from http://www.fitness.gov/

U.S. Department of Health and Human Services, Public Health Service, & Office of the Surgeon General. (2001). *The Surgeon General's Call to Action.* Washington, DC: U.S. Government Printing Office.

U.S. Department of the Interior. *Designation of Pathways to Health.* Retrieved December 15, 2005, from http://www.doi.gov/news/020531.html

U.S. Department of Transportation-Federal Highway Administration. *Safe Routes to Schools Program.* Retrieved December 21, 2005, from http://safety.fhwa.dot.gov/saferoutes/

U.S. Department of Veterans Affairs. *The MOVE weight management program.* Retrieved December 21, 2005, from http://www.va.gov/

United States Government Accountability Office. (2003). *Report to Congressional Requesters, School Lunch Program: Efforts Needed to Improve Nutrition and ncourage Health Eating* (No. 03-506). Washington, DC: Government ccountability Office.

United States Government Accountability Office. (2005). *Report to Congressional Requesters, School Meal Programs: Competitive Foods Are Widely Available and Generate Substantial Revenues for Schools* (No. 04-673). Washington, DC: U.S. Government Accountability Office.

United States Government Accountability Office (Office of the General Counsel). (January 2004). *Principles of Federal Appropriations Law, Volume I (Third Edition).* Washington, DC: U.S. Government Accountability Office.

University of Baltimore Obesity Initiative. (2006). Retrieved February 17, 2006, from http://www.ubalt.edu/experts/obesity/initiative.html

U.S. Food and Drug Administration. *Report of the Working Group on Obesity.* Retrieved December 15, 2005, from http://www.cfsan.fda.gov/~dms/owg-toc.html#trans

USDA Food and Nutrition Service. (2006). *Team Nutrition.* Retrieved December 16, 2005, from http://www.fns.usda.gov/tn/

Womach, J. (2005). *Previewing a 2007 Farm Bill.* Retrieved December 22, 2005, from http://digital.library.unt.edu/govdocs/crs/

World Health Organization. (2002). *Global strategy on diet, physical activity, and health.* Retrieved December 10, 2005, from http://www.who.int/dietphysicalactivity/en/

Chapter 8

Planning and the Built Environment: Implications for Obesity Prevention

Susan Handy and Kelly Clifton

Introduction

The built environment – the physical form of our communities – plays an important role in the obesity epidemic (Frank et al. 2003; Institute of Medicine 2005). An understanding of the built environment and ways of influencing it has, therefore, become essential for any one interested in furthering environments conducive to obesity prevention. The built environment consists of two essential elements: land use patterns, the location of activities across space; and the transportation system, the facilities and services that link one location to another. These elements together determine access to opportunities for physical activity and healthy eating. Access to opportunities, in turn, influences physical activity and nutrition behavior, with implications for obesity. It is increasingly clear that the built environment that predominates in most U.S. cities provides limited opportunities for physical activity and easy access to less healthful food choices, and it is increasingly clear that this situation is contributing to caloric imbalances for many. Indeed, recent studies show a link between suburban sprawl and obesity (Ewing et al. 2003; Lopez 2004), between mix of land uses and obesity (Frank et al. 2004), between access to fast food outlets and obesity (Maddock 2004), and between overweight and absence of community infrastructure for both physical activity and healthy eating (Catlin et al. 2003). In the socio-ecological model of behavior (described in Chapter 13), widely applied in the health community, the built environment is a part of the community level of influence on health (McLeroy et al. 1988; Sallis et al. 2006).

The goal of this chapter is to provide readers with a brief introduction to land use and transportation planning. Although traditional approaches to planning have contributed to the obesity problem, perhaps to the greatest degree in low-income areas, new approaches in both domains open up important opportunities for obesity prevention. Several larger efforts that integrate transportation and land use planning with both planning and public health perspectives offer substantial promise for obesity prevention efforts. The chapter ends with an overview of the ways in which a concern for obesity prevention can be inserted into these planning processes.

Rationale

If the built environment contributes to obesity, then reshaping the built environment is potentially an important intervention in efforts to prevent obesity. The built environment is shaped through the land use planning and the transportation planning processes. In very broad terms, land use planning helps determine the location, intensity and type of development in an urban area. The transportation planning process influences the provision of infrastructure and services that link these urban activities. Together, these two planning domains can act to create communities that support physical activity by increasing access to places where physical activity occurs such as parks, green space, trails and recreation centers, or by providing the opportunity for active travel, such as walking and bicycling, as well as public transit services that are accessed by these non-motorized modes. Urban planning may also impact health outcomes by influencing the nature of access to food resources (James et al. 1997; Sharpe 1999). If obesity concerns are incorporated into land use and transportation planning processes, the outcome can be an environment that fosters healthful eating and physical activity behaviors and supports lifestyle choices conducive to obesity prevention.

Although one affects the other, land use and transportation planning processes as they are structured in the United States are largely separate, with different agencies responsible for each and with power concentrated at different levels of government. The coordination of land use and transportation planning has been hampered by the "bottom up" and "top down" approaches of the respective domains. Local governments and private developers are primarily responsible for land use planning decisions; the role of the federal government tends to be limited to regulations focused on environmental protection; and states fall somewhere in between, exerting their influence in the areas of growth management, environmental regulation and conservation, and regulation of the planning process. Conversely, the transportation planning agenda and processes are set largely by the federal government through requirements tied to federal transportation funding, but with much responsibility for specific decisions delegated to state and regional agencies. Recent efforts to improve coordination between land use and transportation planning are helping to overcome this separation and are also improving the outlook for creating healthy environments.

Local Land Use Planning

How it Works and Who Does What

In the United States, the power to regulate land use resides with state governments and derives from the more general power of a government entity to "restrict private activity in order to achieve a broad public benefit" (Fulton 1999). Most states have delegated this power to local governments – cities, counties, and, in some states, townships or other local entities. As a condition of applying this power, however, most states also impose certain requirements on local governments with respect to land use planning. The requirements vary from state to state, with some states retaining more of a role in land use planning than others. In most places, decisions about land use are made at the local

Table 8.1 Local land use planning tools.

	Purpose	Responsibility	Implications for obesity
Comprehensive Plan	Long-range vision for the community and strategies for achieving vision	Planning Department – Long-Range Planning Section	Determines priority given to health concerns in planning efforts
Land Development Code	Legal regulations that implement the comprehensive plan; includes zoning and subdivision ordinances	Planning Department – Development Review Section	Determines distance to destinations, access to food retailers, layout of street network, availability of bicycle and pedestrian infrastructure in new developments
Capital Improvement Program	Program of public infrastructure projects scheduled for next few years	Public Works Department	Determines improvements in bicycle and pedestrian infrastructure and in parks and playgrounds, mostly in existing areas

level through a process dictated by the state. In this section, we describe the traditional approach to land use planning for cities while recognizing that exceptions to this approach are abundant.

In most cities, land use planning consists of three key elements: the comprehensive plan, the land development code, and the capital improvement program (CIP) (Table 8.1). The comprehensive plan provides a long-term vision for the community and outlines strategies for achieving that vision. The land use map is usually a central part of the comprehensive plan: it shows what kinds of land uses are to be located where in the city in the future. The comprehensive plan is implemented through the land development code, which regulates private activities, and the capital improvement program, which dictates public investments. The land development code encompasses the zoning ordinance and the subdivision ordinance. The zoning ordinance specifies what land uses are allowed on each parcel of land within the city and sets restrictions on the size of buildings and their location on the parcel. The subdivision ordinance guides the process by which large parcels (usually at least five acres but ranging up to hundreds of acres) are divided into smaller lots; it usually includes requirements with respect to street layout and design, such as the provision of sidewalks, and may include requirements for parks and other green space. In its CIP a city specifies the public infrastructure projects it will build within the next few years; the CIP includes such things as sidewalk improvements, bicycle facilities, parks and playgrounds.

Different players have responsibility for different parts of the planning process. City planning departments are traditionally split between development review and long-range planning. The staff of the development review section is responsible for ensuring the consistency of development proposals by private land owners with the land development code and the comprehensive plan. In the long-range planning section, the staff is responsible for initially developing and updating the comprehensive plan and often undertakes special studies for particular areas within the city or to address particular problems. The planning commission, whose members are appointed by the city council, makes discretionary decisions about the application of policy, for example, by granting exceptions to the zoning ordinance. The city council, the elected legislature for the city, has responsibility for legislative acts, including the adoption of the comprehensive plan and amendments to the zoning ordinance. The public has an opportunity to participate in these activities through meetings, hearings and other processes designed to elicit pubic input.

Other local agencies also play important roles in land use planning. Many cities have created redevelopment agencies to plan and carry out the rebuilding of blighted and economically depressed areas of the city. Although the rules that guide these agencies vary from state to state, they generally have the power to assemble land through eminent domain (the power of government to purchase private land for public good without the consent of the land owner) and to apply a variety of public financing techniques to fund investments, infrastructure and other improvements. With these tools, they facilitate private real estate investments in the targeted areas and may fund public improvements to infrastructure (e.g. sidewalks, parks, lighting) that help to attract private investments (Fulton 1999). These agencies are created by cities, and the cities retain some control over their activities, for example, through the appointment of agency board members by the city council. In many cities, special districts also have an important influence over land use. School districts and park districts, for example, control the location and design of these public facilities. Though autonomous, they often work in cooperation with the city planning department.

Although not public agencies, community development corporations (CDCs) play an important role in the implementation of land use plans, particularly in the realm of economic development and housing production in distressed areas and low- to moderate-income neighborhoods. These non-profit organizations, funded through a combination of government grants, private companies, foundations, and other sources, are initiated by the community itself and are characterized by community-based leadership that includes local residents, business owners, community leaders, and other stakeholders. Occupying a gap normally filled by private developers, CDCs often compete for public funding opportunities to attract needed businesses to low-income communities, develop affordable housing, or provide education and skills opportunities to residents. As of the mid-1990s, an estimated 2,200 CDCs nationwide worked to improve physical, social, and economic conditions in low-income areas (Cowan et al. 1999).

Over its history, local planning has grown to encompass more than just land use planning. A typical comprehensive plan, for example, will include a land use element but also address environmental and economic concerns. In California, the state requires cities to include elements for land use, circulation (i.e. transportation), housing, conservation, open-space, noise, and safety (California 2003); cities often choose to include optional elements for public facilities, design, parks and recreation, and air quality, among others (Fulton 1999). Through the comprehensive plan, planning for the local transportation system (local streets as well as bicycle and pedestrian facilities) thus often occurs in conjunction with land use planning; planning for regional transportation system (highways, freeways, transit systems) takes place through a separate process, described below.

It is no accident that public health concerns are explicitly addressed in most comprehensive plans. The "broad public benefit" that first justified planning efforts in the early decades of the 20th century was health. The earliest zoning ordinances aimed to improve conditions for residents of crowded, polluted cities by keeping industrial activities away from residential areas. Before long, however, the legal rationale for zoning evolved to emphasize protection of property rights and residential neighborhoods rather than health (Schilling and Linton 2005). The concern over property values led to even greater separation of uses: stores, offices, and other non-industrial uses were also kept away from residential areas through zoning. More generally, the nascent planning profession actively encouraged suburban development as a way to avoid infectious diseases easily spread in urban environments. No one foresaw that suburban development could play a role in an epidemic of chronic disease by the end of the 20th century. As a result, common land use planning practices inadvertently contributed to increased rates of obesity by limiting opportunities for physical activity and healthy eating.

Today's comprehensive plans still address general health concerns but are not usually focused directly on issues surrounding obesity. Comprehensive plan elements commonly address noise, safety, and air quality, which have direct implications for human health. In the broadest sense, these plans aim to improve quality of life in the community, a goal that surely encompasses health. However, this does not mean that planning decisions are always in the best interests of health: other goals (particularly economic ones) may take precedence, indirect health implications may not be considered, and difficult trade-offs may be ignored. The growing concern over obesity is providing additional impetus for changes in the planning process.

Implications for Obesity of Traditional Approach

The traditional approach to zoning ensures the separation of land uses. Within defined zoning districts, a limited range of land uses is allowed. In general, residential areas are segregated from commercial and industrial areas. More specific classifications restrict what kinds of residential or commercial or industrial activities are found in each area. For example, most cities have a zoning designation in which only detached single-family homes are allowed, one to a lot. Newer areas built under these rules have a greater separation of land uses than older areas built before more restrictive zoning ordinances. While some separation can be justified on health grounds (e.g. locating factories away from schools and homes), the degree of separation built into zoning codes in the United States is probably much greater than it needs to be, with negative implications for health. The greater the separation of land uses, the greater the distances between home and destinations such as school, the grocery store, the post office. The greater the distances to such destinations, the less likely it is that residents will choose to walk or bike. Less walking and biking mean less physical activity and more time in the car.

Because of less restrictive zoning and in part because lower income areas tend to be located in older and more central parts of cities, land uses tend to be less separated in lower income than in higher income areas. This puts residents within closer distance of possible destinations, making walking and transit more of an option. But residents of these areas still have fewer options when it comes to healthy food (Morland et al. 2002; Project for Public Spaces 2003; Flournoy and Treuhaft 2005). One factor is their more limited access to a car, which makes them dependent on stores within close proximity to home. Another factor is market forces that determine the kinds of stores operating in these areas. In the past 30 years, the supermarket industry has become increasingly more centralized; the total number of food stores has declined while at the same time the average store size has increased steadily (Dunkely et al. 2004). The new larger stores have disproportionately been sited in suburban areas, while existing stores in poor urban areas closed or were sold. The result is an urban grocery store gap: low income areas have smaller, higher priced groceries or convenience stores that do not have the same choice of quality, price and selection as found in more suburban supermarkets (Chung and Myers, 1999; Gottlieb et al., 1996; SFC, 1995) or in upper-income urban areas (Horowitz et al. 2004). As a result, low-income neighborhoods tend to have a dearth of healthy food options, such as access to supermarkets that carry good quality fresh produce.

On the other hand, less restrictive zoning in low-income areas may have contributed to an abundance of unhealthy food options, particularly fast food (Block et al. 2004; Morland et al. 2002). Although fast food restaurants aren't usually labeled undesirable as a land use, living close to such restaurants may be undesirable from the standpoint of obesity prevention if fast food restaurants encourage over-consumption of large quantities of high calorie foods and beverages. More affluent neighborhoods tend to restrict the number and location of these outlets through the formal land use planning process, often citing concerns that the design of these establishments does not fit with the character of the neighborhood and raising concerns about the additional automobile traffic generated. The abundance of fast food restaurants affects other vulnerable populations as well. A recent study shows that fast food restaurants tend to locate around schools, targeting their products to children and adolescents (Austin et al. 2005); as long as the zoning code allows fast food establishments in these areas, there is little to stop them.

The problem of land use separation is often compounded by the layout and design of the local street network. In their land development code, cities have traditionally adopted the concept of a street hierarchy, in which streets are distinguished by the degree to which they serve access or movement functions (ASCE et al. 1990). At one end of the hierarchy are freeways, which provide for movement, with limited access; at the other are cul-de-sacs, which provide access to the houses but do not allow for through traffic. This concept underlies the design of residential subdivisions dominated by cul-de-sacs. Although this approach means lower levels of traffic within neighborhoods, it also makes for convoluted routes through neighborhoods for drivers as well as pedestrians and bicyclists. Standards for street design have also been problematic. For decades, residential streets have been built at wider widths than are necessary to accommodate the low volume of cars using these streets (Southworth and Ben-Joseph 1997). Not only does this practice increase the extent of asphalt within a neighborhood, it increases the tendency for drivers to speed. Both of these effects reduce the quality of the walking environment and discourage active travel.

New Approaches with Benefits for Obesity

Cities throughout the United States are increasingly recognizing the negative implications of traditional approaches to land use planning. They are using new approaches to increase the viability of active travel in new developments as well as existing areas, and adopting strategies to improve access to healthy food in low-income areas.

Active Travel

Cities throughout the United States are changing the ordinances that guide the layout and design of new developments. Many cities have designated mixed-use zoning districts, in which residential, commercial, and other uses are allowed or even required. In some mixed-use districts, retail is required on the ground floor of multi-story buildings, with office and residential uses allowed on upper floors. Land use mixing may also occur on a building-to-building basis, for example, where single-family homes sit next to small stores or offices. In these areas, residents are in close proximity to places to work, shop, and recreate, and the potential for walking and biking is greater (Smart Growth Network 2005). A more dramatic approach is to replace the traditional zoning ordinance with a form-based code. A relatively new innovation, form-based codes focus on the form of buildings rather than the uses to which they are put (LGC 2005): building heights and facades, the relation of the building to the street, the location of parking. These codes emphasize the appearance of the street setting and other public spaces. Where adopted, these codes have encouraged a greater mixing of housing types and a greater mixing of residential and commercial uses.

Cities are also using their land development codes to better accommodate active travel. A growing number of cities have adopted ordinances designed to increase street connectivity, often defined in terms of the density of intersections in the street network (Handy et al. 2003). Although the primary aim of these ordinances is to spread vehicle traffic more evenly through the network, the potential benefits for other modes have also been recognized. In a street network with high connectivity, routes from one point to another are more direct, making walking and biking more feasible. Also, more intersections mean smaller blocks; smaller blocks generally mean more human scale development and less auto oriented development. Cities can also ensure adequate infrastructure for active travel through more aggressive application of their land development code. For example, as a condition of subdivision approval, cities can require developers to provide amenities such as sidewalks, bus stops, recreational trails, parks, and sites for schools. These "exactions" are important in building a local infrastructure conducive to active travel and other forms of physical activity.

For existing communities, the challenges are greater. According to one estimate, half of the buildings used by Americans in 2030 will have been built after 2000, meaning that more than half are already on the ground as of this writing (Nelson 2004). Land use plans that seek to retain the character of the traditional mixed-use development pattern can help to facilitate the retention of existing businesses or attract new ones to targeted locations. Many communities have programs that are specific to these older areas. For example, Main Street programs aim to revitalize older commercial corridors or neighborhood centers (e.g. Metro 1996). Infill development and redevelopment programs provide incentives for developers to use parcels within an existing urban area and can help with the adaptation of older buildings for new uses, such as urban lofts, office space, or shopping centers. Designation of selected areas as historic districts helps to protect the neighborhood character through design controls, architectural review, and limits on the nature and scale of development. In suburban areas, older strip malls have been rebuilt as mixed-use projects, with retail, office, and residential on one site, an approach called "grayfield" redevelopment. Each of these programs aims to retain or attract work, shopping, and leisure activities in or near residential areas and foster attractive and interesting environments, thereby supporting active travel.

Traffic calming programs, usually run by city public works departments, seek to address problems with road design in existing developments. These programs attempt to slow down or discourage automobile traffic and thus make streets safer and more attractive for pedestrians and others. Traffic calming techniques emphasize the physical design of streets and their surroundings, including widening sidewalks, narrowing the width of streets at pedestrian crossings, adding landscaping, adding measures to slow vehicles such as speed bumps, altering road alignments, adding traffic circles, or installing pavement treatments. The concept of traffic calming emerged in Europe several decades ago and has been widely adopted by cities across the United States. In some communities, however, traffic calming measures have raised concerns about response time for emergency vehicles. As a result, public works departments often work together with emergency service providers in designing and implementing these programs.

Restoring the ability of children to walk or bike to school has been the focus of two different types of efforts around the country. Safe routes to schools or SR2S programs aim to increase walking and biking to existing schools through education and promotion, enforcement of traffic laws, and improvements to the physical environment that increase safety. In 2000, the California Department of Transportation launched its Safe Routes to School program, which provides $20 to $25 million each year in grants to local communities for improvements to sidewalks, traffic calming and speed reduction, improvements to crossings, and bicycle lanes. An evaluation of this program showed increases in the number of children walking and bicycling at five out of the ten schools studied (Boarnet et al. 2005). Another type of effort takes on school siting policies and aims to ensure that new schools are located in close proximity to residential areas, such that students will have the option to walk or bike. In many places, the policies of state boards of education, local school boards, and local governments combine to favor new schools located on large tracts of land at the edge of newly developing areas at the same time that they encourage the abandonment of smaller neighborhood schools in older parts of the community (NTHP no date). The U.S. Environmental Protection Agency (EPA), the National Trust for Historic Preservation, and many other national organizations are encouraging a rethinking of school siting policies.

Food Access

Some cities have attempted to address the problem of "food deserts" and the prevalence of unhealthy consumer goods in low-income neighborhoods through land use planning tools, although more direct approaches are often needed.

Incentives such as tax breaks and streamlined processes for obtaining permits help to direct supermarkets to locate in urban neighborhoods, and some cities have worked directly with existing food stores to provide better food. Most successful examples involve the leadership of non-governmental organizations, however. The non-profit New Community Corporation garnered much praise for its success in bringing a Pathmark supermarket to Newark, NJ in 1989. The Pennsylvania Fresh Food Financing Initiative, supported with state and private funding, is working to improve access to fresh foods in low-income neighborhoods by providing grants and loans to owners of food stores in these areas (The Reinvestment Fund 2003).

Other efforts focus on access to fresh produce through farmers markets and community gardens. The Sustainable Food Center in Austin, TX, for example, has established several community gardens in low-income areas (SFC 2002). Farmers markets have grown increasingly popular in recent years, expanding in numbers 111% from 1994 to 2004 (USDA 2004). Public markets have potential to increase the supply of healthy food in low-income neighborhoods and have been linked with larger efforts to revitalize communities (PPS 2003; Spitzer and Baum 1995). Planners can play a direct role in facilitating the establishment of markets by securing locations that are visible, accessible and attractive to the public.

Some observers have argued for limiting fast food restaurants, liquor stores, and other retailers of unhealthy food products by zoning them out of selected areas, limiting the number of stores permitted in a neighborhood, or requiring a special permit process for these establishments (Ashe et al. 2003, Mair et al. 2005). This strategy could be especially important in low-income areas, where these kinds of establishments are the most accessible source of food, though it has not been widely applied so far. But this strategy can also have the unintended consequence of further hindering access to retail and services for low-income residents with limited access to cars. The City of Baltimore, for example, had designated corner stores and other neighborhood retail as "non-conforming" land uses according to the zoning code in an attempt to reduce their numbers but is now re-evaluating this approach. The city's efforts now center on preserving the local business establishments that are compatible with the needs of local residents.

On a larger scale, food systems planning, which considers the production, distribution, and retailing of food, offers potential for improving food access in low income area and intersects with several domains of planning, including transportation, land use, environment, and economic development (Pothukuchi and Kaufman 2000). Although regulating the price and quality of food items sold is largely out of the direct control of city planners, they can help to improve the food environment by influencing the siting of food retailers and public markets and the transportation systems that connect both suppliers and customers to these markets. In addition, several federal and state initiatives act to protect and preserve the agricultural land used for farming and food production, which in turn support efforts to promote sustainable and healthy, local food supply (Holtzman 2002, Collins 1976). Agricultural preservation programs can also provide tax benefits and incentives to help farming remain a viable economic activity. The Maryland Agricultural Land Preservation Foundation (MALPF), one of the oldest farmland protection programs in the country, was established in 1977 in part to provide sources of agricultural products within the state for the citizens of the state. Such programs also help to control low density expansion of urban areas and thus complement efforts to create higher density, mixed-used areas conducive to walking.

Regional Transportation Planning

How it Works and Who Does What

Although the federal government leaves land use planning to the states, it plays a strong role in transportation planning by dictating the kinds of projects on which federal funds can be spent and the process by which specific projects are selected (Table 8.2). Since the 1960s, federal transportation authorization bills have specified funding categories as well as requirements for state and regional transportation planning. A turning point in transportation planning came in 1991 when Congress passed the Intermodal Surface Transportation Efficiency Act (ISTEA). This act represented a significant shift in federal policy, with more flexibility to spend funds on projects other than highways and giving more power to regional agencies. The most recent federal transportation bill, the Safe, Accountable, Flexible, Efficient Transportation Equity Act: A Legacy for Users (SAFETEA-LU), signed into law in August 2005, continued these trends and now dictates federal transportation policy through at least 2009.

Federal law requires the establishment of a metropolitan planning organization (MPO) in all metropolitan areas of 50,000 population or more (FHWA no date). The MPO is responsible for long-range regional transportation plans. These plans include a broad vision for the region as well as specific projects and policies proposed for addressing transportation needs for the next 20 or

Table 8.2 Transportation planning agencies and responsibilities.

Level	Agency	Responsibilities
Federal	Federal Highway Administration	Funding and categories
		Planning requirements
State	State Department of Transportation	State transportation plan
		Project selection outside of metro areas
		Implementation of highway projects
		Environmental impact assessment
		Environmental justice requirements
Regional	Metropolitan Planning Organization	Regional transportation plan
		Project selection inside metro area
		Environmental justice requirements
	Public Transit Agency	Implementation of transit projects
		Environmental impact assessment
		Environmental justice requirements
Local	City Department of Public Works	Capital improvement program for local streets
		Traffic operations for local streets

more years. MPOs must update these plans every four to five years. MPOs are also responsible for the short-range transportation improvement program (TIP), a list of projects funded and slated for construction in the next three to five years. Projects included in the TIP must come from the long-range plan. To choose projects for the TIP, MPOs apply a prioritization process that considers a variety of criteria in ranking proposed projects; these criteria often include cost-effectiveness, environmental benefits, and safety impacts. Federal law imposes other requirements on regional transportation planning as well. The Clean Air Act requires consistency – or "conformity" – between the regional transportation plan and air quality planning in areas that do not meet federal standards for selected pollutants. For all of these activities, the federal government has explicit requirements for public involvement. As a result of President Clinton's 1994 executive order on environmental justice, MPOs must consider the implications of their plans and programs for disadvantaged communities and communities of color and must ensure the meaningful involvement of these communities in the planning process.

Although federal law requires the establishment of MPOs and dictates their activities, the boundaries of the MPO's planning area and the membership of its board are designated by agreement between local officials and the governor. The board of the MPO typically includes representatives of the cities and the counties within the region, usually elected officials from the legislative bodies of these local governments. Local interests are represented in the activities of the MPO through this mechanism. In most cases the regional transit agency also has a representative on the board, and an official from the state department of transportation (DOT) may serve as an ex officio member. The size and structure of these boards vary considerably, but for only one MPO in the United States is the board directly elected by the citizens of the region. Federal law states that MPOs should work together with the state DOT in its activities, but the nature of power sharing varies from state to state. The work of the MPO is carried out by the staff, sometimes housed within a city or other local agency. The board typically holds monthly meetings to consider and vote on staff recommendations, including amendments to the regional transportation plan or updates to the TIP; these meetings include some time for public comment.

The MPO does not have responsibility for implementing the plan. Instead, projects are designed and built by the state Department of Transportation (for highways), the public transit agency (for bus and rail projects), or sometimes local governments (for a recreational trail, for example). The design of transportation facilities adheres to professional guidelines, most notably "the Greenbook" published by the American Association of State Highway and Transportation Officials (AASHTO). The "implementing agencies" must also follow federal requirements for projects that involve federal funds, most importantly the National Environmental Protection Act (NEPA). Under this law, the implementing agency must assess the environmental impacts of the proposed project, compare these impacts for a variety of project alternatives including a "no build" alternative, and must identify strategies to mitigate the impacts for the "preferred alternative." Included in these analyses are economic and social impacts, such as the impact of air and noise pollution on schools or the need for displacing houses to make room for the new facility. NEPA requires public involvement in this process.

Agencies responsible for the planning of public transit modes vary in their placement in the government hierarchy. Some are regional entities that span multiple jurisdictions, such as the Washington Metropolitan Area Transit Authority in Washington, DC, which plans for rail and bus transit in Washington, DC, and surrounding areas in Virginia and Maryland. Others are located within city or county government. In some cases, the transit agency is a part of a state-level agency, such as the Maryland Transit Administration, which plans for public transit needs at the state level and operates transit within the City of Baltimore and surrounding counties. Regardless of where they are administratively situated, local and state transit agencies are heavily dependent upon the federal government for financial support to improve, maintain, and operate existing systems and develop new services. The Federal Transit Administration oversees grants to local transit providers and ensures that they follow the federal planning guidelines.

From its beginnings in the 1960s, transportation planning has reflected an overriding concern with traffic congestion. With the exception of air quality and traffic safety, health has not been a significant consideration in regional transportation planning efforts. In recent decades, however, many regions have turned to walking and biking as alternatives to driving and thus as a strategy for addressing both traffic congestion and air quality. The idea that streets belong to pedestrians and bicyclists and not just to drivers has also taken hold in many places. Although obesity concerns have not been the motivation for these efforts, they help to increase opportunities for physical activity.

Implications of Traditional Approach for Obesity

Regional transportation planning has traditionally focused on highways. In part, this focus is driven by the division of federal funding between highways and public transit. Although the federal government began funding highways in the 1930s, federal funding for transit did not begin until the 1960s. In SAFETEA-LU, the most recent federal transportation authorization bill, funding for the highway programs averages $40 billion per year, of which $8.2 billion is in categories that can be spent on projects other than highways and $200 million is designated for bicycle and pedestrian related activities. In contrast, funding for transit averages $8.9 billion per year. Transit advocates have argued that there is an "uneven playing field" for transit, with more hurdles for securing federal funding and a greater share of costs covered by local sources of revenues (e.g. Beimborn and Puentes 2003).

The concern with traffic congestion is embedded in the tools used to carry out regional transportation planning. The performance of the transportation system is measured using the concept of "level-of-service". As defined by the Highway Capacity Manual (TRB 2000), level of service for a highway depends on the ratio of volume to capacity: a high ratio means more congestion and a lower level of service. This measure has traditionally been used to determine the additional highway capacity needed to accommodate future volumes of traffic. As a result, highways and intersections have been widened as much as possible, creating inhospitable environments for bicyclists, pedestrians, and transit users. Until recently, little thought was given to strategies that might improve level of service for vehicles by reducing traffic volumes, including strategies that would encourage walking, biking, and transit use. Trade-offs between level-of-service for vehicles and levels-of-service for other users are not usually considered.

New Approaches with Benefits for Obesity

The overriding concern of federal policy with highways began to abate with the passage of ISTEA in 1991. This landmark piece of legislation, pushed by advocacy groups concerned about automobile dependence and its social and environmental impacts, called for a system that balances different modes of transportation and that integrates land development and transportation planning decisions. For the first time, the federal government provided funding for pedestrian-oriented projects. The Transportation Enhancements program set aside $2.8 billion for projects that complemented highways projects, including hike-and-bike trails and other bicycle and pedestrian facilities. Although not all states responded with the same enthusiasm (McCann et al. 2000), spending on bicycle and pedestrian facilities went from less than $7 million per year before ISTEA to over $400 million annually by 2003, and all states have by now designated a bicycle-pedestrian coordinator. SAFETEA-LU, the most recent federal bill, added new programs that support active modes of travel, including a $612 million Safe Routes to School program, a $100 million Nonmotorized Transportation Pilot Program, and a $370 million Recreational Trails Program that supports the development and maintenance of trails for both motorized and nonmotorized uses.

Recent decades have also seen more emphasis on managing the demand for transportation as a cost-effective alternative to increasing capacity through road expansions. A variety of strategies have been developed. Employer-based transportation demand management (TDM) strategies include flexible work hours, telecommuting options, ride matching services, and transit incentives. These programs are beginning to converge with employer-based programs that encourage healthy behaviors. Another strategy is to get more employees living closer to work. In 1997, the State of Maryland implemented a Live Near Your Work incentive program that gave homebuyers $3,000 toward the purchase of a home if they bought within a certain distance of work. Similarly, Location Efficient Mortgages (LEMs) allow homebuyers to qualify for larger mortgages than they otherwise would if they buy a house in an area that is conducive to walking, biking, and transit on the assumption that they will spend less on driving. In voluntary travel reduction programs, households receive one-on-one counseling on ways to drive less and thus save time and money; the health benefits of driving less and walking, biking, or using transit more are now being promoted as a further incentive for behavior change in these programs. Pricing can also be used to manage demand. For example, in 2003, London implemented a "congestion pricing" program that charges drivers for entering the central city during specified times of day; this program has significantly reduced traffic congestion and increased active travel. Although motivated by concerns over congestion and air quality, these efforts all have the potential to increase physical activity.

Integrated Efforts

The ties between planning and health are becoming more institutionalized as each domain integrates concerns about obesity and the built environment into their practice. Planners are increasingly adding improved health to the list of potential benefits of their activities, in an effort to build further support for

Table 8.3 Finding out more about integrated efforts.

Effort	Organizations	Websites
Smart Growth	Smart Growth America	http://www.smartgrowthamerica.com/
	Smart Growth Network	http://www.smartgrowth.org/
	Environmental Protection Agency	http://www.epa.gov/smartgrowth/about_sg.htm
New Urbanism	Congress for the New Urbanism	http://www.cnu.org/
Healthy Cities	World Health Organization	http://www.who.dk/healthy-cities
	International Healthy Cities Foundation	http://www.healthycities.org/
	Center for Civic Partnerships	http://www.civicpartnerships.org/
Active Living by Design	Active Living by Design	http://www.albd.org/
Health Impact Assessments	World Health Organization	http://www.who.int/hia/en/
	Centers for Disease Control	http://www.cdc.gov/healthyplaces/hia.htm
State Obesity Plans	Centers for Disease Control	http://www.cdc.gov/nccdphp/dnpa/obesity/ state_programs/

these activities. Public health officials are increasingly including planning activities in the list of strategies for addressing obesity at the population level, in an effort to build more effective programs. The result is a promising convergence of interests and efforts (Table 8.3).

Planning-Based Efforts

Two examples where planning efforts have strengthened ties to health include Smart Growth and the New Urbanism. Both of these movements attempt to address some of the ills caused by past planning approaches that produced suburban-style development with separated land uses, little connection to the larger urban fabric, and prioritization of the automobile. However, the approaches differ somewhat in the scale and focus of their efforts, with Smart Growth aiming at implementation at the state, regional, or municipal level and New Urbanism targeting new development or redevelopment of subdivisions, neighborhoods, or even individual parcels. Smart Growth and New Urbanist principles can be a part of an obesity prevention effort to the extent that they provide more choices for active travel and create environments that support physical activity and healthy eating.

Smart Growth practices encourage new development that is more conscious of the environmental, economic and social needs of new and existing communities. Smart Growth practice is guided by ten principles: (1) mix land uses, (2) use compact building design, (3) create a range of housing opportunities and choices, (4) foster communities with a strong sense of place, (5) preserve open space and farmland, (6) direct development toward existing communities, (7) make development decisions predictable, fair and cost-effective, (8) encourage community and stakeholder collaboration, (9) make communities more walkable, and (10) encourage a range of transportation choices (EPA no date). The last two principles relate directly to the provision of active travel opportunities; the others do so by creating environments that support active travel and access to open space. When implemented, the guiding principles of

Smart Growth have the potential to address many of the land use and transportation planning issues raised in this chapter in a more systematic and comprehensive way.

New Urbanism has similar goals to Smart Growth, although the focus of these efforts tends to be at the scale of new development or redevelopment projects rather than the larger regional scale that characterizes Smart Growth. This movement is influenced by the character of more traditional communities, built before the automobile dominated the landscape. In its charter, the Congress for the New Urbanism outlines 27 guiding principles grouped at the level of the region, the neighborhood, and the block, street, and building. These principles emphasize transportation alternatives at each of these levels and state that activities of daily living should be within walking distance and that streets should be safe, comfortable, and interesting to the pedestrian (CNU 1997-2007). The charter also emphasizes population diversity within neighborhoods, though critics have charged the movement with contributing to gentrification in established low-income neighborhoods and with fostering income segregation as a result of high-priced new developments. To counter these charges, the movement has emphasized the importance of creating a range of housing types within every development, including apartments and "granny flats." In addition, New Urbanist principles have been applied in the HOPE VI program of the U.S. Department of Housing and Urban Development, in which distressed housing projects are converted into walkable, mixed-income neighborhoods. Although not all New Urbanist developments adhere to all of these ideals, the movement has brought renewed attention to the ways in which architectural, engineering, and planning practices shape the quality of the walking environment.

Health-Based Efforts

Health-based efforts to shape the built environment as an obesity prevention strategy are also growing. Notable movements include Healthy Cities programs and the Active Living by Design program. Interest in the concept of Health Impact Assessments is growing, and many states are incorporating land use and transportation planning in their statewide health plans.

The international Healthy Cities movement emerged in the 1980s and now includes projects in well over 1,000 cities throughout the world. With ties to community-based public health efforts, this movement has only recently begun to address the role of the built environment in obesity prevention. The World Health Organization's Healthy Cities program, focused on the European region, adopted healthy urban planning as one of three core themes in its Phase IV efforts, with the complementary theme of physical activity and active living. These efforts consciously go beyond the traditional focus on individual lifestyle choices to emphasize the physical environments that influence the ability and motivation of individuals to be physically active (WHO 2000) and the role of urban planning in creating these environments (Barton and Tsourou 2000; Barton et al. 2003). The Healthy Cities movement is also spreading in the United States. In California, the Center for Civic Partnerships has established a Healthy Cities and Communities program that promotes a positive physical environment that supports healthy choices for nutrition and physical activity (Center for Civic Partnerships 2002). Through such efforts, the Healthy Cities movement is building collaborative relationships between public health officials, local planners, and others.

In 2000, the Robert Wood Johnson Foundation convened a meeting of experts to discuss the role of community design in promoting physical activity and public health (RWJF 2000). These discussions led to the establishment of the Active Living by Design program, based at the University of North Carolina. The purpose of this program is to create environments that encourage physical activity as a part of daily life (ALbD 2005). In 2003, the program funded 25 community partnerships across the United States to develop and implement strategies for increasing routine physical activity. These partnerships involve public health officials, local planners, and others in efforts to influence policy and advocate for projects that will create an environment supportive of active living. Two years later, the foundation launched the Healthy Eating by Design program that aims to increase access to healthy foods in low-income communities and schools. In 2005, 12 of the Active Living by Design partnerships were selected to expand their efforts to the creation of healthy eating environments through this program.

Health Impact Assessments (HIAs) are another approach that grew out of the public health field that has the potential to bring obesity concerns into the planning realm (Cole et al. 2004). Modeled after environmental impact assessments, described earlier, these assessments consider the implications of policies, programs, and projects for the health of a population. Promoted by the World Health Organization (WHO 2006), HIAs are gaining ground in the United States through the efforts of the Centers for Disease Control and Prevention (CDC 2005) and others. If applied to land use and transportation planning, this approach could help to ensure that the built environment supports both physical activity and healthy eating. General plans, for example, could be evaluated as to their impact on the quality of the pedestrian environment, access to parks and other recreational areas, proximity to shopping and services, and the distribution of grocery stores. Similarly, regional transportation plans could be evaluated as to improvements in alternatives to driving. Although HIAs are not currently required for these activities, states have the power to require them for local land use plans, and the federal government could require them for regional transportation plans.

Many states are developing health plans that include planning-related interventions to address obesity. The Nutrition and Physical Activity Program to Prevent Obesity and Other Chronic Diseases funded by the Centers for Disease Control and Prevention supports states in their efforts to combat the obesity epidemic (CDC 2006). In the initial implementation phase, states develop interventions, collect data, and support existing programs throughout the state. In the capacity building step of this program, states forge partnerships between appropriate agencies, analyze data, and develop statewide health plans. In 2005, 28 states were funded as a part of this program and many are partnering with planning agencies to develop built environment interventions. For example, the State of Washington is focusing its efforts on increasing physical activity through environmental change, including improvements to the bicycle and pedestrian environment, and has partnered with several planning organizations including the state Department of Transportation.

Opportunities

Changing the built environment to provide more and better choices for physical activity and healthy eating patterns will provide lasting contributions to obesity prevention across the population. Decisions about land use and transportation are most directly influenced at the local and regional levels, but the federal and state governments could have an influential role in prompting local communities to respond through funding opportunities, policies, and guidance. Advocacy groups operate at local, regional, state, federal levels and can facilitate partnerships across disciplines and public agencies. Specific opportunities for advocating for planning approaches that will potentially help to prevent obesity can be found at all these levels (Table 8.4). Working with the private sector, there also are significant opportunities to understand the health effects of changes in the built environment through evaluation of ongoing development projects.

* Because land use decisions reside primarily at the local level, cities have an important role to play in addressing deficiencies in the built environment. Obesity concerns can be explicitly incorporated into goals and strategies of comprehensive plans, providing guidance for current and future decisions. As new development or redevelopment projects are proposed, plans can be reviewed for their obesity implications. Health concerns can be included among the criteria for selecting projects for inclusion in a capital improvement program (CIP). Obesity can be targeted within specific neighborhoods by working with redevelopment agencies or creating special planning districts.
* At the regional level, transportation planning provides the best prospect for contributing to obesity prevention. Health agencies can participate in development of the regional transportation plan and advocate for goals that reflect obesity concerns. The forecasting models used to evaluate these plans can be modified to better represent walking and bicycling as modes of transportation, and new measures of system performance can be adopted. As with CIPs at the local level, obesity concerns can be incorporated into the process for prioritizing projects for the transportation improvement programs (TIP).
* Policies at the state level can provide the impetus for communities to consider obesity in local transportation and land use planning efforts. Obesity concerns can be incorporated into the goals of the state transportation plan. States can themselves provide funding for active transportation projects, in addition to those funds provided by the federal government. On the land use side, states can require a consideration of obesity concerns in local land use planning or provide incentives for adopting land use policies that work towards obesity prevention. Many states, like Maryland, have embraced a non-motorized agenda in their own transportation and land use policies, but there is significant variation across the states in the scope and magnitude of the reach of regulations, programs, funding opportunities, and other incentives.
* The federal government can exert powerful influence in the transportation planning process at lower levels of government through their funding programs and policy requirements. The programs outlined in SAFETEA-LU that address active transportation can be implemented at the local level.

Table 8.4 Examples of opportunities for built environment interventions.

Level	Opportunities
Local	• Incorporate obesity concerns into general plan and criteria for prioritizing projects in capital improvement program
	• Change zoning and subdivision ordinances to increase viability of walking and biking
	• Require amenities supportive of physical activity in new developments
	• Adopt traffic calming programs to improve street environment
	• Develop safe routes to school program
	• Change school siting policies to put schools within walking distances
	• Implement transportation demand management policies
	• Adopt Main Street programs to preserve and revitalize local shopping
	• Offer incentives for supermarkets in low-income neighborhoods
	• Support farmers' markets and community gardens
	• Change zoning to limit fast food outlets and liquor stores in low-income areas
	• Participate in food systems planning
Regional	• Incorporate obesity concerns into regional transportation plan and criteria for prioritizing projects in transportation improvement program
	• Improve representation of active travel in forecasting models
	• Adopt new measures of system performance
	• Shift funding from highways to bicycle and pedestrian projects
	• Implement transportation demand management policies
State	• Require local planning to consider obesity implications
	• Provide incentives for local planning to consider obesity implications
	• Require Health Impact Assessments for land use planning
	• Provide state funding for bicycle and pedestrian projects
	• Support a state Bicycle-Pedestrian coordinator
	• Incorporate planning concerns in state health plan
	• Implement agricultural preservation programs
Federal	• Provide federal funding for bicycle and pedestrian projects
	• Require Health Impact Assessments for transportation planning
Disparities	• Focus local planning efforts on low-income areas
	• Enhance environmental justice efforts at regional and state levels and ensure adherence to requirements
	• Establish state mandates to consider health disparities in local land use planning and regional and state transportation plans
	• Take the built environment into consideration in federal programs targeting low-income households

Future authorization bills can incorporate more funding for bicycle, pedestrian and transit projects that improve opportunities for physical activity through active transportation. Requiring health impact assessments for transportation projects and establishing requirements for conformity with health plans would have a significant impact on regional transportation planning.
• Health disparities can be addressed through activities at each of these levels. Local planning efforts can give priority to needs in low-income areas,

particularly when it comes to capital improvements. Metropolitan Planning Organizations are already required to adhere to federal requirements on environmental justice; their efforts can be monitored and enhanced through the public involvement process. State governments can mandate attention to health disparities in local planning requirements and in their own transportation plans. Ensuring adherence to environmental justice requirements for all relevant federal policies, transportation and otherwise, could help to address health disparities. Federal programs already targeted at health disparities could take into consideration the role of the built environment.

• Most land development, whether in new areas or involving redevelopment of existing areas, is undertaken by private developers. Private developers can lead the way in bringing about healthier communities, even in the absence of support from local government. Although land development must abide by the rules set by local governments, private developers usually have some flexibility to follow the principles of Smart Growth and New Urbanism. Where local codes do not allow for adherence to these principles, developers can push for changes. Successful development projects provide a model for other developers in the area and serve as important laboratories for measuring the effectiveness of these strategies in preventing obesity.

Conclusion

Changing the built environment to provide more and better choices for physical activity and healthy eating will require action at all levels of government in concert with initiatives from citizens and advocacy groups, health professionals, and private developers (IOM 2005). Many of the agencies involved in the transportation and land use planning processes are already moving in this direction (IOM and TRB 2005), providing important opportunities for bringing the goal of obesity prevention into the planning process. The fact that the built environment is fixed in the short run and durable over time, and thus relatively slow and often costly to change, represents both the challenge of this approach and its great promise.

References

Active Living by Design (ALbD). About ALbD. Available: http://www.activelivingbydesign.org/ (accessed 1/4/06).

American Society of Civil Engineers (ASCE), National Association of Home Builders (NAHB), and Urban Land Institute (ULI). (1990). *Residential Streets* (2nd ed). New York and Washington, DC: ASCE, NAHB, and ULI.

Ashe, M., Jernigan, D., Kline, R., & Galaz, R. (2003). Land use planning and the control of alcohol, tobacco, firearms, and fast food restaurants. *American Journal of Public Health*, 93(9), 1404–1408.

Austin, S. B., Melly, S. J., Brisa, N., Sanchez, B. N, Patel, A., Buka, S., & Gortmaker, S. L. (2005). Clustering of fast-food restaurants around schools: A novel application of spatial statistics to the study of food environments. *American Journal of Public Health*, 95(9), 1575–1581.

Barton, H., & Catherine, T. (2000). *Healthy urban planning*. London: Spon Press.

Barton, H., Claire M., & Catherine, T., (Eds.). (2003). *Healthy urban planning in practice: Experience of European cities*. Copenhagen: Regional office for Europe of the World Health Organization.

Beimborn, E., & Puentes, R. (2003). Highways and transit: Leveling the playing field in federal transportation policy, brookings institute. Available: http://www.brookings.edu (accessed 4/4/07).

Boarnet, M. G., Anderson, C. L., Day, K., McMillan, T., & Alfonzo, M. (2005). Evaluation of the California safe routes to school legislation: Urban form changes and children's active transportation to school. *American Journal of Preventive Medicine, 28*(Suppl. 2), 134–140.

Block, J. P., Scribner, R. A., & DeSalvo, K. B. (2004). Fast food, race/ethnicity, and income: A geographic analysis. *American Journal of Preventive Medicine, 27*(3), 211–217.

California, State of. (2003). *General Plan Guidelines*. Sacramento, CA: Governor's Office of Planning and Research.

Catlin, T. K., Simoes, E. J., & Brownson, R. C. (2003). Environmental and policy factors associated with overweight among adults in missouri. *American Journal of Health Promotion, 17*, 249–258.

Center for Civic Partnerships. (2002). *Fresh ideas for community nutrition and physical activity*. Sacramento, CA: Public Health Institute.

Centers for Disease Control and Prevention (CDC). (2005). Health impact assessment. Available: http://www.cdc.gov/healthyplaces/hia.htm (accessed 1/4/06).

Centers for Disease Control and Prevention (CDC). (2006). Overweight and Obesity: State-Based Programs. Available: http://www.cdc.gov/nccdphp/dnpa/obesity/state_programs (accessed 1/4/06).

Chung, C., & Myers, Jr. S. L. (1999). Do the poor pay more for food: An analysis of grocery store availability and food price disparities. *The Journal of Consumer Affairs, 33*(2), 276–296.

Cole, B. L., Wilhelm, M., Long, P. V., Fielding, J. E., Kominski, G., & Morgenstern, H. (2004). Prospects for health impact assessment in the united states: New and improved environmental impact assessment or something different? *Journal of Health Politics, Policy, and Law, 29*(6), 1153–1186.

Collins, R. (1976). Agricultural land preservation in a land use planning perspective. *Journal of Soil and Water Conservation, 31*(5), 182–189.

Congress for the New Urbanism (CNU). (1997–2007). Charter for the New Urbanism. Available: http://www.cnu.org/charter (accessed 4/4/07).

Cowan, S. M., Rohe, W., & Baku, E. (1999). Factors influencing the performance of community development corporations. *Journal of Urban Affairs, 21*(3), 325–340.

Dunkley, B., Helling, A., & Sawicki, D. S. (2004). Acessibility versus scale: Examining the tradeoffs in grocery stores. *Journal of Planning Education and Research, 23*, 387–401.

Environmental Protection Agency (EPA). No date. About Smart Growth. Available: http://www.epa.gov/smartgrowth/about_sg.htm (accessed 1/06/05).

Ewing, R., Schmid, T., Killingsworth, R., Zlot, A., & Raudenbush, S. (2003). Relationship between urban sprawl and physical activity, obesity, and morbidity. *American Journal of Health Promotion, 18*(1), 47–57.

Federal Highway Administration (FHWA). (2005). SAFETEA-LU: Funding Tables. Available: http://www.fhwa.dot.gov/safetealu/fundtables.htm (accessed 12/18/05).

Federal Highway Administration (FHWA). No date. A Citizen's Guide to Transportation Decision Making. Available: http://www.fhwa.dot.gov/planning/citizen/index.htm (accessed 1/4/06).

Flournoy, R., & Treuhaft, S. (2005 Fall). *Healthy food, healthy communities: Improving access and opportunities through food retailing*. Oakland, CA: PolicyLink and the California Endowment.

Frank, L., Andresen, M., & Schmid, T. (2004). Obesity relationships with community design, physical activity, and time spent in cars. *American Journal of Preventive Medicine, 27*, 87–96.

Frank, L. D., Engelke, P. O., & Schmid, T. L. (2003). *Health and community design: The impact of the built environment on physical activity*. Washington, DC: Island Press.

Fulton, W. (1999). *Guide to california planning* (2nd ed.). Point Arena, CA: Solano Press Books.

Gottlieb, R., Fisher, A., Dohan, M., O'Connor, L., & Parks, L. (1996). Homeward bound: Food-Related strategies in low income and transit dependent communities. Working Paper, UCTC No. 336. The university of california transportation center, University of California at Berkeley.

Handy, S., Paterson, R., & Butler, K. (2003). *Planning for street connectivity: Getting from here to there*. Planning advisory service report Number 515. Chicago, IL: American Planning Association.

Holtzman, B. (2002). Agricultural districts: A tool for protecting local agriculture. *Connection*, 5(3): 2,4,8.

Horowitz, C. R., Colson, K. A., Hebert, P. L., & Lancaster, K. (2004). Barriers to buying healthy foods for people with diabetes: Evidence of environmental disparities. *American Journal of Public Health*, 94(9), 1549–1554.

Institute of Medicine. (2005). *Preventing childhood obesity: Health in the balance*. Washington, DC: National Academies Press.

James, W. P., Nelson, M., Ralph, A., & Leather, S. (1997). Socioeconomic determinants of health: The contribution of nutrition to inequalities in health. *British Medical Journal*, 24, 1545–1549.

Lopez, R. (2004). Urban sprawl and risk for being overweight or obese. *American Journal of Public Health*, 94(9), 1574–1579.

Maddock, J. (2004). The Relationship between obesity and the prevalence of fast food restaurants: State-level analysis. *American Journal of Health Promotion*, 19(2), 137–143.

Mair, J. S., Pierce, M. W., & Teret, S. P. (2005). The use of zoning to restrict fast food outlets: A potential strategy to combat obesity. Monograph, center for law and the public's health at johns hopkins and georgetown universities. Available http://www.publichealthlaw.net/Research/Affprojects.htm#Zoning (accessed 4/4/07).

McCann B, Klenitz R, DeLille B. (2000 March). *Changing direction: Federal transportation spending in the 1990s*. Surface Transportation Policy Project.

McLeroy, K. R., Bibeau, D., Steckler, A., & Glantz, K. (1988). An ecological perspective on health promotion programs. *Health Education Quarterly*, 15(4), 351–373.

Metro. (1996). *Main street handbook: A user's guide to main street*. Portland, OR: Metro. Available:
http://www.metro-region.org/library_docs/land_use/main_streets.pdf (accessed 4/4/07).

Morland, K., Wing, S., Diez Roux, A., & Poole, C. (2002). Neighborhood characteristics associated with the location of food stores and food service places. *American Journal of Preventive Medicine*, 22, 23–29.

National Trust for Historic Preservation. No date. Smart growth schools: A fact sheet. Washington, DC. Available:
http://www.nationaltrust.org/issues/schools/schools_smartgrowth_facts.pdf. (accessed 3/17/06).

Nelson, A. (2004 December). *Toward a new metropolis: The opportunity to rebuild america*. Washington, DC: The Brookings Institution.

Pothukuchi, K., & Jerome L. K. (2000). The food system: A stranger to the planning field. *Journal of the American Planning Association*, 66(2), 113–124.

Project for Public Spaces (PPS). (2003). Public markets and community based food systems: Making them work in low income neighborhoods, report to the kellogg foundation, project for public spaces, Inc., New York. Available
http://www.pps.org/pdf/kellogg_report.pdf (accessed 2/28/06).

Robert Wood Johnson Foundation. (2000). *Healthy places, healthy people: Promoting public health & physical activity through community design*. Princeton, NJ.

Sallis, J. F., Cervero, R. B., Ascher, W., Henderson, K. A., Kraft, M. K., & Kerr, J. (2006). An ecological approach to creating active living communities. *Annual Review of Public Health, 27,* 297–322.

Sharpe, D. L., & Abdel-Ghany, M. (1999). Identifying the poor and their consumption patterns. *Family Economics & Nutrition Review, 12,* 15–25.

Schilling, J., & Linton, L. S. (2005). The public health roots of zoning: In search of active living's legal genealogy. *American Journal of Preventive Medicine, 28*(Suppl. 2), 96–104.

Smart Growth Network. (2005). Principles of smart growth: Mixed land uses. Available: http://www.smartgrowth.org/about/principles/principles.asp?prin=1 (accessed 1/4/06).

Southworth, M., & Ben-Joseph, E. (1997). *Streets and the shaping of towns and cities.* New York: McGraw-Hill.

Spitzer, T.M., & Baum, H. (1995). *Public markets and community revitalization.* Washington, DC: Urban Land Institute and Project for Public Spaces.

Sustainable Food Center (SFC). (2002). Programs: community gardens. Available: http://www.sustainablefoodcenter.org/programs_community_gardens.asp (accessed 1/4/06).

Sustainable Food Center (SFC). (1995). Access denied. Available: http://www.sustainablefoodcenter.org/publications_access_denied.asp (accessed 3/17/06).

The Reinvestment Fund. (2003). Pennsylvania fresh food financing initiative. Available at: http://www.trfund.com/financing/fffi/fffi.htm (accessed 1/6/05).

Transportation Research Board (TRB). (2000). Highway capacity manual. Washington, DC: The National Academies.

Transportation Research Board (TRB) and Institute of Medicine (IOM). (2005). *Does the built environment influence physical activity? Examining the evidence.* TRB Special Report 282. Washington, DC: Transportation Research Board.

United States Department of Agriculture (USDA). (2004). Farmers market growth. Agricultural marketing service, United States Department of Agriculture, Washington, DC. http://www.ams.usda.gov/farmersmarkets/FarmersMarketGrowth.htm. (accessed 2/22/06).

United States Environmental Protection Agency (EPA). (2006). Smart growth and schools. Available at: http://www.epa.gov/dced/schools.htm. (accessed 3/17/06).

World Health Organization (WHO). (2000). *Active living in the city.* Copenhagen: Regional Office for Europe of the World Health Organization.

World Health Organization (WHO). (2006). Health impact assessment. Available http://www.who.int/hia/en/ (accessed 1/4/06).

Chapter 9

The Food Industry Role in Obesity Prevention

Brian Wansink and John C. Peters

Introduction

At least once during the last century nearly every country in the world has had to fight food shortages or starvation (Wansink 2006). Examples include Belgium in 1918, America in the Depression, and almost every European and Asian country during World War II. Today the food table has turned. Critics now blame low-cost, easily available food for making us obese (Nestle 2002). In particular, food companies have been accused of contributing to the growing problem of obesity in the United States (Brownell and Horgen 2004). Although food companies perform a vital function in society, they cater to the strong biological drive to eat whenever food is available, and the food supply currently provides a level of calories per capita that exceed caloric needs for most U.S. adults (Harnack et al, 2000; Gerrier and Bente, 2002)

Nearly *every* industry plays some role in creating our obesogenic environment. In the last 100 years, the vast agriculture, manufacturing, energy, and technology industries have all consistently pushed themselves to build production and distribution systems that are more and more efficient and which require less and less physical labor. With food, for instance, these combined efforts have resulted in lower prices and higher availability of many foods in every corner of the United States, whether it be a Subway restaurant in Correctionville, Iowa or the ubiquitous vending machine in the basement of most buildings.

Over the past several decades, technology has significantly reduced the number of jobs that require physical labor. Technology – in the form of electric mowers, garage door openers, and remote controls – has reduced the physical labor we need to expend at home. Thus, the overall energy expenditure of the population has dropped substantially, and there are more and more sedentary entertainment choices to occupy our leisure time.

Another product of these systemic industrialization and technological improvements has been a change in the food supply. In 75 years we have gone from the bread lines of the Great Depression to a system that provides a huge variety of high calorie foods, nearly everywhere in our environment and at relatively low cost, both in terms of money and effort to obtain and prepare.

Because food is such a large part of this modern obesogenic environment, it is not surprising that the food "industry" has become the focus of intense scrutiny. While some see it as the architect of the obesity epidemic (Nestle 2002), others see it as holding the positive solution for future generations (Wansink and Huckabee 2006). This chapter will focus on what the food industry can do to help combat obesity. Specifically in this chapter we examine the main principles that drive the food industry and what the food industry can do to help de-market obesity. As background, we characterize phases in the obesity evolution of the food industry and explain basic principles that drive food acquisition and consumption. We then explain basic principles that govern the behavior of food companies and describe five general drivers that can be reversed to profitably de-market obesity.

A focus on food here is not meant to ignore or under-appreciate the roles of other industries in contributing to the behaviors leading to obesity (e.g., the physical "inactivity industries,") but rather it is to highlight what is happening in the industry that has been "in the bulls eye" since the obesity crisis first began garnering public attention. The potential role of other industries in reversing obesity has been given much less attention to date. The lessons learned from observing the food industry response to obesity will likely apply to these other industries. Eventually they will need to become involved if we are to make meaningful progress toward meeting this public health challenge.

The Evolution of Response

The food industry's response to allegations that it is the culprit in the obesity epidemic appears to be evolving through three phases: (1) denial, (2) appealing to consumer sovereignty, and (3) developing win-win opportunities. In the first phase, many food companies and trade associations denied their role in obesity by noting that rising obesity can also be associated with rising levels of inactivity (Hill et al. 2005). The contention has been that if the food industry is to be blamed for obesity, so are automobiles, cable TV, video games, remote controls, elevators, attached garages, and the internet (Hill and Peters 1998). The second phase of response to obesity criticisms is a free market appeal to consumer sovereignty – let the customer decide. This has often involved an emphasis on moderation and choice (Horovitz 2004). In this phase, many food companies (particularly quick service restaurants) offered to customize current offerings for their patrons (veggie burgers became hamburgers without the burger) while advocating an increase in physical activity.

The third, evolutionary phase of response to these allegations involves developing profitable win-win solutions (where both industry and the public health benefit) to help consumers better control what they want to eat. Clearly no company would want to modify a product in a way that discourages consumers from purchasing it or consuming it. However, it may be in a company's best interest to help consumers better control *how much* they consume in a single setting. Consider the indulgent "C" foods – cookies, cake, crackers, chips, and candy. Overconsuming an indulgent food can not only lead a person to gain weight, but it might also lead them to become satiated and to temporarily "burn out," not repurchasing the food as soon as they otherwise might (Inman 2001). Reducing the per occasion consumption volume of a food may provide a "win-win" solution for both companies and consumers. Not only would this help consumers better control their single occasion consumption, but it could also help promote more favorable attitudes toward the brand and company (Wansink 2005). Collectively, these benefits for consumers may constitute the basic elements of a new value equation such that more and more people will seek those features in products that help them manage their intake.

The win-win solutions in this third phase offer a wide range of profitable segmentation opportunities for companies. Take the notion of single-serving packaging. Although such packaging would increase production costs, the $40 billion spent each year on diet-related products is evidence that there is a portion-predisposed segment that would be willing to pay a premium for packaging that enabled them to eat less of a food in a single serving and to enjoy it more. For instance, results from a survey of 770 North Americans indicated that 57% of respondents would be willing to pay up to 15% more for these portion-controlled items (Wansink 2006). Although targeting this "portion-prone" segment will not initially address the immediate needs of all consumers, it can provide one key driver that companies need to develop profitable win-win changes.

The assumption here is that the effects of food companies' actions on obesity are unintentional, that is, that food companies are focused on making money rather than on making people obese. Following this line of reasoning suggests that the answer to the obesity issue will be found not in increased regulation, but rather in market-based changes that help consumers develop a new appetite for healthy foods (Wansink and Huckabee 2005). The most innovative solutions for de-marketing obesity will be solutions that leverage the basic reasons why we eat the way we eat.

Two Principles that Drive Food Acquisition and Consumption

Until the beginning of the industrial age, food acquisition was a major activity for most people. The efficiency and prosperity of industrialization made it easier and more efficient for us to do our "hunting and gathering." Food became plentiful, tasty, and relatively inexpensive. An outcome of the industrialization of the food supply is that the highest dietary energy sources preferred by humans, sugar and fat, are among the cheapest commodities in the market (Drewnowski and Darmon 2005; Drewnowski, Darmon, and Briend 2004). In addition, shelf stability became important to further reduce the cost of producing and distributing foods and to add other consumer benefits (e.g., convenience). From a food technology perspective, shelf stable foods must generally be low in water, which often means they are high in fat and carbohydrate and consequently, high in calories and calorie density. Thus, many of today's favorite consumer food brands are high in sugar and fat and are much less expensive, in both cost and time to prepare, than fresh produce or other foods now known to be more healthful.

The Two Principles that Drive Food Consumption

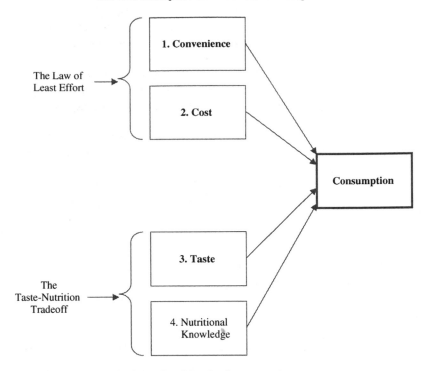

Figure 9.1 The two principles that drive food consumption.

Consumer behavior with respect to food acquisition and consumption can be understood in terms of basic principles: The Law of Least Effort and the Taste-Nutrition Tradeoff (Wansink and Huckabee 2005). The nature of these two principles is shown graphically in Figure 9.1. As explained below, these two principles related to food acquisition and consumption have driven our food acquisition and consumption since the hunter-gatherer days. Understanding these influences informs our understanding of what is realistic to recommend with respect to food industry initiatives and what would be ineffective because of our basic nature.

The Law of Least Effort

The Law of Least Effort holds that people seek the greatest convenience at the lowest cost. Innovations through time have generally reduced the amount of effort it takes to move (e.g., the wheel), to learn (e.g., the printing press), or to communicate (e.g., the telephone). This motivation or tendency to work toward conserving effort also explains why new houses have attached garages with garage door openers, why ice makers and dishwashing machines are never *de*-installed, and why driving is often preferred to walking or biking. Even where people do walk (such as in New York City), bike (as in Amsterdam), or ride mass transit (Washington DC), it is often because it convenient, economically efficient, or socially acceptable. The same principles apply to food – people seek food products that provide them with greater convenience. The drive to acquire food at lower cost is related to basic principles of both economics and psychology (Wansink 2006).

This desire to follow the path of least effort results in a number of changes to our food distribution system that are market-driven and which also create food environments that make it easy for any consumer with average willpower to overeat. Because of this "Law of Least Effort," we get convenient, easy-to-open (and consume) packaging, vending machines, drive-through restaurants, and free pizza delivery. We get the chance to buy foods ready to eat instead of having to prepare them.

The Taste-Nutrition Tradeoff

Three strong taste preferences have been genetically passed on to us over the generations, specifically the tastes for fat, salt, and sugar. By giving us the taste for fat, sugar, and salt, our genes led us to prefer the foods that were most likely to keep us alive. Fatty foods helped our ancestor's weather food shortages. Salt helped them maintain an appropriate water balance in their cells, to avoid dehydration. Sugar and the sweetness associated with it helped them distinguish edible berries from poisonous ones. Having this taste has also led us to desire a wide variety of foods. Eating a greater variety of foods increased the likelihood of consuming the wide range of the, then-unknown nutrients we needed. Our natural inclination for variety made sure we consumed adequate amounts of essential nutrients without requiring knowledge about specific vitamins, minerals or types of energy sources.

In other words, in times of food scarcity or insecurity "good taste," meant "good health." The more fat, salt, and sugar our ancestors consumed (within limits), the more likely they were to survive. In contrast, the surplus of food in the developed world has lead to current perceptions that taste and health are inversely related. The more fat, salt, and sugar a food contains, the *less* healthy it seems to be perceived when food is abundant. Nevertheless, we are still hardwired to prefer "good tasting" food and all the fat, salt, and sugar it provides. Salt, fat, and sugar have a genetic upper-hand when it comes to food choice. These are not ingredients we eat because of clever marketing. They are ingredients we would seek out regardless of marketing. Yet a predisposition toward them makes marketing even more effective at telling us what we want to hear.

Consider the case of restaurant food, especially "fast food." Market research indicates that burgers, French fries, pizza, and Mexican food comprise about 50% of all restaurant orders and, together, are ordered with much greater frequency than vegetables and side salads (see Figure 9.2) (NPD Group 2003). According to a Burger King official, this chain sells about 100 Whoppers for every Veggie Burger, roughly 10 Whoppers for every salad, and about 10 fried chicken sandwiches for every grilled chicken sandwich (Horovitz 2005).

Fast food is so widely consumed because we are genetically designed to love it. More accurately, it has been designed to love *us* by giving us generations of taste evolution that encourage us to crave fat, salt, and sugar, as just described. The components we love in fast food are things that our hunter-gatherer forefathers sought out for survival. French fries and chips have salt

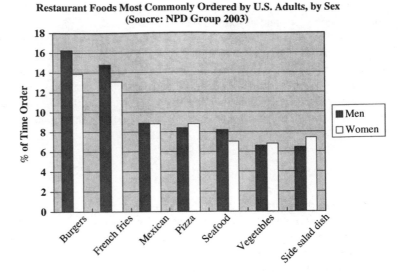

Figure 9.2 Restaurant foods most commonly ordered by U.S. adults, by sex. (*Source:* NPD Group 2003).

and fat, donuts and Pop-tarts have fat and sugar, Coke and Pepsi have sugar and salt, and candy bars pretty much have them all.

Some anti-obesity advocates believe that fast food is addictive (Schlosser 2001; Critser 2003). They believe manipulative companies fill fast food with fat, salt, and sugar because they know we will eat it, love it, and come back again and again. Is this really true? Do food companies put ingredients in their food that they know we will eat and love? The answer is a resounding "yes". However, in a sense, the companies that make fast food are no more guilty than the traditional grandmother who added extra salt and sugar to her secret pasta sauce, loaded her cookies with butter and sugar, who basted the Thanksgiving turkey with its own fat. And the traditional grandmother is no more guilty than anyone else who wants to please their dinner guests: we all add spices, butter, and sugar or other such ingredients so that our friends will enjoy the meal.

Anyone who cooks knows which ingredients make food taste good. Companies know this, and your grandmother knew this. If these ingredients were outlawed, no one would eat fast food anymore, nor would they arrive in time for a meal at grandmother's house. In other words, if we remove the good taste from foods, people will not want to eat them, at least not often or not for long.

Fast food gives us the taste we want, and it gives it to us at a good value and with little effort. The people most critical of fast food are usually not those in this "limited means" market segment. There is no need to defrost the hamburger at noon or to slave over a hot stove when you can say "Value Meal #2 – large" without leaving your car. The typical person pulling in to a fast food parking lot is likely to "have a couple bucks in his pocket and is looking to get as much good food for that money as he can," according to Eric Haviland, Director of Strategy for Taco Johns (2005). Consistent with this, Taco John's rival, Taco Bell, abandoned its Low Calorie menu around 2003, opting to now use the positioning, "Feel Full." For a hungry person with limited means, feeling full is a whole lot more tempting than nibbling on a salad with vinaigrette on the side. In addition fast food is also very predictable and there are no surprises: There are no bad tables, no tipping, and the toppings on a Big Mac are always the same.

Principles that Influence Food Companies

There are also fundamental principles that govern the behavior of food companies. One is that they do not care if you eat the food as long as you repeatedly buy it. The other is that they want to make a profit.

Hence, although it might appear to some that McDonalds, or Kraft, or Haagen-Dazs are only in business to make us fat, in reality, these companies can still make money if we buy a meal or product, eat half, and then throw the other half away. What matters is that we buy their product rather than one from their competitors. The profit is made when the company sells the product to you and this actually applies to any food company or establishment. If we said "We want to buy a dozen heirloom tomatoes, take them home, leave them in the refrigerator for a month, and then throw them out," your local grocery would still sell them to us.

The second principle – that companies are in business to make a profit—can work in favor of the consumer. Two such success stories are in Table 9.1. Similarly, if starting tomorrow at noon, we all went into McDonalds and Burger King and ordered only salads, their menus would change overnight. Within a

Table 9.1 Two success stories of profitably helping de-market obesity.

Company	Action	Result
Kraft	Introduced in 2004, *Nabisco* 100-calorie packs were designed to provide consumers with great-tasting, better-for-you products that helped them stay on track with their sensible eating habits.	The product was considered a success due to positive responses from the consumers, industry, and media, leading to the brand reaching $100M in sales in less than a year.
	The line featured new versions of some *Nabisco* classics, conveniently delivered in pre-portioned packages, each containing 100 calories and 0–3 grams of fat per pack.	
The Family Dining Chain	In 2004, the 90-unit Family Dining Chain began to "lighten up" the menus, creating new dishes with lighter ingredients (in terms of calories and fat) and with more of a Mediterranean flair. One of the chain's biggest successes during this phase has been greater use of vegetables.	Replacing starch with vegetables has caused sales to go up by 10–15% on an item-by-item basis. Entrees with vegetables as a main focus have been selling well also. The chain's overall sales have gone up 4–5% during this period.
	All new entrees are now presented on the menu with vegetables rather than starch (pasta or potatoes) as the standard accompaniment. Customers are explicitly given the option of substituting the starch back in, but roughly 90% of customers go with the vegetables.	

year, people would be able to eat at Taco Salad Bell anytime they wished. Within another year there would be a chain of Broccoli King restaurants. In reality however, for reasons already noted, we are not all going to run down and order salads tomorrow. The earlier cited data on the most frequently ordered restaurant foods demonstrate the relatively low frequency of ordering salads. Cost is not always the issue. Burger King offers a $1 side salad that costs less than medium fries, but the fries win out most of the time. In spite of the salad, it is the burgers, fries, and desserts that keep people coming back.

The perceived benefits for profitability are a factor when companies do respond to consumer preferences along more healthful lines. Just as companies will provide fattening food to eat mindlessly if that is what we want, they will also provide healthy food that we can eat mindfully if they can do so profitably. Improving the corporate image with an important population segment may be one relevant motivation. For example, when McDonalds realized how many vegetarians there were, Veggie Burgers made it onto the menu and the fries were fried in vegetable oil. When the low-carb diet fad grew in popularity, low-carb burgers appeared at Burger King. As a perhaps extreme example of giving an appearance of catering to consumer preferences, each tray liner at Burger King at one time presented the company's version of the Bill of Rights (see Figure 9.3).

De-Marketing Obesity – What Companies Could Do to Profitably Help

So what can food companies do to profitably help us to eat more mindfully? To answer this, we need to look at what is it about food that causes us to gain

---

Burger King Bill of Rights

You have the right to have things your way.
You have the right to hold the pickles and hold the lettuce.
You have the right to mix Coke and Sprite.
You have the right to a Whopper sandwich with extra tomato, extra onion and triple cheese.
You have the right to have that big meal sleepy feeling when you're finished.
You have the right to put a paper crown on your head and pretend you're ruler of "(insert your make believe kingdom here)."
You have the right to have your chicken fire grilled or fried.
You have the right to dip your fries in ketchup, mayonnaise, BBQ sauce or mustard or not.

You have the right to laugh until soda explodes from your nose.
You have the right to stand up and fight for what you believe in.
You have the right to sit down and do nothing.
You have the right to eat a hot and juicy fire-grilled burger prepared just the way you like.
You have the right to crumple this Bill of Rights into a ball and shoot hoops with it.

Have it Your Way

Figure 9.3 Who's deciding what is for dinner? Burger King Bill of Rights.

weight in the first place. Perhaps ironically, the answer can be found in already described factors that enabled our Paleolithic ancestors to maintain enough weight to survive the Ice Age.

Human beings are predisposed to overeat food that is (1) Palatable (tastes good), (2) Convenient (easy to prepare), and (3) Easy (inexpensive) to obtain.

Most of the leading packaged goods companies – like Pepsico, Kraft, and General Mills – are experimenting with new ideas, programs, and products that they think will be win-win solutions for their shareholders and their consumers. As indicated in Figure 9.4, a survey of 28 food and beverage companies indicated these changes can be broadly classified as changing multi-serve packaging, changing single serve packaging, introducing children's sizes, and changing food label information (Nutrition Facts and serving sizes).

These are positive moves forward. Using the "mindless eating" principles outlined in this chapter, let us look at what else an astute, nutrition-conscious marketer could do to profitably offer us food that can mindfully help us lose weight (Wansink 2004; Drewnowski and Rolls 2005), i.e., can "de-market" obesity.

Extra-small and Extra-large Packages

Why do food companies always seem to Super-size? There are two reasons: (1) To satisfy our demand for value, and (2) to match the competition. A large number of people want to be able to buy a lot of food for very little money. If only one restaurant provided supersized value-meals, it would catch both our attention and our $3.59. If the competitor across the street did not quickly do the same, he or she would lose business quickly.

People serve themselves more from larger packages (Wansink 1996). Therefore, one option would be to sell multi-packs with smaller individual

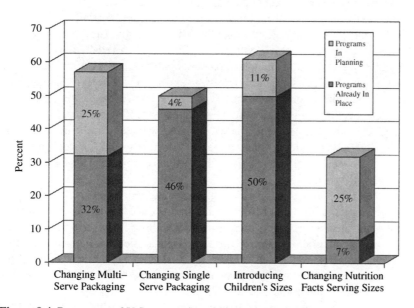

Figure 9.4 Percentage of U.S. companies making packaging changes (2000–2004). (*Source.* Grocery Manufacturers of America 2004).

servings. For instance, instead of selling a large 20 ounce bag of potato chips, the large bag could contain four 5 ounce sleeves inside it. In this way, there would be a natural break point that would give us a chance to pause and decide whether we wanted to stop eating. This was discovered when 124 students were given either a large zip-lock baggie containing 200 M&Ms or a large zip-lock baggie that, in turn, contained 10 smaller zip-lock baggies each containing 20 M&Ms. When there was only one bag to open, people ate an average of 73 M&Ms during an hour. Those with the smaller baggies usually ate a multiple of 10. When the hour was over, they had eaten an average of 42 each from the multi-pack. That is 112 calories less – the mindless margin (Wansink 2006).

Another option would be to offer smaller, premium-priced packages. Although they would be a bit more expensive (per ounce) compared to the larger packages, some people would not mind paying more to eat less . . . or to eat better. Given the millions spent on diet foods and weight loss programs each week, the number of consumers who would pay more is probably substantial. In addition, smaller packages may cater to the ever-growing need for convenience. Consumers seem willing to pay a premium for on-the-go packaging that eliminates the need to either carry a big multi-serving package or to take the time to parcel out single serving portions into other containers.

This does not imply that the industries must abandon the value-priced super-size packages in favor of little boutique-sized, portion packs. There may be sizable markets for both – one that wants value and one that wants portion-control. The introduction of either into the market would give more options to current consumers generally, but particularly to those who are either price-sensitive or portion-sensitive.

Packing Products to Facilitate Portion Control

There are also other profitable packaging changes companies could make that could help us to eat more mindfully. One problem with eating food (such as potato chips) from a large package is that we do not know when to stop. Because we typically get full before we realize it, we can easily continue to eat long after we have eaten enough to meet our caloric needs. Unless we are eating slowly, or unless something interrupts us, we might keep eating until we are past the point where we are full. One way to interrupt the eating process is to create a natural stopping point. This can be done, for instance, by dividing a large container into several smaller containers. It can also be done through the use of internal sleeves that force us to actively make a decision as to whether we want to continue eating after we have finished a sleeve of six (or however many) cookies.

We call this "Thin Mint" packaging. Those familiar with Girl Scout cookies will be aware that the Thin Mint cookies are the ones that have a built-in stopping point. Instead of being presented in a wide-open, no-serving-size-limit tray, they are carefully wrapped in two cellophane sleeves. Finishing the first sleeve creates a pause, which is about all most of us need to stop. One of the more extreme versions of this can be seen with individually packaged cookies, such as many of the brands found in Japan.

These stopping points can take other forms. This was illustrated in the "Red Chip" study. This study used cans of Pringles (potato chips in a tube) in which every 7th chip was dyed red; every 14th chip was dyed red; or no chips were dyed. People (n = 150) were invited to watch a video and to enjoy the new version of chips. Those who ate from the cans where every 14th chip was red ate an average of 15 chips. Those who ate from the cans where every 7th chip was red ate an average of 10. Those with no red chips ate 23. Having something, almost anything, to interrupt our eating gives us the chance to decide if we want to continue (Wansink and Huckabee 2005).

"Silent" Introduction of More Healthful, Good Tasting Formulations

Since 1995, food producers across the U.S. and beyond have instinctively cited the market failure of the McDonald's McLean sandwich as the pre-eminent example of why healthy food does not sell. However, most of them are taking the wrong lesson away from McLean's failure. It was not that there was no market for healthy foods or those companies just can not make good low-fat products. These foods are typically new products that taste new, are advertised as *healthy*, and are expected by consumers to taste bad. In contrast to an approach that draws attention to such new products, companies could quietly alter existing products in modest ways that reduce calorie density. In this way, there would be no negative "I'm sure this low-calorie candy is going to taste terrible" expectations of a healthy food that would prevent it from getting a fair shot.

These silent changes are something we call "stealth health" (Wansink 2005). To generate some initial ideas as to what the current best practices are in this area,[1] an exploratory web-based survey was conducted among 111 restaurant managers, asking them about recent successes in changing recipe formulation (Table 9.2) (Keystone 2006). On average, their successful changes used a "stealth health" approach – they opted to promote these items as fresh and tasty, rather than to use the word "healthy" ($p < .01$). They also had specific ideas as to how to best lower calories. Stealth approaches are facilitated by the fact that consumers will probably not compensate, calorically, when certain types of changes are made to food formulations: (1) When calorie the density of a food is decreased, we eat the same volume we usually do, (2) we think we are just

Table 9.2 How 111 food service operators prefer to reduce the calories in menu items.

How effective are the following techniques in lowering the calories in a successful menu item?	Mean rating (1 = Disagree; 9 = Agree)
Reduce the fat	7.4
Add vegetables	7.2
Add fruit	6.3
Add fiber	5.9
Reduce the carbohydrates	5.7
Reduce the protein	3.8

[1] The survey was done on behalf of an advisory committee which had as its task to provide suggestions to the Food and Drug Administration (FDA) on the nutrition labeling of away-from-home food.

as full, and (3) we think the food tastes the same (as long as it hasn't been labeled as being "reduced calorie"). Studies conducted by Barbara Rolls and colleagues have been the standard of showing how increasing the size of foods with water, air, or less dense ingredient substitutes can make foods more healthy and equally psychologically filling (Rolls et al, 2004a; Ello-Martin et al, 2005; Rolls et al, 2006).

Small modifications in formulations can lead to reduced calorie foods (like candy bars) that are the same size as regular candy bars. High energy density items, such as those with a lot of fat, can be replaced with fruits and vegetables without us even really being aware of it (Rolls 2005; Rolls and Barnett 2002; Rolls et al. 2004). We buy it, and we are happy. We buy it, and the industry is happy. This is now occurring in the marketplace. For example, McDonalds offers the option of having an apple snack with a Happy Meal. For anyone interested in having French dressing instead of French fries, Wendy's offers a small salad for the same price.

In general, we tend to look at the size portion as an indicator of whether it is a good "value." That is, the bigger the food, the better the value. While adding water, or air, or filler may do little to the taste, it helps maintain the perception of value, and it decreases calorie levels (Kral and Rolls 2004). Even if such efforts only reduce calorie levels by 10%, such a decrease in our daily calorie consumption would either slow or reverse the weight gain among most of us. It is important to remember, however, that this would be a slow process. This would be a pound-by-pound reduction, just as it was a pound-by-pound process in which the population has gained weight over the past several decades.

Provide Simple Labeling of Food but with Realistic Expectations about Impact

"Education" is the one-word, ready-answer to anything related to health. Once we say "education," it becomes somebody else's problem – like the government's or industry's. And if the "education" efforts don't work, the answer is "Do more of it."

Although marketing nutrition is a noble enterprise, education – as defined by most – is *not* the answer. See *Marketing Nutrition* (Wansink 2005) for a detailed discussion of this issue. People are generally too busy or distracted to read packages, or are too preoccupied or hungry to care that they should eat a carrot stick rather than a handful of crackers. As noted in other chapters in this book, ecological frameworks would suggest that nutrition education has an important role but only as one component of a multi-level approach to obesity prevention. Once the food environment is re-engineered so that healthy foods are promoted equally with unhealthy foods, labels and nutrition education may become more useful.

Having informational food labels is an important step in helping some consumers understand what they are purchasing and consuming, and accurate labeling of calories and serving sizes is a good idea. However, the impact of labeling on the nutritional quality of the total diet should be viewed realistically. Outside of an artificial laboratory situation – labeling only influences a modest percentage of consumers (Andrews, Netemeyer, and Burton 1998; Kozup, Creyer, and Burton 2003). The question is where should this information stop. How much labeling is helpful and when might labeling information be counterproductive? One issue relates to "health halos" in which a label may backfire because the food becomes too associated with its health benefits (Chandon and Wansink 2007; Wansink and Chandon 2006). Another concern is the potential for overwhelming or confusing the average consumer. A recent report to the FDA made a recommendation that companies should emphasize caloric content when labeling away-from-home food. Caloric content is the one piece of nutrition information most commonly understood by consumers.

Keep it Affordable

Generally, when prices go up, consumption goes down (Drewnowski and Darmon 2005). However, although this may be true for "meat and potatoes" or fruits and vegetables, but it does not seem as true with more tempting foods, like candy, cookies, and ice cream. When the price of these goes up, we either buy it anyway because it is indulgent, or we simply switch to another brand of candy, cookie, or ice cream. One study showed that increasing the price of selected vending machine candy caused people to buy less of that candy (French 2003). However, it is less clear that this would be the case in natural settings. In the real world, if the price of a candy bar doubled, people would either pay it, or they would buy another brand. They would not stop eating candy. Similarly, if a fast food restaurant raised its prices, people would not stop eating fast food, they would simply eat it somewhere else. Raising prices of less healthful foods does not necessarily cause people to consumer more healthful foods that may be lower in cost. They may simply find a less costly form of the same food. In fact, raising prices within a reasonable free-market range does not change purchase behavior, it penalizes the people with the least money.

What is certain is that large increases in food prices make us look for other alternatives for the product in question. The challenge will be to help make the healthier options more attractive and more affordable. We cannot legislate or tax people into eating foods they do not like. However, this is not to say that a smart, well-intentioned marketer cannot help to shift consumer preferences. The two examples in Table 9.1 illustrate that small changes made by Kraft and the Family Dining restaurant chain both helped spark hope for how healthy changes can be profitable changes.

Where Do We Go From Here?

The opportunities and challenges outlined for the food industry also apply to other industries that can help reverse the obesity trend. Certainly, the principles are the same. The most fruitful approaches to changing "business as usual" will involve finding win-win solutions where both the consumer and the industry benefit and find the value equation acceptable. Because eating healthier and being more physically active essentially go against the "biological incentives" programmed into our physiology (i.e., it feels good to eat and rest) it will take a compelling set of circumstances – product, package, placement, education and marketing, price, etc. – to convince today's consumer that they want to change their behavior. However daunting this may seem, it can be done and is happening all the time in the marketplace at least among segments of the population. Our job in promoting the health of the population at large is to help nurture the growth of the market segments comprised of those people most willing to change. Encouraging the "early adopters" may help accelerate the acceptance of change by even larger groups of people so that gradually the majority of the population has embraced and adopted healthier choices.

What strategies are likely to lead toward positive changes and partnerships with the food industries? First, it would be helpful for industry leaders to recognize the role of small positive changes in products, labeling, packaging and so on as meaningful progress in the fight against obesity. All too often we focus more on the larger goal we want to achieve without appreciating *how* we will get there. For example, even though small reductions in the saturated fat, salt or calorie level of a product do not make it "healthy", such changes may in fact help consumers "retrain" their taste preferences toward healthier products. It took over 25 years for a majority of consumers to change their behavior to consume reduced fat or skim milk, and much of this change was made possible by offering many different fat level options over the years, 2%, 1%, skim, which helped people retrain their taste preference for milk.

Second, public health practitioners should help connect consumers to product solutions. People are often worried about conflict-of-interest perceptions if they recommend products, but consumers need credible expert advice about new products on the market. We need to find a way around this barrier so that more consumers will try healthier new things, increasing the chance they might make a more permanent health behavior change.

Third, we need to find better ways for industry and public health to become more engaged and holistic partners. The public health and industry sectors separately are each insufficient to change behavior—they need each other. When health authorities all agree on an objective and when the industry is given a clear goal that is being supported externally, the marketplace can change rapidly. Such was the situation in 1990 when the health and medical community uniformly advocated that the diet should be reduced in total fat. The U.S. Public Health Service's Healthy People 2000 initiative charged industry with launching 5000 new reduced fat foods by the end of the decade. The industry surpassed this goal by 1995. In retrospect, given that the advent of low fat foods did not achieve its intended purpose, one can argue whether fat reduction was the right health goal, but the point is that when a clear goal is set that the health community supports with a single voice, industry can respond rapidly.

Finally, we all must recognize that making healthy eating and active living "business as usual" will take time. The obesity epidemic did not occur overnight and the escape from this problem will also not be immediate. This does not should not mean we continue to advocate for more, faster, and bigger changes. Rather, it means we should embrace those changes that move things in the right direction, however big or small, while at the same time keeping the pressure on for more change, constant, incremental, directional. This strategy will eventually lead to success.

The Future: 21st Century Marketing

The 19th Century has been called the Century of Hygiene (Wansink and Huckabee 2005). That is, in the 19th Century more lives were saved or extended due to an improved understanding of hygiene and public health than to any other single cause. We learned that rats were not house pets and that it is a good idea to wash hands before performing surgery.

The 20th Century was the Century of Medicine and Public Health. Vaccines, antibiotics, transfusions, and chemotherapy all helped to contribute to longer, healthier lives. In 1900, the life expectancy of an American was 49 years. In 2000, it was 77 years.

What about the 21st Century? We believe it will be the Century of Behavior Change. Medicine is still making fundamental discoveries that can extend lives, but changing everyday, long-term behavior is the key to adding years and quality to our lives—changes like reducing risky behavior and improving exercise and nutrition habits. The more we exercise and the better we eat, the longer and more productively we will live. There is not a prescription that can be written for such behavior. Eating better and exercising more are decisions we need to be motivated to make.

When it comes to contributing most to improving the life span and quality of life in the next couple generations, marketers could be important allies. They are in a good position to identify and promote the products that make it easier to exercise and easier to eat more nutritiously. They can also motivate us to do both of these things. Our eating practices would be a good place to start.

References

Andrews J. Craig, Richard G. Netemeyer, and Scot Burton (1998), "Consumer generalization of nutrient content claims in advertising," *Journal of Marketing*, 62 (October): 62–75.

Brownell, Kelly D. and Katherine Battle Horgen (2004), *Food Fight*, Chicago: Contemporary Books.

Chandon, Pierre and Brian Wansink (2007), "Obesity and the calorie underestimation bias: a psychophysical model of fast-food meal size estimation," *Journal of Consumer Research*, forthcoming.

Critser, Greg (2003), *Fat Land: How Americans Became the Fattest People in the World*, New York: Houghton Mifflin Company.

Drewnowski, Adam and Barbara J. Rolls (2005), "How to modify the food environment," *Journal of Nutrition*, 135 (4): 898–899.

Drewnowski, Adam, N. Darmon, and A. Briend (2004), "Replacing fats and sweets with vegetables and fruits – A question of cost," *American Journal of Public Health*, 94 (9): 1555–1559.

Drewnowski, Adam and N. Darmon (2005), "Food choices and diet costs: an economic analysis," *Journal of Nutrition* 135 (4): 900–904.

Ello-Martin, J.A., Ledikwe, J.H., and Rolls, B.J. (2005), "The influence of food portion size and energy density on energy intake: implications for weight management." *Am J Clin Nutr.* Jul; 82 (1 Suppl): 236S–241S.

French, Simone A. (2003), "Pricing effects on food choices," *Journal of Nutrition*, 133: 3 (March): 841S–843S.

Grocery Manufacturers of America (2004). "GMA Members: Part of the Solution," presentation by Collier Shannon Scott (October), cited in MacLeod, W., Samuels, J., Scott, C. S. (2005). Comments of Grocery Manufacturers Association concerning the Federal Trade Commission and Department of Health and Human Services Public Workshop on Marketing, Self-Regulation & Childhood Obesity, Appendix C., page 30. Available at http://www.gmabrands.com/publications/docs/GMACOMMENT.pdf

Harnack, L.J., Jeffery, R.W., and Boutelle, K.N. (2000), "Temporal trends in energy intake in the United States: an ecologic perspective." *Am J Clin Nutr.* Jun; 71 (6): 1478–1484.

Haviland, Eric (2005), Comments at a FDA-sponsored subcommittee of the Keystone Group. Washington, DC, December 14.

Hill James O., Wyatt, H.R. and John C. Peters (2005), "Modifying the environment to reverse obesity," *Environmental Health Perspectives*, SI 108–115.

Hill James, O. and John C. Peters (1998), "Environmental contributions to the obesity epidemic," *Science*, 280 (5368): 1371–1374.

Horovitz Bruce (2004), "You Want it Your Way." *USA Today*, March 5, A.1 + .

Horovitz, Bruce (2005), "Restaurant Sales Climb with Bad-For-You Food," *USA Today*, May 13, A1 + .

Inman, J. Jeffrey (2001), "The Role of Sensory-Specific Satiety in Attribute-Level Variety Seeking," *Journal of Consumer Research*, 28 (June), 105–120.

Keystone Group (2006), "Exploratory Study on Healthy Best Practices in Restaurant," Appendix E.

Kozup, John C., Elizabeth H. Creyer, and Scot Burton (2003), "Making Healthful Food Choices: The Influence of Health Claims and Nutrition Information on Consumers' Evaluations of Packaged Food Products and Restaurant Menu Items," *Journal of Marketing*, 67 (April), 19–34.

Kral, T.V. and Barbara J. Rolls (2004), "Energy density and portion size: their independent and combined effects on energy intake," *Physiology & Behavior*, 82 (1): 131–138.

NPD Group (2003), *Summary of Food Trends – 2002*, www.NPD.com.

Nestle, Marian (2002), *Food Politics: How the Food Industry Influences Nutrition and Health*, Berkeley: University of California Press.

Rolls, Barbara and Robert Barnett (2002), *Volumetrics: The Weight Control Plan*, New York: Torch Books.

Rolls, B.J., Roe, L.S., and Meengs, J.S. (2006), "Reductions in portion size and energy density of foods are additive and lead to sustained decreases in energy intake." *Am J Clin Nutr.* Jan; 83 (1):11–17.

Rolls, B.J., Roe, L.S., and Meengs, J.S. (2004), "Salad and satiety: energy density and portion size of a first-course salad affect energy intake at lunch." *J Am Diet Assoc.* Oct; 104 (10): 1570–1576.

Rolls, Barbara (2005), *The Volumetrics Eating Plan: Techniques and Recipes for Feeling Full on Fewer Calories*, New York: HarperCollins.

Rolls, Barbara, J., Ello-Martin, J.A. and Tohill, B.C. (2004), "What can intervention studies tell us about the relationship between fruit and vegetable consumption and weight management?" *Nutrition Reviews*, 62 (1): 1–17.

Schlosser, Eric (2001), *Fast Food Nation: The Dark Side of the All-American Meal*, New York: Houghton Mifflin Company, 2001.

Wansink, Brian (1996), "Can Package Size Accelerate Usage Volume?" *Journal of Marketing*, Vol. 60: 3 (July), 1–14.

Wansink, Brian (2004), "Environmental Factors that Increase the Food Intake and Consumption Volume of Unknowing Consumers," *Annual Review of Nutrition*, 24: 455–479.

Wansink, Brian (2005), *Marketing Nutrition: Soy, Functional Foods, Biotechnology, and Obesity*, Champaign, IL: University of Illinois Press.

Wansink, Brian (2006), *Mindless Eating: Why We Eat More Than We Think*, New York: Bantam-Dell.

Wansink, Brian and Pierre Chandon (2006), "Do 'Low Fat' Nutrition Labels Lead to Obesity?" *Journal of Marketing Research*, forthcoming.

Wansink, Brian and Mike Huckabee (2005), "De-Marketing Obesity," *California Management Review*, 47: 4 (Summer), 6–18.

Wansink, Brian, Paul Rozin, and Andrew Geiger (2005), "Consumption Interruption and the Red Potato Chip: Packaging Ideas that Help Control Consumption," Working Paper 05–110, Cornell Food and Brand Lab, Ithaca, NY 14853.

Chapter 10

Media, Marketing and Advertising and Obesity

Sarah E. Samuels, Lisa Craypo, Sally Lawrence, Elena O. Lingas and Lori Dorfman

Over the last few decades, while obesity rates in the United States have increased dramatically in both adults and children, there has been a rapid expansion in access to and use of electronic media, for all ages. These trends in media use are frequently blamed for the trends of increasing obesity—at least in part. Media, which here refers to newspapers, magazines, radio, television, movies and videos, electronic video games, and the Internet, have the power to influence both what we know and what we do. Without question these media influence pathways that lead to obesity, in several important ways. Media help to form and to communicate cultural norms and images, provide avenues for health education information, and create channels for food and beverage advertising and product promotion. Most media are used when sitting; hence media use also tends to encourage sedentary behavior. Mechanisms related to the media that contribute to overweight also include commercial marketing and advertising of high-calorie foods and beverages, portrayals of eating, drinking, and body image in both advertising and program or story content, consumption of excess calories during television viewing, and reduced levels of calorie expenditure during periods of inactivity associated with media use.

Recognizing that media are important aspects of the social structure, consideration of how to prevent and control obesity in society at large must include the potential influences of the media on the determinants of and attitudes about obesity and on the ability to mount effective strategies to stabilize and then reduce population weight levels. The purpose of this chapter is to consider both the beneficial and deleterious effects of media on eating and physical activity. We provide a brief overview of the different types of media, demographics of media use, and mass media trends and impacts. We also include information on media regulation and media influence on nutrition, physical activity, and body image. The chapter concludes by describing opportunities for progress in promoting healthy eating and physical activity through the media. In keeping with the focus of this book, the roles of media in the obesity epidemic are discussed in the context of the United States. However, as noted in several chapters in this book (see Chapter 11 in particular), the obesity epidemic is a global phenomenon, and the reach of electronic media into both urban and rural areas throughout the world links the issues discussed in this chapter to a wider, global stage (Hawkes, 2004).

Types of Media and Trends in Use of Media

The media have long played a central role not only in the way people in the United States receive news and information, but also in how they think about politics, culture, family, and leisure activities. Over the years the types of media that people turn to have developed and changed dramatically. This section will provide a brief overview of current media use and trends in the United States and describe how media have been used to convey nutrition and physical activity information.

Print

The primary vehicles for print media in the U.S. are newspapers and magazines. Newspapers, available in the U.S. since the 1700s, remain an important source of local and international news for Americans. However, readership of newspapers has significantly decreased in recent years, with only sixty-two percent of Americans reporting reading the Sunday newspaper and only about 50 percent reporting reading a newspaper during the rest of the week (Editor and Publisher Yearbook, 2003). Many younger adults are shifting away from newspapers and turning to the Internet for their news. Remaining readers are much more likely to be older, white, and have high education levels (The State of the News Media, 2006). Although ethnic newspaper readership has increased in recent years African American, Asian, and Hispanic newspaper readership remains much lower then white newspaper readership (The State of the News Media, 2006).

Unlike newspapers, the readership for magazines is holding steady and in some cases increasing (The State of the News Media, 2006). There has been an increase in readership for entertainment, lifestyle and pop culture magazines (The State of the News Media, 2006). Data indicate that in 2003 pop culture magazines, such as *People*, *Us*, and *The Star*, were read by roughly 180 million people. News magazines were read by nearly 70 million, and business magazines by slightly less then 40 million (Mediamark Research, 2003). The audience for news magazines tends to be aging and more affluent. Fewer news magazine titles have been released in recent years for younger generations (The State of the News Media, 2004). In 2003, readers of news magazines tended to be 29 percent more affluent then the overall population (Mediamark Research, 2003).

Magazines reach readers of all demographics with general news and a wide range of special interest material (The State of the News Media, 2006). Magazines are also a source of health, beauty, and fitness information for women and men. There are a number of magazines that focus specifically on health and fitness issues and reach narrowly defined target audiences. These magazines cover everything from the latest nutrition research and diet fads to workout routines for weight loss.

Radio

Radio was introduced to American households in the 1920s and by 1994, ninety-nine percent of U.S. households had radios (U.S. Department of State, 1997). Radio has held its audience numbers over the years, providing a source of both news and entertainment. Ninety-three percent of Americans 12 years and older report listening to the radio at least weekly (Arbitron, 2006). The recent introduction of satellite radio, Internet radio stations, ipods, podcasts, and mp3 players has contributed to a 45 minute decrease in radio listening per week, but the average radio user still spends roughly 19 hours per week listening to the radio (Arbitron, 2006).

Radio advertising is often considered an inexpensive way to reach audiences, and young audiences in particular. Public health officials have also used the radio to spread healthful messages through Public Service Announcements (PSAs). For example, the Food and Nutrition Services Division of the United States Department of Agriculture (USDA) has created radio PSAs to promote the food stamp program to specific low-income ethnic populations. Many of the radio PSAs created by the USDA were in Spanish and played on Spanish language news and music stations (USDA, 2006).

Television

Since its introduction in the 1940s, television has become one of the most popular forms of media in the United States (Baughman, 1992). Data indicate that television viewing among both adults and children has increased dramatically in the past few decades. According to Nielsen Media Research, over 100 million homes in the United States currently have televisions, and in the average American home, the television is viewed for 8 hours and 11 minutes per day (Nielsen Media Research, 2005). It is estimated that children born during the television age will watch an average of seven years of television during their lives, spending more time watching television than any other activity, except sleeping (Kubey & Csikszentmihalyi, 1990). A study by Rideout, Foehr, Roberts, and Brodie (1999) on children and the media found that on a daily basis, 36 percent of children watch less then one hour of television, 31 percent watch one to three hours, 16 percent watch three to five hours, and 17 percent watch more then 5 hours of television (Figure 10.1).

A Henry J. Kaiser Family Foundation report revealed that African American and Hispanic children spend more time then white children watching television, videos, and playing video games (Rideout et al., 1999). Low income children are also heavier television viewers than their wealthier counterparts (Roberts, 2004). Detailed information on the demographics of television use can be purchased from Nielsen Media Research.

With increasing rates of television viewing there has been a concurrent increase in exposure to food and physical activity messages on television, and the

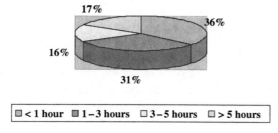

Figure 10.1 Daily television viewing hours of children and youth.

Source: Rideout et al., 1999.

higher rates of television usage among minority and low-income children expose them to an even greater amount of food and physical activity messages. Food and physical activity messages take many forms on television, including: in television news, television show storylines and product placements, advertisements, and public service announcements. In 1997 over 75 percent of the $7 billion spent by food manufacturers on advertising went to television advertisements (Gallo, 1999). Nearly 95 percent of the advertising budget for fast food restaurants also went to advertising on television (Gallo, 1999).

Internet

The early 1990s marked the beginning of wide-spread use of the Internet. Since the early 1990s popularity of the Internet has skyrocketed. In 2004 it was estimated that 70 million people went online daily (Pew Internet & American Life Project, 2005). Americans currently use the Internet for a variety of purposes, including: accessing news, weather, paying bills, shopping, email, and meeting people. However, Internet usage is not equal across the population. Data from the 2003 U.S. Census indicate that only 62 percent of American homes have computers and only 55 percent have Internet access (U.S. Census Bureau, 2003). The census also revealed that higher income families are more likely than low income families to own computers and have Internet access; African American and Latino families are less likely to own computers or have access to the Internet than non-Hispanic whites. For children, roughly 76 percent had access to a computer and the Internet at home and 83 percent of children enrolled in school had access to a computer and the Internet at school (U.S. Census Bureau, 2003).

Advertisers and commercial marketers target the rapidly growing number of people using the Internet with a variety of new interactive techniques that can seamlessly integrate advertising and Web site content (Montgomery, 1996, 2001). For example, almost all of the major companies that advertise and market to children have created their own Web sites, designed as "branded environments" (Montgomery, 2000; 2001). New technologies and software can also collect data about the viewing habits and specific interests of children without the knowledge or consent of either the children or their parents. Interactive Web sites, or "advergames," ask children about their interests, habits, and preferences through surveys or quizzes embedded in the games or activities featured on the sites. Marketers can use this information to tailor their commercial marketing messages and to encourage impulse buying of products featured in programming or advertising.

Interactive television, which allows TV viewers to link directly to a Web site from a television program, allows advertisers to target individual viewers with personalized ads, increasing the likelihood of impulse purchasing (Center for Digital Democracy, 2001). Eventually, broadcasters hope to integrate television programming content, commercial marketing, and data collection. Advertisers will be able to target viewers whenever they are watching and to transmit advertisements for products that are designed to appeal to a target audience—or more specifically, people of a certain gender, age, household income, race/ethnicity, or with certain interests.

In addition, product placements are increasingly incorporated into the sets or even the plots of television programs, movies, video games, and Web sites.

This practice is on the increase as commercial marketers for products of all kinds seek to integrate product advertising directly into program content, thereby confounding viewers' attempts to avoid commercials (Center for Digital Democracy, 2001).

Exposure to media is complex, involving multiple channels and multiple messages, with the potential for positive and negative effects. The media landscape is evolving quickly. With the introduction of new media technology, the way that Americans receive news and information has changed dramatically. Television, cable and digital media now play a dominant role in the lives of many Americans. Realizing the change in media use, commercial marketers have also changed the focus of how they advertise. Commercial marketing and advertising through these newer forms of media can be influential in setting norms and encouraging behaviors.

Media Regulation

In the United States, regulation of the media is primarily a federal function. The two main bodies given authority over the mass media are the Federal Communications Commission (FCC) and the Federal Trade Commission (FTC).

The Communications Act of 1934 established the FCC, and this independent government agency reports to Congress and is "charged with regulating interstate and international communications by radio, television, wire, satellite and cable" (FCC, 2006). The FCC regulates media ownership and has required broadcasters to include a certain amount of programming that benefits the public, in exchange for being granted licenses to the public airwaves.

The FTC was created in 1914, and like the FCC, is an independent government body reporting to Congress. When created, the FTC's purpose was to "prevent unfair methods of competition in commerce" (FTC, 2006). Over the years, acts of Congress have also given the FTC the responsibility to protect consumers against "unfair and deceptive practices" (FTC, 2006). The FTC consists of three bureaus with multiple offices per bureau. Under the Bureau of Consumer Protection is the Division of Advertising Practices, which enforces laws regarding truth in advertising across multiple types of media (FTC, 2006).

Together, these two agencies have domain over multiple aspects of the daily lives of Americans. Among the areas of media regulation of particular relevance to public health are the FTC's authority to regulate commercial marketing and advertising, including health claims, and the FCC's authority over media consolidation and the responsibilities to the public of those licensed to use the public airwaves, such as providing time for educational programming.

In the 1970s, the FTC made an unsuccessful attempt to regulate advertising and commercial marketing to children (Applbaum & Gould, 1981). Also in the 1970s, advertisers and commercial marketers began to take voluntary measures to police their own members, through the Council of Better Business Bureau's National Advertising Review Council. There is a special unit dedicated to self-policing children's advertising, the Children's Advertising Review Unit (CARU) (CARU, 2006). Critics characterize CARU as ineffective, noting that it lacks monitoring and enforcement mechanisms in addition to being funded by the very companies it is supposed to regulate, such as McDonald's Corporation and the Grocery Manufacturers of America (Kelly, 2005).

Media Effects on Health

Media have an important role to play in stimulating and enhancing change in local communities and societies at large. The media, particularly the news media, can place subjects onto the public and policy maker agendas (McCombs and Shaw, 1972–1973), thereby introducing new topics or encouraging new ways of viewing issues. Entertainment media and advertising can also play a role in societal knowledge and understanding of life.

The mass media can exert positive and negative effects on both individuals and populations, and these impacts may be either intended or not (Brown & Walsh-Childers, 2002). The media may provide information on health conditions and treatments, such as that available on health Web sites as well as in newspaper and magazine health columns and articles, and this information can have positive benefits for those who receive the information and are in a position to understand and act on it for themselves or family and friends. The media may also convey negative health messages, such as promotions for alcohol and tobacco products, especially when targeted to children (Brown & Walsh-Childers, 2002). Portrayals of alcohol use on television, in movies, music videos and music can have a particular impact on children and teens, because young people have little or no real-world experience within which to assess or countervail the messages they are exposed to in the media (Brown & Walsh-Childers, 2002). Overall, media have been shown to have effects on the acceptability and understanding of public health issues as diverse as substance use and abuse (tobacco, alcohol, prescription and illegal drugs), violence, sexuality, nutrition, body image, and mental health (Brown & Walsh-Childers, 2002).

One strategy to help people increase their understanding of the media is improving their media literacy, which can be characterized as a process of "informed inquiry" consisting of "awareness, analysis, reflection and action" on the media (Center for Media Literacy, 2006). The aim of media literacy is to both understand the messages communicated by the media and why the messages are present; to "help people become sophisticated citizens rather than sophisticated consumers" (Lewis & Jhally, 1998, pg. 1). Media literacy training provides a means for people to critically examine and reflect on the pervasive messages with which we are constantly bombarded. On other public health topics, such as tobacco and alcohol consumption, media literacy has been useful in helping to inoculate consumers against the illeffects of advertising and marketing and programming by deconstructing the message. This could potentially be a useful tool around food and beverage advertising and programming, particularly that aimed at teenagers.

Media Influence on Obesity

As obesity rates climb, there is both growing concern about the role media may be playing in contributing to the obesity epidemic and increasing support for finding ways media can help stimulate public action to address it. A recent study found that young children who were exposed to two or more hours of television per day were more likely then those with less exposure to be overweight, regardless of home environment or socioeconomic status (Lumeng, Rahnama, Appugliese, Kaciroti, & Bradley, 2006). A report by the Henry J. Kaiser Family Foundation concluded that television and the media in general may contribute to childhood obesity in a number of ways. The time children spend using media displaces time that could be spent engaged in physical activity. Children's food choices are influenced by food and beverage advertisements for high calorie-low nutrition foods. Children snack while using the media, often on relatively less healthful foods, and may consume more of these foods while eating in front of the television. Television may also lower children's metabolic rates, although this line of research is not conclusive (Henry J. Kaiser Family Foundation, 2004).

Over the last several years, the public health issue of obesity has gained prominence among the news media, the public, and also in scholarly journals. The number of news stories about the public policy aspects of the obesity problem rose from a few dozen in the last quarter of 1999 to over 1,000 stories in the last quarter of 2003 (Kersh & Morone, 2005). In addition to an increase in media coverage of obesity in the United States, the International Food Information Council (2004) has found an increase in the amount and depth of coverage of obesity issues in international media (Figure 10.2). By 2004, public opinion polls revealed that obesity was second only to cancer among the most important health problems in the United States (Schlesinger, 2005). Furthermore, a search for the term "obesity" using Google Scholar for the year 1995 returned 3,600 citations, compared to a return of 20,300 citations for the same search for the year 2004, a 464 percent increase (Dorfman & Wallack, 2007). Clearly, the problem of obesity has gained widespread attention throughout the United States.

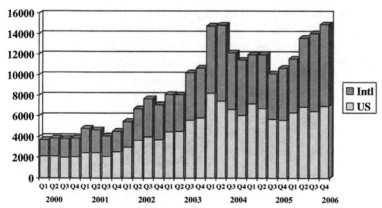

Global Trends in Obsity-Related Media Coverage

Figure 10.2 Global trends in obesity-related media coverage.

Source: The International Food Information Council, 2004.

Media, Food Intake, and Obesity

Food and beverage marketers spend billions of dollars on advertising to encourage consumers to buy their products. Research has shown that (1) the majority of foods advertised are not healthful (i.e., are high in calories and low in essential nutrients) and that (2) advertising has the power to influence food preferences and purchases, especially in children.

Food Advertisements and Commercial Marketing

Americans view tens of thousands of television commercials and see hundreds of billboard and poster advertisements every year. The majority of these advertisements promote food and beverage products (Gantz et al., 2007). As a result, both children and adults are targeted and exposed to multiple food advertisements every day—including promotion of highly sweetened cereals, cookies, candy, fast foods, and soda— that are predominantly high in calories, sugar, and fat. In 2004 the food industry (eating and drinking establishments, food retailers, and food manufacturers combined) reportedly spent $11 billion on advertising, including $5 billion on television ads alone (Commitee on Food Marketing and the Diets of Children and Youth, 2006). A study that reviewed commercials aired during Saturday morning children's programming found that roughly 50 percent of the commercials were for food (Kotz, 1994).

For children, television is the largest media source of advertisements. In 1999, money spent on children's television advertising amounted to roughly $1 billion (Nestle, 2003). For every five hours of television watched, children are exposed to an hour of commercials (Hastings et al., 2003). In addition, food preferences and advertising recall ability among children indicate that advertising is achieving its intended effects.

Commercial Marketing to Ethnic Groups

Though currently no data link food and beverage product marketing to obesity in communities of color, we do know that obesity affects Latinos and African Americans disproportionately to their white peers and that food marketers disproportionately target these population groups. Commercial marketers have demonstrated that within the communities of African American and Latino urban youth, this target marketing creates a loyal "super consumer" (Juzang, 2003).

To target communities of color, commercial marketers use specific images that are meaningful to the audience: celebrities such as entertainers, rap singers, athletes; models in fashionable dress; models using specific cultural associations expressed in language and mannerisms; youth representing peer approval; popular music that is uniquely identified with a specific group of children of color (Juzang, 2003).

Recent research studying the amount and type of advertising on prime-time television programs oriented to African American audiences compared to those for general audiences found that far more food commercials appeared on shows with large African American audiences and a larger percentage of these commercials were for high calorie-low nutrient foods (Tirodkar & Jain, 2003; Henderson & Kelly, 2005). African American prime-time TV also showed food items in non-advertising minutes or during the actual program more often than did prime-time TV programs for general audiences (Tirodkar & Jain, 2003). A content analysis of advertisements during after school television programming for children also revealed that there were a greater number of high calorie-low nutrition foods and beverages advertised on BET (Black Entertainment Television) in comparison to the WB (Warner Brothers) and the Disney Channel (Outley & Taddess, 2006).

Magazines are another major vehicle used by food and beverage advertisers (Gallo, 1999), and magazines aimed at certain ethnic audiences carry a large amount of advertising for high calorie-low nutrient foods. For example, a study of health-related advertising in 12 women's magazines was conducted to determine if magazine advertisements have an effect on health disparities between African American, Latina, and white women. The study compared eight "mainstream" women's magazines (targeted at Caucasian women) to the four highest circulating, general interest magazines targeted to African American and Latina women. Results indicated that in the African American and Latina oriented magazines, there were a greater number of ads for products that could harm health and fewer for products that promote health (Duerksen et al., 2005). High calorie-low nutrient food and drink ads made up 52 percent of food and beverage advertisements in Hispanic magazines, 32% in African American magazines and 29 percent in mainstream magazines (Duerksen et al., 2005).

Media Advertising Influence on Eating and Shopping Behavior

The large amount of food advertising and commercial marketing in the media can have an influence on eating and shopping behaviors in both children and adults. Increased exposure to advertising through the media can influence selection of higher calorie and higher fat foods.

A review conducted by Hastings et al. at the University of Strathclyde, Glasgow (2003) found strong evidence that commercial food marketing and specifically television advertising has been shown to influence children's knowledge and food purchases. This review found that food advertising can, in specific contexts, decrease elementary school-aged children's ability to differentiate healthful products from non-healthful ones. Commercial food marketing also impacts children's food preferences. One study reviewed by Hastings et al. found that exposure to food advertising influenced children's self-reported food preferences, and a number of the studies reviewed by Hastings et al., have shown that food advertising influences children's food selection, either in school or at the grocery store.

Children's food preferences, influenced by advertising, can also influence purchasing and eating habits for their entire family (Center for Science in the Public Interest, 2003). The Center for Science in the Public Interest found that the amount of time a child spends watching television was a predictor of how often they requested a food or beverage product at the grocery store. A study conducted by the USA Weekend/Roper Report on Consumer Decision Making in American Families indicated that 78 percent of children influence where their family purchases fast food, 50 percent influence what their family consumes at home and 31 percent influence which brands their family purchase at the grocery store. When children strongly influence their family's purchasing and eating habits, foods selected tend to be less healthy (USA Weekend/Roper Report, 1989).

Food content in television shows and movies can also have an impact on adult and child eating behavior. High calorie-low nutrient food choices are much more likely than other types of food to be portrayed on television and in the movies, encouraging consumers to eat a diet that contributes to diabetes and obesity. A study of prime time television shows in 1998 revealed that references to food occurred nearly 10 times per hour and that the majority of references were for high calorie-low nutrient foods and beverages (Byrd-Bredbenner et al., 2003). Likewise, one study indicated that foods high in fat and sugar are disproportionately shown over fruits and vegetables in high grossing films (Bell, Berger, & Townsend, 2003).

Television and Food Intake

In addition to influencing food preferences and purchasing, television may also contribute to an increase in snacking while viewing. Preliminary studies in this area have shown that there may be a link between increased calorie intake and television viewing. One study found that families who watch more television are also more likely to consume a greater amount of their calories from junk foods than from fruits and vegetables (Coon, Goldberg, Rogers, & Tucker, 2001). Girls who have the television on during meal time have also been found to have higher calorie intakes than girls who did not watch television during meal time (McNutt et al., 1997).

Media and Body Image

Media play a role in shaping many cultural norms and has great influence on shaping norms around physical attractiveness. Overweight and obese television characters tend to be portrayed as unpopular and unsuccessful, while thin characters are portrayed as having more positive characteristics (Kaufman, 1980). There are fewer overweight and obese characters on television than exist in real life, and nearly a third of women on television are underweight (Greenberg, Eastin, Hofschire, Lachlan, & Brownell, 2003). However, depictions of overweight and obese television characters may vary by ethnicity. A study of four sitcoms with a predominately African American audience found a much higher prevalence of overweight or obese characters and a higher number of food commercials than sitcoms with a general audience (Tirodkar & Jain, 2003).

While there is little evidence that there is a direct association between television viewing and eating disorders, studies have shown that increased exposure to media is associated with higher levels of body dissatisfaction (Borzekowski, Robinson, & Killen, 2000). Since body dissatisfaction is associated with eating disorders, media may be indirectly linked to eating disorders. For example, Borzekowski et al. found that frequent music video viewing among adolescent girls may be a factor in increased perceived importance of appearance and an increase in weight concerns. In another study of girls in 5th through 12th grade, pictures in magazines had a strong impact on perceptions of weight and body shape (Field et al., 1999).

Media Promotion of Diets and Diet Products

Feelings of body dissatisfaction may cause many women and girls to turn to diets and diet products promoted by the media. Commercial marketing and advertising of diets and diet products is a major industry in the United States that can have an effect on body image and overweight status. Commercial marketers and advertisers promote everything from books to weight-loss shakes and bars. Commercials for these products often contain ultra-thin models and portray overweight people as unhealthy and lazy (Padgett & Biro, 2003).

Media and Physical Activity

The large amounts of time spent watching television or engaging in other sedentary media activities can decrease the time spent engaged in physical activity. Data from 1999 Nielsen surveys found that the average American over 12 years old watched television for more then 28 hours per week (Nielsen Media Research, 2000), but only 26.2 percent of U.S. adults are engaging in the recommended 30 minutes of moderate-intensity physical activity for five or more days per week (Brownson et al., 2005). While the research linking television viewing to physical activity levels is limited, we do have evidence that both youth and adults are not achieving the recommended levels of physical activity each day. According to the Youth Risk Behavior Surveillance System (YRBSS) roughly 24 percent of male and 38 percent of female high school students are inactive (Brownson et al., 2005; CDC, 2006). It is recommended that children and adolescents engage in 60 minutes of physical activity on most days of the week (CDC, 2006).

Media and Obesity Prevention

Using the media to raise public awareness, widely disseminate health education messages and advocate for changes in public policy have proven to be useful strategies for public health professionals. Major sources of news information about the obesity epidemic have helped to raise public awareness about the consequences of rapidly rising obesity rates. A poll of Californians conducted by Field Research for The California Endowment found that nearly all residents (92%) consider rising rates of obesity among children and teens to be a problem (Field Research Corporation, 2003). Social marketing and media advocacy are two public health strategies that use the media and may be important for obesity prevention.

Social Marketing

Social marketing involves the application of tools and techniques developed from private sector commercial marketing (Economos et al., 2001; Grier & Bryant, 2005). By using techniques like market research, product positioning, pricing, physical distribution and promotion, social marketing programs seek to influence the behavior of target audiences to improve their personal health. The VERB campaign is an example of a nationwide social marketing campaign focused on increasing the levels of physical activity among children (Wong et al., 2004)

Several social marketing campaigns, like the 5 A Day media campaign, the 1% Milk Campaign, and the national Project LEAN campaign have focused on promoting healthy eating. For example, the national Project LEAN campaign promoted low fat eating through public service announcements (PSAs) and various other communication channels. Findings from the campaign indicate that PSAs alone can generate increased awareness and demand for additional information. PSAs in combination with other public relations and communication strategies can generate greater media attention and awareness of the problem (Samuels, 1993). California Children's 5 A Day-Power Play! was a social marketing campaign aimed at increasing fruit and vegetable consumption among children and their families. The campaign used media in both schools and the community during a one year time frame (Foerster et al., 1998). At the end of the intervention there was an increase in the number of children who believed that they should be consuming more servings of fruits and vegetables per day and a slight increase in reported fruit and vegetable consumption among children in the intervention groups.

Similar to promoting healthy eating, mass media and social marketing campaigns have the potential to influence cultural norms and trends around physical activity. The VERB campaign, launched in 2002 by the Centers for Disease Control and Prevention (CDC), focused on reaching 9 to 13 year old children with the message that physical activity is "fun, cool, and socially appealing" (Huhman et al., 2005). Evaluation results indicated that the VERB campaign produced high levels of awareness and that many subgroups of children in the 9 to 13 age range reported increased levels of free-time physical activity (Huhman et al., 2005). Despite these promising results, long term funding for the VERB Campaign has not been obtained.

While social marketing campaigns have shown some effect in promoting healthy eating and activity in children (i.e., during developmental stages when habits are forming), success of social marketing interventions with adults have been limited (Alcalay & Bell, 2000). In addition, social marketing campaigns are costly, and their funding agencies usually have limited budgets in comparison to food marketers and advertisers. For example, Coca Cola spent $277 million on advertising in 1997 (Jacobson, 1998), while the National Institutes of Health/National Cancer Institute had a total budget of $1 million to promote the 5 A Day media message (Gallo, 1999).

Alcalay and Bell (2000), in their report on *Promoting Nutrition and Physical Activity through Social Marketing*, present several recommendations for improving social marketing interventions. These authors suggest that social marketing interventions are most effectively used to promote prevention to individuals who have not yet formed unhealthy habits, should focus on the environmental influence on people's health, and should work to promote environments more conducive to healthy eating and activity. Carroll, Craypo, and Samuels (2000) also suggest that due to the challenges of changing individual behaviors through social marketing, interventions should be of substantial duration and complemented with policy approaches to maximize the possible impact and benefits.

Media Advocacy

Media advocacy is the strategic use of mass media to support community organizing and advance healthy public policy (Chapman & Lupton, 1994; Wallack et al., 1993, 1999). It differs fundamentally from traditional public health campaigns and social marketing. However, in practice, media advocacy uses some of the same media relations techniques that practitioners of social marketing or public information campaigns might use: sending out news releases, pitching stories to journalists, monitoring the media and keeping a list of media contacts, and paying attention to what is newsworthy. Winett and Wallack (1996) note that media advocacy's purpose is to put pressure on policy makers and reframe public debate on key public health issues. The focus of a media advocacy campaign is to set the agenda and shape the debate to include policy solutions in news coverage of health issues. Media advocacy targets policy makers, other advocates, and community members who can become active in the political process of making change. In the case of preventing obesity, media advocacy has been used for advocating for policy change in schools or neighborhoods to increase access to healthy foods and reduce access to high calorie-low nutrient foods, as opposed to promoting consumption of healthier foods directly to students or residents, which would be better suited to social marketing. For example, in 2000, the release of a report on the prevalence of fast foods on California high school campuses (Craypo et al., 2002) brought the issue to the attention of state law makers and resulted in the introduction and passage of legislation to reduce access to high calorie-low nutrient foods on school campuses.

Media advocacy differs from other types of health communication because it seeks change in the social, physical, or policy environment surrounding individuals, rather than seeking change in individual behavior. Thus, the "target audience" for media advocacy efforts will be a policy maker or body who has decision-making capabilities, such as a school board determining whether to allow sodas to be sold in campus vending machines. This is a fundamentally different understanding of the target than is used in most health communications where the target is the person with the problem. It is often the best media strategy choice when the overall strategy involves changing policy (Dorfman, 2003).

In fact, because most public health problems are complicated and deeply imbedded in social organization and behavior routines, they require long-term and evolving communications strategies. Preventing obesity will require motivation for individuals to adopt healthy eating behavior and active living; social marketing campaigns may help inform them about the most effective ways to do that. But to be successful, people will need affordable access to healthy food, and environments that encourage activity, conditions that will require policy change in many communities. Media advocacy is likely to be a very useful tool to help public health advocates make the case to policy makers for those policies. Public health practitioners need to know which communication strategies are suited to which goals.

Working with Entertainment Media

The media environment is both diverse and specialized, and there are many places for public health professionals to try to leverage opportunities for improving individual and population health. In addition to using social marketing and media advocacy, health organizations have partnered with the entertainment industry to incorporate healthful behaviors into television programs around topics such as pregnancy prevention, substance abuse prevention, and HIV/AIDS. The Henry J. Kaiser Family Foundation (KFF) has partnered with television entertainment programming in order to convey health messages to television viewers; KFF partnered with the hospital-based drama ER to get factual health information into episode story lines (Brodie et al., 2001). KFF also worked with MTV to produce programming that included health messages for youth.

Media and Public Policy

Policy strategies to address the role of media in the obesity epidemic are under consideration in Congress and state legislatures across the country. For example, Senator Tom Harkin introduced legislation in May 2005 that would, among other provisions, restore the authority of the FTC to regulate the advertising and marketing of food and beverage products to children (U.S. Senate, May 18, 2005). Also in 2005, Senator Joseph Lieberman introduced a bill to establish a research program in the National Institute of Child Health and Human Development "to study the role and impact of electronic media in the development of children" (U.S. Senate, March 9, 2005). Increasing the understanding of the impact of both newer and older types of media on children may provide further avenues for intervening to protect and promote child health and wellness. Organizations, like Children Now, maintain active programs in media as it specifically affects children and seek regulatory and policy changes to make sure media interactions are healthful and not harmful (Children Now, 2006).

Conclusions

While many efforts have attempted to use media to positively impact physical activity and nutrition behaviors, media play a large role in promoting overeating and sedentary behavior. Both children and adults are targets of intensive commercial marketing campaigns promoting soda, fast foods, and high-calorie snacks, along with passive leisure-time activities, including TV, movies, and video games. Portrayals of food, physical activity, and body image in news and entertainment media also have an influence on poor nutrition choices and sedentary behavior.

On the health promotion and policy sides, strategies, like social marketing and media advocacy, have been used to influence individual health behaviors and broader policy adoption to sustain environmental changes that support good health. Strategies for creating a media environment more supportive of health and wellness will take sustained efforts on the part of public health practitioners and other professionals and community advocates, acting at local, state, and national levels to address the spectrum and variety of media influences in our daily lives. With increased awareness and understanding of the presence and impact of media, increased opportunities abound for public health to be proactive and engaged with this important component of the broader social environment.

References

Alcalay, R., & Bell, R. (2000). *Promoting nutrition and physical activity through social marketing: Current practices and recommendations*. Davis, CA: Center for Advanced Studies in Nutrition and Social Marketing, University of California.

Applbaum, A., & Gould, S. (1981). *Mike Pertschuk and the Federal Trade Commission*. Kennedy School of Government; President and Fellows of Harvard College. Cambridge, MA

Arbitron. (2006). Radio today: How America listens to radio. http://www.arbitron.com/downloads/radiotoday06.pdf.

Baughman, J. L. (1992). *The republic of mass culture: Journalism, filmmaking and broadcasting in American since 1941*. Baltimore, MD: Johns Hopkins University Press.

Bell, R., Berger, C., & Townsend, M. (2003). *Portrayals of nutritional practices and exercise behavior in popular American films, 1991–2000*. Davis, CA: Center for Advanced Studies of Nutrition and Social Marketing, University of California.

Brodie, M., Foehr, U., Rideout, V., Baer, N., Miller, C., & Flournoy, R., et al. (2001). Communicating health information through the entertainment media; A study of the television drama ER lends support to the notion that Americans pick up information while being entertained. *Health Affairs, 20*(1), 192–199.

Borzekowski, D. L., Robinson, T., & Killen, J. (2000). Does the camera add 10 pounds? Media use, perceived importance of appearance, and weight concerns among teenage girls. *Journal of Adolescent Health, 26*, 36–41.

Brown, J. D., & Walsh-Childers, K. (2002). Effects of media on personal and public health. In J. Bryant, & D. Zillman (Eds.), *Media effects: Advances in theory and research* (2nd ed., pp. 453–488). Mahwah, NJ: Lawrence Erlbaum Associates.

Brownson, R. C., Boehmer, T. K., & Luke, D. A. (2005). Declining rates of physical activity in the United States. *Annual Review of Public Health, 26,* 421–443.

Byrd-Bredbenner, C., Finkenor, M., & Grasso, D. (2003). Health related content in prime-time television programming. *Journal of Health Communication, 8,* 329–341.

Carroll, A., Craypo, L., & Samuels, S. (2000). *Evaluating nutrition and physical activity social marketing campaigns: A review of the literature for use in community campaigns.* Davis, CA: University of California, Center for Advanced Studies in Nutrition and Social Marketing.

Center for Digital Democracy. (2001). *TV that watches you: The prying eyes of interactive television.* http://www.democraticmedia.org/privacyreport.pdf.

Center for Media Literacy. (2006). About CML. Retrieved April 13, 2006, from http://www.medialit.org.

Center for Science in the Public Interest. (2003). *Pestering parents: How food companies market obesity to children.* http://www.cspinet.org/pesteringparents.

Centers for Disease Control and Prevention. (2006). http://www.cdc.gov/nccdphp/dnpa/physical/recommendations/young.htm.

Children's Advertising Review Unit (CARU). (2006). Retrieved March 3, 2006, from http://www.caru.org.

Chapman, S., & Lupton, D. (1994). *The fight for public health: Principles and practice of media advocacy.* London: BMJ Publishing Group.

Children Now. (2006). http://www.childrennow.org/.

Committee on Food Marketing and the Diets of Children and Youth, Food and Nutrition Board, Board on Children, Youth, and Families. (2006). Food marketing to children and youth: Threat or opportunity? Washington, DC: Institute of Medicine, National Academies Press.

Coon, K. A., Goldberg, J., Rogers, B. L., & Tucker, K. L. (2001). Relationships between use of television during meals and children's food consumption patterns. *Pediatrics, 107*(1), E7.

Coon, K. A., & Tucker, K. L. (2002). Television and children's consumption patterns. A review of the literature. *Minerva Pediatr, 54,* 423–436.

Crapyo, L., Purcell, A., Samuels, S. E., Agron, P., Bell, E., & Takada, E. (2002). Fast food sales on high school campuses: Results from the 2000 Californian high school fast food survey. *Journal of School Health, 72*(2), 78–82.

Dorfman, L. (2003). Using media advocacy to influence policy. In R. J. Bensley, & J. Brookins-Fisher (Eds.), *Community health education methods: A practitioner's guide* (2nd ed., chapter 15). Sudbury, MA: Jones & Bartlett Publishers.

Dorfman, L., & Wallack, L. (1993, November–December). Advertising health: The case for counter-ads. *Public Health Reports, 108*(6), 716–726

Dorfman, L., & Wallack, L. (2007, March–April). Moving nutrition upstream: The case for reframing obesity. *Journal of Nutrition Education and Behavior, 39*(suppl. 2), S45–50..

Duerksen, S. C., Mikail, A., Tom, L., Patton, A., & Lopez, J. (2005). Health disparities and advertising content of women's magazines: A cross-sectional study. *BMC Public Health, 5*(85). http://www.biomedcentral.com/1471-2458/5/85.

Economos, C. D., Brownson, R. C., DeAngelis, M. A., Novelli, P., Foerster, S. B., & Foreman, C. T., et al. (2001). What lessons have been learned from other attempts to guide social change? *Nutrition Reviews, 59*(3, Pt. 2), S40–S56; discussion S57–S65.

Editor and Publisher Yearbook. (2003). http://www.editorandpublisher.com/eandp/resources/yearbook.jsp

Federal Communications Commission (FCC). Retrieved March 3, 2006, from http://www.fcc.gov.

Federal Trade Commission (FTC). Retrieved March 3, 2006, from http://www.ftc.gov.

Field, A. E., Cheung, L., Wolf, A. M., Herzog, D. B., Gortmaker, S. L., & Colditz, G. A. (1999). Exposure to the mass media and weight concerns among girls. *Pediatrics*, *103*, e36.

Field Research Corporation. (2003). *A survey of Californians about the problem of childhood obesity*. Conducted for the California Endowment. http://www.calendow.org/reference/publications/pdf/disparities/TCE1126-2003_A_Survey_of_Ca.pdf

Foerster, S. B., Gregson, J., Beall, D. L., Hudes, M., Magnuson, H., Livingston, S., et al. (1998). The California children's 5 a day-power play! campaign: Evaluation of a large scale social marketing initiative. *Family and Community Health*, *21*(1), 46–64.

Gantz, W., Schwartz, N., Angelini, J. R., Rideout, V. (2007). Food for thought: Television food advertising to children in the United States. Menlo Park, CA: The Henry J. Kaiser Family Foundation.

Gallo, A. E. (1999). Food advertising in the United States. In E. Frazao (Ed.), *America's eating habits: Changes and consequences* (pp. 173–180). Washington, DC: USDA, Economic Research Service.

Greenberg, B., Eastin, M., Hofschire, L., Lachlan, K., & Brownell, K. (2003). Portrayals of overweight and obese individuals on commercial television. *American Journal of Public Health*, *8*, 1342–1348.

Grier, S., & Bryant, C. A. (2005). Social marketing in public health. *Annu Rev Public Health*, *26*, 319–339.

Hastings, G., Stead, M., McDermott, L., Forsyth, A., Macintosh, A. M., Rayner, M., et al. (2003). *Review of research on the effects of food promotion to children. Prepared for the food standards agency*. Glasgow, Scotland UK: Center for Social Marketing, University of Strathclyde.

Hawkes, C. (2004). Marketing food to children: The global regulatory environment. Geneva, Switzerland: World Health Organization. http://whqlibdoc.who.int/publications/2004/9241591579.pdf

Henderson, V. R., & Kelly, B. (2005). Food advertising in the age of obesity: Content analysis of food advertising on general market and African American television. *J Nutr Educ Behav*, *37*(4), 191–196.

Henry J. Kaiser Family Foundation. (2004, February). *The role of media in childhood obesity*. http://www.kff.org/entmedia/upload/The-Role-Of-Media-in-Childhood-Obesity.pdf

Huhman, M., Potter, L. D., Wong, F. L., Banspach, S. W., Duke, J. C., & Heitzler, C. D. (2005). Effects of a mass media campaign to increase physical activity among children: Year-1 results of the VERB campaign. *Pediatrics*, *116*(2), e277–e284.

International Food Information Council. (2004). *Trends in obesity-related media coverage*. Washington, DC: International Food Information Council. http://www.ific.org/research/obesitytrends.cfm.

Jacobson, M. (1998). Liquid candy: How soft drinks are harming Americans health. http://www.cspinet.org/sodapop.

Kaufman, L. (1980). Prime-time nutrition. *Journal of Communication*, *30*, 37–46.

Kelly, B. (2005). To quell obesity, who should regulate food marketing to children? *Globalization and Health*, *1*, 9. http://www.globalizationandhealth.com/content/1/1/9.

Kersh, R., & Morone, J. A. (2005, October). Obesity, courts, and the new politics of public health. *Journal of Health Politics, Policy and Law*, *30*(5), 839–868.

Kotz, K., & Story, M. (1994). Food advertisements during children's Saturday morning television programming: Are they consistent with dietary recommendations? *Journal of the American Dietetic Association*, *94*, 1296–1300.

Kubey, R., & Csikszentmihalyi, M. (1990). *Television and the quality of life: How viewing shapes everyday experience*. Hillsdale, NJ: Lawrence Erlbaum Associates.

Lewis, J., & Jhally, S. (1998, Winter). The struggle over media literacy. *Journal of Communication, 48*, 1.

Lumeng, J., Rahnama, S., Appugliese, D., Kaciroti, N., & Bradley, R. (2006). Television exposure and overweight risk in preschoolers. *Archives of Pediatric and Adolescent Medicine, 160*, 417–422.

McCombs, M., & Shaw, D. (1972–1973). The agenda setting function of mass media. *Public Opinion Quarterly, 36*, 176–187.

McNutt, S. W., Hu, Y., Schreiber, G. B., Crawford, P. B., Obarzanek, E., & Mellin, L. A. (1997). Longitudinal study of dietary practice of black and white girls 9- and 10-year-old at enrollment: The NHLBI growth and health study. *Adolescent Health, 20*, 27–7.

Mediamark Research. (2006). Magazine Audience Estimates 1995–2003. http://www.mediamark.com.

Montgomery, K., & Pasnik, S. (1996). *Web of deception*. Washington, DC: Center for Media Education.

Montgomery, K. C. (2000). Children's media culture in the new millennium: Mapping the digital landscape. *The Future of Children, 10*, 145–167.

Montgomery, K. C. (2001). Digital kids: The new online children's consumer culture. In D. G. Singer & J. L. Singer (Eds.), *Handbook of children and the media* (pp. 635–650). Thousand Oaks, CA: Sage Publications.

Nestle, M. (2003). *Food politics: How the food industry influences nutrition and health*. Berkeley, CA: University of California Press.

Nielsen Media Research, Inc. (2000). *2000 Report on television*. http://www.nielsenmedia.com

Nielson Media Research, Inc. (2005). *Nielsen reports American watch TV at record levels. News release*. http://www.nielsenmedia.com/newsrelease/2005/AvgHoursMinutes92905.pdf

Outley, C., & Taddess, A. (2006). A content analysis of health and physical activity messages marketed to African American children during after-school television programming. *Archives of Pediatric and Adolescent Medicine, 160*, 432–435.

Padgett, J., & Biro, F. (2003). Different shapes in different cultures: Body dissatisfaction, overweight, and obesity in African-American and Caucasian females. *Journal of Pediatric Adolescent Gynecology, 16*, 349–354.

Pew Internet & American Life Project. (2005). *Internet: The mainstreaming of online life*. http://www.pewinternet.org/pdfs/Internet_Status_2005.pdf.

Rideout, V., & Hoff, T. (2002). *Shouting to be heard: Public service advertising in a new media age*. Menlo Park, CA: Kaiser Family Foundation. Publication #3152.

Rideout, V., Foehr, U., Roberts, D., & Brodie, M. (1999). *Kids and media at the new millennium*. Menlo Park, CA: Kaiser Family Foundation.

Roberts, D. (2004). *Kids and media in America*. New York: Cambridge University Press.

Samuels, S. E., Craypo, L., Dorfman, L., Purciel, M., & Standish, M. B. (2003, November). Food and beverage industry marketing practices aimed at children: Developing strategies for preventing obesity and diabetes. A report on the proceedings from a meeting sponsored by the California Endowment held in San Francisco in June of 2003. http://www.calendow.org/reference/publications/pdf/disparities/TCE1101-2003_Food_and_Bever.pdf

Samuels, S. E. (1993). Project LEAN-lessons learned from a national social marketing campaign. *Public Health Reports, 108*, 45–53.

Schlesinger, M. (2005, October). Editor's note: Weighting for Godot. *Journal of Health Politics, Policy and Law, 30*(5), 785–801.

The State of the News Media, (2004). Journalism.org. http://www.stateofthenewsmedia.org/

The State of the News Media, (2006). Journalism.org. http://www.stateofthemedia.org/2006

Tirodkar, M., & Jain, A. (2003). Food messages on African American television show. *American Journal of Public Health*, *93*(3), 439–441.

USA Weekend/The Roper Organization. (1989). *A USA Weekend/Roper report on consumer decision-making in American families*. New York, NY.

U.S. Census Bureau. (2003). Computer and Internet Use in the United States. http://www.census.gov/prod/2005pubs/p23-208.pdf.

U.S. Department of Agriculture, Food and Nutrition Services. (2006). Newsroom, Radio Features. http://www.fns.usda.gov/cga/radio/radio.htm.

U.S. Department of State. (1997). Chapter 12: The media and their messages. In *Portrait of America*. http://usinfo.state.gov/usa/infousa/facts/factover/ch12.htm

U.S. Senate. 109th Congress, 1st Session. S. 579, A Bill to amend the Public Health Service Act to authorize funding for the establishment of a program on children and the media within the National Institute of Child Health and Human Development to study the role and impact of electronic media in the development of children. [Introduced in the U.S. Senate; March 9, 2005]. Congressional Bills, Library of Congress, Thomas. http://thomas.loc.gov/cgi-bin/query/z?c109:S.579.

U.S. Senate. 109th Congress, 1st Seassion. S. 1074, A Bill to improve the health of Americans and reduce health care costs by reorienting the Nation's health care system toward prevention, wellness, and self care. [Introduced in the U.S. Senate; May 18, 2005]. Congressional Bills, Library of Congress, Thomas. http://thomas.loc.gov/cgi-bn/query/z?c109:S.1074.

Wallack, L., Dorfman, L., Jernigan, D., & Themba, M. (1993). *Media advocacy and public health: Power for prevention*. Newbury Park, CA: Sage Publications.

Wallack, L., Woodruff, K., Dorfman, L., & Diaz, I. (1999). *News for a change: An advocates' guide to working with the media*. Thousand Oaks, CA: Sage Publications.

Winett, L., & Wallack, L. (1996). Advancing public health goals through the mass media. *Journal of Health Communication*, 1, 173–196.

Wong, F., Huhman, M., Heitzler, C., Asbury, L., Bretthauer-Mueller, R., & McCarthy, S., et al. (2004, July). VERB – A social marketing campaign to increase physical activity among youth. *Prev Chronic Dis*, *1*(3), A10. Epub 2004 Jun 15.

Chapter 11

Global Context of Obesity

Barry M. Popkin

Introduction

The rapid shifts in diet and physical activity and obesity that are occurring are not unique to the United States though they might have begun a bit earlier here than in other regions of the world. However both in the United States and globally we have seen an acceleration in these shifts in the past 15–20 years (Popkin, 2002; Popkin et al., 2005). With such rapid change occurring across the world—both in the higher income more industrialized countries as well as in the set of transitional middle income and lower income developing countries—we can look to the global situation to understand broader changes and consequently, to better understand what might be changing in the U.S. and why. Essentially what appears to be happening is that global forces are more and more dictating our food prices, the technology available for work, transport and leisure, and a great deal of other forces that affect the nature of our diet.

Globalization is a concept that very much relates to the focus on freer and more rapid movement of capital, technology, goods, and services. It captures the profound effects on lifestyles that are linked with diet, activity, and subsequent imbalances that have led to the obesity epidemic (Popkin, 2006). The freer movement of these factors is linked in quite complex ways, with very rapid shifts in dietary and activity patterns seen on a global level (Popkin, 2003). These globalization-related changes are taking place particularly fast in the low- and middle-income countries of the developing world. Adult obesity levels are increasing far more rapidly than in the higher-income countries; overweight and obesity levels of some lower-income developing countries match, or exceed, those of the United States (Popkin, 2003). Currently, child obesity is reaching high levels at a rapid rate in many higher-income countries, but is still relatively less common in the lower- and middle-income developing countries (Lobstein et al., 2004).

While many researchers have placed the global food production, marketing, and distribution sector (including soft drinks, fast food, and other multinational food companies) at the center of blame for these changes, there are other profound, and equally responsible factors that must be understood to enact effective public policy to address them (Brownell & Horgan, 2004). Moreover, there is much heterogeneity in the nature of changes in diets and activity patterns across the globe, though the results of a more energy dense, higher added sugar diet and more sedentarianism might be common to all (Popkin, 1998; Popkin & Adair, 2005). These other factors include: (a) the worldwide shifts in trade of technology innovations that affect energy expenditures during leisure, transportation, and work; (b) globalization of modern food processing, marketing and distribution techniques (most frequently linked with western-ization of the world's diet); (c) vast expansion of the global mass media; and (d) other changes that constitute the rubric of impacts resulting from an increased opening of our world economy.

Globalization has certainly enhanced the interconnectedness of the world in terms of trade in goods, technology, services, and spread of the modern mass media. These changes occurred in the last half of the previous century and were accelerated by the push from the higher-income countries for more open markets for these items. During this period, international agencies (e.g., the International Monetary Fund (IMF) and the World Bank) and most of the higher-income countries, have promoted a "free trade" agenda as the panacea for the ills of the developing world. This chapter does not focus on the exact linkages between each aspect of globalization and how it affects the increased trade in services, commodities, processed products, technology, and invest-ments; rather, the focus is on understanding how technological and other shifts are linked to, and affect diet, activity, and obesity throughout the world. It is impossible at this time, with the available databases, to fully link each aspect of globalization exactly to each one of these elements. We can, however, doc-ument many threads of change that clearly relate to their global shifts.

A range of studies published during the last few years have laid out the basic patterns of change globally. Briefly we summarize some of the key dimensions of global obesity shifts. The vast majority of the nationally representative data is on adults but we do add some information on children. The chapter then addresses some of the major global forces underlying these changes. Else-where we have addressed the dietary changes (Drewnowski & Popkin, 1997; Popkin & Nielsen, 2003; Popkin & Adair, 2005) and physical activity patterns (Popkin, 1999; Bell et al., 2001; Bell et al., 2002).

The Global Obesity Pandemic

Not only is the high prevalence of overweight and obesity in many developing countries of particular importance, but also the quite rapid rate of change. There are few developing countries that have comparable, nationally-representative or random samples of adults who have been directly weighed and measured. Figure 11.1, Panel A presents the prevalence rates for a few countries showing varying levels of development; countries such as Egypt, Mexico, and the Black (African) population of South Africa have a similar overweight and obesity profile with the United States. Figure 11.1, Panel B presents, for a set of coun-tries with comparable data at two points in time, the percentage of the adult population that is becoming overweight in each year (if a linear pattern of growth in overweight prevalence is assumed). For instance, Panel B shows that 2.4% of the adult Mexican female population becomes overweight each year, while among U.S. adult women, only 0.39% become overweight each year. The shifts in becoming overweight for the larger countries with populations over a

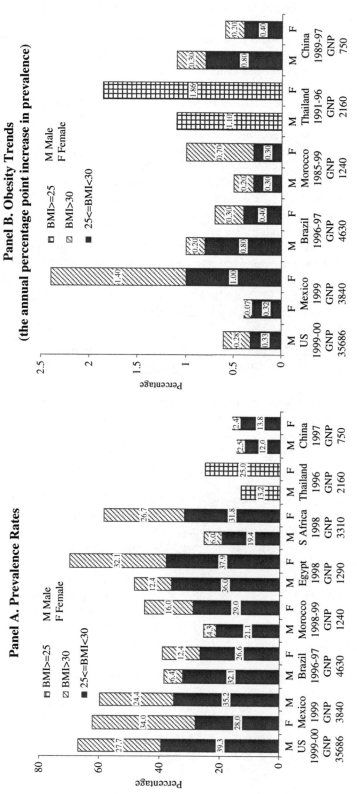

Figure 11.1 Obesity Patterns and Trends Across the World, Adults Aged 20 and Older.

Source: Popkin (2002a).

hundred million (e.g., Brazil, China, and Thailand) are also much greater than for the United States. The gross national incomes per capita are added to show for Panel A and B how the U.S. compares with these other countries. The situation is so different in the Eastern Europe and the former Soviet Union that we do not present these data here (Wang et al., 2002; Jahns et al., 2003). Identically manipulated data for Western Europe and Australia show very high rates of change for both the United Kingdom and Australia (Popkin et al., 2006).

While many scholars have felt that these shifts in obesity were limited to urban areas and that most of the developing world faces much greater underweight than overweight problems of malnutrition, this is no longer the case (at least among women of child-bearing age) (Mendez et al., 2005). Data on the body mass index (BMI) distribution are the only nutrition-related data available on a nationally representative comparable basis for many countries; dietary intake and physical activity patterns and trends are available for few countries. Figure 11.2 presents (for a set of countries with identical methods of measuring weight and height for women of child-bearing age) data on underweight and overweight. As shown, far more obesity (than underweight) is found in rural and urban areas in most countries; however, underweight in rural regions of Haiti, India, and a few subSaharan countries exceeds obesity (Mendez et al., 2005).

A Rapid Shift in Technology Innovations for Work and Transportation is Occurring

In the higher income fully industrialized countries, we have increasingly become aware of the vast set of changes in how we move and work. Included are seemingly small changes such as the use of elevators and escalators instead of stairs, the use of electric food mixers, food processors, and blenders instead of hand preparation of food, the purchase of prepared dishes that replace home preparation of food, the use of television remote controls, and many other such minor changes (Lanningham-Foster et al., 2003). Similarly, we can imagine how a farmer or factory worker undertook his/her work in the 1940s. It was arduous and very energy intensive. Today these tasks are automated—both occupations are more sedentary than many in the service sector. Similarly, the computer, internet, and many other technological changes have diminished the energy expenditures of all service sector and professional employees. The same is true for travel—the car replaced the bus which replaced walking and leisure—where television and computer games and other sedentary activities dominate and have replaced more active activities (note: leisure has increased as a proportion of the day and replaced food preparation, cleaning, and many other physical activities and also has become more sedentary in itself).

The middle income transitional and lower income developing economies are going through similar shifts. However, the changes are occurring very rapidly. Even in 1980 most lower income country farmers did all activities by hand, people walked or biked everywhere, and all aspects of food preparation required extensive time and energy. In the new millennium, jobs in urban areas are comparable often in use of technology to those in the United States and some cities around the developing world are as modern as any in the United States (e.g., Shanghai, China). Food in urban areas is processed as often as in

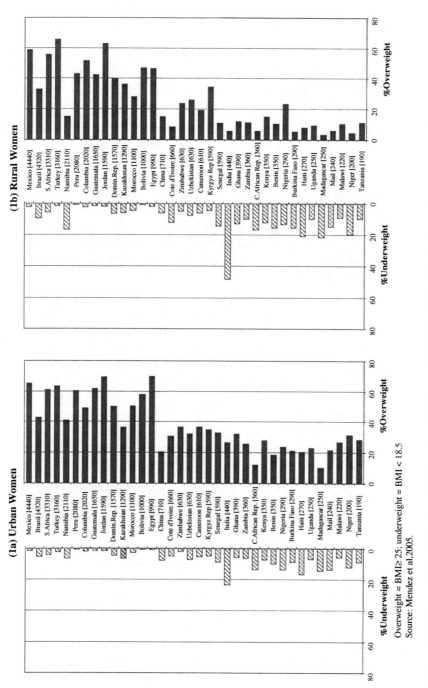

Figure 11.2 Overweight and Underweight Prevalence in Women 20–49y in 36 Developing Countries Ranked by Gross National Income (GNI) Per Capita.

Overweight = BMI ≥25; underweight = BMI <18.5

Source: Mendez et al, 2005.

Europe and the United States, walking is being limited, and television and computers abound. In rural areas, mechanization of most farming activities from the spreading of fertilizer and insecticides to plowing with tiny powered plows to the use of tractors and trucks has replaced most labor intensive activities (which also tend to use much higher level of energy expenditure per minute). There are a few countries with data that allow scholars to document these changes and examine their impact. For example, the China Health and Nutrition Survey has been longitudinally observing 16,000 adults and children since 1989 with repeated surveys in 1991, 1993, 1997, 2000, 2004, and 2006 of the same communities and individuals. The following relationships have been observed in China:

– Adults who purchased motor scooters/motor bikes or cars to travel to work doubled their likelihood of becoming overweight, in comparison to those that made no change in their mode of transportation (Bell et al., 2002).
– Occupational changes accounted for a significant proportion of the weight gain and incident overweight of Chinese adults, especially in urban areas (Bell et al., 2001).
– In a four year period, 16% of Chinese adults' overall work-related physical activity patterns in urban areas shifted significantly to lighter activity, a shift related to significant increases in BMI and overweight (Paeratakul et al., 1998; Popkin, 1999).

Among all adults in the developing world, there was a significant increase in the proportion working in service sector jobs and a large decrease in those involved in farming, forestry and mining—very strenuous occupations (Popkin, 1999). Several recent very thorough secondary analyses of trends in the United States show some of the shifts in occupations linked with activity patterns (Sturm, 2004; Brownson et al., 2005). There is limited evidence on adult physical activity trends in other countries, but what evidence does exist, seems to mirror the Chinese and lesser documented U.S. experience.

The Food System has Changed Equally Fast

Two important examples of the changes in the global food system are found in (a) the rapid increase in consumption of low-cost edible vegetable oils and (b) the way large supermarkets and supermarket chains have gained control of food distribution. One of the earliest food system changes provided inexpensive, readily available oils and related commodities to the developing world; the result being that lower-income countries can now consume fat levels equivalent to the consumption in higher-income countries (Drewnowski & Popkin, 1997).

The edible vegetable oils story is particularly important as its effects have been quite profound. Until the decade following World War II, the majority of fats available for human consumption were animal fats, milk, butter, and meat. Subsequently, a revolution in the production and processing of oilseed-based fats occurred. Principal vegetable oils include soybean, sunflower, rapeseed, palm, and peanut oil. Technological breakthroughs in the development of high-yield oilseeds and in the refining of high-quality vegetable oils greatly reduced the cost of baking and frying fats, margarine, butter-like spreads, salad oils, and cooking oils in relation to animal-based products (Williams, 1984).

Worldwide demand for vegetable fats was fueled by health concerns regarding the consumption of animal fats and cholesterol. Furthermore, a number of major economic and political initiatives led to the development of oil crops, not only in Europe and the United States, but in South East Asia (palm oils), in Brazil, and in Argentina (soybean oils). The net effect was that from 1945 to 1965, there was almost a fourfold increase in the U.S. production of vegetable oils, while animal fat production increased by only 11% (USDA, 1966).

In developing nations, one of the earliest shifts toward a higher-fat diet began with major increases in the domestic production and imports of oilseeds and vegetable oils, rather than increased imports of meat and milk. With the exception of peanut oil, global availability of the vegetable oils (i.e., soybean, sunflower, rapeseed, and palm) has approximately tripled from 1961 to 1990. Soybeans now account for the bulk of vegetable oil consumption worldwide. An additional concern related to the consumption of these oils is that some contain high levels of transfatty acids as in India. In China, many of these oils are highly pathogenic, containing high levels of rapeseed oil (or $C22:1w9$ *cis*, erucic acid) (Wallingford et al., 2004).

The other important change in the global food system is occurring in food distribution. The fresh market (in the agricultural field these are termed "wet markets", as none of the food is processed or sealed and often even the animal portions are live) is disappearing as the major source of supply for food in the developing world. Fresh food markets are being replaced by multinational, regional, and local large supermarkets – supermarkets which are usually part of larger chains (e.g., Carrefour or Wal-Mart) or, in other countries such as South Africa and China, by local domestic chains patterned to function and look like these global chains (Reardon et al., 2004). Increasingly, large megastores are found. For example, in Latin America, supermarkets' share of all retail food sales increased from 15% in 1990 to 60% by 2000 (Reardon, 2003). For comparison, 80% of retail food sales in the United States in 2000 occurred in supermarkets. In one decade, the role of supermarkets in Latin America has expanded equivalent to about a half century of expansion in the United States. Supermarket use has spread across both large and small countries, from capital cities to rural villages, and from upper- and middle-class families to the working class (Hu, 2004). This same process is also occurring at varying rates and different stages in Asia, Eastern Europe, and Africa.

There are many factors causing this food system phenomenon (Wilkinson, 2004). Consumer demand for processed and safer foods is on the rise in developing countries. Additionally, as countries modernize, the opportunity cost of women's time has grown; building a market for time-saving, prepared foods has become more important. Transportation and access to technology, such as refrigerators, have also played a role in the demand for, and access to, supermarkets. Other factors include the liberalization of direct foreign investment, trade liberalization, and the saturation of Western markets that has pushed growing companies into other locales. Furthermore, improvements in the logistics and procurement systems used by the supermarkets have allowed them to compete on cost with the more typical outlets in developing countries: the small "mom-and-pop" stores and wet markets (open public markets) for fruits, vegetables, and all other products.

Supermarkets are large providers of processed higher-fat, added-sugar, and salt-laden foods in developing countries, but they have also been the purveyors of some good. For example, supermarkets (a) were instrumental in the development of radioactively treated milk, giving it a long shelf life and providing a safe source of milk for all income groups and (b) were key players in establishing food safety standards (Balsevich et al., 2003). Most importantly, they have solved the cold chain and in many instances have brought higher-quality produce to the urban consumer throughout the year.

Mass Media Changes are Equally Profound

One of the least discussed and least understood areas of change affecting dietary and physical activity patterns is the role of the modern mass media. Throughout the developing world, there has been a profound increase in the ownership of television sets and the penetration of modern television programming (International Broadcasting Audience Research, 2004). This has been accompanied by a proliferation of modern magazines and ready access to DVDs of Western movies. To date, documentation of the health implications of this phenomenon is limited. Examples from China are used to illustrate this set of changes.

Television (TV) set ownership and modern TV programmings are recent phenomena in China. In China, less than two-thirds (63%) of households owned a TV in 1989, and most (49%) owned a black and white set. By 2000, more than 91% of Chinese households owned a TV, with most (68%) owning a color set (Du et al., 2002).

TV use in China is still lower than in the United States. While the majority of American children watched more than five hours of TV a day in the late 1990s, the average Chinese child spent about an hour a day watching TV and/ or playing video games. Only about 10% watched TV more than one hour a day, and fewer than 5% played video games for more than one hour (Tudor-Locke et al., 2003).

Programming and advertisements have been rapidly shifting toward more modern and Western content. For instance, the first TV advertisements in China began with one advertisement in 1979 on a Shanghai TV station and only began in earnest with a large increase in the 1990s. Today, China is considered the world's fastest growing advertising market (Weber, 2000).

Similar increases in TV ownership and viewership are noted throughout the developing world (International Broadcasting Audience Research, 2004).

What About Multinational "Fast Food" and Soft-Drink Companies–Do These Sectors of the Food Industry Have any Responsibility?

There is a view among some researchers that the U.S. fast food sector and soft drink industry have led to the declines of diets throughout the developing world (Brownell and Horgan, 2004; Lobstein et al., 2004). The growth of American food companies has certainly spread across the globe. Coca-Cola is sold in more than 200 countries and more than half of McDonald's sales are made outside the United States. Many other examples can be found to show that the McDonald's, Pizza Huts, and Kentucky Fried Chicken restaurants are rapidly spreading across the globe. They are quickly followed, or even preceded, by local food chains that follow their models, even to the point of serving the same dishes and being equally hygienic and efficient.

Major questions include: What are these companies doing to impact the diet of the developing world? Are they leading people away from their healthy traditional diets to higher-fat and added sugar-laden away-from-home prepared food products? Are they leading to increased portion sizes worldwide, as they have in the United States? The answer might be "yes" or "no", depending on which country you study and how you examine the data.

On one hand, research which collected individual dietary intake data in detailed, precise ways for large representative samples of children from the Philippines, Russia, and China (together with U.S. data), shows very mixed results (Popkin and Adair, 2005). The most noticeable difference among these countries is in the intake of away from home food. United States and Filipino youth consume more than a third of their total daily calories from foods prepared away-from-home (see Figure 11.3). More meals are purchased away-from-home, and either eaten away (in restaurants or fast food establishments in the United States), or brought home from small cafeterias and street vendors as in the Philippine city of Cebu. In contrast, Chinese children consume very little of their total energy from foods prepared or eaten away-from-home, although more snack foods are purchased away-from-home. Chinese snack foods are typically a biscuit, some peanuts, or fruit. Eating in restaurants is rare among Chinese families and there is not a tradition of purchasing inexpensive foods from street vendors, as is the case of Cebu. Similarly, in Russia, there is not yet a tradition of bringing ready-prepared foods into the home, nor is there a prevalent practice of taking children to eat in restaurants.

The Philippines is not alone in its high consumption of soft drinks. There are other countries, such as Mexico, where supersized U.S. soft drinks have had a major effect on diets (Arroyo et al., 2004).

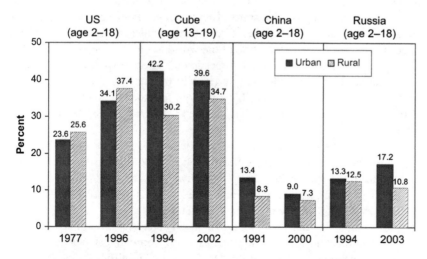

Figure 11.3 The Proportion of Energy Consumed From Foods Prepared Away from Home by Urban-Rural Residence.

Source: Adair and Popkin, 2005.

On the other hand, anthropologists who have tried to understand the impact of McDonald's from the consumer's perspective find a very complex picture. Despite widespread criticism of McDonald's as a symbol of global homogeneity and environmental degradation in East Asia, it was discovered that not all of these changes attributed to McDonald's have been negative (Watson, 1997). In Hong Kong and China, for instance, McDonald's has actually contributed to improving standards of bathroom cleanliness and table manners. The transformation has also affected McDonald's as well as the consumers; McDonald's itself has been forced to adapt to local culture and tastes and has undergone a complex process of cultural accommodation, compromise, and change in its assimilation into Asian societies.

Conclusions

This book focuses on obesity and obesity prevention in U.S. populations, but as explained in this chapter, obesity in the United States is influenced by a complex set of factors with many determinants that are global in nature. In addition, the U.S. is part of the global problem and bears some responsibility for helping to craft solutions worldwide. Further, we can learn from understanding the causes of these changes in other countries.

We truly live in one world today, where persons living in any major city in a low or moderate income country can eat and move in a manner akin to that of the higher-income cities of the world. The systematic spread of these changes across the globe illustrates the huge impact of these global economic and technology forces on the daily lives of millions of people. Moreover, these provide a very strong argument for focusing on larger food policy issues such as food price policies (e.g., Schmidhuber, 2004).

Has globalization mattered? The edible oil story and the examples of shifts in activity levels at work, travel, and leisure in China provide a few examples of the manner in which rapid technological shifts have influenced the adults in a country of more than one billion people; but, it is impossible to ascribe any one factor to any one of these shifts. These changes have been very rapid and certainly the shift to unimpeded direct foreign investment has opened the opportunities for the super markets of the world to rapidly become established in any country and have required domestic equivalent responses. These large supermarket chains ease the way to globally produce and sell modern food stuffs but so many other forces have worked together to create these shifts. Further, there is great heterogeneity in these changes across the developing world.

Essentially, this means that for obesity control, a one sized shoe will not fit all. There will need to be many different policy responses for different regions and countries to improve their dietary and physical activity patterns in a marked manner. Ultimately, a major global response is needed to create the evidence to base the array of food price policies, shifts in the food supply, and ways of moving foodstuffs so we can stem this global obesity pandemic. As of yet, at a time when the global health system is focused on communicable and parasitic diseases and malnutrition which still face hundreds of millions, this new silent global killer is growing rapidly and will require a similar focus (Commission on Macroeconomics and Health, 2001; Hotez et al., 2006).

References

Arroyo, P., Loria, A., & Mendez, O. (2004). Changes in the household calorie supply during the 1994 economic crisis in Mexico and its implications on the obesity epidemic. *Nutrition Reviews, 62*, S163–S168.

Balsevich, F., Berdegué, J. A., Flores, L., Mainville, D., & Reardon, T. (2003). Supermarkets and produce quality and safety standards in Latin America. *American Journal of Agricultural Economics, 85*, 1147–1154.

Bell, A. C., Ge, K., & Popkin, B. M. (2001). Weight gain and its predictors in Chinese adults. *International Journal of Obesity and related metabolic disorders, 25*(7), 1079–1086.

Bell, A. C., Ge, K., & Popkin, B. M. (2002). The road to obesity or the path to prevention: Motorized transportation and obesity in China. *Obesity Research, 10*(4), 277–283.

Brownell, K., & Horgan, K. (2004). *Food fight: The inside story of the food industry, America's obesity crisis, and what we can do about it.* New York: Contemporary Books.

Brownson, R. C., Boehmer, T. K., Luke, D. A. (2005). Declining rates of physical activity in the United States: What are the contributors? *Annual Review Public Health, 26*, 421–443.

Commission on Macroeconomics and Health. (2001). *Macroeconomics and health: Investing in health for economic development.* Geneva: World Health Organization.

Drewnowski, A., & Popkin, B. M. (1997). The nutrition transition: New trends in the global diet. *Nutrition Reviews, 55*(2), 31–43.

Du, S., Bing, L., Zhai, F., Popkin, B. M. (2002). The nutrition transition in China: A new stage of the Chinese diet. In B. Caballero, & B. Popkin (Eds.), *The nutrition transition: Diet and disease in the developing world* (pp. 205–222). London: Academic Press.

Hotez, P. J., Molyneux, D. H., Fenwick, A., Ottesen, E., Ehrlich Sachs, S., Sachs, J. D. (2006). Incorporating a rapid-impact package for neglected tropical diseases with programs for HIV/AIDS, tuberculosis, and malaria. *PLoS Medicine, 3*(5), e102.

Hu, D. et al. (2004). The emergence of supermarkets with Chinese characteristics: Challenges and opportunities for China's Agricultural Development. *Development Policy Review, 22*(5): 557–586.

International Broadcasting Audience Research. (2004). *World radio and television receivers international broadcasting audience research library.* London: BBC World Service.

Jahns, L., Baturin, A., & Popkin, B. M. (2003). Obesity, diet, and poverty: Trends in the Russian transition to market economy. *European Journal of Clinical Nutrition, 57*(10), 1295–1302.

Lanningham-Foster, L., Nysse, L. J., Levine, J. A. (2003). Labor saved, calories lost: The energetic impact of domestic labor-saving devices. *Obesity Research, 11*(10), 1178–1181.

Lobstein, T., Baur, L., Uauy, R., IASO International Obesity Task Force. (2004). Obesity in children and young people: A crisis in public health. *Obesity Reviews, 5*(Suppl. 1), 4–104.

Mendez, M. A., Monteiro, C. A., & Popkin, B. M (2005). Overweight exceeds underweight among women in most developing countries. *American Journal of Clinical Nutrition, 81*(3), 714–721.

Paeratakul, S., Popkin, B. M., Keyou, G., Adair, L. S., & Stevens, J. (1998). Changes in diet and physical activity affect the body mass index of Chinese adults. *International Journal of Obesity and related metabolic disorders, 22*(5), 424–431.

Popkin, B. (2003). The nutrition transition in the developing world. *Development Policy Review, 21*(5), 581–597.

Popkin, B., & Adair, L. (2005). Are child eating patterns being transformed globally? *Obesity Research, 13,* 1281–1299.

Popkin, B. M. (1998). The nutrition transition and its health implications in lower-income countries. *Public Health & Nutrition, 1*(1), 5–21.

Popkin, B. M. (1999). Urbanization, lifestyle changes and the nutrition transition. *World Development, 27*, 1905–1916.

Popkin, B. M. (2002). The shift in stages of the nutrition transition in the developing world differs from past experiences! *Public Health & Nutrition, 5*(1A), 205–214.

Popkin, B. M. (2006). Technology, transport, globalization and the nutrition transition. *Food Policy, 31,* 554–569.

Popkin, B. M., Conde, W., Hou, N., & Monteiro, C. (2006). *Why the lag globally in obesity trends for children as compared to adults?* Unpublished manuscript.

Popkin, B. M., & Nielsen, S. J. (2003). The sweetening of the world's diet. *Obesity. Research. 11*(11), 1325–1332.

Popkin, B. M., Wolney, C., Ningqi, H., & Carlos, M. (2005). *Why the lag globally in obesity trends for children as compared to adults?* Unpublished manuscript.

Reardon, T., Timmer, C. P., Barrett, C. B., & Berdegue, J. A. (2003). The rise of supermarkets in Africa, Asia, and Latin America. *American Journal of Agricultural Economics, 85*, 1140–1146.

Reardon, T., Timmer, P., & Berdegue, J. (2004). The rapid rise of supermarkets in developing countries: Induced organizational, institutional, and technological change in agrifood systems. *The Electronic Journal of Agricultural and Development Economics, 1*, 168–183.

Schmidhuber, J. (2004). The growing global obesity problem: Some policy options to address it. *The Electronic Journal of Agricultural and Development Economics, 1*, 272–290.

Sturm, R. (2004). The economics of physical activity: Societal trends and rationales for interventions. *American Journal of Preventive Medicine, 27*(3, Suppl. 1), 126–135.

Tudor-Locke, C., Ainsworth B. E., Adair, L. S., Du, S., Popkin, B. M. (2003). Physical activity and inactivity in Chinese school-aged youth: The China Health and Nutrition Survey. *International Journal of Obesity and related metabolic disorders, 27*(9), 1093–1099.

USDA (1966). U.S. fats and oils statistics, 1909–65. *Statistical Bulletin, 376*, pp. 1–222.

Wallingford, J. C., Yuhas, R., Du, S., Zhai, F., Popkin, B. M. (2004). Fatty acids in Chinese edible oils: Value of direct analysis as a basis for labeling. = *Food and Nutrition Bulletin, 25*(4), 330–336.

Wang, Y., Monteiro, C., & Popkin, B. M. (2002). Trends of obesity and underweight in older children and adolescents in the United States, Brazil, China, and Russia. *American Journal of Clinical Nutrition, 75*(6), 971–977.

Watson, J. L. (1997). *Golden arches East: McDonald's in East Asia.* Palo Alto: Stanford University Press.

Weber, I. G. (2000). Challenges facing China's television advertising industry in the age of spiritual civilization: An industry analysis. *International Journal of Advertising*, 259–281.

Wilkinson, J. (2004). The food processing industry, globalization and developing countries. *Electronic Journal of Agricultural Developmental Economics, 1*, 184–201.

Williams, G. W. (1984). Development and future direction of the world soybean market. *Quarterly Journal International Agriculture, 23*, 319–337.

Chapter 12

Organizational Change for Obesity Prevention—Perspectives, Possibilities and Potential Pitfalls

Barbara L. Riley, John M. Garcia and Nancy C. Edwards

Introduction

This section is about crafting solutions to address the complex problems associated with obesity prevention – solutions that will involve the ability to influence organizational settings (Part 1) as well as individuals and families (Part 2). Most of the chapters in Part 1 (chapters 13–16) focus on opportunities for changing environments and policies for obesity prevention in specific *organizational settings* (e.g., communities at large, health care systems, worksites, schools or child care centers, or social institutions such as churches). This introductory chapter for Part 1 is a primer on the concepts and approaches needed to influence change at the *organizational* level. In it, we emphasize changing organizational environments and policies since these approaches are generally less well understood and practiced compared to more individually-focused and clinical programs. They are also potentially potent interventions since they shape social and physical environments. In addition, when appropriately conceived, organizational environments and policies can promote equity, whereas individually-oriented interventions may selectively help those with pre-existing advantages (e.g., greater access to environments supporting obesity prevention). A goal of Part 1 is to promote quality and depth in this sphere of intervention for obesity prevention.

This chapter will be useful for individuals who want to facilitate organizational change to support obesity prevention. It may be within their own organization or in another organization (e.g., state or local public health practitioners working with workplace personnel or staff of a health care office). The chapter mainly focuses on change *within* organizations but also addresses some concepts related to change *across* organizations.

We cover two main topics:

1. **Making the Case: Organizational Environments and Policies to Support Obesity Prevention.** The chapter begins with a rationale for changing organizational environments and policies rather than only using

organizations as locations to reach individuals. Organizations that can make significant contributions to prevent obesity are then briefly described, along with examples of how the environments and policies within these organizations can contribute to obesity prevention.

2. **Making it Happen: Changing Organizational Environments and Policies to Support Obesity Prevention.** Next, we describe features of organizations and types of organizational change that are most pertinent to obesity prevention. Organizational change processes are then addressed, presented as a general problem-solving framework with five interacting processes. Opportunities to enhance organizational change and overcome potential pitfalls are also discussed.

The chapter concludes by summarizing key messages. These messages are intended to facilitate application of evidence-informed interventions, including those that follow in chapters 13–16.

Making the Case: Organizational Environments and Policies to Support Obesity Prevention

"Organizations have become the pivotal focus for wide-scale change" (Bradbury & Waage, 2005, p.133)

An Ecological Perspective

Physical activity and eating behaviors are developed and shaped in social and physical settings (Doak, Visscher, Renders & Seidell, 2006; Kumanyika, Jeffery, Morabia et al., 2002). These settings, such as recreation facilities, living conditions, and workplaces, are significant determinants of health, including obesity (Dubois, 2006; Hamilton & Bhatti, 1996). In addition, interventions aimed at improving physical activity and eating behaviors, when conducted in isolation of environmental and policy interventions tend to have limited success (Kumanyika et al., 2002). Based on these realities, population-level obesity prevention requires effective interventions in multiple settings that target change at multiple levels (e.g., individual, social network, organization, community) (Doak et al., 2006; Kumanyika, 2001).

Such multi-setting, and multi-level approaches are defining features of social ecological intervention models (Edwards, Mill & Kothari, 2004; Green, Richard & Potvin, 1996; Riley, Taylor & Elliott, 2001; Sallis & Owen, 1996; Stokols, 1992) (described in chapter 5), which emphasize the interaction between individuals and their environments. Individuals are seen as being nested within the context of various social networks (e.g., families, work groups, neighborhoods), organizations, social institutions, communities and society-at-large. And within these contexts, many structural (e.g., legislation, geo-political boundaries), social and cultural forces can influence health and behavior (Green et al., 1996; Green & Kreuter, 2005).

Population-based tobacco control has demonstrated success by using a social ecological approach (Siegel, 2002; Wilcox, 2003). Leaders in health promotion have suggested that such approaches could be adapted for application to obesity prevention (cf. Mercer, Green, Rosenthal et al., 2003; Yach, McKee, Lopez & Novotny, 2005). For this reason and others, the applicability of an ecological perspective to obesity prevention has been widely recognized. In fact, the case for obesity prevention (especially as it applies to children) with its clear and very compelling environmental and policy elements, has probably helped to "sell" the social ecological model to those who had previously tried to address the problem with the individual as the sole target of interventions (Institute of Medicine, 2005; Kumanyika et al., 2002). As part of an ecological approach to obesity prevention, organizational environments and policies provide important opportunities to promote physical activity, healthy eating and healthy weights (Kumanyika, 2001; McLaren, Sheill, Ghali, Lorenzetti, & Huculak, 2004; Raine, 2004). These environments and policies are the main focus of this chapter.

A 'Whole Setting' Approach

A main focus on environmental and policy interventions does not mean ignoring other types of interventions (e.g., educational). Indeed, the success of environmental and policy changes often depends on educational and other initiatives that create support for policy change among those affected. Consistent with a social ecological framework, such complementary interventions should target other levels such as individual workers, social networks (e.g., work teams, union, management), and partnerships with other organizations (e.g., health-related coalitions). Such a multi-level approach used by an organization is what we refer to as a 'whole setting' approach. Table 12.1 illustrates a whole setting approach for obesity prevention. Interventions at the various levels are implemented by a single organization.

Table 12.1 Example of a 'whole setting' approach for obesity prevention, by level of intervention.

Level of intervention	Examples
Individual	• Health risk assessments • Self-help materials • Behavioral counseling • Vouchers for food supplements
Social Network	• Walking clubs • Family physical activity challenge • Group self help programs on meal preparation, strategies to effectively balance work and family life
Organizational	• Food service policy: healthy foods in vending machines; healthy choices available in cafeterias; healthy food for meetings • Subsidies for gym membership • Curricula requirements for daily, quality physical activity in schools • Health impact assessments for all policies (i.e., evaluating health consequences of all policies) • Workplace providing showers for those who bike to work • Recreational facilities
Inter-organizational	• Extending and maintaining walking and bicycle paths • Workplace wellness challenge across several workplaces • Networks or coalitions of organizations to promote healthy eating and physical activity • Advocacy for state-level educational policy on daily physical activity for all students

A whole setting approach is used to maximize impact. In general, interventions implemented on their own (at any level) tend not to work, but together they do (e.g., Doak et al., 2006). The combined effects may be additive or they may multiply. The overall aim of such combinations of interventions is to enhance or enable the impact of single interventions (Edwards et al., 2004; Smedley & Syme, 2001) – sometimes referred to as 'synergistic effects'. Synergy within a setting can be created with two or more interventions at one level (e.g., built environment and media campaign that both support physical activity in the community setting), or two or more interventions across levels (e.g., workplace health risk assessments for individuals combined with organizational policies to provide access to healthy foods). In addition to complementary interventions within a single organizational setting, organizations should also try to align their efforts in a manner that complements and takes advantage of interventions delivered in other settings (e.g., workplaces, schools, etc.). While the concept of synergistic effects is powerful, research on combinations of interventions is very limited. This is a priority for future research (Edwards et al., 2004).

Organizational Settings to Support Obesity Prevention

Many settings, such as workplaces, schools, physician offices, and the community-at-large all have roles to play in preventing obesity (Bracht & Kingsbury, 1990; Green et al., 1996). For example, to promote physical activity, planning departments in local government can enhance opportunities for physical activity (e.g., bike lanes, pedestrian pathways, parks), access to healthy foods (e.g., grocery store locations) and social interaction (e.g., safe and walk-able communities). Schools can provide health education in the curriculum and provide an environment that supports healthy eating choices (e.g., healthy foods in vending machines and cafeterias, intramural activities). Workplaces can provide opportunities for employees to make healthy food choices in the cafeteria, work flexible hours, participate in decision-making, and promote healthy work-related policies. In some communities, churches provide communal meals, day care, and recreational facilities that could be targets for policy changes to support obesity prevention. Numerous promising interventions in these settings are provided in chapters 13–16. To maximize synergy, all of these organizational settings would consistently support healthy eating and physical activity.

The above examples illustrate different roles of organizations. Organizations can contribute to obesity prevention in three general roles.

1. Organizations are *workplaces*: they employ people to fulfill a particular mission (e.g., manufacture cars, provide business training, manage health care);
2. Organizations are *service locations*: they provide something of value (product or service) to a defined audience (e.g., literacy training for adults, recreational services for families, spiritual and social guidance and support);
3. Organizations *relate to other organizations and systems*: they interface with other organizations, especially those with overlapping mandates (e.g., public health and education, natural resources and agriculture) and provide leadership in the community.

In each of these roles, there are opportunities for organizations to contribute to making the healthy choices the easier choices. For example, schools are a workplace for teachers; they provide education, social activities and food services for students; and have relationships with parents (home), and providers in health, social services, and educational sectors (e.g., those responsible for state-wide curriculum design). School communities can also be healthy environments for employees, students and others. These organizational roles emerge from a view of organizations as social systems. We describe this view of organizations in the next section.

Making it Happen: Changing Organizational Environments and Policies to Support Obesity Prevention

Organizations as Social Systems

Long gone is the view of organizations as machines (Meynell, 2005), now replaced by organizations as social systems (Anderson, Guthrie & Schirle, 2002). Organizations as social systems emphasize interaction, adaptation and learning – all of which influence organizational efforts to prevent obesity.

With respect to interaction, when organizations are viewed as social systems, patterns of relationships are emphasized (cf. Jackson, 2005). This includes patterns of interactions among internal organizational components (e.g., people, administrative processes, information technology, communication processes) and among these internal components and the external environment (e.g., social, economic and political context; external change agents). Adaptation is an organization's ability to respond incrementally to changes in the environment or changes in goals; whereas organizational learning occurs from insight, knowledge about action and consequences derived from experience, and learning from changes introduced by organizations (Fiol & Lyles, 1985; Rosenheck, 2001).

Central to each of these features is the assumption (consistent with social systems) that learning and change are social processes. This assumption is supported by organizational learning theorists who suggest that we need to understand the importance of psychological, social, policy and broader contextual factors that affect organizational behavior (Kimberly & Bouchikhi, 1995; Lipshitz, Popper & Friedman, 2002). People learn from each other in organizations, including understanding their commitments to organizational goals, their identities and roles in organizations (Kogut & Zander, 1996). Role differentiation allows for organizations to have multiple areas of expertise and it may even be desirable to have this diversity of knowledge and experience in order for organizations to have enough variety to generate creative responses to meet their goals in changing environments (cf. Bandura, 2000 or 2001 for discussions of collective and proxy efficacy). Creating a culture concerned with and enabling people to be creative with solutions in their own environment is critical.

Obesity prevention and control will require organizations to be creative in looking at aspects of their organizational systems that either contribute to the problem in the first place or could be part of the solution. It will also require that organizations act on what they think will fit best in their own context, understand whether their interventions are working, and share this learning within their organization and with other individuals and organizations who share a concern for obesity prevention (sometimes referred to as a 'community of practice'; see Wenger, McDermott & Snyder, 2002).

Characteristics of Organizations

Organizations are multi-layered, complex systems. Both structural and cultural characteristics of organizations need to be considered in obesity prevention efforts (cf. Lipshitz et al., 2002). Structures generally refer to the 'hardware' of organizations (e.g., mandate, rules and regulations, accountabilities). Culture refers to the 'software' of organizations (e.g., norms, patterns of interaction, shared beliefs). Each organizational characteristic provides clues as to where one might begin to shift the organizational context to one that is more supportive of healthy eating, active living and the prevention and control of overweight and obesity. Table 12.2 gives some examples of how various structural and cultural features can support obesity prevention.

We elaborate on a few characteristics that may be most relevant to organizational change for obesity prevention. One is organizational levels or 'layers'. Goodman, Steckler and Kegler (1997) describe the nested hierarchy within organizations.

Table 12.2 Examples of organizational characteristics that support obesity prevention.

Examples of organizational features	Examples supporting obesity prevention
Structures or 'hardware'	
Mandate	• School board commitment to promote regular daily physical activity
Regulations	• Decisions to make healthy food choices more prevalent by eliminating marketing practices that encourage unhealthy behavior (e.g., preventing easy access to high-calorie low nutrient value foods through promotions, placement and price discounting)
Accountability	• Schools reporting on actions taken to increase physical activity that is reported to parent–teacher associations.
Human resource policies	• Flexible work schedules to accommodate for physical activity breaks and programs • Benefit programs to encourage fitness club or weight management programs, with positive rewards for those who take advantage
Culture or 'software'	
Patterns of interaction	• Information shared across departments about organizational opportunities to prevent obesity • Shared governance within an organization
Norms	• Health and productivity valued in the workplace • Occupational health and safety committees of workers and managers see chronic disease prevention as critical and promote organization-wide understanding about how this relates to organization health and well functioning • Employees encouraged to maintain balance of family and work life

"Organizations are layered. Their strata range from the surrounding environment at the broadest level, to the overall organizational structure, to the management within, to work groups, to each individual member." (p. 287)

As we described in a previous section, these layers help to identify targets of intervention (e.g., individual workers, work teams, management, organizational environment). Layers are also relevant to decision-making and communication within organizations, both of which influence organizational change efforts. With respect to decision-making, organizations with hierarchical (bureaucratic) structures tend to maintain vertical lines of authority. Under these circumstances, support from senior administration is often an important prerequisite for introducing and sustaining organizational change. This is the traditional 'top-down' approach, and may compromise support for and compliance with a change in policy. A 'bottom-up' approach is more common in organizations with horizontal, collaborative structures for decision-making. Under these circumstances, leadership and champions for change are more likely to emerge from different levels in the organization, and to have influence on the change (Rogers, 2004).

The organizational learning literature suggests the need for alternative organizational structures that can facilitate learning across and within levels of organizations (Nonaka & Takeuchi, 1995; Wenger et al., 2002). These structures complement (and serve a different function than) the inherent hierarchical set of subsystems that are necessary for organizations to be viable (cf. Beer, 1981; Beer, 1984; and discussion of implementation, coordination, operational control, development and policy subsystems by Jackson, 2005). One alternative structure that facilitates learning across an organization, regardless of hierarchical position, is a 'community of practice' – a group of people who share a common concern, a set of problems, or a passion about a topic (e.g., health), and who deepen their knowledge and expertise in this area by interacting on an ongoing basis (Wenger et al., 2002). These people may come from a single organization, but typically they span sectors and organizations.

An example of a community of practice specific to obesity prevention is "O-Net," an emerging forum in Canada. Initiated by the Chronic Disease Prevention Alliance of Canada, O-Net is a virtual community of professionals (researchers, advocates, practitioners, policy-makers) that provides opportunities for sharing information, central access to resources, discussion forums, web conferences and other forms of e-learning and interactions (www.cdpac.ca/content/initiatives/onet.asp). Another example of a community of practice, with a broader focus on community health, is CHNET-works! (Edwards & Kothari, 2004; www.chnet-works.ca). CHNET_works! is a pilot infrastructure to support a network of community health professionals across Canada.

Four Types of Organizational Change

Whereas it may be tempting to consider organizational change as a single entity, it is useful to understand different types of change undertaken by organizations (cf. Kaluzny & Hernandez, 1988). The type of change influences the nature of the change process.

Organizational change refers to any modification *within* an organization that relates to operations, structure, or ends (i.e., goals, mandate), and any modification

Table 12.3 Definitions and examples of different types of organizational change.

Types of organizational change	Definition	Examples
Operational	Some modification in the means by which the activities of the organization are carried out (e.g., technology, program, communication mechanism)	Physical activity offered during lunch breaks Outdoor recreation/activity encouraged during school recess Pricing of cafeteria food makes healthy choices the less expensive choices
Structural	Some modification in the way the organization is structured (e.g., governance, management, accountability mechanisms, departments and committees) strategies offered in the school	School management responsible for contracting out to catering Accountability (reporting back) to parent teacher association regarding physical activity
Transformational	Change occurs in both means (e.g., planning and evaluation, teams) and ends of the organization (e.g., mandate)	Schools taking on day care responsibility Schools become the hub for recreational activities in less affluent neighborhoods
Inter-organizational	A modification in the relationship between an organization and one or more other organizations	Contractual arrangements with vending machine company to provide healthy choice labeling on food products sold in vending machines and to offer a wider range of healthy choices in vending machines

between an organization and its environment (e.g., other organizations). These four types of organizational change (respectively) are: operational, structural, transformational, and inter-organizational. Table 12.3 provides definitions and some examples of these changes.

Most environmental and policy conditions to support obesity prevention require operational or structural change. For example, an organization might offer healthy food choices on cafeteria menus, or a school board might ban the sale of high calorie-low nutrition foods and beverages in vending machines. This is good news from an organizational change perspective because compared to other types of organizational change, operational and structural changes are less extreme changes, and thus easier to accomplish.

Organizational Change Processes – A Brief Overview

Organizational change has been the subject of much research and debate over the years. Perspectives on change are numerous and as varied as the disciplines from which they come – business and management, organizational psychology, education, health, planning, economics, political science, ecology, sociology, engineering, and more (c.f. Brown & Zavestoski, 2004; DeJoy & Wilson, 2003; Frankish & Green, 1994; Paton, Sengupta & Hassan 2005; Rogers, 1995). Despite diverse perspectives, organizational specialists converge on one main point: that organizational theory is complex and difficult to apply.

Even so, some useful guidance is available. Consistent with the types of change most common for obesity prevention, this chapter focuses mainly on making operational and structural changes.

Components and processes vary, but at the core of most models of planned organizational change is a problem-solving process. We present a problem-solving framework with five interacting processes and apply these processes to environmental and policy change for obesity prevention at the organizational level. The problem-solving process draws on various theoretical perspectives (e.g., diffusion of innovations, organizational learning) (Cain & Mittman, 2002; Greenhalgh, Robert, Macfarlane et al., 2004; Greenhalgh, Collard & Begum, 2005; Rogers, 1995; Sanson-Fisher, 2004), and procedural models for planning and evaluation (e.g., Bryson, 1988; RE-AIM in Glasgow, Vogt & Boles, 1999; PRECEDE-PROCEED in Green & Kreuter, 2005).

An Organizational Problem-solving Process for Obesity Prevention

Figure 12.1 provides an overview of a general problem-solving framework for organizational change. It involves five interacting processes, variations of which have been described by others as 'issues' (e.g., Swinburn, Gill & Kumanyika, 2005) and as 'stages' (Rogers, 1995). Some objectives, activities and considerations for each process are described following Figure 12.1, tailored to organizational change to support obesity prevention.

Identify Needs and Opportunities
Possible outputs:

• Obesity is identified as a problem in an organizational setting.
• The reasons for the obesity problem and how the organization is contributing to the problem are understood.
• The need to address obesity in an organizational setting is recognized, especially by influential individuals and senior decision-makers in the organization.
• The audience for organizational change to prevent obesity is identified.

Making the case for obesity prevention has been developed extensively by others (cf. Swinburn et al., 2005) including types of evidence that can help make the case. To complement this work, we focus on developing an understanding of why organizations change – by choice or otherwise – to prevent obesity.

Organizations generally change to deal with an identified problem confronting the organization, or to take advantage of a new opportunity. The idea for change may come from within the organization (e.g., staff or manager

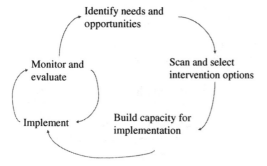

Figure 12.1: Problem-solving process for organizational change.

champions the cause of a healthy workplace), or from outside the organization (e.g., health and safety association identifies organizational features that contribute to obesity, media attention on the dangers of obesity). The change may be triggered by some new information (e.g., citizen support for healthy workplaces, government funding incentives for preventive health care practice, health 'report card'), an event (e.g., local hero dies prematurely from a heart attack, transportation plan is up for renewal), an emerging and important trend (e.g., increased worker absenteeism), or recognition of the problem by a credible authority. For example, the World Health Organization has recognized the global pandemic of obesity as a major challenge to world health (World Health Organization, 2003).

The most powerful triggers for organizational change usually relate to organizational goals, performance and reputation. Thus, organizations that perceive obesity prevention initiatives as helping them to achieve their goals (e.g., increased revenue, education, product sales, maintaining a loyal congregation), or to enhance their image or profile (e.g., recognized as good corporate citizens or as a model organization) are typically more receptive to change and willing to undertake a change process. In addition, healthy eating, active living and obesity prevention may be a primary goal directly related to the mandate – for example in the case of school boards responsible for implementing curricula and other programs for school children addressing healthy eating and physical activity. Otherwise, it might be necessary to address obesity as a major concern to the organization on other grounds, including absenteeism, health costs or less than desirable productivity. Management and/or union members may agree, for example, that coordinating socially related physical activities such as team sports or group hiking or dancing might go a long way to increase morale and a sense of community in the office.

This discussion illustrates that a wide range of possible triggers for organizational change exists. One or more of these triggers can help to make the case for obesity prevention. In addition to a rationale for taking action, there should be at least a preliminary theory of the causes of the problem, as well as possible interventions that could be used to address these. Drawing on communication and behavior change principles, a persuasive case can be made to inform organizations about the need for change; their role in change; and their ability to make change.

Scan for Interventions, Obtain Stakeholder Input and Select Intervention Options

Possible outputs:

- The criteria for selecting organizational interventions to prevent obesity are identified.
- Possible intervention options are identified.
- The type and scope of supporting evidence for various intervention options is documented.
- Relevant organizational members and other individuals, as appropriate, are engaged in the planning process.
- Possible interventions are evaluated in relation to the criteria for selection.
- One or more interventions are selected to implement in the organizational setting, and a plan for implementation is developed.

A final output for this process is selection of the interventions and their combinations that are likely to have an optimal effect in the organization(s) of interest. As discussed, a single intervention is unlikely to be effective in isolation (see earlier section on 'A whole setting approach'). In addition, sustained effects require a combination of educational, behavioral, and environmental interventions. Additionally, the overall impact of these combined interventions will be a function of the efficacy of each individual intervention chosen, how successfully interventions can be adapted to fit the organization, the number of people reached with the intervention, and how these interventions interact or support each other (e.g., cafeteria food choices should reflect company policy on healthy eating and educational and promotion programs) (cf. Glasgow, Klesges & Dzewaltowski et al., 2004 for a discussion of their RE-AIM framework, and Green & Kreuter, 2005, for their principles for administrative diagnosis). We now turn to the processes to achieve the most suitable interventions.

In the general context of evidence-based public health, scanning for and selecting interventions are the subject of considerable reflection (e.g., Anderson, Brownson, Fullilove et al., 2005; Briss, Brownson, Fielding & Zaza, 2004). Organizational interventions to prevent obesity are part of the broader debate. It is generally accepted that in order to optimize efficiency and impact of organizational interventions, best available evidence should be considered. To this end, many intervention options have been identified for obesity prevention. Thus, although innovative approaches can emerge, a useful starting point is with existing intervention ideas and models for action, and preferably those with demonstrated effectiveness (for particular audiences and settings).

This handbook contains many ideas for action. Another rich source is the Guide to Community Preventive Services (the "Community Guide") (e.g., Briss et al., 2004; Zaza, Briss & Harris, 2005). Poor nutrition, physical inactivity, diabetes, and sociocultural environments are some topics addressed in the Community Guide that are relevant to obesity prevention (Anderson et al., 2005).

The Community Guide (and other similar analytic tools – see for example www.cancercontrolplanet.gov) contains recommendations for the use of public health programs and policies based on scientific evidence about what practices have worked to improve health. Interventions recommended for use are those that were judged to be effective based on well-established criteria to assess strength and consistency of evidence. Typically, interventions are also identified that have some evidence of promise, but require more research to address gaps in evidence. Ideally, sources would also identify interventions that have been proven *in*effective (which is different from a lack of evidence). However, in some cases, interventions that are ineffective in a context that does not provide for complementary programs or policies at other ecological levels may be worth consideration for inclusion in multi-level approaches.

Environmental and policy interventions are least likely to meet the traditional criteria for effective interventions, in part, because evaluation of these interventions is difficult due to the general infeasibility of experimental 'control' (Koepsell, Wagner, Cheadle et al., 1992; Potvin, 1996). In addition, research often lags behind innovative and exemplary interventions. As a result, not all promising interventions will be included in systematic reviews. Organizations, therefore, need sources in addition to systematic reviews to find out about promising interventions and about interventions that they should avoid.

Several other sources exist to identify obesity prevention interventions. Some include: grey literature, conferences, peer-review publications, and interpersonal networks (e.g., communities of practice, Listservs). Experience suggests that scanning is most typically done through interpersonal networks. Indeed, social modeling is a powerful stimulus for change; a concept grounded in social learning theory, which states that individuals learn from others who they recognize as being similar to themselves, and then imitate by following similar (but not necessarily identical) behavior (Bandura, 2001).

Another issue in selecting interventions on effectiveness alone is that interventions that are proven effective in other jurisdictions may not be practical to implement in a particular organizational setting (Goodman, 2000; Green, 2001). This reality has broadened the debate about factors, in addition to effectiveness, to consider when selecting interventions. An emerging set of more inclusive criteria includes effectiveness, plausibility and practicality (Table 12.4).

Due to the limited evidence base on environmental and policy interventions, plausibility is an important criterion to consider. A useful tool to assess plausibility is logic frameworks (e.g., Goodman, 2000) (also called logic models or analytic frameworks) – a diagram that makes the assumed links explicit between intervention(s), short- and long-term outcomes, and pathways for these effects. The stronger the theoretical support for the assumed linkages, the higher the plausibility. Plausibility is also enhanced by synergy (e.g., education about healthy food choices combined with healthy food choices in vending machines and cafeterias).

Additionally, environmental and policy interventions, like others, will only be effective if they are practical to implement – resources are available, staff have the

Table 12.4 Some definitions for effectiveness, plausibility and practicality criteria[a].

Criteria	Definition	Assessment of criteria
Effectiveness	Effectiveness criteria assess whether the intervention did or did not work. Both results of reported evaluations of the intervention and the quality of study designs are considered.	Strongest evidence is provided by positive results (e.g., change in behaviors or environments) using a good impact or outcome study design. Weaker evidence is provided by positive results using a process evaluation only.
Plausibility	Plausibility criteria assess whether an intervention will likely be effective based on its attributes (e.g., content, evaluation, process attributes); its probable reach; and the existence of other complementary interventions or conditions of success.	The assessment of plausibility does not necessarily reflect what happened but the potential of the intervention (i.e., "could the intervention . . ." rather than "did the intervention . . ."). Plausibility can be assessed using many forms of evidence, such as: theory, process evaluations, experience, and parallel evidence (from other issue areas).
Practicality	Practicality criteria determine: (a) the readiness of the organizational setting to address the perceived need of the intervention being considered; and (b) the availability of the necessary technical, financial, and personnel resources to implement the intervention.	Practicality criteria are generally applied by those responsible for implementing or administering the intervention. Assessments are typically based on experiential evidence (e.g., tacit knowledge).

[a] Definitions integrate ideas from several sources, mainly: Cameron, Walker & Jolin, 1998 and Swinburn et al., 2005.

necessary knowledge and skills, the interventions are relatively easy to understand and use, and if other interventions (e.g., education, enforcement) are available to support policy change. Favorable conditions are often essential for environmental and policy change. These include community values, social norms, and policy-related "windows of opportunity" that may be supported by politics and public opinion (Kingdon, 2003). Incentives, such as expected benefits that result directly from participation (e.g., flavorful food, enjoyable social and physical activity), and compatibility of the intervention with the organization's mandate and practices, are powerful motivators for adoption. A high need relative to other priorities is also helpful (Swinburn et al., 2005). These issues of practicality relate directly to capacity for implementation, to which we now turn.

Build Capacity for Implementation
Possible outputs:

- The necessary skills, resources and conditions for making the organizational change are understood.
- Individual, organizational and environmental capacities required for the organizational change are assessed, and strengths and limitations of these capacities are identified.
- The appropriate capacities exist to implement and sustain environmental or policy interventions and other complementary interventions, as appropriate.

In our efforts to move towards evidence-based public health, the emphasis (understandably) has been on collating, evaluating, and disseminating evidence (Speller, Wimbush & Morgan, 2005). The evidence, however, can only be used under favorable conditions. These favorable conditions include capacities at individual, organizational and environmental levels and have been the subject of considerable research in the last 10 years (e.g., Germann & Wilson, 2004; Goodman, Speers, McLeroy et al., 1998; Joffres, Heath, Farquharson et al., 2004; NSW Health, 2001; Riley et al., 2001; Yeatman & Nove, 2002). The presence of favorable conditions signals a 'readiness for change'. Readiness is required for successful organizational change and can be assessed using the dimensions shown in Figure 12.2.

Individual capacity means that those individuals responsible for implementation are motivated; have sufficient human, material and financial resources for implementation; and have the necessary knowledge and skills to undertake the selected obesity prevention interventions (McLean et al., 2005).

Organizational capacity begins with commitment; the desired environmental or policy change is a priority for the organization (e.g., in a business plan; supported by senior administrators). Structures, such as working groups, need to exist and have sufficient authority to ensure appropriate planning, delivery and evaluation of the organizational changes. Structures need adequate financial and human resources (e.g., to survey organizational members, purchase bike racks), and they need to facilitate interaction. Culture is the most intangible yet perhaps the most powerful dimension of organizational capacity. It is the 'character' of the organization. Does the organization take risks? Can it adapt to change? Do members anticipate positive results from their efforts? The culture must support change and learning from action (McLean et al., 2005).

One or more 'champions' for change are also needed (Economos, Brownson, DeAngelis et al., 2001). Opinion leaders and champions are just as, if not

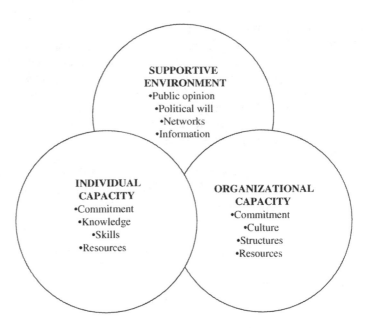

Figure 12.2 Dimensions of readiness for organizational change[a].

[a] Based in part on McLean, Feather and Butler-Jones, 2005.

more, important than positional leaders (e.g., administrators). These more informal leaders can emerge from any level in the organization (Nissen, Merrigan & Kraft, 2005; Rogers, 1995) and their influence can be powerful.

A supportive environment is also needed for successful organizational change. This domain focuses on factors external to the organization. These factors, such as citizen support (e.g., parents volunteering to coach sports teams), political will (e.g., elected officials who are champions for obesity prevention), networks or coalitions of organizations that identify obesity as a priority for action, information (e.g., evidence of effectiveness, public opinion surveys demonstrating support), and significant events interact with other dimensions of capacity. Significant community, state or national events can be especially useful to catalyze action for health and social movements (including tobacco control) (Raymond & Moon, 2003).

Initial and Sustained Implementation
Possible outputs:

- The one or more selected interventions are implemented in the organization. Interventions are adapted to accommodate organizational needs and structures and/or organizations may be changed to fit the interventions.
- As appropriate, implementation of interventions increases over time and interventions are incorporated into the regular activities of organizations (i.e., variably referred to as routinized, maintained, sustained or institutionalized).

Implementing an intervention idea that already exists covers a wide spectrum from straightforward borrowing or adoption of the intervention (application of an intervention developed in some other setting with little modification) to substantial adaptation (application of some prototype intervention developed outside the organization but modified to fit organizational goals and circumstances). By far, adaptation is more common and is a key aspect of implementation (Green, 2001; Smedley & Syme, 2001).

Adaptation generally means modification of interventions. Modifications may be needed for at least two reasons. One reason is contextual adaptation – tailoring an intervention so that it 'fits' within the organizational structure and culture (e.g., centrality of health in the mandate, degree of social interaction among colleagues). Broader social, economic and political factors (i.e., beyond the organization) may also need to be considered (e.g., time required to commute, problems of access due to geography or a variety of financial considerations) (e.g., Johns, 2001; McCormack, Kitson, Harvey et al., 2002).

Interventions may also be modified for practical reasons. Most often, this type of adaptation results from a need to 'downscale' an intervention when funding is lacking or other aspects of capacity are lacking. The risk with modification of interventions is a potential dilution (watering down) of the effect or removal of active ingredients (e.g., signage on stairs as environmental cues for physical activity). Any guidelines available on these active ingredients for interventions should be considered during the implementation process.

Another issue related to implementation is the 'newness' of the intervention within a particular set of similar organizations (e.g., large workplaces, physician offices). Informed by diffusion theory (Rogers, 1995, 2004), new ideas (such as a food service policy) are typically picked up slowly at first; the rate of adoption increases as the majority of organizations adopt; and then adoption tapers off when the majority of organizations has adopted the environmental or policy change. Adoption may be enhanced in situations where partnerships and supportive relationships are present, as in the diffusion of church-based lifestyle interventions in African American communities (Peterson, Atwood & Yates, 2002).

A final consideration is the sustainability of organizational change. A potential strength of environmental and policy changes is their durability. They may be challenging to introduce, but once in place, they may also be difficult to reverse. Nevertheless, factors that support sustainability need to be considered, including monitoring of compliance with policies (e.g., monitoring availability of food choices) and evaluation to refine the implementation process and to determine changes that result from the new organizational policy. In the next section, we discuss some additional considerations for monitoring and evaluation.

Monitoring and Evaluation
Possible outputs:

- An organizational commitment is made to 'learning from practice'.
- Plans are established to monitor and evaluate the organizational change. The plan includes examining the process of implementation and results (or outcomes).
- Evaluation findings are used to inform decisions about continuation and modification of the obesity prevention intervention(s).

Evaluation is an essential mechanism for individual and organizational learning. Feedback on performance – processes and outcomes – has solid foundations in social learning theory (Bandura, 1986). And it is the most influential of Green and Kreuter's (2005) reinforcing factors, which exert their influence during and after implementation. Characteristic of a self-correcting system, feedback loops are essential to adapt to changing circumstances within the organization and in the surrounding environment. These are essential system characteristics for a learning organization (Argyris & Schon, 1978; Beer 1981; Preskill & Torres, 1999; Senge, 1999), and can be used to inform obesity prevention interventions. For example, some useful feedback may be information on changes in revenue from vending machines in high schools that switched to healthy choices. In general, information on various aspects of policy implementation (e.g., support, compliance) and consequences (e.g., increased concern for obesity, healthier food choices) is needed to inform decisions about continuation and modification of interventions.

Environmental, policy and multi-level interventions have unique evaluation challenges. Increasingly, it is recognized that the classical evidence hierarchies (and study designs) are less suitable or valuable in assessing effectiveness of these interventions. In this context, we offer some general evaluation guidelines:

- Steps should be taken, as appropriate, to ensure that implementation of the intervention is undertaken as planned and coordinated with other programs and services to achieve synergy (Edwards et al., 2004).
- Monitoring (e.g., audience reach, barriers to implementation, compliance) should be put in place to ensure that implementation of the intervention is sustained, as appropriate.
- Organizational 'outcomes' can be usefully conceived as intervention impact measures. Possible measures include: policy statements, legislation, regulation, resource allocation, and organizational practices (e.g., yearly health assessments for all employees).
- Organizational and institutional change can take a long time to put in place and even longer to yield results (Kumanyika et al., 2002). Evaluation planning needs to consider realistic outcomes and a realistic rate of change. The problem-solving process for organizational change can serve as a useful framework to identify meaningful indicators of progress. For example, some early indicators of progress could be an awareness among senior administrators of the obesity problem and their organization's contributions to the problem; obesity prevention is identified as an organizational priority; staff are assigned to search for promising interventions that may be suitable for their organization; and a plan is developed with specific obesity preventive interventions, a time line for implementation, resource needs and accountabilities.
- High priority needs to be given to evaluation of obesity prevention interventions. Agreement is widespread that a significant investment is needed in sustained, theory-based healthy eating and physical activity interventions, which are designed as applied research initiatives (or emerge as 'natural experiments') with rigorous formative and outcome evaluation components (McAmmond, 2001). This call was reinforced by the 2005 Institute of Medicine report 'Preventing Childhood Obesity: Health in the Balance' (Institute of Medicine, 2005). The call for enhanced evaluation, however, does not stop there. Other recent calls are for evaluation to contribute to 'practice-based evidence' (Green, 2006; Marmot, 2004); that is, information that is relevant to intervention design and implementation issues. Evaluations, therefore, need to be guided by all three selection criteria (i.e., effectiveness, plausibility, practicality), and resulting studies will include strong assessments of the implementation process, contextual analyses and economic evaluations (e.g., cost-effectiveness), to name a few.

Resistance to Organizational Change . . . and Ways to Overcome it

"Current patterns of behavior among individuals and within institutions and organizations have proven durable and quite difficult to change." (Bradbury & Waage, 2005, p. 131)

Resistance to change needs to be an expected part of the process. Change is unsettling and resistance to it is both natural and protective. Diamond (1995) pinpoints the problem as a denial of change and innovation as a human process. Most often, change is approached in a technical and rational manner. Technical approaches ignore the psychological and emotional attachment to prevailing ways of working and to bureaucratic organizational cultures. The result is defensiveness – a resistance to change and learning (cf. also Arygris, 2004 regarding defensive routines).

The goal in a change process is workers or organizational members to develop ownership and to endorse the rationale behind the change. This is more likely to happen if the loss experienced by organizational participants (e.g., cognitive and emotional losses introduced by change) is acknowledged and explicitly addressed in the change process. Some kind of 'transitional space' is needed to separate from the old way of doing things in order to embrace the new way. Transitional space might be announcing a change in food policy six months before it is implemented, and having samples of the new healthy choices during this time period.

It might be unrealistic to think that resistance will be eliminated altogether, but it can be minimized and overcome. A key strategy is to match the rate of organizational change with the ability of the organization to cope (i.e., not exceed it). On a change course, the basic goal of leaders and change agents is to strive to achieve a rate of change that leads to 'dynamic equilibrium'. This state is achieved when the rate of change within an organization is matched to the organization's ability to cope with change (Rogers, 1995). To achieve this balance requires capitalizing on opportunities as they present. It also requires an understanding of the organization's 'readiness for change' and setting expectations for change that consider that readiness.

Organizational and institutional change can take a long time – to implement and for results. Expectations for rapid change may only feed perceptions of failure. Often it is optimal to move ahead and allow for a period of adjustment after change is introduced. People within organizations are generally in the best position to decide what changes should be introduced and how rapidly.

Summary and Conclusions

Knowing *what* to do and *how* to do it will make a difference if this knowledge is applied in organizational settings. To facilitate this application, we reinforce some key points from this chapter, including the need for attention to:

• *An ecological approach to obesity prevention*: Environmental and policy interventions at an organizational level will be most effective if supported by complementary interventions targeting other levels of change (e.g., individual workers; social networks such as work teams, management; committees or circles within faith organizations).

- *Organizational roles to support obesity prevention*: Organizations are complex social systems. They can contribute to obesity prevention as workplaces, service locations and in their relationship with other organizations and systems.
- *'Hardware' and 'software' of organizations that support obesity prevention*: Many features of organizations – including structures (or hardware) and culture (or software) – can support obesity prevention. Some powerful supports are interaction and exchange of ideas among those working on obesity prevention (within and outside an organization); a mandate and/or senior administrative or leadership support for obesity prevention; opportunities for organizational benefits such as reduced absenteeism and cost-savings; and champions for obesity prevention (who can emerge from any position in an organization).
- *Types of organizational change to support obesity prevention*: Introducing and sustaining organizational policies to prevent obesity typically require operational or structural changes. Less frequently they require transformational and inter-organizational change, which are more difficult to achieve.
- *An organizational problem-solving process for obesity prevention*: A general problem-solving process with five interacting processes can guide organizational change: (1) identify needs and opportunities; (2) scan for interventions, obtain stakeholder input, and select intervention options; (3) build capacity for implementation; (4) implement; and (5) monitor and evaluate. The processes are to enable organizations to select an appropriate mix of interventions to support obesity prevention, and to tailor those interventions to the organizational setting. In this chapter, we encouraged an emphasis on environmental and policy interventions to maximize effectiveness and sustainability of impacts.
- *Advances in evaluation and other 'practice-based' research*: We reinforced the importance of monitoring and evaluation in the organizational change process as a key learning mechanism. One reason is the limited evidence base on environmental and policy interventions. Other reasons are that organizations need to continually adapt their activities to dynamic contextual and organizational environments; and they need to know what works in their particular context. Feedback from monitoring and evaluation allows for appropriate reflection and response.
- *Understanding resistance to organizational change*: Resistance to change is a natural part of the organizational change process. Typically, the greater the change, the greater the resistance.

Conclusions

This chapter reinforced the importance of change within and across organizations as part of a comprehensive approach to prevent obesity. A key message in this chapter and its companions (chapters 13–16) is the need for obesity prevention to become part of our organizational cultures; for incentives and opportunities for physical activity and healthy eating to be the norm in all organizational settings (not just in health-related settings); and to make healthy choices the easy and preferred choices. Many organizations have features that contribute to obesity (e.g., barriers to physical activity, limited access to healthy foods) and other features that support obesity prevention (e.g., worksite incentives, support from leadership, other types of health or wellness programs). Both large-scale and incremental changes to increase the relative proportion of features that support obesity prevention can make healthy eating and active living the norm throughout our organizations and our society. Another important message is the need to start any change process with understanding: understanding of the organizational setting; understanding of the desired change; understanding of the change process; and understanding of the environment within which organizations operate. This foundation of understanding is essential for planning and implementing successful environmental and policy interventions to support obesity prevention.

We integrated change perspectives into five processes for organizational problem-solving. Although no standard protocol exists to initiate, facilitate, and sustain organizational change, the chapter equips the reader with some tools – concepts, principles and guidelines – for the journey. The tools emphasize understanding: perspectives, possibilities and potential pitfalls. These tools are intended for use in various settings, including those addressed in chapters 13–16. Nevertheless, their relevance, importance and form will be unique to every time and place.

We believe that there is reason to be optimistic and to try to effect change. Experience with other issues (e.g., tobacco control, seat belt use, vaccines) has shown that persistence and vision in organizational change can have major benefits to public health. By taking advantage of the natural talents currently residing in organizations, it is highly likely that important changes can come about – to create environments conducive to active living and healthy living – thus, achieving and maintaining healthy weights.

Acknowledgments. The Preparation of this chapter was supported by a personnel award to Dr. Riley from the Heart and Stroke Foundation of Canada and the Canadian Institutes of Health Research, and a Nursing Chair to Dr. Edwards funded by the Canadian Health Services Research Foundation, Canadian Institutes of Health Research, and the Ontario Ministry of Health and Long-term Care.

References

Anderson, D., Guthrie, T., & Schirle, R. (2002). A nursing model of community organization for change. *Public Health Nursing, 19*(1), 40–46.

Anderson, L. M., Brownson, R. C., Fullilove, M. T., Teutsch, S. M., Novick, L. F., & Fielding, J. et al. (2005). Evidence-based public health policy and practice: Promises and limits. *American Journal of Preventive Medicine, 28*(Suppl. 5), 226–230.

Argyris, C. (2004). *Reasons and rationalizations: The limits to organizational knowledge.* New York: Oxford University Press.

Argyris, C., & Schon, D. A. (1978). *Organizational learning: A theory of action perspective.* Reading, MA: Addison-Wesley.

Bandura, A. (1986). *Social foundations of thought and action: A social cognition theory.* Englewood Cliffs, NJ: Prentice-Hall.

Bandura, A. (2000). Exercise of human agency through collective efficacy. *Current Directions in Psychological Science, 9*(3), 75–78.

Bandura, A. (2001). Social cognitive theory: An agentic perspective. *Annual Review of Psychology, 52*, 1–26.

Beer, S. (1981). *The brain of the firm* (2nd ed.). West Sussex, England: John Wiley and Sons.

Beer, S. (1984). The viable system model: Its provenance, development, methodology, and pathology. *Journal of the Operational Research Society, 35*(1), 7–35.

Bracht, N., & Kingsbury, L. (1990). Community organization principles in health promotion: A five-stage model. In N. Bracht (Ed.), *Health promotion at the community level* (pp. 66–88). Newbury Park, CA: Sage.

Bradbury, H., & Waage, S. (2005). Editorial. *Action Research, 3*(2), 131–134.

Briss, P. A., Brownson, R. C., Fielding, J. E., & Zaza, S. (2004). Developing and using the guide to community preventive services: Lessons learned about evidence-based public health. *Annual Review of Public Health, 25*, 281–302.

Brown, P., & Zavestoski, S. (2004). Social movements in health: An introduction. *Sociology of Health & Illness, 26*(6), 679–694.

Bryson, J. M. (1988). *Strategic planning for public and non-profit organizations* (1st ed.). San Franscisco, CA: Jossey-Bass.

Cain, M., & Mittman, R. (2002). *Diffusion of innovation in health care.* Oakland, CA: Institute for the Future.

Cameron, R., Walker, R., & Jolin, M. A. (1998). *International best practices in heart health.* Toronto, ON: Ontario Public Health Association.

DeJoy, D. M., & Wilson, M. G. (2003). Organizational health promotion: Broadening the horizon of workplace health promotion. *American Journal of Health Promotion, 17*(5), 337–341.

Diamond, M. A. (1995). Organizational change as human process, not technique. *NIDA Research Monograph, 155*, 119–131.

Doak, C. M., Visscher, T. L. S., Renders, C. M. & Seidell, J. C. (2006). The prevention of overweight and obesity in children and adolescents: A review of interventions and programmes. *Obesity Reviews, 7*, 111–136.

Dubois, L. (2006). Food, nutrition, and population health: From scarcity to social inequalities. Chapter 6. In J. Heyman, C. Hertzman, M. L. Barer, & R. G. Evans (Eds.), *Healthier societies: From analysis to action.* New York: Oxford University Press.

Economos, C. D., Brownson, R. C., DeAngelis, M. A., Novelli, P., Foerster, S. B., & Foreman, C. T. et al. (2001). What lessons have been learned from other attempts to guide social change? *Nutrition Reviews, 59*, S40–S56.

Edwards, N., & Kothari, A. (2004). CHNET-Works! A Networking infrastructure for community health nurse researchers and decision-makers. *Canadian Journal of Nursing Research, 36*(4), 203–207.

Edwards, N., Mill, J., & Kothari, A. R. (2004). Multiple intervention research programs in community health. *The Canadian Journal of Nursing Research = Revue Canadienne De Recherche En Sciences Infirmieres, 36*(1), 40–54.

Fiol, C. M., & Lyles, M. A. (1985). Organizational learning. *Academy of Management Review, 10*(4), 803–813.

Frankish, C. J., & Green, L. W. (1994). Organizational and community change as the social scientific basis for disease prevention and health promotion policy. *Advances in Medical Sociology, 4*, 209–233.

Germann, K., & Wilson, D. (2004). Organizational capacity for community development in regional health authorities: A conceptual model. *Health Promotion International, 19*(3), 289–298.

Glasgow, R. E., Vogt, T. M., & Boles, S. M. (1999). Evaluating the public health impact of health promotion interventions: The RE-AIM framework. *American Journal of Public Health, 89*(9), 1322–1327.

Glasgow, R. E., Klesges, L. M., Dzewaltowski, D. A., Bull, S. S., & Estabrooks, P. (2004). The future of health behavior change research: What is needed to improve translation of research into health promotion practice? *Annals of Behavioral Medicine, 27*(1), 3–12.

Goodman, R. M., Steckler, A. B., & Kegler. (1997). Mobilizing organizations for health enhancement: Theories of organizational change. In K. Glanz, F. M. Lewis, & B. K. Rimer (Eds.), *Health behavior and health education: Theory, research, and practice.* San Francisco: Jossey-Bass.

Goodman, R. M. (2000). Bridging the gap in effective program implementation: From Concept to Application. *Journal of Community Psychology, 28*(3), 309–321.

Goodman, R. M., Speers, M. A., McLeroy, K., Fawcett, S., Kegler, M., & Parker, E. et al. (1998). Identifying and defining the dimensions of community capacity to provide a basis for measurement. *Health Education Behavior, 25*(3), 258–278.

Green, L. W. (2006). Public health asks of systems science: to advance our evidence-based practice, can you help us get more practice-based evidence? *American Journal of Public Health, 96*(3), 406–409.

Green, L. W. (2001). From research to "best practices" in other settings and populations. *American Journal of Health Behavior, 25*(3), 165–178.

Green, L. W., & Kreuter, M. W. (2005). *Health program planning: An educational and ecological approach* (4th ed.). New York: McGraw-Hill.

Green, L. W., Richard, L., & Potvin, L. (1996). Ecological foundations of health promotion. *American Journal of Health Promotion, 10*(4), 270–281.

Greenhalgh, T., Robert, G., Macfarlane, F., Bate, P., & Kyriakidou, O. (2004). Diffusion of innovations in service organizations: Systematic review and recommendations. *Milbank Quarterly, 82*(4), 581–629.

Greenhalgh, T., Collard, A., & Begum, N. (2005). Sharing stories: Complex intervention for diabetes education in minority ethnic groups who do not speak English. *British Medical Journal (Clinical Research Edition), 330*(7492), 628.

Hamilton, N., & Bhatti, T. (1996). *Population health promotion: An integrated model of population health and health promotion.* Ottawa, ON, Canada: Health Promotion Department Division, Health Canada.

Institute of Medicine (2005). Committee on prevention of obesity in children and youth. *Preventing childhood obesity: Health in the balance.* Washington, DC: National Academies Press.

Jackson, M. C. (2005). *Systems thinking: Creative holism for managers* (1st ed.). Chicester, UK: John Wiley and Sons.

Joffres, C., Heath, S., Farquharson, J., Barkhouse, K., Latter, C., & MacLean, D. R. (2004). Facilitators and challenges to organizational capacity building in heart health promotion. *Qualitative Health Research, 14*(1), 39–60.

Johns, G. (2001). In praise of context. *Journal of Organizational Behaviour, 22*, 31–42.

Kaluzny, A. D., & Hernandez, S. R. (1988). Organizational change and innovation. In S. M. Shortell, & A. D. Kaluzny (Eds.), *Health care management: A text in organizational theory and behavior* (2nd ed.) (pp. 379–417). New York: Wiley.

Kingdon, J. W. (2003). *Agendas, alternatives, and public policies.* New York: Longman.

Kimberly, J. R., & Bouchikhi, H. (1995). The dynamics of organizational development and change: How the past shapes the present and constrains the future. *Organizational Science, 6*(1), 9–18.

Koepsell, T. D., Wagner, E. H., Cheadle, A. C., Patrick, D. L., Martin, D. C., & Diehr, P. H. et al. (1992). Selected methodological issues in evaluating community-based health promotion and disease prevention programs. *Annual Review of Public Health, 13*, 31–57.

Kogut, B., & Zander, U. (1996). What firms do? coordination, identity, and learning. *Organization Science, 7*(5), 502–518.

Kumanyika, S., Jeffery, R. W., Morabia, A., Ritenbaugh, C., Antipatis, V. J., & Public Health Approaches to the Prevention of Obesity (PHAPO), Working Group of the International Obesity Task Force (IOTF). (2002). Obesity prevention: The case for action. *International Journal of Obesity and Related Metabolic Disorders, Journal of the International Association for the Study of Obesity, 26*(3), 425–436.

Kumanyika, S. K. (2001). Minisymposium on obesity: Overview and some strategic considerations. *Annual Review of Public Health, 22*, 293–308.

Lipshitz, R., Popper, M., & Friedman, V. J. (2002). A multifacet model of organizational learning. *Journal of Applied Behavioral Science, 38*(1), 78–98.

Marmot, M. G. (2004). Evidence based policy or policy based evidence? *British Medical Journal (Clinical Research Edition), 328*(7445), 906–907.

McAmmond, D. (2001). *Promotion and support of healthy eating: An initial overview of knowledge gaps and research needs.* Ottawa: Office of Nutrition Policy and Promotion, Health Canada.

McCormack, B., Kitson, A., Harvey, G., Rycroft-Malone, J., Titchen, A., & Seers, K. (2002). Getting evidence into practice: The meaning of 'context'. *Journal of Advanced Nursing, 38*(1), 94–104.

McLaren, L., Sheill, A., Ghali, L., Lorenzetti, R. M., & Huculak, S. (2004). *Are integrated approaches working to promote healthy weights and prevent obesity and chronic disease?* Ottawa, ON: Health Canada.

McLean, S., Feather, J., & Butler-Jones, D. (2005). *Building health promotion capacity: Action for learning, learning from action* (1st ed.). Vancouver, Canada: UBC Press.

Mercer, S. L., Green, L. W., Rosenthal, A. C., Husten, C. G., Kettel Khan, L., & Dietz, W. H. (2003). Possible lessons from the tobacco experience for obesity control. *American Journal of Clinical Nutrition, 77*(Suppl. 4), 1073S–1082S.

Meynell, F. (2005). A second-order approach to evaluating and facilitating organizational change. *Action Research, 3*(2), 211–231.

Nissen, L. B., Merrigan, D. M., & Kraft, M. K. (2005). Moving mountains together: Strategic community leadership and systems change. *Child welfare* (pp. 123–140) Child Welfare League of America.

Nonaka, I., & Takeuchi, H. (1995). *The knowledge-creating company: How japanese companies create the dynamics of innovation* (1st ed.). New York: Oxford University Press.

NSW Health. (2001). *A framework for building capacity to improve health.*Sydney: NSW Health Department.

Paton, K., Sengupta, S., & Hassan, L. (2005). Settings, systems and organization development: The healthy living and working model. *Health Promotion International, 20*(1), 81–89.

Peterson, J., Atwood, J. R., & Yates, B. (2002). Key elements for church-based health promotion programs: Outcome-based literature review. *Public Health Nursing, 19*(6), 401–411.

Potvin, L. (1996). Methodological challenges in evaluation of dissemination programs. *Canadian Journal of Public Health. Revue Canadienne De Sante Publique, 87*(Suppl. 2), S79–S83.

Preskill, H., & Torres, R. T. (1999). *Evaluative inquiry for learning in organizations.* Thousand Oakes, CA: Sage Publications.

Raine, K. D. (for the Canadian Population Health Initiative). (2004). *Overweight and obesity in Canada – A population health perspective.* Ottawa: The Canadian Institute for Health Information.

Raymond, B., & Moon, C. (2003). Prevention and treatment of overweight and obesity: Toward a roadmap for advocacy and action. *The Permanente Journal, 7*(4), 6–8.

Riley, B. L., Taylor, S. M., & Elliott, S. J. (2001). Determinants of implementing heart health: Promotion activities in Ontario public health units: A social ecological perspective. *Health Education Research, 16*(4), 425–441.

Rogers, E. M. (Ed.). (1995). *Diffusion of innovations* (4th ed.). New York: The Free Press.

Rogers, E. M. (2004). A prospective and retrospective look at the diffusion model. *Journal of Health Communication, 9*(Suppl. 1), 13–19.

Rosenheck, R. A. (2001). Organizational process: A missing link between research and practice. *Psychiatric Services (Washington, DC), 52*(12), 1607–1612.

Sallis, J. F., & Owen, N. (1996). Ecological models. In K. Glanz, F. M. Lewis, & B. K. Rimer (Eds.), *Health education and health behavior*, (pp. 403–424). San Francisco: Jossey-Bass.

Sanson-Fisher, R. W. (2004 March 15). Diffusion of innovation theory for clinical change. *Medical Journal of Australia, 180*, S55–S56.

Senge, P (1999). *The dance of change: The challenges of sustaining momentum in learning organizations.* New York: Doubleday.

Siegel, M. (2002). The effectiveness of state-level tobacco control interventions: A review of program implementation and behavioral outcomes. *Annual Review of Public Health, 23,* 45–71.

Smedley, B. D., Syme, S. L., & Committee on Capitalizing on Social Science and Behavioral Research to Improve the Public's Health. (2001). Promoting health: Intervention strategies from social and behavioral research. *American Journal of Health Promotion, 15*(3), 149–166.

Speller, V., Wimbush, E., & Morgan, A. (2005). Evidence-based health promotion practice: How to make it work. *Promotion & Education,* (Suppl. 1), 15–20.

Stokols, D. (1992). Establishing and maintaining healthy environments: Toward a social ecology of health promotion. *American Psychologist, 47*(1), 6–22.

Stokols, D. (1996). Translating social ecological theory into guidelines for community health promotion. *American Journal of Health Promotion, 10*(4), 282–298.

Swinburn, B., Gill, T., & Kumanyika, S. (2005). Obesity prevention: A proposed framework for translating evidence into action. *Obesity Review, 6*(1), 23–33.

Wenger, E., McDermott, R., & Snyder, W. M. (2002). *Cultivating communities of practice: A guide to managing knowledge* (1st ed.). Boston, MA: Harvard Business.

Wilcox, P. (2003). An ecological approach to understanding youth smoking trajectories: Problems and prospects. *Addiction, 98*(Suppl. 1), 57–77.

World Health Organization. (2003). *Diet, nutrition and the prevention of chronic diseases.* Geneva: Joint FAO/WHO Expert Consultation.

Yach, D., McKee, M., Lopez, A. D., & Novotny, T. for Oxford Vision 2020. (2005). Improving diet and physical activity: 12 lessons from controlling tobacco smoking. *British Medical Journal, 330,* 898–900.

Yeatman, H. R., & Nove, T. (2002). Reorienting health services with capacity building: A case study of the core skills in health promotion project. *Health Promotion International, 17*(4), 341–350.

Zaza, S., Briss, P. A., & Harris, K. W. (Eds.). (2005). *The guide to community preventive services: what works to promote health?* New York: Oxford University Press.

Chapter 13

Community-Based Approaches to Obesity Prevention: The Role of Environmental and Policy Change

Alice S. Ammerman, Carmen D. Samuel-Hodge, Janice K. Sommers, May May Leung, Amy E. Paxton, and Maihan B. Vu

Introduction

One could argue that it was environmental and policy change that "got us into this mess" regarding the obesity epidemic. The built environment is perhaps the most obvious example, where urban sprawl and increasing dependence on the automobile have been linked with prevalence of obesity in adults (see Chapter 8). The cars on which we depend have ever expanding numbers and sizes of beverage holders, making it easy for us to accommodate the oversized calorie-laden drinks now available on nearly every corner in many urban areas. Meanwhile, state level school policies related to high stakes testing and increasing pressure for instructional time have squeezed out opportunities for physical activity by limiting recess and physical education classes in many schools (National Association for Sport and Physical Education & American Heart Association, 2006).

Obesity is a complex and multi-factorial problem, and preventing it will require multi-level change. Just as environmental and policy changes over time have contributed to exacerbating the obesity epidemic; if handled properly, such changes can also greatly contribute to the reversal of this public health epidemic. There are many common elements in the strategies needed to overcome society-wide public health problems such as automotive safety, tobacco, and gun control (Economos, Brownson, DeAngelis, Novelli, Foerster, Foreman, Gregson, Kumanyika, & Pate, 2001; Institute of Medicine, 2005).

However, in certain ways food and physical activity are very different from these other public health issues with respect to environmental and policy change. Behaviors associated with obesity prevention are not ones that can be accomplished with a 'swift arm motion and click' —like fastening a seat belt— or controlled by the cessation of a discrete behavior, such as the use of cigarettes. While legal approaches to tobacco, alcohol, and gun control have had a positive public health impact, litigation for dietary change associated with fast food has not been widely used or accepted as a direct approach to environmental or policy change (Evans, Finkelstein, Kamerow, & Renaud, 2005; Evans, Renaud, Finkelstein, Kamerow, & Brown, 2006). While it's not easy to institute strict controls on any industry, it is relatively easier when one can identify "bad guys," as with tobacco, but much riskier to use strategies that "demonize" the people who produce or prepare our food (Kersh & Morone, 2002).

Implementing environmental and policy changes may have mixed results and does not guarantee that positive behavior change will result. Policies to remove soft drinks and vending machines from schools may, ironically, negatively impact schools' ability to provide opportunities for physical activity through financial support of recreation and sports programming. Costly efforts to provide parks, bike paths, and walking trails do not guarantee that they will be used. It seems clear that while individual and organizational level interventions to prevent and control obesity are not enough, neither will changing environments and policies alone be likely to succeed in the absence of supportive individual level intervention efforts.

Despite the implementation challenges, environmental and policy changes at the local and state levels have the potential for a broader and more sustainable societal impact than more individually-oriented approaches to obesity prevention (Brownson, Haire-Joshu, & Luke, 2006). This may make it possible, ultimately, to reduce obesity-related health disparities affecting lower income and minority populations who are currently at highest risk (see Chapter 3). However, this will not occur without careful planning and attention. To date, for example, efforts to enhance communities' conduciveness to walking and biking have occurred primarily in higher income neighborhoods, where there are more resources to change the physical infrastructure. In addition, it is often in higher income neighborhoods where the political will exists to adopt policies to increase physical activity, for example, ordinances requiring sidewalks in all new developments. Even as opportunities to obtain fresh fruits and vegetables are increasing through marketing innovations, it has been shown repeatedly that lower income and communities of color continue to have the least access to affordable healthy foods (Diez-Roux, Nieto, Caulfield, Tyroler, Watson, & Szklo, 1999; King, Leibtag, & Behl, 2004; Morland, Wing, Diez Roux, & Poole, 2002; Sallis, Nader, Rupp, Atkins, & Wilson, 1986; Zenk, Schulz, Israel, James, Bao, & Wilson, 2006).

The goal of this chapter is to provide an overview of the role of community-level interventions in the prevention of obesity. We begin by defining key concepts related to community action for environmental and policy change. Next, we briefly review the existing literature on environmental and policy approaches to promoting physical activity and healthy eating. We conclude by identifying key issues in planning and evaluating community-level interventions to prevent obesity.

Key Concepts for Community Action

Socio-Ecologic Framework

The **socio-ecologic framework** (McLeroy, Bibeau, Strecker, & Glanz, 1988) is a general way of depicting the layering of micro and macro-influences on individual behavior, using concentric circles (see Figure 13.1 and Chapter 5). This type of framework provides an intuitive understanding of how policy and environmental change can affect availability and accessibility in order to facilitate individual and collective behaviors. While there are many versions of the socio-ecologic framework (see Chapter 5), McLeroy's model will be used in

Socio-Ecologic Model

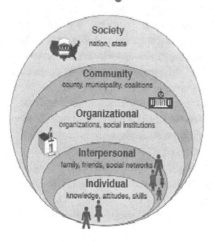

Source: Adapted from McLeroy, et, al, an ecological perspective on health promotion program a
Health Education Quarterly 1968, 15:351-77

Figure 13.1 Socio-ecological model.

this chapter. The socio-ecologic model stresses the importance of addressing public health problems at multiple levels and conveys the dynamic relationship across and within the various levels (McLeroy et al., 1988). However, it is important to remember that policy and environmental change can take place in all but the individual level of the model. For example, worksites can encourage healthier food and exercise breaks at meetings by adopting relevant organizational policy; and families can decide they will purchase only one liter of soda a week, or only have the television on at certain times.

Multi-level interventions that include several layers of the socio-ecologic framework help create a context in which the individual and interpersonal impacts are facilitated by changes at the organizational, community, and societal levels. Brownson et al. (2005) demonstrated the effectiveness of promoting physical activity in rural communities with a multi-level ecological approach. Three levels of the socio-ecologic framework were addressed in the intervention; individual, interpersonal and community. Tailored newsletters addressed the individual level; interpersonal activities focused on social support and the patient-health provider relationship; and community-wide events such as walking groups, festivals and health fairs would be considered organizational and community level interventions. In this study, the greater the exposure to multi-level intervention activities, the more people were likely to be physically active. This demonstrates the impact of combining environmental changes in the outer rings of the socio-ecologic framework (e.g., building walking trails) with behavioral and social interventions to reach the desired health outcome.

Similarly, Peterson et al. (2002) designed an intervention using the individual, interpersonal, and organizational levels of the socio-ecologic model to address barriers of proper nutrition in low-income, multi-ethnic women. Behavior change was the primary focus at the individual level through education and skills training to improve diet and physical activity for weight loss, while efforts to increase social support through home visits and group classes addressed the interpersonal level. Organizational support from federal programs such as WIC (The Supplemental Nutrition Program for Women, Infants, and Children) and the Expanded Food and Nutrition Education Program was needed during the developmental process of the intervention and to ensure its future sustainability. These interventions, at multiple levels, provide examples of designing interventions that are guided by the socio-ecologic framework, which allows one to address the comprehensive nature of the barriers and risks involved, by integrating multiple behavior change strategies.

An excellent illustration of a socio-ecologic framework is found in the IOTF Obesity Causal Web (see Chapter 5 and Chapter 7). A toolkit on childhood obesity sponsored by the American Public Health Association allows users to access intervention ideas by clicking on different elements of this multi-level model (http://www.apha.org/ppp/obesity_toolkit/007_how.htm).

Community-Based Participatory Research, Coalitions and Partnerships

Achieving policy and environmental change is not simply a matter of writing a grant for the funding to design and implement a program. Environments are often, though not always, changed by policy, which is in turn dependent on the right combination of political will, social momentum, and often media advocacy to identify the issues, create partnerships, rally support, and influence decision makers. Often the most effective way to influence policy is through coalitions of stakeholders who may represent diverse interests yet share a common policy goal.

Community-Based Participatory Research (CBPR)
Community-based participatory research (CBPR) is designed to increase the relevance of research to community needs by involving members of that community in identification of the problem and at every step of the research process through intervention design, data collection, and ultimately interpretation of the data and application to addressing the initial problem identified (Israel, Eng, Schulz, & Parker, 2005; Minkler & Wallerstein, 2003). Because effective policy change is best achieved through broad community support guided by research-based evidence of the most effective approaches, CBPR can facilitate the bringing together of researchers and community members in a way that builds on the strengths of each (Kreuter, & Lezin, 2002; Kreuter, Lezin, & Young, 2000; Roussos & Fawcett, 2000).

Researchers can apply their methods to both identifying the most promising evidence-based approaches and then evaluating the impact of policy and environmental change. Community members bring networks of influence and the political will to accomplish meaningful change.

Coalitions and Partnerships
By whatever name they are called, coalitions, partnerships, task forces, networks, or consortia, are groups of individuals, often simultaneously representing other organizations, who come together around a shared cause in the belief that they can have a greater impact collectively. Benefits of a partnership approach are that they: (a) span boundaries between populations and organizations; (b) minimize duplication of effort and services; (c) build trust and

Table 13.1 Characteristics and challenges of effective partnerships.

Characteristics of effective partnerships	Challenges of partnership approaches
• Well defined, specific focus • Agreed upon vision and goal • Solidarity among members	• Time is needed to build partnerships that respond effectively to public health issues
• Unambiguous adversary or health problem	• Ownership of issues and power ultimately rests with partners
• Strong leadership	• Health issue must resonate with stakeholders and take priority over other issues

Source: Butterfoss, 2006a.

respect among organizations; (d) effectively pool innovative talent and resources; (e) reach previously untapped community assets; and (f) implement some strategies (e.g., policy and media advocacy) better than public health or social service agencies (Butterfoss, 2006a; Kegler, Steckler, Malek, & McLeroy, 1998). Characteristics and challenges of effective partnerships are highlighted in Table 13.1, which are followed by a case study to illustrate a successful coalition effort to change policy related to obesity prevention. Effective partnerships are focused and cohesive but they take time to develop and often require significant negotiation and compromise to achieve the desired level of functioning.

Example: Combating Childhood Obesity in North Carolina-7 Steps

Butterfoss (2006b) has suggested seven steps to coalition success. We list these seven steps below, illustrating each step as it contributed to an effort in North Carolina to influence school nutrition and physical activity policy. (http://www. healthwellnc.com/hwtfc/pdffiles/FitFamilies-StudyCommitteeReport05.pdf.) In this case the Coalition is Fit Families NC: A Study Committee for Childhood Overweight/Obesity established by the Lieutenant Governor and funded by tobacco settlement money through the North Carolina Health and Wellness Trust Fund Commission. Formation of the Study Committee resulted in part from longstanding collaborative efforts on the part of multiple coalitions and interest groups to influence nutrition policy. Recommendations from the Study Committee were instrumental in the passage of two pieces of legislation related to beverage vending and school nutrition standards, and one regulation passed by the State Board of Education requiring 30 minutes of daily physical activity for all K-8 children.

Step 1: Clarify or reaffirm vision and mission: After the Study Committee was appointed, the Co-Chairs (2 legislators and a prominent pediatrician) met with a small sub-group of obesity researchers and the Study Committee staff person to clearly define the issues and craft a mission statement that included the objective to influence policy change.

Step 2: Create community ownership of partnership: The Study Committee was announced as part of a kick-off event that was well publicized and involved many stakeholders in the area of child health and particularly nutrition and physical activity. Early meetings involved identifying key issues to address and topics about which the Study Committee needed additional information and guidance from outside experts. All Study Committee meetings were open to the public with observers invited to offer input on all topics. Meetings were well attended by stakeholders involved with childhood obesity prevention efforts.

Step 3: Solidify partnership structure and processes: This committee was fortunate to have a full time staff person who worked closely with the co-chairs and committee members to create a mission statement and goals and, over time, to create additional sub-committees to address important issues that emerged, such as the practice of charging indirect costs to child nutrition services and resulting impact on their ability to serve healthy meals to children in schools. Meetings were organized to provide the committee with in-depth education regarding child obesity topics, particularly nutrition and physical activity in the schools. The committee went through an organized process of drafting a long list of legislative recommendations and then refining these as well as determining the most politically feasible approach to moving them to the legislature or the state board of education.

Step 4: Recruit and retain an active diverse membership: The Study Committee was carefully selected to include broad representation from community organizations both directly and indirectly involved with public education. This included school administrators, business leaders, child nutrition staff, physical activity advocates, clergy, academics, and state health leaders. Representatives of the vending industry were also brought to the table. Excellent communication and well run meetings kept Study Committee members involved and engaged. Co-chairs, staff, and committee members clearly communicated that the opinions of all members of the group were valued. Well publicized legislative successes contributed to retention and continued investment of committee members.

Step 5: Develop collaborative leadership: In this case, the leadership was appointed at the time of committee formation. Committee leadership included two highly respected legislators committed to child health and a pediatrician known throughout the state with a track record of advocacy around pediatric obesity. Despite the "high level" nature of the leadership, they were very successful in conducting meetings in a way that drew on the expertise of all committee members and empowered them to play an active role in discussions and policy recommendations.

Step 6: Focus on action and advocacy: Study Committees can be used by legislative bodies to either kill a legislative issue by taking it off the table, or to mobilize the necessary effort to achieve policy change. This Study Committee clearly accomplished the latter. Despite the rather passive sounding name of "Study Committee," this group defined its mission early as impacting policy. However, this was done in such a way as to gain broad community support, due to the credibility of committee members and deliberate process by which the work was done.

Step 7: Market your partnership: The Study Committee staff moved quickly to keep the committee informed of legislative actions and successes as well as working with the media to publicize these accomplishments. Committee publications detailing the recommendations and resulting regulations and policies made the work of the committee visible and highlighted its impact.

Evidence of the Impact of Policy and Environmental Change to Date

Brownson et al. (2006) have developed a specific framework to address the prevention of chronic diseases through environmental and policy change (see Figure 13.2). This framework illustrates how environmental and policy interventions altering the physical, economic, and communication environments combined with shifts toward more supportive social norms and necessary human resources and capital input can result in positive health behavior changes ultimately leading to reduced risk for chronic disease and increased quality of life. The following sections present evidence for the relative strength of different elements of this model based on research to date in the area of physical activity and healthy eating. The strength of evidence in each area was rated by Brownson and colleagues as strong, sufficient, or insufficient to warrant strong recommendation without further research. In the case of interventions with high face validity or supportive evidence from another area of public health yet where the evidence of effectiveness has not been clearly documented, the intervention is labeled as a "promising practice."

Physical Activity

Relative to tobacco policy and environmental change efforts, efforts to promote physical activity and healthy eating through this approach are relatively new and untested. However, there is a growing body of evidence helping to direct future intervention approaches. Brownson et al. (2006) present the evidence in six specific categories that bridge the domains in Figure 13.2.

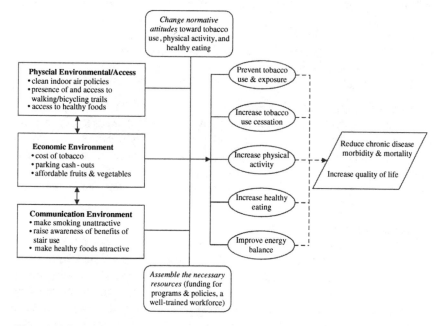

Figure 13.2 Framework for Addressing the Prevention of Chronic Diseases through Environmental and Policy Change.

Source: Brownson et al., 2006.

Further details and references regarding this evidence review can be obtained from the article in the Annual Review of Public Health (Brownson et al., 2006). The methods of the Guide to Community Services were used to evaluate the set of physical activity interventions according to their study design and execution (Zaza, Briss, & Harris, 2005).

Access to Facilities

According to Brownson's review, there appears to be a consistent association between level of physical activity in a community and accessibility of recreational facilities, opportunities to be active, and aesthetic qualities of the facilities, such as appealing scenery on walking trails. Interventions designed to increase facilities use either through training or health communication have achieved some success.

Urban Planning and Policy

Changes in the urban landscape over the last half century moving us into the "freeway era" have been among the most profound in terms of limiting the opportunities and need for physical activity related to transportation (see Chapter 8). Given the cost and relative permanence of this type of environmental design, reversing these trends will not happen easily. There is consistent evidence now documenting the fact that higher residential density, mixed land use (e.g., shopping within walking distance from homes) and connected streets (vs. cul-de-sacs) are associated with higher rates of walking and cycling. Interventions through urban planning and policy have showed some positive impact on these forms of physical activity. A limitation of studies in this area is that few address communities with ethnically diverse populations.

Transportation Policy

Changes in transportation policy have the potential to impact travel choice (walking vs. driving) as well as improving air quality and traffic congestion which may ultimately encourage more non-motorized transport. To date, there is insufficient evidence to make specific recommendations regarding the best approaches to transportation, but this appears to be a promising area of research and action.

School-Based Physical Education

There is strong evidence that policy and environmental changes to increase the number and length of PE classes as well as the intensity of activity (e.g., substituting soccer for softball, modifying game rules to increase activity levels) are associated with increased energy expenditure among children. There is also promising evidence for the sustainability of these interventions after the research period has ended.

Economic Incentives

The adverse economic impact of physical inactivity has been widely estimated and publicized ($76 billion in year 2000) in the U.S. associated with direct medical expenses (Pratt, Macera, & Wang, 2000). There has been some effort to study how financial incentives and disincentives may influence level of activity but as yet there are few empirical data showing the impact of such interventions. However, this represents a promising area of policy intervention and research.

Point of Decision Prompts

While often thought of as an environmental approach to changing food purchases, point of decision prompts have also been quite useful in promoting increased physical activity. There is now sufficient evidence to recommend the use of prompts to encourage the use of stairs, and recent studies are beginning to refine the specific recommended approaches. This represents an unusually low cost approach to environmental change that holds promise and could also impact future building design decisions by creating a demand for easier access to stairwells.

Promotion of Healthy Eating

There are also a number of policies and environmental change approaches to improved nutrition that have been evaluated. Brownson and colleagues (2006) divide them into 5 specific areas within the broader context of physical, economic, and communication environments.

Food and Beverage Availability in Schools

This has been an area of significant recent interest as schools across the country participating in the federal child nutrition reimbursement programs are now required to submit wellness policies for their districts. Interventions tested to date have included changes in the food service, including menu planning, staff training, and purchasing. Improved health curricula and classroom snacks are other targets of change. Evidence across these studies shows positive results, but in general the effect is small. An important area of research will be to evaluate the degree to which school nutrition policies are implemented, enforced, and have an impact on children's dietary intake.

Access to Healthy Ready-to-Eat Foods

Ready-to-eat foods typically offer portion sizes two to five times larger than the norm over the last 20–30 years and account for over one third of the total energy intake in the U.S. (Ledikwe, Ello-Martin, & Rolls, 2005; Wansink, 2004; Young & Nestle, 2003). To date, there is promising evidence that worksite and school programs can improve ready-to-eat foods in cafeterias and vending machines. Community-based programs in churches, hotels, and restaurants have also improved food preparation and access to healthier options, and have increased customer requests for healthier entrees. Little work has been done to evaluate the impact of interventions in fast food restaurants.

Food Pricing and Incentives

There also appears to be promising, though limited, evidence regarding food pricing and incentives such as reduced pricing of healthy vending machine offerings. These studies have taken place primarily in schools and worksites. Additional efforts could test policies within specific settings that increase the price for unhealthier foods while lowering the cost of healthier items.

Nutrition Labeling and information

This approach to policy and environmental change generally involves point of purchase labeling in restaurants, grocery stores, cafeterias, and worksites, including snack bars, cafeterias, and vending machines. According to Brownson's review, there is sufficient evidence that such interventions can lead to improvements in the selection and intake of healthy foods. Just as point-of-decision prompts can promote increased physical activity without major structural change, point of purchase prompts for foods also appear to be a relatively low cost approach to environmental change to promote healthier eating.

Media and Marketing Policies

Included in this category are policy and environmental intervention campaign efforts promoting education and awareness of healthy foods, and limiting advertisements for foods of minimal nutritional value. Also included are approaches to regulating food through advertising, particularly when targeting youth. This is a challenging area of study, and, to date, there is some evidence suggesting benefits in terms of awareness, intention to improve intake, and modest improvements in reported intake associated with media and marketing approaches promoting healthier foods. There is, as yet, limited evidence of the impact of nutrition policies regulating media messages that address unhealthy food intake. However, given the success of this approach in other areas such as tobacco control, regulation of media messages regarding unhealthy food remains a promising area for future work.

Planning and Implementation

There are a number of planning models designed for public health interventions, but most are aimed at the individual and organizational levels, so must be adapted for or refocused on policy and environmental changes in communities. Because of the critical role of partnerships and coalitions in the process of identifying and influencing policy, planning and evaluation models that address community engagement and empowerment can also be useful. In this case, "community" is more broadly defined as the stakeholders sharing a common policy-related interest. This could include parents who desire better food served in schools as well as legislators who believe healthier food is necessary for improved academic performance.

Earlier in this chapter we reviewed the key elements of coalition building (see Table 13.1). The success of coalitions is largely determined by their ability to engage in continuous planning and evaluation, i.e., to assess progress, identify facilitators and barriers to progress from inside and outside their ranks, and use this information to adjust their approach and move forward. Therefore, perhaps even more than most public health planning and implementation models, formative evaluation (sometimes called participatory evaluation using an action research cycle) (Fetterman, Wandersman, & Kafterian, 1995) is critical to the ongoing process. We will therefore, discuss this in tandem with approaches to planning and empowerment. A considerable body of literature now addresses successful approaches for community engagement and/or empowerment. While most of this literature is not specific to obesity prevention, the key principles apply to public health issues generally.

Community Engagement

Involving communities and coalitions in national, state, or local actions to address health issues can be viewed as taking place in 3 stages: (a) Community

Engagement and Assessment; (b) Deliberation and Planning; and (c) Implementation (Thompson, Minkler, Bell, Rose, & Butler, 2003). During the **community engagement and assessment stage**, the main objectives are to: (1) identify the level of concern and awareness of the health issue; (2) identify stakeholders and create a forum for partnership; (3) provide opportunities for individuals and organizations to share their values, attitudes and beliefs; and (4) create opportunities for building trust between partners. In this initial stage it is critical that the diversity of voices is heard and that issues are identified and framed by coalition members who know the social, political, and cultural context. The **deliberation and planning stage** creates the basis for identifying potential solutions and their associated costs and benefits. The goal of deliberations is to find common ground for action. Finally, the **implementation stage** involves decision-making and compromise to identify and begin working on a manageable number of priority areas with achievable (and measurable) outcomes. Good communication between coalition partners is essential. These or similar stages have been applied to a variety of public health issues and settings including asthma, tobacco, and school health (Butterfoss et al., 2006; Kegler et al., 1998; Moore, 1998; Smith, Howell, & McCann, 1990).

Development of Community Partnerships and Coalitions

As described earlier, the role of the coalition is to identify and mobilize individuals and organizations in the community that are committed to a similar issue (although not necessarily for similar reasons) and have the ability, either through affiliations or persuasiveness, to contribute toward affecting the desired change. In the case of obesity prevention or any other public health issue, early steps in the planning process are to identify existing organizations and coalitions as well as individuals who share a common concern regarding obesity. A focused mission and "winnable" objectives should be identified early in the process, followed by further efforts to assure that important players are "at the table." For example, if the objective is to increase physical activity in the schools, key school administrators as well as representative teachers should be involved.

Butterfoss (2006b) identifies key factors that influence community empowerment: leadership identification and/or development; problem assessment and identification; organizational structures and management; and resource mobilization. In the text below, we use these factors to guide a discussion of how the process of coalition building and empowerment can be used to plan and implement policy and environmental change for obesity prevention. We also use these factors to frame approaches to evaluation that are designed to both guide the planning process and help to measure its effectiveness.

Leadership Identification and/or Development

Coalitions must identify leaders who are skilled at recognizing the priorities, motivations, skills, and liabilities of coalition members and be able to guide the efforts of these individuals so that they contribute most and detract least from the work of the group. Group members contribute by helping to identify and support the leadership efforts of those who have these abilities, while redirecting the energies of individuals who might want to claim a leadership role but who are less likely to be successful. Because coalitions often depend on leaders who are already overcommitted, opportunities to nurture the development of new leaders should be sought.

Problem Assessment and Identification

It is common for coalitions, in their enthusiasm for the issue that brought them together, to identify too large a task and then fail in trying to achieve it. Initial work of the group should involve discussion of potential directions and approaches to achieving goals in order to identify key stakeholders and gradually focus on a problem and potential policy or environmental change solution which is achievable. Early in the life of a coalition, it is wise to look for "low hanging fruit," i.e., to select readily achievable objectives in order to demonstrate to coalition members that they are capable of having an impact. For example, in the North Carolina Childhood Obesity Study Committee example discussed earlier, although a long list of possible policy actions was identified initially, careful thought was given to those for which the current climate and levels of stakeholder interest offered the greatest chance of achieving legislative action. Early successes in these areas created both positive media coverage for the committee and renewed energy on the part of its members to tackle some of the more intractable problems.

Organizational Structures and Management

Coalitions are generally in the position of making up their organizational and management structures as they go along. Since the lack of time and the commitment of coalition members to other duties are often major barriers to moving forward toward action, identifying an individual whose duty is to "staff" the coalition (whether paid or in kind) can often be key to success. It is important to assure that this individual takes a broad interest in coalition members and their needs rather than appearing to favor their own organization or a select few. All members of the coalition should be involved in discussing and implementing management approaches, such as frequency of meetings, communication systems, and decision making approaches.

Resource Mobilization

An underlying intent of policy and environmental change is to achieve a longer term impact than what can usually be accomplished by intervention programs targeting individuals. Such programs are often dependent on year to year appropriations of funding and are at risk for termination due to budget cuts. Individual level counseling and education programs also require a significant "dose" in terms of staff time and intervention materials, and the behavioral effects generally diminish after the program ends. On the other hand, policies such as seat belt laws require few resources for implementation and are largely self enforcing once they become a habit. Policy alternatives that are "passive" (require limited action on the part of the individual), such as lowering of trans fats in the food supply, can have a broad impact with limited resources required beyond initial implementation. Overdependence on grant funding is a common problem in public health, resulting in 1–3 year program cycles with little hope of sustainability.

Perhaps most frustrating to those in the position of implementing policy is the "unfunded mandate." If not accompanied by any funding or structure for implementation, such policies can have a limited, or perhaps even adverse impact. For example, schools are already under a great deal of pressure regarding academic achievement. Principals' and teachers' evaluations and salaries are increasingly tied to the academic achievements of their students. Food and nutrition policies that are seen to detract from the academic focus (like devoting more time for recess or other physical activity) are often viewed negatively and sometimes actively resisted. This creates a climate where promoting healthy eating and physical activity becomes viewed as yet another burden and a distraction rather than something embraced as integral to children's formative development. Thus, it is key to think beyond passing a piece of legislation to its potential impact. A smaller legislative step that has both funding and "teeth" may ultimately be far more effective than what appears to be a major policy success, but, in reality, has little hope for implementation.

Evaluating Outcomes

Measuring the impact of policy and environmental change is a relatively new and evolving area of evaluation with many potential approaches. In this chapter, we will first discuss the use of process measures to evaluate coalition success, and then address broader approaches to assessing community-level change in support of nutrition and physical activity. Key to successful evaluation is the recognition that it is integrally connected with broader program planning and implementation processes.

Evaluating Coalition Success

Given the importance of coalitions in achieving policy and environmental changes, explicit evaluation of the success of coalitions can be very useful. Butterfoss (2006b) outlines seven steps to successful partnership evaluation in Table 13.2 and describes key indicators that have been widely used by researchers and practitioners to gauge community participation levels (Butterfoss, 2006a).

Strategies to measure community participation and coalition success include: **participant surveys**; event or activity logs to document coalition actions and accomplishments relative to goals and objectives; **key informant interviews** to assess contextual coalition information, such as the formation, structure, operations, resources, and linkages; **focus groups** to identify and explore barriers,

Table 13.2 Partnership evaluation steps.

Seven steps to successful partnership evaluation
1. Establish evaluation plan from the onset of the program
2. Obtain buy-in from community and coalition partners to build commitment to evaluation
3. Allot staff time to make evaluation a priority
4. Match methods to evaluation questions
5. Engage priority populations to help create measures that generate reliable data
6. Report results clearly and often to the community (coalition)
7. Be flexible and creative

Source: Butterfoss, 2006b.

Table 13.3 Key indicators to gauge community and coalition participation.

Measures of community/coalition participation
1. Diversity of participants/organizations
2. Recruitment/retention of new members
3. Role in the coalition or its activities
4. Number and type of coalition events attended
5. Amount of time spent in and outside coalition activities
6. Benefits and challenges of participation
7. Satisfaction with the work or process of participation
8. Balance of power and leadership

Source: Butterfoss, 2006a.

facilitators, and coalition roles; **observation of meetings** to determine quality, participation, and productivity of meeting interactions; **and review of existing documents,** such as meeting agendas, minutes, and annual reports. Publications by Butterfoss (2006a) and Granner and Sharpe (2003, 2004) include extensive references to and inventories of measurement tools for assessing coalition effectiveness. Table 13.3 gives examples of key indicators that are widely used by researchers and practitioners to gauge community and coalition participation.

Evaluating the Broader Impact of Policy and Environmental Changes

Goodman (1998) and Israel et al. (2005) offer models for evaluating community-based programs which can serve as a helpful guide to evaluate intervention approaches to policy and environmental change. Others are developing and testing measurement tools for this relatively new area of evaluation. Key elements and potential measurement strategies to evaluate policy and environmental change are described in this section.

Use Logic Models or Causal Pathways to Identify Evaluation Focus

A frequent challenge of evaluating policy and environmental change is the expectation of measuring the impact on improved health outcomes at the individual level. Because this type of intervention is designed to change environments and reach populations rather than individuals, it is often not feasible or even possible to track the impact to this level. Instead, a logic model can be used to specify the full range of causal factors and outcomes associated with achieving the health outcome of interest. By identifying the elements of the pathway where evidence based associations exist, we can narrow the focus of evaluation for policy and environmental change. For example, there is strong evidence that increased physical activity is associated with obesity prevention and control in children (see Figure 13.3). This change in physical activity and BMI are far to the right on logical models designed to show the causal chain from left to right. Therefore, to evaluate the impact of a policy change designed to prevent and control obesity by increasing physical activity time at school outside of the traditional PE class setting, we do not necessarily need to measure whether children lose or maintain weight, but rather whether they become more active as a result of the policy. If these measures are not possible, it is still useful to move further to the left on the logic model to measure intermediate steps, such as the degree to which the policy is implemented and enforced in schools.

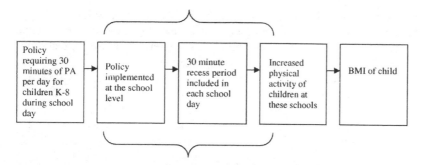

Figure 13.3 Logic model: Areas of measurement to assess impact of policy change.

Adapt Evaluation Methods to Fit the Context: Political, Economic, Cultural Characteristics

Usually a combination of qualitative and quantitative methods is necessary to fully understand the impact of a policy or environmental change. Unlike measuring behavioral change at the individual level where a validated instrument can be used in a wide variety of settings, most policy and environmental changes are developed around a specific political and social context and thus should be evaluated within that context. Therefore, evaluation instruments must be adapted to capture relevant information. If, for example, one wants to measure the impact of removing soft drinks from vending machines in high school, it will be important to determine whether this results in new behaviors that might maintain the level of soft drink consumption, such as more students going off campus for lunch or increased soft drink sales by clubs. Anecdotal reports suggest that implementation of nutrition standards in schools has sometimes resulted in student and even teacher run "black market" sales of candy and other snack foods. Failing to understand such unintended consequences of a policy can result in an inaccurate evaluation of its impact.

Assess Multiple Types of Change Including Process, Impact, and Outcome

As discussed earlier, process evaluation is critical to understanding the success of coalitions and focuses on the process of how an outcome is achieved. Such evaluation is most useful if data are collected and analyzed in conjunction with impact or outcome data. Regarding environmental changes at the community level, some important questions to ask and process data to collect through community surveys, logs, coding of minutes, and observation include: (1) were the goals of the environmental change important to the community?; (2) was the project implemented as planned?; (3) what population was most impacted and was it the one intended?; (4) were there unintended consequences?; and (5) what might be done differently in future implementation to achieve greater success? Often ongoing process measures are key to helping design additional qualitative and quantitative assessment to understand impact of policy and environmental change.

Impact and outcome measures are designed to assess the effects of policy and environmental change and have been variously defined. According to Israel et al. (2005), impact evaluation assesses effectiveness in achieving desired change in targeted mediators that precede the outcome, focusing on what the intervention is designed to alter. While outcome measures are traditionally defined as a physiologic health indicator, as described earlier, this may not be necessary if there is an evidence base linking a behavior with a health outcome. For example, if the purpose of a state level nutrition policy change is to prevent obesity in children, impact assessment might involve determining the number and type of schools that implement the policy; while outcome measures might assess the impact (in a sub-sample of students) on a selected set of dietary practices known to be associated with obesity. The distinction between impact and outcome measures is often blurred. Perhaps most important is to measure variables at multiple points along the causal chain in order to understand the effect at various levels and to inform future change efforts.

Tools to Assess Environmental and Policy Change
Several researchers have developed and tested measures specifically designed to assess the impact and outcomes associated with policy and environmental change. Each must be adapted to the particular context, but these tools offer insight into evaluation options.

Ecobehavioral Measures
Richter and colleagues (2000) describe their approach as an ecobehavioral perspective, with "units of analysis" as the "social, physical, and cultural circumstances that affect the aggregate behavior of groups or classes of individuals." Applying this theory to the health environment for physical activity and nutrition among youth, they identify a variety of relevant environmental measures and then present an evaluation case study applying some of these methods (Richter et al., 2000). The types of measures reviewed include:

1. **written surveys:** such as a national non-random sample of park and recreation directors regarding the number and type of exercise facilities, programs, and personnel
2. **written reports, logs, and interviews:** including city, county and state levels; completed by project staff, organization representatives, owners, and leaders; church, supermarket, school, restaurant, and labor unions; documentation of the frequency, type, and extent of health promotion activities, policies, or environmental features, such as eating out options and recreation opportunities
3. **direct observation:** completed in grocery stores, supermarkets, bodegas, community exercise facilities, family settings, neighborhoods; documenting types of food available (e.g., proportion of milk available that is low fat, bread that is whole wheat), shelf space or menu offerings for healthier options, number of sporting goods stores, parental modeling of healthy behaviors, presence or absence of healthy and unhealthy foods in family pantry.

Among the 16 instruments identified and reviewed by Richter, nearly three quarters reported some level of reliability, typically inter-rater reliability and somewhat fewer reported a comparison with health behaviors.

In a case study of a school intervention initiative designed to improve school lunches and nutrition education, enhance opportunities of school and community fitness activities, and involve a variety of stakeholders to create broader community change, Richter and colleagues (2000) illustrate how measures of process, environmental change, and individual level outcomes can be combined to assess project effectiveness.

Process measures included community surveys and teacher logs to document community and school buy-in and the quality and integrity of intervention delivery; while environmental level outcomes, such as change in school lunches and community-based opportunities for physical activity, were documented by tracking systems and analyzing school lunch menus. Finally, individual level outcomes such as child nutrition knowledge and fitness levels were measured by survey and fitness assessments.

Richter and colleagues note the critical role of partnerships and coalitions in environmental and policy change, and that community change data not only provides an outcome evaluation but can be used during the life of the project to improve partnership functioning and to focus on "what matters" to the community. In suggesting future research, they call for: identification of additional environmental factors for measurement; studies to validate environmental assessments against behavioral measures (vs. health status inputs); and efforts to determine causal relationships between measures of environment and behavior using innovative study designs. Finally, they encourage the use of environmental measures to advocate for environmental and policy change, arguing that this type of "creative epidemiology" can catch the attention of both policy makers and consumers, and "combined with tactics from diffusion theory and media advocacy may help policy makers engender backing for widespread environmental changes to support physical activity and nutrition in children" (Richter et al., 2000).

Community-Level Indicators

The CDC convened a panel of experts knowledgeable about community-based program evaluation and chronic disease prevention to generate a list of Community Level Indicators (CLIs), which are based on observations/ measures to assess a variety of outcomes at the community rather than the individual health behavior level. These measures were designed to be lower cost alternatives and an approach to assessing environmental level change in the areas of tobacco use, physical activity, and diet (Cheadle, Sterling, Schmid, & Fawcett, 2000). Cheadle and colleagues grouped the CLIs as measuring: (1) information, (2) behavioral outcomes, (3) policy and regulation, and (4) environmental change. Table 13.4 illustrates some of the measures identified for nutrition and physical activity in these four categories. Note that while we would normally think of education (information) and behavioral outcomes as individual level indicators, these are measured at the community level.

Cheadle and colleagues (2000) note that advantages of these measures are: (1) they may be much less expensive to collect (in some cases less than one-tenth the cost) with roughly the same relative power as individual surveys (Cheadle et al., 2000); (2) they tend to reflect intermediate measures that are often the specific target of community level interventions, thus provide monitoring and feedback on progress; and (3) they tend to be unobtrusive and therefore non-reactive measures, and thus are less susceptible to social desirability bias.

Limitations of these measures are that the information is not always readily available, numerous assumptions and definitions must be specified, and they are not easily standardized across settings.

Tracking Programs

A final form of evaluation for environmental and policy change involves tracking programs to document community actions and changes over time. Led by Steve Fawcett, one system was developed by the Kansas Workgroup on Health

Table 13.4 Summary of community level indicators (CLI).

CLI category	Physical activity	Nutrition
Information	• Percent of health care providers routinely advising patients to exercise • Availability of education materials at worksites linking PA to health	• Point of purchase information provided in cafeterias • Presence of nutrition posters in learning environments
Behavioral outcome	• Observation of usage (walking trails, mall walk programs) • Memberships in YMCAs, health clubs • Sales of sports equipment, exercise videos	• Bar code sales data • Inventory control data (e.g., school and worksite cafeterias) for food usage • Proportion of low-fat items in stores (via use of marker items like low fat milk)
Environmental change	• Miles of walking trails per capita • # of PA facilities per capita in schools • Availability of PA facilities to community members (hours, fees, etc.)	• Presence of healthy foods in school vending machines • Healthy menus in schools, worksites, etc. • Number of low-fat items in restaurants (menu analysis)
Policy and regulation	• Presence of local policies to include PE in public K-12 curriculum • Amount/percent of local budget per capita for PA/recreation • Presence of policies promoting inclusion of recreation facilities with new construction	• Percent of schools with lunch options congruent with dietary guidelines • Commodity food programs-presence of low fat foods • Policy to monitor nutrition claims made by local food retailers

Source: Cheadle et al., 2000.

Promotion and Community Development and the Centers for Disease Control and Prevention (Fawcett, Paine-Andrews, Harris, Francisco, Richter, & Lewis, 1995). This system can be used as part of a larger and very useful "Community Tool Box" developed by Fawcett and colleagues, http://ctb.ku.edu/. Such tracking systems monitor community-based efforts to effect policy and environmental changes that support healthy eating and promote physical activity. Adapted from this model, the Progress Check System is a Microsoft Access based evaluation tool that has the capacity to track the process and outcomes of community efforts. In addition to the Fawcett program, Progress Check was adapted from progress documentation systems used by the North Carolina Cardiovascular Health Program, and the New York State Department of Health.

Important features of Progress Check and other tracking programs are that they capture: (1) local agency efforts toward accomplishing environmental and policy level changes; (2) actual changes accomplished; and (3) unique information about local programs while at the same time providing statewide data. This facilitates: (1) tracking local environment and policy level changes over time across the state; (2) data-based decisions on program planning and development by local programs; and (3) identifying and implementing best practices for local programs in achieving policy and environment level changes.

These systems are based on a logic model (see Figure 13.4) that illustrates the development of a program from groundwork to program outcomes. This

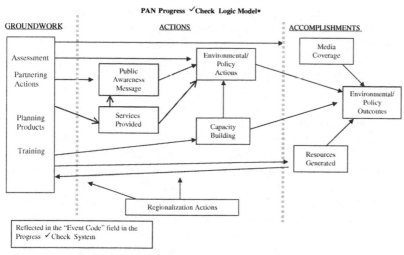

Source: Adapted from the User's Guide to PAN Progress ✓Check System, 2006

Figure 13.4 ProgressCheck logic model.

Source: Adapted from the User's Guide to PAN ProgressCheck System, 2006.

logic model includes the elements of successful programs designed to bring about policy and environment level changes.

Data recorded include actual events and their immediate outcomes, funding source(s) for the initiative, types of agencies that collaborated for the event, risk factor(s) addressed, geographic area(s) served, setting(s) targeted by the initiative, population(s) served, and the specific outcome objective the event relates to. Each event is then coded as to which part of the logic model it addresses. While the ultimate goal is to improve health by increasing healthy lifestyle behaviors and improving individual risk factors, tracking programs document efforts by community-based organizations in initiating policies and practices that create healthier environments. The systems stop short of evaluating the impact of these efforts on individual behaviors and risk factors in communities.

Summary and Conclusions

Environment and policy change for obesity prevention at the community level is an area of rapid growth and exciting development. It is not for the faint of heart, however, in that it requires risk taking, comfort with ambiguity, a long time horizon, and uncertainty about outcomes and strategies for evaluation. At the same time, it may hold the greatest promise for broad and sustainable impact that can benefit all members of the community. Lessons learned to date can help us better address the challenges that remain in this field.

One of the most significant challenges facing researchers and practitioners regarding environmental and policy change is assuring that these interventions reach the most vulnerable and underserved. While an advantage of this type of broad change is generally greater population reach, to date many changes in the built environment have benefited mostly those living in communities that have the resources and political will to make changes. One way to better address disparities is through more creative partnering, with organizations and state or federal agencies related to housing and transportation, for example, that have mandates to address the needs of the underserved.

Another significant challenge related to environmental and policy change is rigorously addressing the question, "If you build it, will they come?" This relates both to structural changes in the environment and "building" policies designed to improve nutrition and physical activity. As discussed in the chapter, there is substantial evidence that multi-level approaches to environmental and policy change are more likely to be successful than those taking place at one level only. Building a walking trail alone (community level of the socio-ecologic model) will likely have more impact on physical activity if supported by efforts to increase social support and motivation through walking clubs and incentive programs. Similarly, we are already seeing that the national requirement for school wellness policies needed to qualify for child nutrition program reimbursement, while a far reaching policy change, has little in the way of "teeth" for enforcement and will likely require other multi-level supportive interventions in order to be successful.

It has become increasingly important for success in accessing and retaining resources to support obesity prevention interventions to demonstrate the evidence base. Most often such interventions are asked to demonstrate efficacy or effectiveness in achieving weight loss or maintenance. This can be a daunting or even impossible task when evaluating environmental and policy change that is designed to reach entire communities and to be one component of a multi-level approach. As we have discussed in this chapter, we need to "think outside the box" in terms of outcomes to be assessed and not assume that data on health-related outcomes is critical, especially if there is a good evidence base connecting the behavior targeted with health improvement. Intermediate variables related to "community level indicators" can increase our evaluation flexibility in terms of cost and feasibility and also serve as important checks for community partners on the implementation process (see also Chapter 5). We have seen that it is critical to consider unintended or negative outcomes associated with environmental and policy change. It is also clear that economic analyses will be needed to help us justify this approach to obesity treatment and prevention in the long term.

When designing and implementing environmental and policy change, we need to build broad coalitions with new and unusual partners and to think entrepreneurially. This represents a different way of thinking for many in public health. It is both exciting and perhaps unsettling. Creating partnerships with the department of transportation or the vending industry will require thoughtful planning and careful attention to both compromise and sustainability. It will also require persistence and innovation and the ability to learn from both our successes and failures. Just as environmental and policy changes over the last 50 years have significantly contributed to "getting us into this mess" of the obesity epidemic, we now have the opportunity to use these same forces to begin working our way out of it.

References

Brownson, R. C., Hagood, L., Lovegreen, S. L., Britton, B., Caito, N. M., & Elliott, M. B. et al. (2005). A multilevel ecological approach to promoting walking in rural communities. *Preventive Medicine, 41*, 837–842.

Brownson, R. C., Haire-Joshu, D., & Luke, D. A. (2006). Shaping the context of health: A review of environmental and policy approaches in the prevention of chronic diseases. *Annual Review of Public Health, 27*, 341–370.

Butterfoss, F. D. (2006a). Process evaluation for community participation. *Annual Review of Public Health, 27*, 323–340.

Butterfoss, F. D. (2006b). Building, maintaining and evaluating state HDSP partnerships. Plenary session 5 at CDC's Heart disease and stroke prevention program management and evaluation training: State programs, Atlanta, GA.

Butterfoss, F. D., Gilmore, L. A., Krieger, J. W., Lachance, L. L., Lara, M., & Meurer, J. R., (2006). From formation to action: How allies against asthma coalitions are getting the job done. *Health Promotion Practice, 7*(Suppl. 2), 34S–43S.

Cheadle, A., Sterling, T. D., Schmid, T. L., & Fawcett, S. B. (2000). Promising community-level indicators for evaluating cardiovascular health-promotion programs. *Health Education Research, 15*, 109–116.

Diez-Roux, A. V., Nieto, F. J., Caulfield, L., Tyroler, H. A., Watson, R. L., & Szklo, M. (1999). Neighbourhood differences in diet: The Atherosclerosis Risk in Communities (ARIC) Study. *Journal of Epidemiology and Community Health, 53*, 55–63.

Economos, C. D., Brownson, R. C., DeAngelis, M. A., Novelli, P., Foerster, S. B., & Foreman, C. T. et al. (2001). What lessons have been learned from other attempts to guide social change? *Nutrition Reviews, 59*, S40–S56; discussion S57–S65.

Evans, W. D., Finkelstein, E. A., Kamerow, D. B., & Renaud, J. M. (2005). Public perceptions of childhood obesity. *American Journal of Preventive Medicine, 28*, 26–32.

Evans, W. D., Renaud, J. M., Finkelstein, E., Kamerow, D. B., & Brown, D. S. (2006). Changing perceptions of the childhood obesity epidemic. *American Journal of Health Behavior, 30*, 167–176.

Fawcett, S. B., Paine-Andrews, A., Harris, K. J., Francisco, V. T., Richter, K. P., & Lewis, R. K. (1995). *Evaluating community efforts to prevent cardiovascular diseases*. Atlanta, GA: Centers for Disease Control and Prevention.

Fetterman, D. M., Wandersman, A., & Kafterian, S. (1995). Empowerment evaluation: Knowledge and tools for self-assessment and accountability. Thousand Oaks, CA: Sage.

Goodman, R. M. (1998). Principals and tools for evaluating community-based prevention and health promotion programs. *Journal of Public Health Management and Practice, 4*, 37–47.

Granner, M. L., & Sharpe, P. A. (2003). An inventory of measurement tools for evaluating community coalition characteristics and functioning. Retrieved October 26, 2006, from University of South Carolina Web site: http://prevention.sph.sc.edu/tools/CoalitionEvalInvent.pdf

Granner, M. L., & Sharpe, P. A. (2004). Evaluating community coalition characteristics and functioning: A summary of measurement tools. *Health Education Research, 19*, 514–532.

Institute of Medicine. (2005). *Preventing childhood obesity: Health in the balance*. Washington, DC: National Academies Press.

Israel, B. A., Eng, E., Schulz, A. J., & Parker, E. A. (2005). *Methods in community-based participatory research for health*. San Francisco: Jossey-Bass.

Kegler, M. C., Steckler, A., Malek, S. H., & McLeroy, K. (1998). A multiple case study of implementation in 10 local Project ASSIST coalitions in North Carolina. *Health Education Research, 13*, 225–238.

Kersh, R., & Morone, J. (2002). The politics of obesity: Seven steps to government action. *Health Affairs, 21*, 142–153.

King, R. P., Leibtag, E. S., & Behl, A. S. (2004). *Supermarket characteristics and operating costs in low income areas.* Washington, DC: U.S. Department of Agriculture Economic Report 839.

Kreuter, M., & Lezin, N. (2002). Coalitions, consortia and partnerships. In J. Last, L. Breslow, & L. W. Green (Eds.), *Encyclopedia of public health.* London: MacMillan.

Kreuter, M. W., Lezin, N. A., & Young, L. A. (2000). Evaluating community-based collaborative mechanisms: Implications for practitioners. *Health Promotion Practice, 1*, 49–63.

Ledikwe, J. H., Ello-Martin, J. A., & Rolls, B. J. (2005). Portion sizes and the obesity epidemic. *Journal of Nutrition, 135*, 905–909.

McLeroy, K., Bibeau, D., Strecker, A., & Glanz, K. (1988). An ecologic perspective on health promotion programs. *Health Education Quarterly, 15*, 351–377.

Minkler, M., & Wallerstein, N. (2003). *Community based participatory research for health.* San Francisco: Jossey-Bass.

Moore, J. M. (1998). Designing an effective statewide tobacco control program—Oregon. *Cancer, 83*(Suppl. 12), 2733–2735.

Morland, K., Wing, S., Diez Roux, A., & Poole, C. (2002). Neighborhood characteristics associated with the location of food stores and food service places. *American Journal of Preventive Medicine, 22*, 23–29.

National Association for Sport and Physical Education & American Heart Association. (2006). *2006 Shape of the nation report: Status of physical education in the USA.* Reston, VA: National Association for Sport and Physical Education.

Peterson, K. E., Sorensen, G., Pearson, M., Hebert, J. R., Gottlieb, B. R., & McCormick, M. C. (2002). Design of an intervention addressing multiple levels of influence on dietary and activity patterns of low-income, postpartum women. *Health Education Research, 17*, 531–540.

Pratt, M., Macera, C. A., & Wang, G., (2000). Higher direct medical costs associated with physical inactivity. *Physician and Sportsmedicine, 28*, 63–70.

Richter, K. P., Harris, K. J., Paine-Andrews, A., Fawcett, S. B., Schmid, T. L., Lankenau, B. H., & Johnston, J. (2000). Measuring the health environment for physical activity and nutrition among youth: A review of the literature and applications for community initiatives. *Preventive Medicine, 31*, S98–S111.

Roussos, S. T., & Fawcett, S. B. (2000). A review of collaborative partnerships as a strategy for improving community health. *Annual Review of Public Health, 21*, 369–402.

Sallis, J. F., Nader, P. R., Rupp, J. W., Atkins, C. J., & Wilson, W. C. (1986). San Diego surveyed for heart-healthy foods and exercise facilities. *Public Health Reports, 101*, 216–219.

Smith, D. W., Howell, K. A., & McCann, K. M. (1990). Evaluation of the coalition index: A guide to school health education materials. *Journal of School Health, 60*, 49–52.

Thompson, M., Minkler, M., Bell, J., Rose, K., & Butler, L. (2003). Facilitators of well-functioning consortia: National Healthy Start program lessons. *Health and Social Work, 28*, 185–195.

Wansink, B. (2004). Environmental factors that increase the food intake and consumption volume of unknowing consumers. *Annual Review of Nutrition, 24*, 455–479.

Young, L. R., & Nestle, M. (2003). Expanding portion sizes in the U.S. marketplace: Implications for nutrition counseling. *Journal of the American Dietetic Association, 103*, 231–234.

Zaza, S., Briss, P. A., & Harris, K. W. (2005). *The guide to community preventive services: What works to promote health?* New York: Oxford University Press.

Zenk, S. N., Schulz, A. J., Israel, B. A., James, S. A., Bao, S., & Wilson, M. L. (2006). Fruit and vegetable access differs by community racial composition and socioeconomic position in Detroit, Michigan. *Ethnicity and Disease, 16*, 275–280.

Chapter 14

Health Care System Approaches to Obesity Prevention and Control

David L. Katz and Zubaida Faridi

Introduction

A health care system may be one of those things that we know when we see, but have a hard time defining. Challenges in defining the scope of the health care system have long been noted (Rodwin, 1990). It has been suggested by some that such systems encompass all societal activities designed to protect or restore health; others have suggested a more limited definition, related expressly to medical care but interacting with heredity, lifestyle and environmental influences.

Defined narrowly or broadly, the health care system represents an array of resources and activities with considerable potential to influence health-related behavioral patterns and outcomes over time. This is of course germane to the challenge of obesity prevention and control, which is ultimately a matter of dietary and activity patterns over the course of a lifetime. The role of the health care system in weight management has obvious implications for other conditions, including the most prevalent chronic diseases in our society – cardiovascular diseases, diabetes mellitus, cancer, arthritis – which represents an incomplete list of the potential metabolic sequelae of obesity.

Obesity and overweight are among the most common conditions seen in adult primary care, and are increasingly prevalent in pediatric and adolescent patients (Hedley *et al.*, 2004; M. Noel *et al.*, 1998a; O'Brien *et al.*, 2004; Ogden *et al.*, 2006). The number of children in the United States who are overweight has tripled over the last two decades. Also, despite a conservative definition of overweight, at least 15% (over 9 million) of children aged 6–19 years are considered overweight (Grundy, 2000; Hassink, 2003; Richard, 2003). Independent of any other considerations, the epidemiology of obesity makes weight management efforts by the health care system a priority.

Health care efforts directed toward weight management (implying both obesity prevention and control) should be universal and anticipatory, meaning prevention-oriented. While there is certainly a place in obesity management for various specialists (e.g., endocrinologists, cardiologists, etc.), obesity prevention is largely a task for primary care providers, including the disciplines of pediatrics, family practice, obstetrics and gynecology, and internal medicine

(Cifuentes *et al.*, 2005; Leermakers *et al.*, 1998; P. D. Martin *et al.*, 2003; McCallum & Gerner, 2005; O'Brien et al., 2004; Olson *et al.*, 2004; Polley *et al.*, 2002; Scott *et al.*, 2004).

While there is little direct evidence for the efficacy of obesity-prevention counseling, or for counseling to foster sustained weight loss, (U.S. Preventive Services Task Force, 2003b) the rationale for such counseling is strong on theoretical grounds. Weight control is contingent upon the quality and quantity of dietary intake (calories in), and the pattern of physical activity (calories out). Both these factors – prudent dietary choices and regular physical activity – are also important to health (Fulton *et al.*, 2004; D. L. Katz, 2001b; Wahlqvist, 2005). Thus, weight control counseling is, in essence, counseling to encourage healthful lifestyle practices. The fact that counseling directed toward improvement in diet (U.S. Preventive Services Task Force, 2003a) and physical activity (U.S. Preventive Services Task Force, 2002) patterns is as yet of unproved effectiveness is an invitation to improve the delivery and evaluation of such counseling, rather than a reason to abandon it.

Such considerations make attention to weight management in the health care system setting a question of "how" rather than of "whether." But the "how" is a challenging and perhaps even daunting question. Understanding how to enhance, revise, expand, extend or coordinate the complex components of the health care system so that weight management is consistently fostered at an acceptable cost is inchoate at best. The health care system offers enormous potential contributions to obesity prevention and control efforts, but is encumbered by obstacles to many of the most promising applications. This chapter is devoted to a consideration of the obstacles to, and opportunities for, obesity prevention and control in the health care system. A case is made for cautious optimism.

Components of the Health Care System

There is no single, definitive source to characterize a comprehensive inventory of health care system components, as they relate to weight control or any other condition. The Healthcare Systems Bureau of the *Health Resources and Services Administration* of the U.S. Government encompasses programs related to health care access for the underserved; organ donation; emergency preparedness; and vaccine injury compensation (Health Resources and Services Administration). Rather than establishing the bounds of the health care system, this programmatic cluster seems to highlight that the term is open to interpretation. Therefore, the inventory of health care system components included in **Table 14.1**, which also suggests how each component might contribute to obesity prevention and control, should be considered illustrative rather than definitive.

Obesity Prevention and Management in the U.S. Health Care System: Obstacles and Opportunities

Current efforts to promote adoption and institutionalization of obesity prevention and management are fragmented and disparate at best. A considerable gap exists between what we think optimal obesity prevention and control efforts

Table 14.1 Discrete components of the health care system with potential application to obesity prevention and control. (Note: *Components are categorized into micro, meso, and macro domains with micro relating to the patient/provider encounter; meso relating to health care service delivery in general; and macro relating to the situation of health care services within a societal context.*[*])

Micro Level

Component	Application
Patient	The attitudes, beliefs, knowledge and capacities the patient brings into the health care setting (e.g., health literacy) influence the productivity of the encounter. Obesity control could be pursued through efforts to enhance patient self-efficacy prior to accessing the health care system.
Provider	Traditionally, efforts to enhance the provision of clinical services have focused on enhancing the knowledge, proficiency, and performance of providers. In the case of obesity prevention and control, this entails enhancing the capacity of the provider to deliver effective counseling. Improving provider personal self efficacy for a healthy lifestyle translates into increased rates of counseling (Crawford *et al.*, 2004)
Non-clinical support staff (i.e., administrative and clerical staff)	To the extent time pressures limit the interaction between patient and provider, practice staff in the health care setting may compensate by contributing to information exchange and monitoring. Obesity prevention and control could be advanced by increasing the contributions of support staff to patient self-efficacy.
Human interactions/ relationships	Obesity is a stigmatizing condition, and thus a sensitive topic of discussion. Specific efforts to improve provider/patient relationships so that the topic is addressed comfortably and productively could enhance control efforts.

Meso Level – Organizational

Component	Application
Infrastructure/facilities	Everything from the availability and placement of scales and other devices for assessing weight/adiposity to the space available for encounters, may contribute to the productivity of encounters pertaining to weight management.
Medical technology & resources (diagnostic, therapeutic)	The availability and use of technology for the assessment of anthropometrics; pharmacy services; and even surgical services all potentially contribute to obesity prevention and control.
Networking capacity/ coordination	Improvements in referral patterns to dietitians, physical therapists/trainers, and/or specialists could enhance the efficacy of weight control efforts. Expansion of the provision of weight control guidance into more clinical encounters, such as dental encounters, could contribute to the reinforcement of key messages.
Repeated communication	Enhancements in longitudinal reinforcement of messages delivered during clinical encounters by use of telephone, Internet, or print materials have the potential to enhance the effectiveness of obesity prevention and control efforts.

(Continued)

Table 14.1 (Continued)

Meso Level – Organizational

Component	Application
Information technology	Provider access to state-of-the-art weight control guidance during and between encounters, and patient access to analogous lay materials, could enhance the quality and efficiency of clinical weight control efforts.
Patient flow management/logistics	Innovations in patient management, such as group encounters to extend contact time with providers, could be used to enhance obesity control efforts.

Meso Level – Community

Component	Application
Outreach activities	Clinical sites can engage in efforts to attract patients for services related to weight management (e.g., seminars), and can attempt to influence non-clinical resources in the community (e.g., schools, restaurants).
Inreach activities	Coordinated community efforts for weight control may encompass efforts by non-clinical entities to obtain support and information from the health care system. The availability of resources from health care to enhance information exchange or services in schools or worksites could contribute to obesity prevention and control.

Macro Level – Policy

Component	Application
Financing	Changes in reimbursement mechanisms can alter clinical priorities and could be used to encourage greater clinical attention to weight control.
Accountability/regulation	Various approaches to the monitoring and regulation of weight control activities in the clinical setting may reinforce commitment to them. These include pay-for-performance; monitoring of pertinent HEDIS measures; documentation of BMI and risk assessment for overweight and obesity; direct incentives/disincentives to patients; etc.

*Based on the classification scheme outlined in WHO (World Health Organization, 2001). The content of the table is otherwise original.

§ Health Plan Employer Data and Information Set (HEDIS) (Corrigan & Nielsen, 1993)

should look like and actual patterns of care. Indeed, much of the discussion of weight management has focused on the growing realization of the distance between normative standards of care and actual practice. While the list of obstacles to effective weight management in primary care can appear daunting, each obstacle represents a potential opportunity to intervene in distinct components of the health care system elucidated in Table 14.1. As noted below, neither the components of the health care system, nor the application of each to the goal of weight management, is truly independent of the entire system.

Efforts to enhance the receptiveness of patients to provider counseling are dependent partly on the nature of that counseling; the effectiveness of providers requires active participation by the patient, and by payers. Nonetheless, a delineation of system components is a useful framework for illustration of both obstacles and opportunities, along the way toward resynthesizing those elements back into a better-functioning whole.

The health care setting offers nearly universal, if episodic, access to the population. Approximately 40 million Americans are hospitalized at least once each year (Agency for Healthcare Research and Quality, 2002). More than 70% of the U.S. population visits a health care provider in any given year for a check up (Center for Disease Control and Prevention, 2004). When visits for all reasons are considered, the health care setting provides annual access to nearly the entire population; this access alone constitutes an important reason why weight control efforts in this setting should be a priority.

Patient

The patient is an important element in the functioning of the health care system. With regard to addressing weight management effectively, the ideal patient would present to a clinical encounter with a good working knowledge of determinants of weight control; knowledge of and interest in both physical activity and healthful diet; motivation to engage in these behaviors, and the resources to incorporate these into daily life. Further, an ideal patient would be receptive to provider advice about lifestyle, and would readily understand such advice whether spoken or in print.

The reality is often quite discrepant from this ideal, however. Knowledge of a healthful diet is limited at best in our society (Popkin et al., 2005). While recognition of the value of physical activity is widespread, knowledge of how to make physical activity a part of daily life and motivation for doing so are not (Fenton, 2005; Keim et al., 2004). Literacy levels in general, and health literacy levels in particular, are far from ideal. This increases the time providers must spend explaining lifestyle guidance, and increases the risk of misunderstanding and non compliance (National Academy on an Aging Society/Center for Health Care Strategies, 1998).

Several studies have documented strategies and interventions to address these barriers effectively. These include providing information and raising awareness of obesity and its consequences through community venues such as schools, shopping malls, supermarkets and both print and electronic media (Caldwell et al., 2005; Potter et al., 2001).

Also, use of patient communication models (Epstein et al., 2005; Glasgow et al., 2001a; Irving & Dickson, 2004; Makoul, 2003) helps prepare the patient for the medical visit and facilitate effective communication and discussion.

Efforts to cultivate health literacy regarding weight management include the provision of tailored information specific to patient needs, summarizing the instructions by asking the patient to repeat the instructions, providing clear and concise instructions on next steps, offering small amounts of information at a time, and using educational materials written at the appropriate reading level. Also useful would be the inclusion of instruction in nutrition and practical approaches to routine physical activity in both primary and secondary education (Ad Hoc Committee on Health Literacy for the American Council on Scientific Affairs, 1999; Ezenwaka & Offiah, 2003; Gerber et al., 2005; Kennen et al., 2005; P. H. Noel et al., 1998b; Williams et al., 1998; Rothman et al., 2004).

Support of patient self management skills is a key component of effective weight management and improved patient outcomes. Self-management support goes beyond traditional knowledge-based patient education to include processes that develop patient problem-solving skills, improve self-efficacy, and guide application of knowledge in real-life situations. A more collaborative approach between the patient and provider is recommended to help patients come to their own decisions by exploring their uncertainties and identifying their personal barriers to change (Baker et al., 2005; Barlow et al., 2005; Caldwell et al., 2005; Deakin et al., 2005; Norris et al., 2001; Wantland et al., 2004).

Patient families remain an undervalued asset in obesity control efforts. Yet their potential to affect outcomes is considerable and their role should be fully incorporated into any model designed to address obesity. Also, social support and participation in collaborative chronic care groups has been shown to improve outcomes in chronic conditions such as diabetes and heart failure and may be equally applicable to weight loss programs (Nthangeni et al., 2002).

Provider

The ideal provider would be knowledgeable and trained in the essentials of behavioral counseling, possess the necessary self efficacy and motivation for counseling, and be equipped with the necessary tools and materials to counsel patients on weight management effectively, persuasively, and efficiently.

In a recent survey by Zogby, most people surveyed thought that their doctors should play a more active role in promoting a healthy lifestyle, and two thirds thought it important for a doctor to focus on preventive measures, such as diet and physical activity, rather than just diagnosing and treating illnesses (Truswell, 1999). Also, patients who were advised to lose weight were nearly three times more likely to report an attempt to do so than those who did not receive such advice (Galuska et al., 1999). However, it appears that the most common experience by patients of any weight is that their physician does not bring up the issue. Multiple studies confirm this observation (de Fine Olivarius et al., 2005; Maheux et al., 1999; Wee et al., 1999). More disturbingly recent studies indicate that disparities in professional advice to lose weight associated with income and educational attainment increased from 1994 to 2000 (Honda, 2004; J. E. Jackson et al., 2005; Lin & Larson, 2005; Wee et al., 1999).

The barriers to effective counseling by primary care providers are well documented and include lack of brief and effective counseling techniques, lack of self efficacy for counseling, lack of validated tools and materials for counseling, lack of evidence of effectiveness of counseling and lack of reimbursement. The demands and limitations of a busy primary care practice preclude any meaningful discussion about lifestyle behaviors by the clinician. The typical primary care physician cares for 1,500 to 3,000 people in a community, depending on its demographics. This visit-dependent model of care allows a physician about an hour per year per patient and limits the clinician's ability to provide adequate preventive care. More importantly, clinicians express little confidence in the utility of behavioral counseling. Although clinical guidelines for obesity management are widely available (HSTAT, Evidence Syntheses, formerly Systematic Evidence Reviews 21) they have not resulted in significant changes in practice patterns pertaining to weight counseling (N. Campbell & McAlister, 2006; Genuis, 2005; Glasgow *et al.*, 2001b; Goolsby, 2001; Klardie *et al.*, 2004; Larsen *et al.*, 2006; Mazza & Russell, 2001; R. S. Thompson, 1996).

Historically, weight management counseling has been sporadic and largely limited to knowledge based instruction based on the belief that increasing a patient's knowledge about obesity would lead to behavior change and improved health outcomes. Eliciting information about patient's personal assessment of risk and barriers to change is neglected and the advice is prescriptive and generic in nature with a focus on clinical outcomes rather than day to day strategies of dealing with overweight or obesity. These efforts are further hampered by the inability of clinicians to assess patient's readiness to change and functional health literacy. The dearth of culturally appropriate materials and resources to inform the discussion contribute to the lack of success of weight counseling efforts (Nawaz *et al.*, 1999; Nawaz & Katz, 2001; Nawaz *et al.*, 2000; Nicolucci *et al.*, 2000). Many strategies to help optimize provider performance are based on behavior change theories and models that describe the social, cognitive, psychosocial and environmental determinants of health behaviors. Broadly speaking, the Health Belief Model, the Theory of Reasoned Action and the Stages of Change Theory focus on the effect of individual factors such as knowledge, attitudes, beliefs, prior experience and personality on behavioral choices, while the Social Cognitive Theory, the Community Organizing Theory and the Social Marketing Theory focus on the processes between the individual and the groups that provide the necessary support. Applied as originally developed, these models tend to be time consuming, resource intensive and tailored to psychological models of care; however, they can be adapted to the requirements and limitations of the primary care setting (Abrams *et al.*, 1999; Elder *et al.*, 1999; Glanz *et al.*, 1999; Heaney & Israil, 1999; Institute of Medicine, 2001; National Cancer Institute, 1995; Prochaska & DiClemente, 1983; Stokols *et al.*, 1996).

Thus, several counseling programs have adapted the constructs of these theories to fit the primary care context. Most of these programs use a general approach to assisting patients that includes *the five A's: Assess, Advise, Agree, Assist and Arrange*. The Worcester Area Trial for Counseling in Hyperlipidemia (WATCH), Patient-centered Assessment Counseling for Exercise and Nutrition (PACE) (Albright *et al.*, 2000; Patrick *et al.*, 2001) Activity Counseling Trial (ACT) (King *et al.*, 1998), Physically Active for Life (PAL) (Keim *et al.*, 2004; Pinto *et al.*, 1998) the Step Test Exercise Prescription (STEP) (Petrella *et al.*, 2003) and the Pressure System Model (PSM) (DL. Katz, 2001a) developed by one of the authors (DLK), have provided early evidence for the efficacy of counseling in the primary care setting. Elements that can increase applicability and ease of implementation of a model include enhanced provider training, explicit guidance on counseling strategies, brevity of the counseling script, standardized, validated instruments to assess the patient, and clear delineation of provider response and responsibility. The clinician should be encouraged to use directive questions and reflective listening to encourage patient goal-setting, action-planning and problem-solving that is tailored to the patient's unique situation (DL Katz *et al.*, 2002; D. L. Katz, 2002; B. Marcus *et al.*, 1997; Ockene *et al.*, 1995; Yeh *et al.*, 2003).

Shifting part of the burden of care to support staff is particularly relevant for poorer communities. Encouragingly, there is ample evidence of successful nurse led programs for managing chronic diseases in developing countries. By optimizing the use of human resources, appropriate obesity control and management programs can also be implemented in resource poor regions in the United States (Barlow *et al.*, 2005; Dickey *et al.*, 1999; Rothman *et al.*, 2005; Yarmo, 1998).

Physicians' health behavior characteristics and personal self efficacy for targeted health behaviors has been associated with reported lifestyle counseling of patients. Therefore promoting healthy lifestyle behaviors among primary healthcare providers may potentially improve physician counseling rates (Abramson *et al.*, 2000; Frank *et al.*, 2003; Frank *et al.*, 2002; Livaudais *et al.*, 2005).

Non-Clinical Support Staff

Like the primary care provider, the practice staff should also be knowledgeable, motivated and equipped with the necessary tools to support the clinician in his/her counseling efforts. As mentioned above, time pressures severely limit the interaction between patient and provider on non-acute care matters. Thus, it is advisable to share the burden of counseling between the clinician and support staff. However, such an approach requires not only a change in how practices are organized, but some basic training for the support staff in lifestyle counseling.

Use of ancillary support staff to augment or substitute physician counseling has shown promise in several studies. In the PACE program (Calfas *et al.*, 1996; Long *et al.*, 1996; Peiss *et al.*, 1995) the receptionist initiated the counseling process by asking the patient to complete various assessment forms. This was followed by a discussion with the provider. The practice nurse then took responsibility for scheduling follow up visits and reminders. Similarly, the PSM program is supported by office staff other than the primary care provider (DL. Katz, 2001a; D. L. Katz *et al.*, 2006). Follow up and telephone reminders can be assigned to the support staff while other designated members of the practice staff can be given specific roles to support counseling efforts (Friedman, 1998; Piette *et al.*, 2000; Ramelson *et al.*, 1999; Schofferman *et al.*, 1977; Taylor *et al.*, 2005). There are various approaches to engagement of support staff in weight management, allowing for tailoring to the needs and resources of a given practice.

Human Interactions/Relationships

Addressing obesity in a healthcare setting requires the cultivation of empathetic, understanding and interactive relationships between the patient and the provider team. Such a relationship based approach is important because obesity and overweight are stigmatizing conditions (see Chapter 6). Indeed, obese subjects experience a pattern of denigration and condemnation that is so pervasive as to constitute civilized oppression (Harvey, 1999; Levy & Williamson, 1988; Rogge *et al.*, 2004).

The term "relationship based care" refers to both the philosophical founda-tion of the model and its operational framework and focuses on three crucial interactions: care provider's relationship with patients and families, care provider's relationship with self, and care provider's relationship with colleagues. At the heart of relationship based care is the creation of healing associations by gaining an understanding of the other's experience, leading to the delivery of compassionate care. Barriers to widespread adoption of the relationship model include lack of education and training of practice staff, costs associated with the training, and the cultural and process change required to implement such a model (Beach & Inui, 2006; Tresolini, 1994).

Relationship-Based Care has been implemented in clinical settings with tan-gible benefits for the patients and the care givers. The caring experience, inter-active style and healing environment provided by the model can be effective in weight management in primary care practices. There are three Rs of the Relationship-Based Care model – roles, responsibilities and resources. Effective application of the model involves the creation of interdependent, collaborative, multidisciplinary teams where each member has clearly articu-lated roles and responsibilities commensurate with their skills and knowledge. In addition, resources at the point of care delivery are managed judiciously and authoritatively by the managers and clinical staff responsible for care.

Based on these three Rs the operating culture of the practice can potentially be reorganized to address obesity sensitively and compassionately. The I^2E^2 formula is a practical measure that defines four elements required to change the environment of care. The formula is widely used to assess the implemen-tation of relationship based care processes. Using the I^2E^2 formula (inspira-tion, infrastructure, education and evidence) as a guide, the patient provider relationship, staff personal skills and competencies, and interpersonal relation-ships between the healthcare team can be transformed to establish and culti-vate ongoing therapeutic relationships with patients and their families (De Camargo & Coeli, 2006; Forman, 2004; Scott et al., 2004; Kearney et al., 2000). Both patients and providers are apt to address weight management more constructively when the topic is comfortable for both groups, and the relationship between them strong and positive.

Infrastructure/Facilities

The ideal waiting area in a practice would provide ample information on obesity prevention and control and encourage the patient to learn more about healthy living. Larger practices would offer more facilities. Barriers to redesigning the practice include lack of resources, competing demands on space and lack of suitable health information to provide to patients. Furthermore, there is no comprehensive multimedia patient education program available as a single package that creatively utilizes the opportunity to educate the patient (McVea et al., 2000; Oermann et al., 2003; Shiroyama et al., 1997; Stanley & Tongue, 1991; Wicke et al., 1994).

Some of these barriers can be overcome easily. A simple step would be to place scales and other devices for assessing weight/adiposity in a convenient place in the office and then actively encouraging their use. This can be supple-mented by the availability of patient education material pertaining to weight management for the entire family and access to interactive, computerized assessment tools in the waiting area, with suitable arrangements to protect privacy. Provision of skill building exercises such as planning a healthy meal, interpreting food labels, or identifying credible sources of information on the internet, is likely to lead to increased patient understanding and receptivity to a discussion of weight control with their healthcare providers (Collings *et al.*, 1991; Elliott & Polkinhorn, 1994; Koperski, 1989; Philipp *et al.*, 1990; *Stanley & Tongue*, 1991; Varnavides *et al.*, 1984). Larger practices may offer a community classroom with interactive computer kiosks, space for group meetings, a teaching kitchen and perhaps even a small fitness center free to patients. These approaches can be piloted in managed care or group practices to assess their feasibility and utility (Gerber et al., 2005).

Medical Technology/Resources

Ideally, providers would use the latest medical technologies in obesity prevention and control. Although advanced medical technologies for measuring fat distribution are now available (Goodpaster, 2002) they are generally not used by clinicians. The main barriers to widespread utilization of these services – including computed tomography, magnetic resonance imaging, and underwater weighing for total body fat content- is cost and limited evidence to date of added value commensurate with that cost. The putative value of such anthropometric measures would encompass enhanced risk stratification, and enhanced motivation for behavior change.

Creative use of medical assessments such as medical imaging of body fat or measurement of body composition may be used to convey the magnitude and severity of the health risk. These technologies may have the potential to serve as a powerful basis for individualized advice, and a powerful motivator of behavior change. Strategic use of these diagnostic technologies may facilitate lifestyle modification and should be explored further. Some useful guidelines for comprehensive evaluation of obesity-related risks are available in the literature on bariatric surgery (Blackburn *et al.*, 2005; Saltzman *et al.*, 2005). There is some evidence that imaging modalities may influence behavior in ways that other measures of personal risk do not (Lederman *et al.*, 2006).

Networking Capacity/Coordination

A model obesity prevention and management network would be located either within a managed healthcare plan or a geographic entity or both. It would utilize a family/household based approach and would reinforce the same basic message of healthy lifestyle to all family members through multiple portals and resources such as pediatricians, internists, family practitioners and obstetricians. Specialists such as cardiologists would work in tandem with the generalists to encourage patients to adopt healthy lifestyles, and other providers such as dentists would also provide pertinent advice.

Today there is little coordination between primary providers of patient care and other health professionals. Barriers to formation of such networks include primary care/specialist conflict, lack of incentives to establish networks and improve communication, and lack of local leadership to integrate obesity prevention and management efforts.

The creation of local healthcare networks dedicated to obesity prevention and control efforts can serve to complement and reinforce the clinician's effort at weight management. Increased referrals to dietitians, physical fitness instructors, weight loss programs, and other local resources can augment the counseling efforts of physicians and increase success rates (Katon *et al.*, 2004; Provan *et al.*, 2003; Provan *et al.*, 2004; Rothman et al., 2005). Expanding the provision of weight management advice into other clinical encounters such as dental visits, could further reinforce key messages. These referrals require regular communication between the care providers. Use of a central electronic database can help all the care providers track patient progress and coordinate care efforts (Faulkner *et al.*, 2003; Jacobs & Rauber, 1996; Lee, 1997; Provan *et al.*, 2005; Unutzer *et al.*, 2002; Wager *et al.*, 1997).

Repeated Communication

Under ideal circumstances, practices would provide regular, proactive follow up by mail, telephone or online. The anatomy of follow up counseling would be clearly outlined, staff would be trained in counseling, and the practice would be structured to include reminders and prompts to engage in on-going counseling. Such a vision for coordinated care highlights the inter-dependence of the varied components of the health care system in any meaningful effort to curtail the spread of obesity. Regrettably, the use of such communication tools, and the attendant coordination of services, is limited to date. This may be attributed to untrained staff, cost pressures and the absence of a structured process to facilitate counseling.

Several studies have demonstrated a dose response effect – the greater the number of contacts the more effective the results (Jeffery *et al.*, 2004; Jeffery *et al.*, 2003). The benefits of follow up contact by practice staff between clinical consultations with the physician in the form of email exchanges, mailing of print materials, and brief telephone discussions to assess progress and ensure compliance has been established (Bray *et al.*, 2005; GESICA Investigators, 2005; Kaplan *et al.*, 2003; Kelly *et al.*, 2005; Logue *et al.*, 2005; McBride & Rimer, 1999; Randomised trial of telephone intervention in chronic heart failure: Dial trial, 2005). These methodologies represent an effective and inexpensive way of engaging the patient, addressing barriers to weight loss in a timely fashion, increasing support staff involvement in weight management efforts, and building better patient and provider team relationships. Advances in system automation should allow for greater use of communication technology at lower costs.

Information Technology

An optimal information technology system for weight management in a healthcare setting would include web based behavioral intervention, tailored messaging, interactive provider monitoring and feedback, and maintenance of an electronic database. Barriers to integration of information technology in healthcare systems are cost of implementation, practice reorganization, training of staff, and access and acceptance by patients (Hersh *et al.*, 2001; B. H. Marcus *et al.*, 1998; O'Toole *et al.*, 2005; Revere & Dunbar, 2001; Tate *et al.*, 2001).

A review of the literature indicates that successful behavioral interventions targeting modifiable lifestyle characteristics have several common design attributes. These include offering tailored informational advice, ipsative feedback (assessing present performance against the prior performance) and self monitoring. The use of information technology such as computer assisted obesity interventions, use of web based self help tools in commercial weight loss programs, telephone delivered tailored information, and interpersonal feedback to enhance each of these features has led to improved health outcomes and sustained behavior change. Mobile systems may have clear advantages over computer, telephone, or print communication systems for delivery of tailored health behavior interventions, because of their "anytime, anywhere" messaging and communication capability and other features (Gorman, 2000; Mann, 1998).

The public adoption of cellular phones, wireless PDAs and the Web also permits greater monitoring and feedback by clinical personnel. Application of interactive behavior change technology (IBCT) to deliver behavior change counseling before, during or after the office visit to enhance patient-clinician interaction has shown promise. Similarly, internet usage, clinic based CD-ROMs and interactive voice response telephone calls have been shown to be potentially feasible and valuable adjuncts to clinic based behavioral counseling (Glasgow *et al.*, 2004a; Panniers *et al.*, 2003). Studies show that these ubiquitous technologies can lead to clinically significant and sustainable weight loss among primary care patients. A pertinent example of the use of information technology to improve patient outcomes is the use of cellular phone technology to deliver tailored messages to patients with diabetes. The system analyzes biomedical data such as HBA1c values, fasting blood glucose and blood pressure to generate and transmit tailored text messages to the patient. These timely, personalized reminders serve to enhance patient motivation and compliance to therapeutic regimens. The feasibility of the system for Type 2 diabetes management is currently being evaluated in several community health practices through funding by NIH (Bodenheimer, 2005; Cumbo *et al.*, 2002; Dorr *et al.*, 2006; Helwig *et al.*, 1999; Vickery, 2000; Wantland *et al.*, 2004).

Equally important is provider access to state-of-the art, electronic decision support systems at the time of clinical decision making. Such systems can help raise the standard level of care and have already shown promise in managing conditions like asthma and diabetes (Cherry *et al.*, 2002; Chuang *et al.*, 2000; MacLean *et al.*, 2006; Polniaszek & Klinger, 2004; Tufano & Karras, 2005; Zrebiec, 2005).

Patient Flow Management: Group Visits

Ideally, patient management and interaction would be maximized by the use of innovative strategies such as group visits. Each visit could be led by a physician or could include multiple providers such as a dietitian or a behavioral therapist. The encounter would be longer than the 15 minutes generally allocated to a non acute consultation.

Commonly encountered impediments to group visits include lack of time and conflicts in scheduling. Frequently, practices lack professionals other than the physician to lead group visits. Also, patient resistance to group visits due to privacy concerns has been reported in some studies (Miller *et al.*, 2004; E. Thompson, 2000).

Group visits have been used for a variety of chronic conditions such as osteoporosis, diabetes and coronary heart disease (Bray *et al.*, 2005; Porta & Trento, 2004). They can easily be structured to address weight management in primary care. Strategies to enhance the group visit include the addition of a patient education component to emphasize self-management. Physicians and patients can work together to create behavior-change action plans, which detail achievable and behavior-specific goals that participants aim to accomplish by the next session. Once plans are set, the group may discuss ways to overcome potential obstacles and raise patients' self-efficacy and commitment to behavioral change. Patients' family members can also be included in these group sessions (Houck *et al.*, 2003; Masley *et al.*, 2000; Mathur *et al.*, 2005; Noffsinger *et al.*, 2003).

Group visits can contribute to interactive health literacy by offering opportunities for dialogue, experiential learning and developing personal skills in a supportive environment (Hartman *et al.*, 1994; Nutbeam, 2000; Rothman *et al.*, 2004). In addition, group visits can serve as a vehicle for ongoing social support in weight loss efforts. Participants can offer emotional support by expressing approval or appreciation for the patient's behavior. The group may provide appraisal support by helping the patient understand the implications of obesity and what resources or coping strategies may be used to achieve weight loss (Rickheim *et al.*, 2002; Trento *et al.*, 2001). The role of group visits for weight maintenance has been assessed (DL Katz et al., 2002; Yeh et al., 2003) but remains uncertain.

Outreach Activities

Ideally, primary care practices would engage in a variety of community outreach activities to enhance clinical weight management efforts. Outreach may be defined as efforts by the healthcare providers to actively involve the community in obesity prevention and control. This would include partnering with grassroots community based organizations to offer educational seminars and skill building classes, offering training to non-medical personnel such as peer educators and health advisors, and working with community institutions such as schools, community clinics, local businesses and media outlets to advocate for environmental and policy change. In reality, this does not happen often or in a systematic way. Time and cost pressures limit the ability of the provider to reach out to the community, and the leadership and incentives required for this are generally not there.

A review of collaborative partnerships shows that involving and empowering residents and outreach activities to include the community in health promotion can lead to improved outcomes. An example of a successful outreach activity is the Hochunk Youth Fitness Program which is a partnership among healthcare professionals, youth services, social services and area school districts to reduce the incidence of childhood obesity, prevent adult obesity, and set up an infrastructure to address children at risk for diabetes. Daily communication within the partnership network contributed to the success of the program (Y. Jackson *et al.*, 2002). In another example, family physicians served as community leaders and agents of change to partner with schools to help families deal with asthma. They provided school nurses with asthma action plans and helped organize asthma camps (Butterfoss & Francisco,

2004; Gamm, 1998; Landis *et al.*, 2006; Margolis *et al.*, 2001; Roussos & Fawcett, 2000; Wagner *et al.*, 2001b). Such grass roots strategic models of community inclusion can easily be applied to identify, implement, strengthen and sustain collective efforts for the prevention and management of obesity.

In-reach Activities

In-reach activities, that is initiatives led by the community to engage and inter-act with health care providers and systems, in an ideal setting, would involve a set of coordinated community efforts for weight control and management that are led by non-clinical entities. However, community organizations have disparate missions and the lack of focus and coordination on obesity related issues, compounded by a lack of incentives, limit these activities in reality.

Community resources are required to enhance uptake of clinical counseling. In the case of weight management, this may be especially salient: advice to improve diet and/or increase physical activity requires the availability of foods and fitness facilities that conform to the clinical guidance (Sallis & Glanz, 2006). Since patients and their families spend the majority of their time outside the clinical setting, a supportive community environment may be essential for sustained behavior change (Gordon-Larsen *et al.*, 2006; Morland *et al.*, 2006). Linkages between the primary care system and community organizations can eliminate redundancies in obesity prevention and control efforts. Recognized community structures such as health ministries, commu-nity boards and chambers of commerce can pull in primary care providers and jointly develop programs best suited to support obesity control efforts (Parker *et al.*, 1992).

These efforts can be modeled on an award winning program – Sickness Prevention through Regional Collaboration (SPARC). The program consists of a collaboration between private practitioners, public health nurses, local hospitals and academic centers to increase the delivery of preventive services to the community by creating new points of contact and building activities tailored to the community (Sickness Prevention Achieved through Regional Collaboration). The program can be applied to prevent and control obesity in the community by offering screenings at churches, schools and community clinics to identify individuals at risk for obesity related health conditions. Also, license renewal or voter registration can be linked to a health risk assess-ment. Such innovative strategies that capitalize on existing infrastructure and increase delivery of prevention education and services to the community can prove to be quite effective.

Another area of considerable promise is worksite wellness programs (see Chapter 15). Employers have a clear benefit in having healthy workers and are thus a natural, and usually well funded, potential partner in obesity prevention efforts.

Financing

In an ideal world adequate financing would be available to encourage obesity prevention efforts. However, in the current U.S. health care system, reim-bursement for behavioral counseling is limited at best. The financial under-pinnings of the system lead to commentary that is about "sick" care rather than "health" care, with incentives for pharmacotherapy and procedures rather than prevention.

Creating a reimbursement structure to compensate clinicians for counseling can go a long way towards improving the rate and quality of lifestyle counseling. Encouragingly, recent changes in the Medicare statutes make it possible to identify obesity as a disease, and this opens the door to reimbursement for its management in the federal system. Under the plan, Medicare will "be able to review scientific evidence in order to determine which interventions improve health outcomes for senior disabled Americans who are obese." Also, Congress recently expanded Medicare coverage to offer medical nutrition therapy as a strategy for treating and managing conditions like diabetes, hypertension and heart disease (Fitzner *et al.*, 2003; L. F. Martin *et al.*, 2000; Stern *et al.*, 2005; White, 1999). Private insurers support the classification of obesity as a disease and are looking to Medicare for direction in setting standards of what is effective and what should be covered. These changes are promising and may make a significant difference in obesity prevention and control efforts.

Whether or not it is appropriate to classify obesity as a disease, it is certainly on the causal pathway toward leading chronic diseases. There is thus a strong financial incentive for the provision of effective weight management counseling. If payers have been reticent to reimburse for weight control counseling, it is partly due to the relative lack of evidence that such counseling is, indeed, effective.

In this context, it is worth noting that absence of evidence of effectiveness is not necessarily evidence of an absence of effectiveness. When the best available counseling constructs are applied, particularly in concert with effective outreach and inreach, effective weight management guidance in primary care may well be achievable.

If providers are reluctant to counsel without reimbursement, and payers are reluctant to reimburse without evidence that counseling is effective, an impasse results (Murray & Frenk, 2000). Resolving it requires meeting the needs of both parties simultaneously. In a regional obesity control initiative in New England conducted with support from the New England Coalition for Health Promotion (The New England Coalition for Health Promotion and Disease Prevention) a proposal to resolve the impasse is currently under development. The plan would call for the creation of an on-line weight counseling training program offering continuing medical education (CME) credits, along with credentialing. Providers completing the training and earning credentials would be entered into a database to which insurers would have access.

Insurers would thus be in a position to identify providers suitably trained to offer "state of the art" weight management counseling, and reimburse for their services. The website (construction of which is currently under way) could further house key quality control indicators to be used in the documentation of care, which would be useful for quality audits. Ideally, the program would be restricted access at first so that a controlled evaluation of costs and benefits could be conducted. A pilot period of 2–3 years should be ample to determine if the system is cost-effective, attractive to insurers, and should be made accessible to all.

Accountability/Regulation

Given the obesity epidemic in the United States, one would expect major, coordinated regulatory efforts to attack the scourge. Instead, public policy barriers contribute to the inadequate obesity prevention and management in the United States. Weight management requires stability and continuity of care yet the primary care system remains organized around a "spell of illness" which by definition is time limited. Reimbursement is structured to reward this orientation and there are no incentives for practitioners to deliver systematic and coordinated programs for weight management (Casalino *et al.*, 2003; Wee *et al.*, 2001).

Pay for performance programs in the primary care setting have the potential to reward care coordination, time spent counseling a patient with chronic conditions, and prevention efforts through better financial incentives (Grumbach *et al.*, 1998; Roski *et al.*, 2003). Currently, the Center for Medicare and Medicaid Services compensates physicians on the number and complexity of services provided to patients. Under pay for performance programs, providers will be rewarded for cost savings by focusing on prevention, risk identification and quality of care. This restructuring of payment mechanisms can lead to an increased focus on lifestyle modification and prevention of obesity. Tracking of pertinent HEDIS measures in primary care, such as childhood preventive care, counseling for risk factors, and screening for cholesterol and blood glucose, can help evaluate the effectiveness of obesity prevention, and management and provider incentives can be linked to these performance measures. Direct patient incentives and disincentives can also play an important role in the success of weight management efforts (Baker et al., 2005; Hubbert *et al.*, 2003).

Integrated Systems Approach

The measures and interventions described above represent a veritable menu of opportunities to redesign the existing primary health care system to deliver optimal obesity prevention and control care to patients. Under each of the components of the healthcare system, there are some easy to implement recommendations and others that require more time, effort and resources. Also very important is the integration of these efforts to amplify the total systemic change (Lewis & Dixon, 2004).

Systems thinking approaches to obesity prevention and management, based on systems thinking theory (Senge, 1994) permit the use of diverse methods, resources and strategies to design effective solutions that achieve broad reach and have long term impact. These approaches are designed to facilitate and optimize interrelationships between key stakeholders, data, information sources, theories and principles leading to a single common process intended to generate sustainable solutions (Pronk *et al.*, 2004).

Several promising programs to population health improvement have been outlined in the literature by Pronk & O'Connor, 1997. The authors examined the impact of integration of clinical guidelines with office systems in a managed care setting using diabetes as an example. Specific changes in the office system included provision of clinical guidelines and specific health goals, setting up a clinical database that could identify and monitor patients eligible for guideline based care, and providing guideline directed clinical care based on cues from the database. Successful application of this strategy resulted in improvements in population health.

Similarly, another study by Pronk and Boucher outlined an effective systems approach to childhood obesity prevention and management in a MCO setting. The intervention involved various actors: child/adolescent, family unit, physician and allied health professionals. Salient features included processes to facilitate effective communication, long term support and access to resources. Participants could enter the system at multiple points including the healthcare clinic, school or the home. Once in the system a closed loop process allowed resources to be shared with the patient, the family, as well as the healthcare provider (Pronk & Boucher, 1999).

The authors built on their previous work by developing an integrated system for the implementation of lifestyle and behavior change programs across multiple settings and media. The system had three basic components: organizational staff with clearly delineated roles, computer technology that connected multiple staff, multiple types of service delivery functions and protocols for decision support. The real value of the approach was in the integration and organization of the three components of the system to generate behavior change in the population reached (Pronk et al., 2002).

Pronk et al. revisited health systems design in another study designed to address multiple risk factors in primary care. They generated a series of recommendations at both the patient and the practice level to support counseling for multiple health behaviors. Many of their recommendations are consistent with those outlined earlier in this chapter (Glasgow et al., 2004b).

Another systems approach, the Chronic Care Model (CCM), identifies the essential elements of a health care system that encourage high-quality chronic disease care. These elements are the community, the health system, self-management support, delivery system design, decision support and clinical information systems. Evidence-based change concepts under each element, in combination, foster productive interactions between informed patients who take an active part in their care and providers with resources and expertise. The net outcome is healthier patients, more satisfied providers, and cost savings (Felt Lisk & Kleinman, 2000; McCulloch et al., 1998; Wagner, 2004).

A recent randomized controlled trial by Piatt et al. assessed the applicability of the CCM model to initiate and sustain systems change in group practices serving socio-economically depressed communities. The intervention consisted of an audit chart to establish existing quality of diabetes care. Participating practices were randomized to either CCM group, provider education group or usual care. This pilot study found that a CCM-based intervention was effective in improving clinical, behavioral, psychological/psychosocial, and diabetes knowledge outcomes in patients with diabetes. The CCM group, which received both patient and provider education, demonstrated significantly improved A1C levels, non-HDL cholesterol levels, and rates of self-monitoring of blood glucose compared with the other study groups (Piatt et al., 2006).

The CCM has guided a number of American healthcare organizations to improve their efforts in care for chronic illness (Bodenheimer, 2003; Bodenheimer et al., 2002b; Ferlie & Shortell, 2001; Wagner et al., 2001a).

Most of these organizations have made measurable improvements in the quality of their care. A recent review of the literature reiterates that the most successful chronic disease improvement strategies are consistent with concepts and components identified in the CCM. The systems approach described in this chapter is similar to the CCM approach, but applied also to prevention.

The World Health Organization (WHO) convened a group of health leaders from a number of countries to revise and enlarge the CCM. The resultant effort was the Innovative Care for Chronic Conditions (ICCC) framework. The framework demarcates the various components of the healthcare system into micro (patient and family), meso (healthcare organization and community), and macro (policy) levels (see Table 1) (Bodenheimer *et al.*, 2002a; Epping-Jordan, 2005). It highlights the need for comprehensive system change – and recommends that specific changes in each component be tailored to unique needs and available resources (Barr *et al.*, 2003; Epping-Jordan *et al.*, 2004).

To date many building blocks of the ICCC Framework have been evaluated in healthcare systems globally. These programs have improved biological disease indicators, reduced deaths, saved money and healthcare resources, changed patients' lifestyle and management abilities, led to cost savings and improved processes of care. The building blocks of the ICCC model closely adhere to the elements outlined in this chapter. These components provide the basis for redesigning the existing U.S. healthcare system to provide effective obesity prevention and management (Barr et al., 2003; Casalino et al., 2003).

Systems change is not easy and there is no one size fits all model from previous research and experience that can be responsive to the needs of all practices (Cranney *et al.*, 2001; Mayberry & Gennaro, 2001). Rather healthcare systems that implement a series of small experiments and keep revising and refining these until they get it right are more likely to achieve their stated goals. The Plan-Do-Study-Act (PDSA) cycle is a continuous quality improvement model consisting of a logical sequence of repetitive steps that has been used extensively in the health care field. It consists of small-scale tests of planned actions, followed by assessment and improvement of the initial plan. Numerous small cycles of change accumulate into large effects through synergy. The PDSA evaluation process allows practices to tailor changes to their needs and leads to continuous refinement and improvement (Berwick, 1996, 2003; Berwick & Nolan, 1998; S. M. Campbell *et al.*, 2002; Grol, 2001; Monteleoni & Clark, 2004; Pruitt & Epping-Jordan, 2005; Ramsey *et al.*, 2001; Smith, 2003).

Future Directions

Effective obesity management by health care systems in general, and primary care systems in particular, will require reorienting the system to adequately address the need of the patient and produce the desired outcomes. These differ from those considered important for the acute care system. Dealing with obesity in primary care requires providing patients with broad support not limited to biomedical outcomes. The healthcare system should provide self management skills, planned and patient centered care, and integrated care that cuts across time and settings (Hill, 2005).

The system to address obesity related issues will also require a departure from the physician dominated model. Establishment of multidisciplinary teams, with clear delineation of roles and responsibilities according to capacity and skills, is essential to weight management in primary care (Lawrence, 2002). Changes in medical and information technology should also be leveraged to increase effectiveness and save costs.

Community partners and resources can serve to augment clinical care systems and personnel by taking on functions traditionally assigned to public health workers. Peer educators and lay health advisors can play a key role in obesity prevention. Educated and prepared community partners can reduce the burden of obesity management on clinical personnel and can deliver follow up services and social support to patients and their families (Dohlie *et al.*, 2000; Olden, 2003).

Reimbursement and healthcare insurance programs should be changed to facilitate and sustain integrated, flexible and adaptable healthcare systems that ensure evidence based care with a focus on preventive, quality obesity care. Policy makers should recognize obesity as a serious medical and economic problem, and drive the systemic change that is required with some urgency ("It's time to tackle the high cost of overweight and obesity", 2005; Klein, 2005).

While the components of the health care system can be isolated for purposes of discussion, they are, in fact, parts of a whole, and must be repackaged as such for effective weight management to be widely achieved. Patients must receive prior education in determinants of weight so that the entire burden of such instruction does not fall to the clinical setting. Providers must be schooled in effective counseling methods, and empowered with approaches designed specifically for the clinical care setting. Messages by providers treating different members of the same family, or different aspects of an individual's health, must be consistent, complementary, and reinforcing (Melin *et al.*, 2005). Modifications of the clinical care setting and its practices should allow for multidisciplinary support of patient behavior change. Technology should be used to extend the reach of clinical support beyond the brief span of the encounter. Quality standards for weight management should be established and reinforced, with incorporation into HEDIS measures. Quality monitoring might be used to apply pay-for-performance approaches. Reimbursement strategies linked to quality of care are appropriate (McQuigg *et al.*, 2005).

Conclusion

Epidemic obesity is among the more urgent health threats faced by our population, and should thus be a priority for all health care providers, particularly those delivering primary care. A coordinated systems approach to the problem is likely to yield the best results. While a complete system overhaul may not be necessary, incremental changes should be made quickly in each of the system components outlined in this chapter. Obesity prevention and management deserve the dedicated commitment of health care professionals, community organizations and the policy makers responsible for health care finance. While there will be costs involved in revamping the health care system to deal effectively with the obesity epidemic, the costs of failing to do so will be far greater.

Acknowledgements. The authors gratefully acknowledge the technical assistance of Mrs. Michelle LaRovera.

References

Abrams, D. B., Emmons, K. M., & Linnan, L. A. (1999). Health behavior and health education: The past, present, and future. In K. Glanz, F. Lewis, & B. Rimer (Eds.), *Health behavior and health education: Theory, research and practice* (2nd ed., pp. 453–478). San Francisco, CA: Jossey-Bass.

Abramson, S., Stein, J., Schaufele, M., Frates, E., & Rogan, S. (2000). Personal exercise habits and counseling practices of primary care physicians: A national survey. *Clinical Journal of Sport Medicine, 10*, 40–48.

Ad Hoc Committee on Health Literacy for the American Council on Scientific Affairs. (1999). *Health literacy: Report of the council on scientific affairs. Journal of the American medical association*: American Medical Association.

Agency for Healthcare Research and Quality. (2002). Hcup fact book no. 6: Hospitalization in the United States, 2002 (continued). from http://www.ahrq.gov/data/hcup/factbk6/factbk6c.htm

Albright, C. L., Cohen, S., Gibbons, L., Miller, S., Marcus, B., & Sallis, J., et al. (2000). Incorporating physical activity advice into primary care: Physician-delivered advice within the activity counseling trial. *American Journal of Preventive Medicine, 18*(3), 225–234.

Baker, D. W., Asch, S. M., Keesey, J. W., Brown, J. A., Chan, K. S., & Joyce, G., et al. (2005). Differences in education, knowledge, self-management activities, and health outcomes for patients with heart failure cared for under the chronic disease model: The improving chronic illness care evaluation. *Journal of Cardiac Failure, 11*(6), 405–413.

Barlow, J. H., Wright, C. C., Turner, A. P., & Bancroft, G. V. (2005). A 12-month follow-up study of self-management training for people with chronic disease: Are changes maintained over time? *British Journal of Health Psychology, 10*(Pt 4), 589–599.

Barr, V. J., Robinson, S., Marin-Link, B., Underhill, L., Dotts, A., & Ravensdale, D., et al. (2003). The expanded chronic care model: An integration of concepts and strategies from population health promotion and the chronic care model. *Hospital Quarterly, 7*(1), 73–82.

Beach, M. C., & Inui, T. (2006). Relationship-centered care. A constructive reframing. *Journal of General Internal Medicine, 21*(Suppl. 1), S3–S8.

Berwick, D. M. (1996). A primer on leading the improvement of systems. *British Medical Journal, 312*(7031), 619–622.

Berwick, D. M. (2003). Improvement, trust, and the healthcare workforce. *Quality & Safety in Health Care, 12*(6), 448–452.

Berwick, D. M., & Nolan, T. W. (1998). Physicians as leaders in improving health care: A new series in annals of internal medicine. *Annals of Internal Medicine, 128*(4), 289–292.

Blackburn, G. L., Hu, F. B., & Harvey, A. M. (2005). Evidence-based recommendations for best practices in weight loss surgery. *Obesity Research, 13*(2), 203–204.

Bodenheimer, T. (2003). Interventions to improve chronic illness care: Evaluating their effectiveness. *Disease Management, 6*(2), 63–71.

Bodenheimer, T. (2005). Helping patients improve their health-related behaviors: What system changes do we need? *Disease Management, 8*(5), 319–330.

Bodenheimer, T., Wagner, E. H., & Grumbach, K. (2002a). Improving primary care for patients with chronic illness. *Journal of the American Medical Association, 288*(14), 1775–1779.

Bodenheimer, T., Wagner, E. H., & Grumbach, K. (2002b). Improving primary care for patients with chronic illness: The chronic care model, part 2. *Journal of the American Medical Association, 288*(15), 1909–1914.

Bray, P., Roupe, M., Young, S., Harrell, J., Cummings, D. M., & Whetstone, L. M. (2005). Feasibility and effectiveness of system redesign for diabetes care management in rural areas: The eastern North Carolina experience. *Diabetes Educator, 31*(5), 712–718.

Butterfoss, F. D., & Francisco, V. T. (2004). Evaluating community partnerships and coalitions with practitioners in mind. *Health Promotion Practice, 5*(2), 108–114.

Caldwell, M. A., Peters, K. J., & Dracup, K. A. (2005). A simplified education program improves knowledge, self-care behavior, and disease severity in heart failure patients in rural settings. *American Heart Journal, 150*(5), 983.

Calfas, K., Long, B., Sallis, J., Wooten, W., Pratt, M., & Patrick, K. (1996). A controlled trial of physician counseling to promote the adoption of physical activity. *Preventive Medicine, 25*(3), 225–233.

Campbell, N., & McAlister, F. A. (2006). Not all guidelines are created equal. *Canadian Medical Association Journal, 174*(6), 814–815; discussion 815.

Campbell, S. M., Sheaff, R., Sibbald, B., Marshall, M. N., Pickard, S., & Gask, L., et al. (2002). Implementing clinical governance in English primary care groups/trusts: Reconciling quality improvement and quality assurance. *Quality & Safety in Health Care, 11*(1), 9–14.

Casalino, L., Gillies, R. R., Shortell, S. M., Schmittdiel, J. A., Bodenheimer, T., & Robinson, J. C., et al. (2003). External incentives, information technology, and organized processes to improve health care quality for patients with chronic diseases. *Journal of the American Medical Association, 289*(4), 434–441.

Center for Disease Control and Prevention. (2004). Health, United States, 2004. from http://www.cdc.gov/nchs/data/hus/hus04trend.pdf

Cherry, J. C., Moffatt, T. P., Rodriguez, C., & Dryden, K. (2002). Diabetes disease management program for an indigent population empowered by telemedicine technology. *Diabetes Technology & therapeutics, 4*(6), 783–791.

Chuang, J. H., Hripcsak, G., & Jenders, R. A. (2000). Considering clustering: A methodological review of clinical decision support system studies. *Proceedings. AMIA Symposium*, 146–150.

Cifuentes, M., Fernald, D. H., Green, L. A., Niebauer, L. J., Crabtree, B. F., & Stange, K. C., et al. (2005). Prescription for health: Changing primary care practice to foster healthy behaviors. *Annals of Family Medicine, 3*(Suppl. 2), S4–S11.

Collings, L. H., Pike, L. C., Binder, A. I., McClymont, M. E., & Knight, S. T. (1991). Value of written health information in the general practice setting. *British Journal of General Practice, 41*, 466.

Corrigan, J. M., & Nielsen, D. M. (1993). Toward the development of uniform reporting standards for managed care organizations: The health plan employer data and information set (version 2.0). *Joint Commission Journal on Quality Improvement, 19*(12), 566–575.

Cranney, M., Warren, E., Barton, S., Gardner, K., & Walley, T. (2001). Why do GPs not implement evidence-based guidelines? A descriptive study. *Family Practice, 18*(4), 359–363.

Crawford, P. B., Gosliner, W., Strode, P., Samuels, S. E., Burnett, C., & Craypo, L., et al. (2004). Walking the talk: Fit wic wellness programs improve self-efficacy in pediatric obesity prevention counseling. *American Journal of Public Health, 94*(9), 1480–1485.

Cumbo, A., Agre, P., Dougherty, J., Callery, M., Tetzlaff, L., & Pirone, J., et al. (2002). Online cancer patient education: Evaluating usability and content. *Cancer Practice, 10*(3), 155–161.

De Camargo, Jr. K., & Coeli, C. M. (2006). Theory in practice: Why "good medicine" and "scientific medicine" are not necessarily the same thing. *Advances in Health Sciences Education: Theory & Practice, 11*(1), 77–89.

de Fine Olivarius, N., Palmvig, B., Andreasen, A. H., Thorgersen, J. T., & Hundrup, C. (2005). An educational model for improving diet counseling in primary care a case study of the creative use of doctors' own diet, their attitudes to it and to nutritional counselling of their patients with diabetes. *Patient Education & Counseling, 58*(2), 199–202.

Deakin, T., McShane, C. E., Cade, J. E., & Williams, R. D. (2005). Group based training for self-management strategies in people with type 2 diabetes mellitus. *Cochrane Database Syst Rev*(2), CD003417.

Dickey, L. L., Gemson, D. H., & Carney, P. (1999). Office system interventions supporting primary care-based health behavior change counseling. *American Journal of Preventive Medicine, 17*(4), 299–308.

Dohlie, M. B., Mielke, E., Bwire, T., Adriance, D., & Mumba, F. (2000). Cope (client-oriented, provider-efficient), a model for building community partnerships that improve care in East Africa. *Journal for Healthcare Quality, 22*(5), 34–39.

Dorr, D. A., Wilcox, A., Burns, L., Brunker, C. P., Narus, S. P., & Clayton, P. D. (2006). Implementing a multidisease chronic care model in primary care using people and technology. *Disease Management, 9*(1), 1–15.

Elder, J., Ayala, G., & Harris, S. (1999). Theories and intervention approaches to health-behavior change in primary care. *American Journal of Preventive Medicine, 17*, 275–284.

Elliott, B. J., & Polkinhorn, J. S. (1994). Provision of consumer health information in general practice. *British Medical Journal, 308*, 509–551.

Epping-Jordan, J. E. (2005). Integrated approaches to prevention and control of chronic conditions. *Kidney International. Supplement., 98*, S86–S88.

Epping-Jordan, J. E., Pruitt, S. D., Bengoa, R., & Wagner, E. H. (2004). Improving the quality of health care for chronic conditions. *Quality & Safety in Health Care, 13*(4), 299–305.

Epstein, R. M., Franks, P., Fiscella, K., Shields, C. G., Meldrum, S. C., & Kravitz, R. L., et al. (2005). Measuring patient-centered communication in patient-physician consultations: Theoretical and practical issues. *Social Science & Medicine, 61*(7), 1516–1528.

Ezenwaka, C. E., & Offiah, N. V. (2003). Patients' health education and diabetes control in a developing country. *Acta Diabetol, 40*(4), 173–175.

Faulkner, A., Mills, N., Bainton, D., Baxter, K., Kinnersley, P., & Peters, T. J., et al. (2003). A systematic review of the effect of primary care-based service innovations on quality and patterns of referral to specialist secondary care. *British Journal of General Practice, 53*(496), 878–884.

Felt Lisk, S., & Kleinman, L. (2000). *Effective clinical practices in managed care: Findings from 10 case studies*. New York: Commonwealth Fund.

Fenton, M. (2005). Battling America's epidemic of physical inactivity: Building more walkable, livable communities. *Journal of Nutrition Education and Behavior, 37*(Suppl. 2), S115–S120.

Ferlie, E. B., & Shortell, S. M. (2001). Improving the quality of health care in the United Kingdom and the United States: A framework for change. *Milbank Quarterly, 79*(2), 281–315.

Fitzner, K., Caputo, N., Trendell, W., French, M. V., Bondi, M. A., & Jennings, C. (2003). Recent tax changes may assist treatment of obesity. *Managed Care Interface, 16*(1), 47–51, 55.

Forman, H. (2004). Do we really practice relationship-based care? *J Nurs Adm, 34*(1), 9.

Frank, E., Bhat Schelbert, K., & Elon, L. (2003). Exercise counseling and personal exercise habits of us women physicians. *Journal of the American Medical Women's Association, 58*(3), 178–184.

Frank, E., Wright, E. H., Serdula, M. K., Elon, L. K., & Baldwin, G. (2002). Personal and professional nutrition-related practices of us female physicians. *American Journal of Clinical Nutrition, 75*(2), 326–332.

Friedman, R. H. (1998). Automated telephone conversations to assess health behavior and deliver behavioral interventions. *Journal of Medical Systems, 22*(2), 95–102.

Fulton, J. E., Garg, M., Galuska, D. A., Rattay, K. T., & Caspersen, C. J. (2004). Public health and clinical recommendations for physical activity and physical fitness: Special focus on overweight youth. *Sports Medicine, 34*(9), 581–599.

Galuska, D. A., Will, J. C., Serdula, M. K., & Ford, E. S. (1999). Are health care professionals advising obese patients to lose weight? [see comments]. *Journal of the American Medical Association, 282*(16), 1576–1578.

Gamm, L. D. (1998). Advancing community health through community health partnerships. *Journal of Healthcare Management, 43*(1), 51–66; discussion 57–66.

Genuis, S. J. (2005). The proliferation of clinical practice guidelines: Professional development or medicine-by-numbers? *Jounal of the American Board of Family Practice, 18*(5), 419–425.

Gerber, B. S., Brodsky, I. G., Lawless, K. A., Smolin, L. I., Arozullah, A. M., & Smith, E. V., et al. (2005). Implementation and evaluation of a low-literacy diabetes education computer multimedia application. *Diabetes Care, 28*(7), 1574–1580.

GESICA Investigators. (2005). Randomised trial of telephone intervention in chronic heart failure: Dial trial. *British Medical Journal, 331*(7514), 425.

Glanz, K., Lewis, F., & Rimer, B. (1999). Linking theory, research, and practice. In F. Lewis, K. Glanz, & B. Rimer (Eds.), *Health behavior and health education: Theory, research and practice* (2nd ed.). San Francisco, CA: Jossey-Bass.

Glasgow, R. E., Bull, S. S., Piette, J. D., & Steiner, J. F. (2004a). Interactive behavior change technology. A partial solution to the competing demands of primary care. *American Journal of Preventive Medicine, 27*(Suppl. 2), 80–87.

Glasgow, R. E., Eakin, E. G., Fisher, E. B., Bacak, S. J., & Brownson, R. C. (2001a). Physician advice and support for physical activity: Results from a national survey. *American Journal of Preventive Medicine, 21*(3), 189–196.

Glasgow, R. E., Goldstein, M. G., Ockene, J. K., & Pronk, N. P. (2004b). Translating what we have learned into practice. Principles and hypotheses for interventions addressing multiple behaviors in primary care. *American Journal of Preventive Medicine, 27*(2 Suppl), 88–101.

Glasgow, R. E., Orleans, C. T., & Wagner, E. H. (2001b). Does the chronic care model serve also as a template for improving prevention? *Milbank Quarterly, 79*(4), 579–612, iv–v.

Goodpaster, B. H. (2002). Measuring body fat distribution and content in humans. *Curr Opin Clin Nutr Metab Care, 5*(5), 481–487.

Goolsby, M. J. (2001). Evaluating and applying clinical practice guidelines. *Journal of the American Academy of Nurse Practitioners, 13*(1), 3–6.

Gordon-Larsen, P., Nelson, M. C., Page, P., & Popkin, B. M. (2006). Inequality in the built environment underlies key health disparities in physical activity and obesity. *Pediatrics, 117*(2), 417–424.

Gorman, J. (2000, Sunday, Jun 11). The size of things to come. *NY Times*, 21–22.

Grol, R. (2001). Improving the quality of medical care: Building bridges among professional pride, payer profit, and patient satisfaction. *Journal of the American Medical Association, 286*(20), 2578–2585.

Grumbach, K., Osmond, D., Vranizan, K., Jaffe, D., & Bindman, A. B. (1998). Primary care physicians' experience of financial incentives in managed-care systems. *New England Journal of Medicine, 339*(21), 1516–1521.

Grundy, S. M. (2000). Metabolic complications of obesity. *Endocrine Reviews, 13*, 155–165.

Hartman, T., McCarthy, P., Park, R., Schuster, E., & Kushi, L. (1994). Focus group responses of potential participants in a nutrition education program for individuals with limited literacy skills. *Journal of the American Dietetic Association, 94*, 744–748.

Harvey, J. (1999). *Civilized oppression.* Lanham, Md.: Rowman and Littlefield Publishers, Inc.

Hassink, S. (2003). Problems in childhood obesity. *Primary Care, 30*, 357–374.

Health Resources and Services Administration. National vaccine injury compensation program (VICP). from http://www.hrsa.gov/vaccinecompensation/default.htm

Heaney, C. A., & Israil, B. A. (1999). Social networks and social support. In K. Glanz, F. Lewis, & B. Rimer (Eds.), *Health behavior and health education: Theory, research and practice* (2nd ed., pp. 179–205). San Francisco, CA: Jossey-Bass.

Hedley, A. A., Ogden, C. L., Johnson, C. L., Carroll, M. D., Curtin, L. R., & Flegal, K. M. (2004). Prevalence of overweight and obesity among us children, adolescents, and adults, 1999–2002. *Journal of the American Medical Association, 291*(23), 2847–2850.

Helwig, A. L., Lovelle, A., Guse, C. E., & Gottlieb, M. S. (1999). An office-based internet patient education system: A pilot study. *Jounal of the American Board of Family Practice, 48*(2), 123–127.

Hersh, W. R., Wallace, J. A., Patterson, P. K., Shapiro, S. E., Kraemer, D. F., & Eilers, G. M., et al. (2001). Telemedicine for the medicare population: Pediatric, obstetric, and clinician-indirect home interventions. *Evidence Report/Technology assessment (Summ)* (24 *Suppl*), 1–32.

Hill, J. (2005). Practical management of obesity in primary care. *British Journal for Nursing, 14*(17), 892.

Honda, K. (2004). Factors underlying variation in receipt of physician advice on diet and exercise: Applications of the behavioral model of health care utilization. *American Journal of Health Promotion, 18*(5), 370–377.

Houck, S., Kilo, C., & Scott, J. C. (2003). Improving patient care. Group visits 101. *Family Practice Management, 10*(5), 66–68.

HSTAT. (Evidence Syntheses, formerly Systematic Evidence Reviews 21). *Screening and interventions for overweight and obesity in adults. Guide to clinical preventive services, 3rd edition: Recommendations and systematic evidence reviews, guide to community preventive services.*

Hubbert, K. A., Bussey, B. F., Allison, D. B., Beasley, T. M., Henson, C. S., & Heimburger, D. C. (2003). Effects of outcome-driven insurance reimbursement on short-term weight control. *International Journal of Obesity and Related Metabolic Disorders, 27*(11), 1423–1429.

Institute of Medicine. (2001). *Health and behavior: The interplay of biological, behavioral, and societal influences.* Washington, DC: National Academy Press.

Irving, P., & Dickson, D. (2004). Empathy: Towards a conceptual framework for health professionals. *International Journal of Health Care Quality Assurance Incorporating Leadership in Health Services, 17*(4–5), 212–220.

It's time to tackle the high cost of overweight and obesity. (2005). *Disease Management Advisor, 11*(1), 1–4.

Jackson, J. E., Doescher, M. P., Saver, B. G., & Hart, L. G. (2005). Trends in professional advice to lose weight among obese adults, 1994 to 2000. *Journal of General Internal Medicine, 20*(9), 814–818.

Jackson, Y., Dietz, W. H., Sanders, C., Kolbe, L. J., Whyte, J. J., & Wechsler, H., et al. (2002). Summary of the 2000 surgeon general's listening session: Toward a national action plan on overweight and obesity. *Obesity Research, 10*(12), 1299–1305.

Jacobs, M., & Rauber, R. (1996). Developing a networking strategy for an integrated healthcare delivery system. *Journal of American Health Information Management Association (AHIMA), 67*(1), 56–58.

Jeffery, R. W., McGuire, M. T., Brelje, K. L., Pronk, N. P., Boyle, R. G., & Hase, K. A., et al. (2004). Recruitment to mail and telephone interventions for obesity in a managed care environment: The weigh-to-be project. *American Journal of Managed Care, 10*(6), 378–382.

Jeffery, R. W., Sherwood, N. E., Brelje, K., Pronk, N. P., Boyle, R., & Boucher, J. L., et al. (2003). Mail and phone interventions for weight loss in a managed-care setting: Weigh-to-be one-year outcomes. *International Journal of Obesity and Related Metabolic Disorders, 27*(12), 1584–1592.

Kaplan, B., Farzanfar, R., & Friedman, R. H. (2003). Personal relationships with an intelligent interactive telephone health behavior advisor system: A multimethod study using surveys and ethnographic interviews. *International Journal of Medical Informatics, 71*(1), 33–41.

Katon, W. J., Von Korff, M., Lin, E. H., Simon, G., Ludman, E., & Russo, J., et al. (2004). The pathways study: A randomized trial of collaborative care in patients with diabetes and depression. *Archives of General Psychiatry, 61*(10), 1042–1049.

Katz, D. (2001a). Behavior modification in primary care: The pressure system model. *Preventive Medicine, 32*(1), 66–72.

Katz, D., Chan, W., Gonzalez, M., Larson, D., Nawaz, H., & Abdulrahman, M., et al. (2002). Technical skills for weight loss: Preliminary data from a randomized trial. *Preventive Medicine, 34*, 681–615.

Katz, D. L. (2001b). Dietary recommendations for health promotion and disease prevention. In D. L. Katz, (Ed.), *Nutrition in clinical practice* (pp. 291–298). Philadelphia, PA: Lippincott, Williams & Wilkins.

Katz, D. L. (2002). Effective dietary counseling: Helping patients find and follow "the way" to eat. *West Virginia Medical Journal, 98*(6), 256–259.

Katz, D. L., Suval, K., Comerford, B. P., Faridi, Z., Njike, V. Y. Impact of an educational intervention on internal medicine residents' physical activity counseling: The Pressure System Model. *Journal of Evaluation & Clinical Practice.* In press.

Kearney, M. H., York, R., & Deatrick, J. A. (2000). Effects of home visits to vulnerable young families. *Journal of Nursing Scholarship, 32*(4), 369–376.

Keim, N. L., Blanton, C. A., & Kretsch, M. J. (2004). America's obesity epidemic: Measuring physical activity to promote an active lifestyle. *Journal of the American Dietetic Association, 104*(9), 1398–1409.

Kelly, J., Crowe, P., & Shearer, M. (2005). The good life club project. Telephone coaching for chronic disease self management. *Australian Family Physician, 34*(1–2), 31–34.

Kennen, E. M., Davis, T. C., Huang, J., Yu, H., Carden, D., & Bass, R., et al. (2005). Tipping the scales: The effect of literacy on obese patients' knowledge and readiness to lose weight. *Southern Medical Journal, 98*(1), 15–18.

King, A. C., Sallis, J. F., Dunn, A. L., Simons-Morton, D. G., Albright, C. A., & Cohen, S., et al. (1998). Overview of the activity counseling trial (act) intervention for promoting physical activity in primary health care settings. Activity counseling trial research group. *Medicine and Science in Sports and Exercise, 30*(7), 1086–1096.

Klardie, K. A., Johnson, J., McNaughton, M. A., & Meyers, W. (2004). Integrating the principles of evidence-based practice into clinical practice. *Journal of the American Academy of Nurse Practitioners, 16*(3), 98, 100–102, 104–105.

Klein, S. (2005). Does paying for obesity therapy make cents? *Gastroenterology, 128*(3), 530.

Koperski, M. (1989). Health education using video recordings in a general practice waiting area: An evaluation. *Journal of the Royal College of General Practitioners, 39*, 328–330.

Landis, S. E., Schwarz, M., & Curran, D. R. (2006). North Carolina family medicine residency programs' diabetes learning collaborative. *Family Medicine, 38*(3), 190–195.

Larsen, L., Mandleco, B., Williams, M., & Tiedeman, M. (2006). Childhood obesity: Prevention practices of nurse practitioners. *Journal of the American Academy of Nurse Practitioners, 18*(2), 70–79.

Lawrence, D. (2002). *From chaos to care: The promise of team-based medicine.* Cambridge: Perseus Publishing.

Lederman, J., Ballard, J., Njike, V. Y., Margolies, L., Katz, D. L. (2007). Information given to postmenopausal women on coronary computed tomography may influence cardiac risk reduction efforts. *Journal of Clinical Epidemiology, 60*(4), 389–396.

Lee, F. W. (1997). Evolution of computer-based information systems and networks to support integrated health care delivery systems. *Topics in Health Information Management, 17*(4), 1–10.

Leermakers, E. A., Anglin, K., & Wing, R. R. (1998). Reducing postpartum weight retention through a correspondence intervention. *International Journal of Obesity & Related Metabolic Disorders, 22*(11), 1103–1109.

Levy, B., & Williamson, P. (1988). Patient perceptions and weight loss of obese adults. *Journal of Family Practice, 27*, 285–290.

Lewis, R., & Dixon, J. (2004). Rethinking management of chronic diseases. *British Medical Journal, 328*(7433), 220–222.

Lin, S. X., & Larson, E. (2005). Does provision of health counseling differ by patient race? *Family Medicine, 37*(9), 650–654.

Livaudais, J. C., Kaplan, C. P., Haas, J. S., Perez-Stable, E. J., Stewart, S., & Jarlais, G. D. (2005). Lifestyle behavior counseling for women patients among a sample of California physicians. *Journal of Women's Health, 14*(6), 485–495.

Logue, E., Sutton, K., Jarjoura, D., Smucker, W., Baughman, K., & Capers, C. (2005). Transtheoretical model-chronic disease care for obesity in primary care: A randomized trial. *Obesity Research, 13*(5), 917–927.

Long, B. J., Calfas, K. J., Wooten, W., Sallis, J. F., Patrick, K., & Goldstein, M., et al. (1996). A multisite field test of the acceptability of physical activity counseling in primary care: Project pace. *American Journal of Preventive Medicine, 12*(2), 73–81.

MacLean, C. D., Littenberg, B., & Gagnon, M. (2006). Diabetes decision support: Initial experience with the Vermont diabetes information system. *American Journal of Public Health, 96*(4), 593–595.

Maheux, B., Haley, N., Rivard, M., & Gervais, A. (1999). Do physicians assess lifestyle health risks during general medical examinations? A survey of general practitioners and obstetrician-gynecologists in Quebec. *Canadian Medical Association Journal, 160*(13), 1830–1834.

Makoul, G. (2003). The interplay between education and research about patient-provider communication. *Patient Education & Counseling, 50*(1), 79–84.

Mann, S. (1998). *Wearable computing as a means for personal empowerment.* Paper presented at the Proc 1st Int Conf Wearable Comput (ICWC '98), Los Alamitos, CA.

Marcus, B., Goldstein, M., Jette, A., Simkin-Silverman, L., Pinto, B., & Milan, F., et al. (1997). Training physicians to conduct physical activity counseling. *Preventive Medicine, 26*, 382–388.

Marcus, B. H., Owen, N., Forsyth, L. H., Cavill, N. A., & Fridinger, F. (1998). Physical activity interventions using mass media, print media, and information technology. *American Journal of Preventive Medicine, 15*(4), 362–378.

Margolis, P. A., Stevens, R., Bordley, W. C., Stuart, J., Harlan, C., & Keyes-Elstein, L., et al. (2001). From concept to application: The impact of a community-wide intervention to improve the delivery of preventive services to children. *Pediatrics, 108*(3), E42.

Martin, L. F., Robinson, A., & Moore, B. J. (2000). Socioeconomic issues affecting the treatment of obesity in the new millennium. *Pharmacoeconomics, 18*(4), 335–353.

Martin, P. D., Rhode, P. C., Howe, J. T., & Brantley, P. J. (2003). Primary care weight management counseling: Physician and patient perspectives. *Journal of the Louisiana State Medical Society, 155*(1), 52–56.

Masley, S., Sokoloff, J., & Hawes, C. (2000). Planning group visits for high-risk patients. *Family Practice Management, 7*(6), 33–37.

Mathur, R., Roybal, G. M., & Peters, A. L. (2005). Short and longer term outcomes of a diabetes disease management program in underserved Latino patients. *Current Medical Research and Opinion, 21*(12), 1935–1941.

Mayberry, L. J., & Gennaro, S. (2001). A quality of health outcomes model for guiding obstetrical practice. *Journal of Nursing Scholarship, 33*(2), 141–146.

Mazza, D., & Russell, S. J. (2001). Are GPs using clinical practice guidelines? *Australian Family Physician, 30*(8), 817–821.

McBride, C. M., & Rimer, B. K. (1999). Using the telephone to improve health behavior and health service delivery. *Patient Education & Counseling, 37*(1), 3–18.

McCallum, Z., & Gerner, B. (2005). Weighty matters–an approach to childhood overweight in general practice. *Australian Family Physician, 34*(9), 745–748.

McCulloch, D. K., Price, M. J., Hindmarsh, M., & Wagner, E. H. (1998). A population-based approach to diabetes management in a primary care setting: Early results and lessons learned. *Effective Clinical Practice, 1*(1), 12–22.

McQuigg, M., Brown, J., Broom, J., Laws, R. A., Reckless, J. P., & Noble, P. A., et al. (2005). Empowering primary care to tackle the obesity epidemic: The counterweight programme. *European Journal of Clinical Nutrition, 59*(Suppl. 1), S93–100; discussion S101.

McVea, K., Venugopal, M., Crabtree, B. F., & Aita, V. (2000). The organization and distribution of patient education materials in family medicine practices. *49*(4).

Melin, I., Karlstrom, B., Berglund, L., Zamfir, M., & Rossner, S. (2005). Education and supervision of health care professionals to initiate, implement and improve management of obesity. *Patient Education & Counseling, 58*(2), 127–136.

Miller, D., Zantop, V., Hammer, H., Faust, S., & Grumbach, K. (2004). Group medical visits for low-income women with chronic disease: A feasibility study. *Journal of Women's Health, 13*(2), 217–225.

Monteleoni, C., & Clark, E. (2004). Using rapid-cycle quality improvement methodology to reduce feeding tubes in patients with advanced dementia: Before and after study. *British Medical Journal, 329*(7464), 491–494.

Morland, K., Diez Roux, A. V., & Wing, S. (2006). Supermarkets, other food stores, and obesity: The atherosclerosis risk in communities study. *American Journal of Preventive Medicine, 30*(4), 333–339.

Murray, C. J., & Frenk, J. (2000). A framework for assessing the performance of health systems. *Bulletin of the World Health Organization, 78*(6), 717–731.

National Academy on an Aging Society/Center for Health Care Strategies. (1998). *Low health literacy skills increase annual health care expenditures by $73 billion. Center for health care strategies fact sheet*. Washington DC.

National Cancer Institute. (1995). *Theory at a glance: A guide for health promotion practice* (No. NIH Publication No. 95-3896). Bethesda, MD: National Institutes of Health, National Cancer Institute.

Nawaz, H., Adams, M., & Katz, D. (1999). Weight loss counseling by health care providers. *American Journal of Public Health, 89*, 764–767.

Nawaz, H., & Katz, D. (2001). American college of preventive medicine practice policy statement. Weight management counseling of overweight adults. *American Journal of Preventive Medicine, 21*, 73–78.

Nawaz, H., Katz, D., & Adams, M. (2000). Physician-patient interactions regarding diet, exercise and smoking. *Preventive Medicine, 31*, 652–657.

Nicolucci, A., Ciccarone, E., Consoli, A., Di Martino, G., La Penna, G., & Latorre, A., et al. (2000). Relationship between patient practice-oriented knowledge and metabolic control in intensively treated type 1 diabetic patients: Results of the validation of the knowledge and practices diabetes questionnaire. *Diabetes, Nutrition & Metabolism, 13*(5), 276–283.

Noel, M., Hickner, J., Ettenhofer, T., & Gauthier, B. (1998a). The high prevalence of obesity in Michigan primary care practices. An uprnet study. Upper Peninsula research network. *Journal of Family Practice, 47*, 39–43.

Noel, P. H., Larme, A. C., Meyer, J., Marsh, G., Correa, A., & Pugh, J. A. (1998b). Patient choice in diabetes education curriculum. Nutritional versus standard content for type 2 diabetes. *Diabetes Care, 21*(6), 896–901.

Noffsinger, E. B., Sawyer, D. R., & Scott, J. C. (2003). Group medical visits: A glimpse into the future? *Patient Care, 37*, 18–27.

Norris, S. L., Engelgau, M. M., & Narayan, K. M. (2001). Effectiveness of self-management training in type 2 diabetes: A systematic review of randomized controlled trials. *Diabetes Care, 24*(3), 561–587.

Nthangeni, G., Steyn, N. P., Alberts, M., Steyn, K., Levitt, N. S., & Laubscher, R., et al. (2002). Dietary intake and barriers to dietary compliance in black type 2 diabetic patients attending primary health-care services. *Public Health Nutrition*, 5(2), 329–338.

Nutbeam, D. (2000). Health literacy as a public health goal: A challenge for contemporary health education and communication strategies into the 21st century. *Health Promotion International*, 15(3), 259–267.

O'Brien, S. H., Holubkov, R., & Reis, E. C. (2004). Identification, evaluation, and management of obesity in an academic primary care center. *Pediatrics*, 114, e154–e159.

O'Toole, M. F., Kmetik, K. S., Bossley, H., Cahill, J. M., Kotsos, T. P., & Schwamberger, P. A., et al. (2005). Electronic health record systems: The vehicle for implementing performance measures. *American Heart Hospital Journal*, 3(2), 88–93.

Ockene, J. K., Ockene, I. S., Quirk, M. E., Hebert, J. R., Saperia, G. M., Luippold, R. S., et al. (1995). Physician training for patient-centered nutrition counseling in a lipid intervention trial. *Preventive Medicine*, 24(6), 563–570.

Oermann, M. H., Webb, S. A., & Ashare, J. A. (2003). Outcomes of videotape instruction in clinic waiting area. *Orthopedic Nursing*, 22(2), 102–105.

Ogden, C. L., Carroll, M. D., Curtin, L. R., McDowell, M. A., Tabak, C. J., & Flegal, K. M. (2006). Prevalence of overweight and obesity in the United States, 1999–2004. *Journal of the American Medical Association*, 295(13), 1549–1555.

Olden, P. C. (2003). Hospital and community health: Going from stakeholder management to stakeholder collaboration. *Journal of Health and Human Services Administration*, 26(1), 35–57.

Olson, C. M., Strawderman, M. S., & Reed, R. G. (2004). Efficacy of an intervention to prevent excessive gestational weight gain. *American Journal of Obstetrics and Gynecology*, 191(2), 530–536.

Panniers, T. L., Feuerbach, R. D., & Soeken, K. L. (2003). Methods in informatics: Using data derived from a systematic review of health care texts to develop a concept map for use in the neonatal intensive care setting. *Journal of Biomedical Informatics*, 36(4–5), 232–239.

Parker, K. A., Ressa, M., Skelley, S., & Smith, D. K. (1992). Community resources in obese care. *Journal of the Florida Medical Association*, 79(6), 389–391.

Patrick, K., Sallis, J. F., Prochaska, J. J., Lydston, D. D., Calfas, K. J., & Zabinski, M. F., et al. (2001). A multicomponent program for nutrition and physical activity change in primary care: Pace+ for adolescents. *Archives of Pediatrics & Adolescent Medicine*, 155(8), 940–946.

Peiss, B., Kurleto, B., & Rubenfire, M. (1995). Physicians and nurses can be effective educators in coronary risk reduction. *Journal of General Internal Medicine*, 10(2), 77–81.

Petrella, R. J., Koval, J. J., Cunningham, D. A., & Paterson, D. H. (2003). Can primary care doctors prescribe exercise to improve fitness? The step test exercise prescription (step) project. *American Journal of Preventive Medicine*, 24(4), 316–322.

Philipp, R., Hughes, A., Wood, N., Burns-Cox, C., Cook, N., & Fletcher, G. (1990). Information needs of patients and visitors in a district general hospital. *Journal of the Royal Society of Health*, 1, 10–12.

Piatt, G. A., Orchard, T. J., Emerson, S., Simmons, D., Songer, T. J., & Brooks, M. M., et al. (2006). Translating the chronic care model into the community: Results from a randomized controlled trial of a multifaceted diabetes care intervention. *Diabetes Care*, 29(4), 811–817.

Piette, J. D., Weinberger, M., McPhee, S. J., Mah, C. A., Kraemer, F. B., & Crapo, L. M. (2000). Do automated calls with nurse follow-up improve self-care and glycemic control among vulnerable patients with diabetes? *American Journal of Medicine*, 108(1), 20–27.

Pinto, B., Goldstein, M., DePue, J., & Milan, F. (1998). Acceptability and feasibility of physician-based activity counseling. The pal project. *American Journal of Preventive Medicine*, 15, 95–102.

Polley, B. A., Wing, R. R., & Sims, C. J. (2002). Randomized controlled trial to prevent excessive weight gain in pregnant women. *International Journal of Obesity and Related Metabolic Disorders*, 26(11), 1494–1502.

Polniaszek, S., & Klinger, C. (2004). Long-term care counselor: An electronic decision-support tool. *Care Management Journals*, *5*(3), 139–144.

Popkin, B. M., Barclay, D. V., & Nielsen, S. J. (2005). Water and food consumption patterns of U.S. Adults from 1999 to 2001. *Obesity Research*, *13*(12), 2146–2152.

Porta, M., & Trento, M. (2004). Romeo: Rethink organization to improve education and outcomes. *Diabetic Medicine, 21*(6), 644–645.

Potter, M. B., Vu, J. D., & Croughan-Minihane, M. (2001). Weight management: What patients want from their primary care physicians. *Journal of Family Practice, 50*(6), 513–518.

Prochaska, J., & DiClemente, C. (1983). Stages and processes of self change of smoking: Toward an integrative model of change. *Journal of Consulting and Clinical Psychology*, *51*, 390–395.

Pronk, N. P., & Boucher, J. (1999). Systems approach to childhood and adolescent obesity prevention and treatment in a managed care organization. *International Journal of Obesity and Related Metabolic Disorders*, *23*(Suppl. 2), S38–S42.

Pronk, N. P., Boucher, J. L., Gehling, E., Boyle, R. G., & Jeffery, R. W. (2002). A platform for population-based weight management: Description of a health plan-based integrated systems approach. *American Journal of Managed Care*, *8*(10), 847–857.

Pronk, N. P., & O'Connor, P. J. (1997). Systems approach to population health improvement. *Journal of Ambulatory Care Management*, *20*(4), 24–31.

Pronk, N. P., Peek, C. J., & Goldstein, M. G. (2004). Addressing multiple behavioral risk factors in primary care. A synthesis of current knowledge and stakeholder dialogue sessions. *American Journal of Preventive Medicine*, *27*(Suppl. 2), 4–17.

Provan, K. G., Harvey, J., & de Zapien, J. G. (2003). Building community capacity around chronic disease services through a collaborative interorganizational network. *Health Education & Behavior, 30*(6), 646–662.

Provan, K. G., Harvey, J., & de Zapien, J. G. (2005). Network structure and attitudes toward collaboration in a community partnership for diabetes control on the US-Mexican border. *Journal of Health Organization and Management*, *19*(6), 504–518.

Provan, K. G., Lamb, G., & Doyle, M. (2004). Building legitimacy and the early growth of health networks for the uninsured. *Health Care Manage Rev*, *29*(2), 117–128.

Pruitt, S. D., & Epping-Jordan, J. E. (2005). Preparing the 21st century global health-care workforce. *British Medical Journal*, *330*(7492), 637–639.

Ramelson, H. Z., Friedman, R. H., & Ockene, J. K. (1999). An automated telephone-based smoking cessation education and counseling system. *Patient Education & Counseling*, *36*(2), 131–144.

Ramsey, C., Ormsby, S., & Marsh, T. (2001). Performance-improvement strategies can reduce costs. *Healthcare Financial Management*, (Suppl.), 2–6.

Randomised trial of telephone intervention in chronic heart failure: Dial trial. (2005). *British Medical Journal*, *331*(7514), 425.

Revere, D., & Dunbar, P. J. (2001). Review of computer-generated outpatient health behavior interventions: Clinical encounters "in absentia". *Journal of the American Medical Informatics Association*, *8*(1), 62–79.

Richard, D. (2003). Complications of obesity: The inflammatory link. Introduction. *International Journal of Obesity and Related Metabolic Disorders*, *27*(Suppl. 3), S2–S3.

Rickheim, P. L., Weaver, T. W., Flader, J. L., & Kendall, D. M. (2002). Assessment of group versus individual diabetes education: A randomized study. *Diabetes Care*, *25*(2), 269–274.

Rodwin, V. G. (1990). Comparative health systems: A policy perspective. In A. R. Kovner (Ed.), *Health care delivery in the United States* (pp. 435-465). New York: Springer Publishing Company.

Rogge, M. M., Greenwald, M., & Golden, A. (2004). Obesity, stigma, and civilized oppression. *ANS. Advances in Nursing Science*, *27*(4), 301–315.

Roski, J., Jeddeloh, R., An, L., Lando, H., Hannan, P., & Hall, C., et al. (2003). The impact of financial incentives and a patient registry on preventive care quality:

Increasing provider adherence to evidence-based smoking cessation practice guidelines. *Preventive Medicine, 36*(3), 291–299.

Rothman, R. L., DeWalt, D. A., Malone, R., Bryant, B., Shintani, A., & Crigler, B., et al. (2004). Influence of patient literacy on the effectiveness of a primary care-based diabetes disease management program. *Journal of the American Medical Association, 292*(14), 1711–1716.

Rothman, R. L., Malone, R., Bryant, B., Shintani, A. K., Crigler, B., & Dewalt, D. A., et al. (2005). A randomized trial of a primary care-based disease management program to improve cardiovascular risk factors and glycated hemoglobin levels in patients with diabetes. *American Journal of Medicine, 118*(3), 276–284.

Roussos, S. T., & Fawcett, S. B. (2000). A review of collaborative partnerships as a strategy for improving community health. *Annual Review of Public Health, 21*, 369–402.

Sallis, J. F., & Glanz, K. (2006). The role of built environments in physical activity, eating, and obesity in childhood. *Future of Children, 16*(1), 89–108.

Saltzman, E., Anderson, W., Apovian, C. M., Boulton, H., Chamberlain, A., & Cullum-Dugan, D., et al. (2005). Criteria for patient selection and multidisciplinary evaluation and treatment of the weight loss surgery patient. *Obesity Research, 13*(2), 234–243.

Schofferman, J., Diamond, N., Oill, P. A., & Becker, L. (1977). Use of the telephone for short-term follow-up. *Medical Care, 15*(5), 430–434.

Scott, J. G., Cohen, D., DiCicco-Bloom, B., Orzano, A. J., Gregory, P., & Flocke, S. A., et al. (2004). Speaking of weight: How patients and primary care clinicians initiate weight loss counseling. *Preventive Medicine, 38*(6), 819–827.

Senge, P. (1994). *The fifth discipline: The art & practice of the learning organization.* New York: Doubleday.

Shiroyama, C., Begg, A., Griffiths, J., & McKie, L. (1997). Getting the message across: The development and evaluation of a health education video in general practice. *Health Bulletin, 55*(1), 58–61.

Sickness Prevention Achieved through Regional Collaboration. from http://www.sparc-health.org/

Smith, R. (2003). What doctors and managers can learn from each other. *British Medical Journal, 326*(7390), 610–611.

Stanley, I., & Tongue, B. (1991). Providing information and detecting concerns about health in general practice populations using a computer system in the waiting area. *British Journal of General Practice, 41*(353), 499–503.

Stern, J. S., Kazaks, A., & Downey, M. (2005). Future and implications of reimbursement for obesity treatment. *Journal of the American Dietetic Association, 105*(5 Suppl 1), S104–S109.

Stokols, D., Allen, J., & Bellingham, R. L. (1996). The social ecology of health promotion: Implications for research and practice. *American Journal of Health Promotion, 10*(4), 247–251.

Tate, D. F., Wing, R. R., & Winett, R. A. (2001). Using internet technology to deliver a behavioral weight loss program. *Journal of the American Medical Association, 285*(9), 1172–1177.

Taylor, K. I., Oberle, K. M., Crutcher, R. A., & Norton, P. G. (2005). Promoting health in type 2 diabetes: Nurse-physician collaboration in primary care. *Biological Research for Nursing, 6*(3), 207–215.

The New England Coalition for Health Promotion and Disease Prevention. from http://www.neconinfo.org

Thompson, E. (2000). The power of group visits. Improved quality of care, increased productivity entice physicians to see up to 15 patients at a time. *Modern Healthcare, 30*(23), 54, 56, 62.

Thompson, R. S. (1996). What have HMOS learned about clinical prevention services? An examination of the experience at group health cooperative of puget sound. *Milbank Quarterly, 74*(4), 469–509.

Trento, M., Passera, P., Tomalino, M., Bajardi, M., Pomero, F., & Allione, A., et al. (2001). Group visits improve metabolic control in type 2 diabetes: A 2-year follow-up. *Diabetes Care, 24*(6), 995–1000.

Tresolini, C. (1994). *Report of the pew-fetzer task force on advancing psychosocial health education. Health professions education and relationship centered care.*

Truswell, A. S. (1999). What nutrition knowledge and skills do primary care physicians need to have, and how should this be communicated? *European Journal of Clinical Nutrition, 53*(Suppl. 2), S67–S71.

Tufano, J. T., & Karras, B. T. (2005). Mobile ehealth interventions for obesity: A timely opportunity to leverage convergence trends. *Journal of Medical Internet Research, 7*(5), e58.

U.S. Preventive Services Task Force. (2002). Behavioral counseling in primary care to promote physical activity: Recommendation and rationale. *Annals of Internal Medicine, 137*(3), 205–207.

U.S. Preventive Services Task Force. (2003a). Healthy diet counseling. Retrieved March 4, 2006, from http://www.ahrq.gov/clinic/uspstf/uspsdiet.htm

U.S. Preventive Services Task Force. (2003b). Screening for obesity in adults. Retrieved March 4, 2006, from http://www.ahrq.gov/clinic/uspstf/uspsobes.htm

Unutzer, J., Katon, W., Callahan, C. M., Williams, J. W. J., Hunkeler, E., & Harpole, L., et al. (2002). Impact investigators. Improving mood-promoting access to collaborative treatment. Collaborative care management of late-life depression in the primary care setting: A randomized controlled trial. *Journal of the American Medical Association, 288*(22), 2836–2845.

Varnavides, C. K., Zermansky, A. G., & Pace, C. (1984). Health library for patients in general practice. *British Medical Journal, 288*, 535–537.

Vickery, K. (2000). Going with the flow. Providers expand service to create a smooth continuum of care. *Provider, 26*(10), 34–38, 41–32, 45–36 passim.

Wager, K. A., Heda, S., & Austin, C. J. (1997). Developing a health information network within an integrated delivery system: A case study. *Topics in Health Information Management, 17*(4), 20–31.

Wagner, E. H. (2004). Chronic disease care. *British Medical Journal, 328*(7433), 177–178.

Wagner, E. H., Austin, B. T., Davis, C., Hindmarsh, M., Schaefer, J., & Bonomi, A. (2001a). Improving chronic illness care: Translating evidence into action. *Health Affairs, 20*(6), 64–78.

Wagner, E. H., Glasgow, R. E., Davis, C., Bonomi, A. E., Provost, L., & McCulloch, D., et al. (2001b). Quality improvement in chronic illness care: A collaborative approach. *Joint Commission Journal on Quality Improvement, 27*(2), 63–80.

Wahlqvist, M. L. (2005). Physical activity for health: An overview. *World Review of Nutrition & Dietetics, 95*, 62–72.

Wantland, D. J., Portillo, C. J., Holzemer, W. L., Slaughter, R., & McGhee, E. M. (2004). The effectiveness of web-based vs. Non-web-based interventions: A meta-analysis of behavioral change outcomes. *Journal of Medical Internet Research, 6*(4), e40.

Wee, C. C., McCarthy, E. P., Davis, R. B., & Phillips, R. S. (1999). Physician counseling about exercise. *Journal of the American Medical Association, 282*(16), 1583–1588.

Wee, C. C., Phillips, R. S., Burstin, H. R., Cook, E. F., Puopolo, A. L., & Brennan, T. A., et al. (2001). Influence of financial productivity incentives on the use of preventive care. *American Journal of Medicine, 110*(3), 181–187.

White, J. (1999). Targets and systems of health care cost control. *Journal of Health Politics, Policy and Law, 24*(4), 653–696.

Wicke, D. M., Lorge, R. E., Coppin, R. J., & Jones, K. P. (1994). The effectiveness of waiting room notice-boards as a vehicle for health education. *Family Practice, 11*(3), 292–295.

Williams, M. V., Baker, D. W., Parker, R. M., & Nurss, J. R. (1998). Relationship of functional health literacy to patients' knowledge of their chronic disease. A study of patients with hypertension and diabetes. *Archives of Internal Medicine, 158*(2), 166–172.

World Health Organization. (2001). *Innovative care for chronic conditions: Building blocks for action. Global report.*

Yarmo, D. (1998). Research directions for case management. *Journal of Case Management, 7*(2), 84–91.

Yeh, M. C., Rodriguez, E., Nawaz, H., Gonzalez, M., Nakamoto, D., & Katz, D. L. (2003). Technical skills for weight loss: Two-year follow-up results of a randomized trial. *International Journal of Obesity, 27,* 1500–1506.

Zrebiec, J. F. (2005). Internet communities: Do they improve coping with diabetes? *Diabetes Educator, 31*(6), 825–828, 830–822, 834, 836.

Chapter 15

Workplace Approaches to Obesity Prevention

Antronette K. Yancey, Nico P. Pronk and Brian L. Cole

Introduction

Worksites are extremely important settings for obesity prevention initiatives. Given the large proportion of each day that most adults spend in work settings, and the potentially significant influences of workplace policies and culture on personal weight-related health behaviors, workplaces can play a vital role in promoting more active lifestyles and healthier eating practices that will assist in controlling the obesity epidemic (Peterson & Wilson, 2002). In fact, diffusion of healthy eating and active living practices in socioeconomically and ethnically diverse populations is more likely to occur at work than in any other setting (Sorensen, Barbeau, Stoddard, Hunt, Kaphingst, & Wallace, 2005). In addition, in that many employed individuals are parents, there are many potential synergistic interactions between worksite policies and programs and obesity prevention initiatives in home settings. For example, flexible work hours and telecommuting may decrease automobile commuting time, permitting additional discretionary time for active family leisure activities and food acquisition and preparation for family meals. Perhaps most compelling from an economic perspective, the obesity epidemic has a substantive impact on employers in terms of rising health care costs and productivity losses. Certain industries have additional impetus to invest in the development of effective obesity prevention models, as rising obesity levels in the general public beyond their employee population affect their profitability, e.g., airlines and managed care organizations.

Employers show increasing evidence of receptivity to and utilization of structural approaches to obesity prevention that is, approaches that alter the worksite environment rather than the more traditional approaches that focus solely on individuals (Zernike, 2003). For example, in a recent survey, 75% of business leaders said they would support making healthy foods available at worksite cafeterias, in vending machines and at company meetings (Backman, Carman, & Aldana, 2004). However, studies to formally evaluate such strategies that endeavor to change the organizational fabric of the workplace, particularly those incorporating physical activity into organizational routine, are still relatively few in number.

The purpose of this chapter is to synthesize current thinking on workplace obesity prevention and control interventions, including promising strategies from organizational and policy reports appearing outside of refereed scientific publications. We will highlight the strengths and weaknesses of current approaches and their evaluation, as well as gaps in our knowledge base. We will then identify future directions in policy and programmatic interventions, with an emphasis on those aimed at preventing weight gain rather than those focusing on weight loss (Hill, Thompson, & Wyatt, 2005).

Rationale

Workforce Characteristics

Obesity prevalence rates and corresponding trends vary substantially across occupational groups, though they are rising in all occupational groups— the average annual change increased from +0.6% between 1986 and 1996 to +1.0% between 1997 and 2002 (Caban, Lee, Fleming, Gomez-Marin, LeBlanc, & Pitman, 2005). The highest rates in men have been found among public administrators and officials, motor vehicle operators, and police and fire fighters, while among women, rates were highest in motor vehicle operators, and health service and other protective service personnel (Caban et al., 2005) Consistent with national population averages, obesity rates are higher for female workers than for males within most occupations, and black women workers have the highest obesity prevalence of any ethnicity-gender group (Caban et al., 2005).

The armed services present a special case—the obesity epidemic has reduced the pool of available recruits, and a high percentage of the individuals exceeding military weight-for-height standards at the time of entry into the service leave the military before completing their term of enlistment (Institute of Medicine (U.S.), 2004). People of ethnic minority and lower socioeconomic status are overrepresented in the military, and its structure provides an excellent opportunity for environmental and policy-related interventions.

Economic Consequences

The societal costs of obesity are covered in Chapter 4. The economic consequences of obesity and sedentary lifestyle for employers, business and government are staggering, both in health care costs incurred and in lost productivity, and are estimated to rival those of tobacco (Colditz & Mariani, 2000; Finkelstein E.A., Fiebelkorn, & Wang, 2003; Sturm, 2002; Thompson, Edelsberg, Kinsey, & Oster, 1998). Medical expenditures for obese adults are 36% higher than for normal weight adults (Sturm, 2002). A recent analysis has evaluated the high cost of obesity in the workplace, including an assessment of both increased medical expenditures and the value associated with increased absenteeism (Finkelstein E. A., Fiebelkorn, & Wang, 2004; Wang, McDonald, Champagne, & Edington, 2004). Wang et al. (Wang et al., 2004) demonstrated a $250 savings in health care costs for physically active vs. sedentary employees overall, and $450 in savings among active vs. sedentary obese workers. Expenditures related to overweight, obesity and low levels of physical activity based on NHIS prevalence data were estimated to be 27% of the total costs of health care for the United States (Anderson, Martinson, Crain, Pronk, Whitebird, O'Connor, & Fine, 2005). Disability rates among U.S. residents 30–50 years of age have also increased dramatically during the past two decades, largely linked to increased obesity rates (Lakdawalla, Bhattacharya, & Goldman, 2004). Short-term disability claims attributed to obesity have increased by a factor of 10 during the past decade, costing employers more than $8700 per employee per annum (UnumProvident Corporation, 2006). In fact, Medicare data suggest that obese 70 year olds will spend 40% more time disabled than their normal weight counterparts (Lakdawalla, Goldman, & Shang, 2005).

Limitations of Individually-focused Approaches

Worksite interventions have rarely reached their full potential for employee health improvement. Most have disproportionately engaged younger, more highly educated, non-Hispanic whites in large private corporate settings (Dishman, Oldenburg, O'Neal, & Shephard, 1998; Emmons K. M., Linnan, Abrams, & Lovell, 1996; Goetzel, Ozminkowski, Bruno, Rutter, Isaac, & Wang, 2002; Ozminkowski, Ling, Goetzel, Bruno, Rutter, Isaac, & Wang, 2002). In reviews of the more rigorously constructed studies (involving acceptable levels of study retention, recruitment across job categories/statuses, long-term follow-up), observed effect sizes have been small at best (Dishman et al., 1998; Shephard, 1992) probably because the voluntary nature of these interventions engages primarily the more motivated and fit, usually only 5–15% of the workforce (Glanz & Kristal, 2002). The focus of these interventions has mostly been on individual-level change. Even when the social environment is targeted, e.g., cultivating social support for physical activity by establishing walking groups or conducting exercise classes, it is usually during non-paid employee discretionary time.

As scientific understanding of behavior change has evolved, particularly in culturally diverse organizational settings, there has been a growing preference for environmental modification ("push") strategies that engage most or all staff, including those at early stages in the behavior change continuum, rather than relying exclusively on strategies primarily engaging motivated or high risk volunteers "ready to change" or already lean/fit ("pull"). Workplace obesity prevention and control intervention studies targeting environmental and policy change represent a relatively new and burgeoning area of inquiry. In a recent review, Matson-Koffman and colleagues (Matson-Koffman, Brownstein, Neiner, & Greaney, 2005) found 10 such studies published before 1990, but 23 published since. Only 12 of the 33 included a focus on physical activity. Two older studies targeting organizational practice/policy change and resulting environmental influences demonstrated more favorable outcomes than most worksite interventions (Blair, Piserchia, Wilbur, & Crowder, 1986; Linenger, Chesson, & Nice, 1991).

Definitions and Conceptual Framework

As companies are increasingly interested in the application of worksite health promotion programs for their employees, it is also becoming increasingly important to describe issues and factors that are central to an effective program design and implementation approach. First of all, when considering implementation of worksite-based programs designed to address obesity, it is important to recognize that not all worksites are alike. Large, self-insured corporations may have strong incentives to address the obesity issue, as those companies bear the financial risk related to the excess cost and health burden of unhealthy weight. For example, the Institute on the Cost and Health Effects of Obesity was established by the National Business Group on Health with the explicit goal of addressing obesity at the worksite. This coalition of 175 large employers provides health care benefits to approximately 40 million people. Yet, most people in the United States are employed by much smaller companies. The vast majority of these smaller companies are not self-insured (hence do not assume the financial risk for the health care insurance of their covered workers) and therefore the incentives for the small employer group to address obesity at the worksite will be different—likely much more related to an attempt to boost productivity (Hemp, 2004; Pronk N. P., Martinson, Kessler, Beck, Simon, & Wang, 2004; Riedel, Lynch, Baase, Hymel, & Peterson, 2001). Besides company size, other differences between worksites include such factors as single- or multiple-locations, on-site or remote-programming options, a workforce that is mobile (sales travel, service workers in rural areas, metro transit workers, etc.) as opposed to relatively stationary (administrators, teachers, etc.), union or non-union representation among employees, and the diversity and mix of the employee population in terms of gender, race and ethnicity, education, income and other sociodemographic characteristics. All of these factors are elements of a thorough description of the company profile and are important to understand and take into account when considering the implementation of programs.

Other factors to consider are related to the internal company processes for program implementation. These factors address such issues as the recognition of the company culture in addressing obesity, the inclusion of employees in designing and implementing the program (for example through the creation of employee advisory committees), the level at which programs are implemented (for example, company-wide policies that affect all employees, stage of readiness-to-change specific program options for those who want to participate, on-site fitness center access for those who work at company headquarters versus fitness club fee waivers for those who do not work at the headquarter location, programs entirely paid for by the company versus options that are partially subsidized or entirely paid for by the employee, etc.), and issues dealing with the protection of employee privacy. The employee privacy issue is particularly important and guidelines outlined by the Health Insurance Portability and Accountability Act (HIPAA) should be followed. Safeguards must be put in place to protect individual employee data, and the employees themselves need to be fully informed about the use of their information as they become active participants in these programs.

Adapting the logic frameworks used by the Task Force on Community Preventive Services to assess research evidence on a range of public health interventions in communities, workplaces and schools ("Recommendations to increase physical activity in communities", 2002) we can categorize obesity interventions according to the determinants of health addressed—informational, behavioral/social and environmental (see Table 15.1). These categories correspond closely to the levels of impact—awareness, behavior change and supportive environments—described by O'Donnell, 1986 (O'Donnell, 1986). Combining this with the two topical areas of obesity interventions, physical

Table 15.1 Examples of workplace obesity intervention approaches categorized by topical focus and determinants addressed.

Determinants addressed	Topical focus			
	Physical activity only	Nutrition only	Combined (i.e. nutrition + physical activity)	Indirect (i.e. other than nutrition and physical activity)
Information	*Didactic instruction on the benefits of physical activity	*Didactic instruction on good nutritional practices	*Health Risk (see left)	Appraisal (HRA)
Behavior management skills and social support	*Walking groups *Weight management & monitoring support groups	*Meal planning classes *Weight management & monitoring support groups	(see left)	*Counseling following HRA
Physical and organizational environmental	*Physical activity breaks on paid time *Restricted elevator access	*Healthier foods in vending machines *Healthier refreshments at work functions	(see left)	*Workplace health committees

activity and nutrition, we have a useful way of differentiating various types of workplace interventions used to address obesity.

A number of behavior change theories are embedded in the worksite wellness literature. Social marketing principles, communications theory, stages of change models and many others have been applied to this setting. We have chosen to highlight two, social cognitive and diffusion of innovations theories, as most relevant to environmental and policy intervention in diverse worker populations.

Social Cognitive Theory (SCT)

As noted in Chapter 17, SCT posits, among other assertions, that learning occurs through observation and imitation of role models, individuals perceived as worthy of emulation (Bandura, 1986). A key premise of the theory is that certain sociodemographic similarities exist between individuals and their role model choices, e.g., ethnic, SES and gender congruence. Another central construct is self-efficacy or self-perceived ability to accomplish certain desired outcomes. Observation of sociodemographically similar others carrying out a desired behavior has been shown to increase the self-efficacy of the observer. Application of these concepts to interventions with adult populations using such tools as culturally targeted videos has been effective in other areas of health promotion (Yancey, Tanjasiri, Klein, & Tunder, 1995; Yancey & Walden, 1994). Worksites are ideal settings because they permit a ready means of delivering targeted messages and a "micro-environment" or community, both physically and socioculturally, that may be more malleable by one or a few leaders and permit more rapid change than does the broader societal milieu. Experiential learning ("enactive mastery" in SCT) such as recognizing and tasting healthier foods, sampling moderate intensity aerobic dance with a group of co-workers, and participating in a walking meeting, as well as the aforementioned social/cultural norm change via leadership and role modeling ("vicarious experience" in SCT) by sociodemographically similar and/or high status individuals within the hierarchy are also critical elements of effective weight-related lifestyle intervention supported by SCT.

Diffusion of Innovations; Organizational Institutionalization

Most worksite wellness interventions have been individually-targeted, using organizations mainly as staging venues for intervention delivery, rather than directed at organizational systems themselves. Consequently, critical process features of these strategies and innovations have not been evaluated from an organizational dynamics perspective, e.g., institutionalization and diffusion processes (Glasgow, Vogt, & Boles, 1999; Rogers, 2003; Steckler & Goodman, 1989; Steckler, Goodman, McLeroy, Davis, & Koch, 1992). As outlined in Chapter 12, the diffusion of health behavior change innovations has been described as having five phases (Oldenburg, Sallis, French, & Owen, 1999). The first phase is *innovation development* in which the program is developed and evaluated. The second phase is *dissemination* in which it is communicated widely so the effective program is available for adoption. The third phase is *adoption*, which can be defined as purchasing materials or participating in training. The fourth phase is *implementation* in which users put the program into practice, and fidelity to the procedures used in the original research phase needs to be considered. The final phase is *maintenance*, or the sustained use of the innovation by adopters. In this phase, both the quantity (e.g., proportion of people in a given sector using the program regularly) and quality of implementation (e.g., adherence to the program) need to be considered.

A key implication of diffusion of innovations theory is that mediated information sources (media-driven vs. interpersonal communications) are most important in the early stages of organizational adoption, e.g., awareness and interest building (Glanz & Kristal, 2002; Rogers, 2003). For example, an Australian study utilized telemarketing to facilitate adoption of health promotion initiatives via provision of tool kits, pamphlets and other mediated informational resources and services (Daly, Licata, Gillham, & Wiggers, 2005). Investigators found significant increases in uptake after four years for seven of the eight initiatives selected (only one—alcohol control, however, was even tangentially related to obesity control). Interpersonal communication rises in importance during the active evaluation and trial phases. Thus, consistent with SCT, early implementation activities should create an environment conducive to change and promulgate strategies through successful examples.

Organizational change theory is central to the optimal design of these interventions. Critical features of an innovation can accelerate or hinder the diffusion process (Rogers, 2003) as reflected in the formative evaluation data presented in Box 15.1. From a diffusion process perspective, organizational wellness change strategies with "face validity" have relative advantage (potential health and productivity benefits) compared to current practice. They can generally be implemented on a limited basis (trialability). Furthermore, as more research is conducted, results become known and visible to increasing numbers of work units or organizations (observability)

Box 15.1. Nutrition program dissemination in worksite cafeterias in the Netherlands

A study was undertaken to identify factors facilitating or deterring planned dissemination of a multi-level nutrition intervention (education, labeling, and food supply modification) to increase fruit and vegetable consumption and reduce fat intake in point-of-choice settings, including worksite cafeterias. Twelve key informant interviews were conducted with representatives from companies selected to include those with majority white collar and majority blue collar workforces. Catering or food service managers were queried to assess characteristics of their organizations and these decision makers' attitudes toward nutrition education in general and toward specific program attributes. Unobtrusiveness, minimal time and effort demands on cafeteria personnel and staff consumers, competitive pricing of healthy foods and avoidance of introducing delays in food purchasing at the counter were among the most frequently cited program requirements. Relative advantages mentioned included positive influence on corporate image, increased customer satisfaction and improvements in employee well-being. Potential difficulties included program cost, decreased sales of profitable unhealthy products, the limited shelf life of low-fat products, waste (left-over stock if demand does not match supply), and concerns about restriction of choice and unwanted peer pressure to eat more healthfully(Steenhuis, Van Assema, & Glanz, 2001).

(Yancey, Miles, & Jordan, 1999). Overall, these strategies have the potential to encompass features that favorably influence the speed and extent of the diffusion process.

Social norm change in workplaces may build a foundation for similar changes in the other settings in which these workers study, worship, live, create, advocate and play. Modification of the culture, physical environment and staff behavior within health and social services organizations may also, secondarily, influence client behavior, through changes in priorities in their providers' decision-making, and through physical (e.g., vending machine selections) and social (conformity with social norms, e.g., if others are taking the stairs) environmental changes making healthy choices more available, affordable, accessible and unavoidable. In turn, because these staff members belong to other organizations with similar sociodemographic compositions, these changes may ripple throughout the community. This "spill-over" is even more likely in this area of health promotion, nutrition and physical activity, in which all individuals participate and in which nearly all are touched, either personally or socially, by the highly prevalent obesity epidemic. Many workers, especially those in the human services sector, are not only decision-makers, gatekeepers, role models and change agents for their clients and patients, but also within their own families and social circles. Their organizational missions may produce even greater personal investment in and commitment to creating lasting change. Local government workplaces in urban areas are especially ripe for intervention because they have large (often the largest employers in a community), stable and ethnically diverse workforces, and internal opportunities, infrastructure and resources for changing organizational practices and institutionalizing those changes.

Methodological Issues

Recent studies have increasingly begun to intervene at the organizational level and in more ethnically, socio-economically diverse worksites (Golaszewski & Fisher, 2002; Hunt, Stoddard, Barbeau, Goldman, Wallace, Gutheil, & Sorensen, 2003; Sorensen, Hunt, & Morris, 1990). Methodological quality continues to be an issue, as few studies employ rigorous, randomized controlled designs or recruit truly representative samples of employees. Effect sizes in the most rigorous are generally quite small (Glanz & Kristal, 2002; Marcus, Williams, Dubbert, Sallis, King, Yancey, Franklin, Buchner, Daniels, & Claytor, 2006). As in earlier efforts, nutritional intervention is more common and more fully integrated into workplace routine than is physical activity. This is of particular concern to effective obesity intervention, since physical activity-related programmatic and policy changes generally engender less opposition and resistance than food restriction and regulation (Maibach, 2003). In addition, while the role of nutrition in weight control is well-established, the essential role of physical activity in the prevention of weight gain is increasingly evident but operationally underdeveloped (Donnelly, 2005; Hill & Wyatt, 2005; Jeffery & Utter, 2003; Kimm, Glynn, Obarzanek, Kriska, Daniels, Barton, & Liu, 2005; Mummery, Schofield, Steele, Eakin, & Brown, 2005; Sternfeld, Wang, Quesenberry, Abrams, Everson-Rose, Greendale, Matthews, Torrens, & Sowers, 2004) and is given particular emphasis in this chapter. In fact, the increasing prevalence of overweight may reflect the fact that the majority of the population fails to achieve some threshold level of regular physical activity below which it is difficult for most people to achieve energy balance at a desirable body weight (Hill et al., 2005). Clearly, modest, incremental improvements in both physical activity and eating patterns, sustained over time, will be necessary to stem this epidemic.

Many employers, particularly in the private commercial and public sectors, have begun to implement policies providing economic incentives to employees for healthy weight-related lifestyle adoption/maintenance. Such policies include insurance premium discounts, free/discounted on-site preventive health care services such as nutrition counseling, subsidies for fitness activities and club memberships, disease management benefits, and wellness program reimbursements. However, evaluation studies are rarely conducted, and negligibly few of these reports reach the peer-reviewed literature. Essentially, studies of primary obesity prevention through worksite-based environmental change are lacking (Katz, O'Connell, Yeh, Nawaz, Njike, Anderson, Cory, & Dietz, 2005). At any rate, economic incentives alone, as earlier underscored, are unlikely to result in sustainable behavior change (Yancey, Lewis, Guinyard, Sloane, Nascimento, Galloway-Gilliam, Diamant, & McCarthy, 2006). Thus, insights will be gleaned from the existing literature examining various weight-related lifestyle outcomes.

Insights from Environmental and Policy Initiatives and Research

Overall Evidence Base for System-level Obesity Prevention and Control in the Workplace

Physical Activity

The notion that synergy will occur when "supply" (physical environmental access and facilitation) meets "demand" (individual motivation and skills/interests; sociocultural environmental instigation and support) is implicit in multi-level change models. The importance of sociocultural environmental "demand creation" in physical activity promotion, however, has been even less appreciated than that of physical environmental change (Emmons K.M., 2000; Giles-Corti & Donovan, 2002; McKeever, Faddis, Koroloff, & Henn, 2004; Peltomaki, Johansson, Ahrens, Sala, Wesseling, Brenes, Font, Husman, Janer, Kallas-Tarpila, Kogevinas, Loponen, Sole, Tempel, Vasama-Neuvonen, & Partanen, 2003; Stahl, Rutten, Nutbeam, Bauman, Kannas, Abel, Luschen, Rodriquez, Vinck, & van der Zee, 2001) and the workplace is a primary venue for promulgation of sociocultural norm changes supporting adoption and maintenance of active lifestyles (Linnan, LaMontagne, Stoddard, Emmons, & Sorensen, 2005; Sorensen, Linnan, & Hunt, 2004). The work of Fox and colleagues (Fox, Rejeski, & Gauvin, 2000) suggests the importance of supportive group dynamics on PA enjoyment and probability of future participation. Several investigators have shown that visible commitment of organizational leaders on-site, e.g., as manifested in role modeling by participation in group physical activities, is associated with increasing and institutionalizing PA among employees in government agencies and community-based organizations (Crawford, Gosliner, Strode, Samuels, Burnett, Craypo, & Yancey, 2004; Englberger, 1999; Hammond, Leonard, & Fridinger, 2000; Yancey, Jordan, Bradford, Voas, Eller, Buzzard, Welch, & McCarthy, 2003; Yancey, Lewis, Sloane, Guinyard, Diamant, Nascimento, & McCarthy, 2004a; Yancey et al., 1999).

The more favorable physical activity outcomes have occurred in studies targeting organizational practices and policies, and sociocultural and physical environmental characteristics. Comprehensive approaches melding individual-level approaches (counseling, group health education) with physical environmental access (on-site fitness facilities, shower and changing rooms, accessible stairways) have been shown to be more effective in increasing levels of self-reported exercise than single-component interventions (Matson-Koffman et al., 2005). Features associated with effectiveness and/or sustainability in individual-level intervention may be incorporated, i.e. including resistance training and lifestyle PA in addition to aerobic exercise, encouraging peer group leadership, employing incentives, and utilizing exercise prescriptions (Dishman et al., 1998). Health education and health risk appraisal interventions were associated with smaller effect sizes (Dishman et al., 1998). In particular, inexpensive prompts encouraging stair use, combined with physical improvements to stairwells, have been demonstrated to increase physical activity levels (self-reported and observed) at worksites at least in the short term; little long-term follow-up data, however, are available (Coleman & Gonzalez, 2001; Hammond et al., 2000; Titze, Martin, Seiler, & Marti, 2001).

Emerging models include, for example, demonstration of increased efficacy and sustainability of a peer-led vs. professionally-led PA intervention with factory blue collar workers delivered during regularly-scheduled safety meetings (Elbel, Aldana, Bloswick, & Lyon, 2003), of extended work capacity of convalescent home aides by providing 20-minute exercise sessions three times weekly during paid time (Pohjonen & Ranta, 2001) (in which injury prevention complements health promotion) (Sorensen et al., 2005), and of increased physical activity levels overall with installation of slowed hydraulic or skip-stop elevators and distant parking lots in worksites (expanding the concept of the built environment to include indoor milieus) (Naik, 2005; Nicoll, 2007; Zernike, 2003).

Elbel and colleagues (Elbel et al., 2003) recommended incorporating a performance or skills practice component in the design of workplace lifestyle PA promotion interventions to increase their effectiveness, a component which employer liability concerns had precluded their implementing. Yancey et al. (Yancey, McCarthy, Taylor, Merlo, Gewa, Weber, & Fielding, 2004b) have demonstrated the feasibility of incorporating such an experiential intervention, 10-minute exercise breaks, into the workday among public health department staff in Los Angeles County. More than 90% of workers elected to participate in these breaks during a randomized, controlled trial evaluating these breaks conducted in staff meetings and training seminars. Health-related motivational benefits were apparent in this study, in that *sedentary* intervention participants rated their health or fitness status more realistically (poorly) than did those in control condition meetings with only the usual phone or restroom breaks (Yancey et al., 2004b). Similarly, in a group-randomized, controlled, pre-test/post-test, intervention trial wedding injury prevention and health promotion, employees who assembled computer boards performed a set of 23 flexibility and strength exercises, designed to prevent lower back and carpal tunnel injury, for 10 minutes each day on company time under supervision (Pronk S. J., Pronk, Sisco, Ingalls, & Ochoa, 1995). Daily employee participation rates were 97–100%. After 6 months of program implementation, significant improvements were observed in wrist flexion, wrist extension, low-back flexibility, fatigue, anger, and mood state. Maine sporting goods manufacturer L. L. Bean incorporates three formalized 5-minute mandatory stretch breaks each day led by trained co-workers (California Nutrition Network & California Department of Health Service, 2004). Productivity gains have been shown to offset the time devoted to stretching by 100%; reduced injuries and sick days have also been reported.

Nutrition

Policy and environmental interventions to promote healthy eating in the workplace are further developed and better studied than those for promoting physical activity, though still much less common than the more clinical or individually-targeted behavioral approaches. Three general types of these intervention strategies have been implemented, influencing: food access (increased nutritional value of available foods, healthy catering policies); nutritional information delivery (food labeling, point-of-choice information); and economic strategies (incentives, pricing manipulation) (Glanz & Kristal, 2002).

A review by Matson-Koffman and colleagues (Matson-Koffman et al., 2005) revealed that a number of these approaches were effective in improving such dietary behaviors as fruit and vegetable, dairy, fat, fiber, and total energy intake, including: point-of-purchase labeling of healthier food selections in cafeterias and vending machines; food service preparation modification to decrease fat and sodium, and to incorporate more fruits and vegetables; price reduction on healthier foods; expanded healthy food options; coupon distribution; and creating and reinforcing healthy eating-friendly social norms (see Box 15.2 for example). Complementary educational intervention components, e.g., media, have generally increased intervention effectiveness. Support from management is crucial, both for facilitating implementation of these changes, and for building social support for adoption of healthier eating patterns.

Many environmental nutrition interventions involve changes in workplace vending machines and cafeterias. These interventions may be of limited generalizability since many worksites, especially smaller worksites, do not have on-site food sales (see Box 15.3 for example). Cafeterias and mobile food vendors may also be managed by outside contractors over whom the employer has limited power to determine food choices. There are, however other means through which worksites can encourage consumption of healthier foods. For example, price reductions of 10%, 25%, and 50% of low-fat snacks sold in vending machines in worksites in Minnesota produced relative sales increases of 9%, 39%, and 93% of these foods, respectively (French, Jeffery, Story, Breitlow, Baxter, Hannan, & Snyder, 2001). Employers may also partner with local farmers, produce delivery services and farmers' markets to offer fresh produce during lunch breaks or immediately after working hours for employees to purchase in the immediate after-work hours. This could be especially

---

Box 15.2. Larger worksites with on-site food service:
"Seattle 5 A Day Worksite Program"

Changing the nutrition environment at the workplace was a key component of the Seattle 5 A Day Worksite Program (Beresford, Thompson, Feng, Christianson, McLerran, & Patrick, 2001). The study involved 28 worksites, each with 250 to 2000 workers, with food-serving cafeterias in the Seattle metropolitan area. A range of informational, social support and environmental changes were used to improve nutritional practices of employees at the 14 intervention sites. Worksite cafeteria changes included putting up point-of-purchase displays and signs identifying healthy food choices, and providing incentives for employees eating more fruits and vegetables. These were coupled with activities such as cookbooks for children and healthy food preparation demonstrations to encourage healthier eating practices at home. The study succeeded in increasing the consumption of fresh fruit and vegetables by 0.3 servings per day but the generalizability of this study might be limited by the large size of the worksites and the relatively high educational levels of employees at these sites.

> **Box 15.3.** Smaller worksites with limited or no on-site
> food service: "Treatwell 5-A-Day Study" and
> "Healthy Directions—Small Business Study."
>
> Changing the workplace food environment at worksites has been shown to
> be a part of successful efforts to improve eating patterns even at smaller
> worksites with limited or no on-site food service. Twenty of the 22 com-
> munity health centers participating in the Treatwell 5-A-Day Study in
> Massachusetts had less than 120 employees (Sorensen, Stoddard, Peterson,
> Cohen, Hunt, Stein, Palombo, & Lederman, 1999). The Healthy
> Directions—Small Business Study" involved 26 worksites, each with 50
> to 150 employees (Sorensen et al., 2005). Complementing individual/
> interpersonal interventions, both these studies included environmental and
> organizational changes in the nutrition environment. Without cafeterias,
> these changes were limited to such approaches as modifying policies
> governing the types of foods served at meetings and on special occasions,
> and offering healthier food choices in vending machines. The changes may
> have been minor, but in conjunction with other strategies, including educa-
> tion and support for healthier eating at home, both interventions succeeded
> in improving dietary quality at the intervention sites.

advantageous to workers living in neighborhoods with limited availability of
fresh produce (Algert, Agrawal, & Lewis, 2006).

Weight Management

Most worksite weight management involves individual-level behavioral or clinical intervention. Environmental and policy intervention strategies for weight
management in the workplace generally fall into two categories: (1) financial
incentives for weight loss or maintenance, such as payroll deductions, returns of
monetary deposits, and competitions; and (2) comprehensive health promotion
intervention (Kaplan, Brinkman-Kaplan, & Framer, 2002). The latter will be
discussed in the following section.

Competitions have emerged as among the most promising worksite strategy, though little long-term follow-up data are available. Evidence suggests
that team-based competitions—cooperative efforts among employees making changes—are more effective than individuals competing against each
other (Kaplan et al., 2002). No evaluation data exist on repeat competitions,
i.e. for those who may benefit from additional losses beyond the standard
12-week period. Data on competitions focused on such behavior changes as
physical activity also have yet to be published. For example, "pedometer-
mediated" step competitions are relatively new, and have generally been
evaluated only in the context of comprehensive wellness programs.
Competitions have not been shown to be effective for long-term maintenance
of weight loss.

Deposits/payroll deductions have mainly been used to improve participation and decrease attrition in behavioral or clinical programs. Even without a
formal treatment program, however, incentive participants doubled the

amounts of weight lost and weight losses maintained of control participants (Kaplan et al., 2002).

Combined/Comprehensive Wellness Policy/Programmatic Efforts

Just as effective weight control strategies at the individual level combine healthy eating and physical activity, so, too, can programs at the organizational level be more effective when they promote multiple aspects of wellness. For example, *Health Works for Women*, one of few studies aimed at rural female blue collar workers, produced long-term increases in fruit and vegetable consumption and participation in stretching and flexibility exercises, along with short-term decreases in dietary fat intake with a lay health worker/tailored media intervention (Campbell, Tessaro, DeVellis, Benedict, Kelsey, Belton, & Sanhueza, 2002). Such comprehensive approaches to wellness promotion, offer several advantages over programs that focus on only one aspect. First, they appeal to a broader cross-section of the workforce. Not all workers are interested in exercise or healthier eating. Some may be more interested in stress reduction. A program to reduce stress offers an excellent opportunity to introduce participants to various exercises that reduce stress and increase physical activity. Second, they offer greater opportunities for building participants' sense of self-efficacy for and interest in practicing health-promoting behaviors (changes that come more easily may bolster resolve to persist with others). Third, some health promoting behaviors are mutually reinforcing on a physiological level—practicing one predisposes one to greater success at the other. This effect can be seen in the observed relation between healthy eating and physical activity, as evidenced by exercisers' greater interest in water-dense foods with lower caloric density and beverages of lesser sweetness, compared to non-exercisers, and the relative appetite suppressant effect of exercise (Passe, Horn, & Murray, 2000; Westerterp-Plantenga, Verwegen, Ijedema, Wijckmans, & Saris, 1997). A particularly promising combined approach is integrating injury prevention/occupational safety with health promotion programming (Seabury, Lakdawalla, & Reville, 2005; Sorensen, Stoddard, LaMontagne, Emmons, Hunt, Youngstrom, McLellan, & Christiani, 2002).

Interface with Obesity Prevention Intervention Outside the Workplace

Many of the most successful examples of large-scale health promotion campaigns have employed multi-pronged strategies that targeted multiple sectors and industries. These diverse campaigns, ranging from cardiovascular disease prevention in Finland (Puska, Nissinen, Tuomilehto, Salonen, Koskela, McAlister, Kottke, Maccoby, & Farquhar, 1985) and tobacco control in California (Pierce, White, & Gilpin, 2005) to adolescent pregnancy prevention in South Carolina (Vincent, Clearie, & Schluchter, 1987) to physical activity promotion in Brazil (Matsudo, Matsudo, Araujo, Andrade, Andrade, de Oliveira, & Braggion, 2003), all involved activities in a wide variety of settings, including schools, community organizations, faith communities, public health centers, and workplaces. Following on principles from socio-ecological frameworks (Breslow, 2001; Stokols, Grzywacz, McMahan, & Phillips, 2003), it is likely that successful obesity prevention efforts will combine workplace intervention with other community and policy efforts.

Addressing change in sectors normally outside the purview of public health and medicine is particularly important for efforts to promote increased physical activity and healthier eating, since these behaviors are so deeply intertwined in the activities of daily living. Promoting recreational physical activity, e.g., working with public recreations and parks agency efforts to address inequities in distribution and quality of these spaces and facilities, is important. However, widespread, sustained increases in physical activity levels will require changes in how we commute, shop and work. One means of encouraging such changes is through "Smart Growth" urban planning initiatives, which endeavor to decrease the suburban sprawl associated with ease of access for private transportation, and increase mixed use urban development associated with "walkability"/"bikeability" (Ewing, Schmid, Killingsworth, Zlot, & Raudenbush, 2003) (see Chapter 8). Likewise, widespread, sustained changes in eating practices will require more than public health messages about what constitutes healthy eating patterns. Changes will need to be made in how foods are marketed and distributed in all of the different settings in which people buy, consume and learn about food (see Chapter 9).

For both the energy intake and expenditure sides of the energy balance equation, workplaces control essential elements of the "mosaic" of complementary and synergistic environmental changes necessary to combat obesity. In addition, workplaces can offer a venue for introducing innovative environmental changes before they are disseminated in the wider community, similar to the role played by schools which have been at the forefront of efforts to limit unhealthy foods and beverages in vending machines and introducing farm-to-school programs to increase the availability and affordability of fresh fruit and vegetables. (And schools are workplaces in themselves.) For example, one important dissemination strategy is tailoring messages to workers as parents, as has been done in other areas of health promotion (e.g., Eastman, Corona, Ryan, Warsofsky, & Schuster, 2005).

Interface with Interventions Targeting other Public Health Issues

Besides building synergy in multiple sectors towards a single public health goal, obesity prevention and control efforts can also gain momentum by linking with other health and community promotion efforts. For instance, active commuting and stair use also serve to conserve energy and reduce air pollution. Similarly, efforts to increase the availability of retail outlets selling fresh fruits and vegetables or promote accessibility of school facilities for recreation during after school hours may be framed as environmental justice or economic development issues. Local municipalities conducting food safety inspections in restaurants may find ways to join these efforts with those encouraging restaurants to offer more healthy eating options. Joint employer/employee health and safety committees, whose primary mission is injury prevention, can identify and promote opportunities for increasing physical activity in the workforce.

This "piggybacking" of health promotion efforts has several advantages. First, it can make more efficient use of limited resources. Second, when other health promotion efforts are already in place, such as workplace safety programs, obesity control efforts can draw on the institutional support of these programs. Third, this approach can leverage support from other constituencies as partners in obesity control who would not be among the early adopters of healthy eating/active living innovations. The chief drawback of this approach, particularly in workplaces, is that individuals or groups might see it as an unwanted expansion of or infringement on their current responsibilities. Depending upon site-specific considerations, some of these partnerships may make sense, while others may not.

Evidence Base for Workplace Obesity Prevention and Control Intervention in Ethnic Minority and/or Low-income Populations

Sociocultural and physical environmental interventions that rely less on individual motivation and cultural values prioritizing active leisure pursuits, primarily organizational policy or practice changes incentivizing physical activity, should be implemented and rigorously evaluated in communities of color. Physical environmental intervention is certainly indicated in predominantly African-American and Latino communities and lower income communities, with their few recreational facilities and opportunities (Estabrooks, Lee, & Gyurcsik, 2003; Powell, Slater, & Chaloupka, 2004). Physical structural changes are costly and time-consuming, however, and tend to assume lower priority in low-resource surrounds with so many pressing needs (Kumanyika S. & Grier, 2006; Kumanyika S. K., 2001). In addition, underserved communities experience more substantial cultural and economic barriers to physical activity participation (Galbally, 1997; Kumanyika S., 2002; Yancey, Ory, & Davis, 2006). For instance, among African-American girls and women, arduous hair maintenance is a disincentive to perspire (Katz et al., 2005; Kumanyika S., 2002; Leslie, Yancey, McCarthy, Albert, Wert, Miles, & James, 1999) and the higher levels of perceived exertion associated with their higher rates of obesity may discourage more vigorous activity, e.g., stair-climbing, or longer exercise bouts (Kumanyika, S., 2002; Whitt, DuBose, Ainsworth, & Tudor-Locke, 2004). Perhaps as a result, many environmental interventions, as implemented, have been less effective or ineffective in ethnically or socio-economically marginalized population segments, e.g., the failure of stair prompts to increase stair-climbing among the subset of African Americans in an intervention successful among whites in a suburban Baltimore mall (Andersen, Franckowiak, Snyder, Bartlett, & Fontaine, 1998) or do not include sufficiently large samples of these populations to present sub-group analyses. Thus, immediate attention must be given to the socio-cultural environment to address these barriers ("demand generation"), complementing efforts to change the physical environment ("supply creation").

Workplace approaches, particularly *push* strategies that make physical activity and healthy food choices hard to avoid (e.g., exercise breaks on non-discretionary time, healthier refreshments served in meetings and at events, walking meetings, vending restrictions, elevator and nearby parking restrictions) are especially promising in ethnic minority and lower-income communities. They increase the likelihood of delivering substantial returns on investment to employers (and to local governments, in which public health agencies develop and implement such efforts, and which bear many of the costs of obesity and sedentariness) by engaging the more sedentary and overweight population segments less successfully reached by traditional worksite programs.

They also obviate such barriers as unsafe and unappealing outdoor surroundings, lack of access to high-quality produce and recreational facilities, and copious perspiration during longer bouts of strenuous exercise. Some, in fact, build upon such cultural assets as the normative nature of movement to music throughout adulthood, cultural salience of many plant-based foods (e.g., collard greens, yams, corn, peppers and various legumes), and collectivist versus individualist values (Day, 2006; Yancey et al., 2006).

The aforementioned strategy, that of incorporating brief structured exercise bouts into organizational routine in churches (Wilcox, Laken, Anderson, Bopp, Bryant, Gethers, Jordan, McClorin, O'Rourke, Parrott, Swinton, & Yancey, In press 2006) public agency worksites (Crawford et al., 2004; Yancey et al., 2004b) community-based organizations (Yancey et al., 2004a) private corporate worksites (Pronk S. J. et al., 1995) and elementary schools (Lloyd, Cook, & Kohl, 2005; Metzler & Williams, 2006; Stewart, Dennison, Kohl, & Doyle, 2004), is exemplary as a case study. Yancey and colleagues (Yancey et al., 2006; Yancey et al., 2004a) have demonstrated substantial organizational receptivity to integrating 10-minute exercise breaks into daily routines (involving staff and clients/members) in community-based health and social services organizations serving Latinos and African Americans in Los Angeles (Yancey et al., 2004b). This approach is culturally salient in communities of color, in which leisure time structural integration of group physical activity is valued (e.g., Englberger, 1999; McKeever et al., 2004) (Englberger, 1999; McKeever et al., 2004), e.g., dancing to music at parties and holiday celebrations is normative behavior, even among middle-aged and older adults, as noted above. Further evidence for the cultural salience of this approach comes from the Mexican Ministry of Health. A similar intervention, consisting of 10- to 15-minute daily mid-day group exercise breaks during work time, was developed and implemented in the foyer of one of the main headquarters buildings among their mostly overweight and obese staff. Significant decreases in systolic blood pressure and waist circumference were observed at one year (Lara, 2004) While most interventions operate psychologically to motivate behavior change, social conformity-influenced exercise participation by sedentary and overweight workers adds physiological synergy to the psychological impetus—enjoyment and enhanced feelings of well-being while engaging in short bouts of physical activity, complemented by a reminder, via more than expected perceived exertion, of being a bit "out of shape." (Ekkekakis, Hall, VanLanduyt, & Petruzzello, 2000; Yancey et al., 2004b). Evidence also suggests that physical activity initiated in the workplace may generalize (and innovations may diffuse (Rogers, 2003)), from one setting or type to another (Sevick, Dunn, Morrow, Marcus, Chen, & Blair, 2000; Yancey, McCarthy, Harrison, Wong, Siegel, & Leslie, 2006).

Obesity Prevention and Control Planning and Evaluation

Assessing Needs and Opportunities

Policy Climate for Workplace Obesity Prevention and Control Intervention
Public sector. State and local governments are employers, as well as providers of governance and public service. City and county governments are often the

largest employers in a given locale, with workforces characterized by considerable ethnic and socioeconomic diversity. Los Angeles County, for example, employs more than 80,000 full-time, permanent employees. Fully 70% are people of color, most, women. More than 60% are 40 years of age or older. About half earn less than $40,000 per year. More than half have 12 or more years of service. Thus, mature age, majority "minority" ethnicity and modest average earnings make this an ideal group for weight-related risk reduction efforts. The average length of service of more than one decade ensures not only adequate exposure time to lifestyle intervention, but also time for the employer to reap the economic benefits of improved health status.

For several reasons, these are critical settings for obesity control/wellness promotion: (a) it is in their organizational self-interest, in this climate of shrinking revenues and expanding costs, because they frequently bear the costs associated with obesity-related disease in their residents, in addition to their own staff; (b) among their staff are a disproportionate number of gate-keepers, opinion leaders, and decision-makers within any community at various levels from grassroots to elected/appointed leadership, particularly among direct providers of human services (Crawford et al., 2004; Sorensen et al., 1990)—in fact, a review of the literature by Dishman and colleagues (Dishman et al., 1998) found greater intervention physical activity outcome effect sizes in public agencies and universities than private corporations; and (c) the logistical structure of the workday is more flexible and accommodating than in many private concerns. The recent distribution of federal obesity control intervention grants by the National Association for Equal Opportunity in Higher Education at historically black colleges and universities reflects growing recognition of the utility of public and university settings for worksite wellness efforts—both staff and students may benefit, the latter with presumably more malleable behaviors and prospects for diffusing strategies as they move into their professional lives because of their relative youth and leadership potential (Walker, 2005).

Many cities and counties have initiated small-scale efforts, although these often lack adequate evaluation (e.g. Yancey et al., 2003). For example, Culver City, CA has initiated an employee-driven program releasing up to 60 minutes per week (20 minutes on each of 3 days/week) of paid time during the workday for wellness activities, primarily walking, and creating signage marking distances around city office buildings to facilitate these activity breaks (personal communication, Culver City Mayor Carol Gross, August 1, 2002).

Private sector. The increasing trend in health care costs is such a threat to business profitability and viability that it ranks as the number one rated issue facing American business today. Obesity is a major concern related to this trend as it drove 27% of the medical cost increases between 1987 and 2001 (Thorpe, Florence, Howard, & Joski, 2004). Furthermore, according to the National Business Group on Health, which represents 240 self-insured employers, health-care premiums for families increased by 100% between 2001 and 2006, with obesity accounting for 25% of this increase.(Institute of Medicine (U.S.), 2006) The total obesity-related costs borne by companies across the U.S. is estimated at $13 billion per year. This amount is the aggregate of obesity related expenses in the areas of health insurance ($8 billion), paid sick leave ($2.4 billion), life insurance ($1.8 billion), and disability insurance

($1 billion) (United States. Dept. of Health and Human Services., 2003). Obesity is associated with 39 million lost work days, 239 million restricted activity days, 90 million bed days, and 63 million physician visits (Wolf & Colditz, 1998). In addition, as earlier noted, many industries representing large proportions of the U.S. GNP have further motivation to address obesity rates in the general public, e.g., decreases in fuel efficiency associated with increases in average passenger weights in the airline industry, or the health care industry's increased capital investments in larger wheelchairs, beds and gurneys, along with productivity losses resulting from increased musculoskeletal injury rates among staff lifting and moving heavy patients. Based on such data that directly relate obesity to the bottom line, identification of opportunities for business to influence obesity are actively sought, warranted and justified.

Cost-related outcomes of obesity may be considered indicators of the direct and indirect impact of obesity on employee health and productivity. Hemp (Hemp, 2004) outlined the various components of the total cost of illness for an employer. Six components including medical and pharmacy were considered direct expenditures through medical care-related costs. The remaining four components, worker's compensation, short-term disability, long-term disability, and absenteeism and presenteeism, represented indirect costs considered the result of reductions in productivity. Obesity has been shown to affect all of those components (Finkelstein E., Fiebelkorn, & Wang, 2005; Hertz, Unger, McDonald, Lustik, & Biddulph-Krentar, 2004; Institute of Medicine (U.S.). Committee to Assess Worksite Preventive Health Program Needs for NASA Employees, 2005; Pronk N. P. et al., 2004). Hence, in addition to the direct impact of health care costs on the bottom line, companies must begin to consider the impact of workers' excess weight on their work performance.

The relationships noted between obesity and health care costs, as well as productivity decrements, recognize the influence of obesity on functioning and performance. Indeed, the effects of obesity make a 30 year-old obese worker comparable to a 50 year old normal-weight worker in terms of their medical care expenses (Sturm, 2002) and work limitations (Hertz et al., 2004)— obesity may be equated to 20 years of aging. This affects small, mid-sized, and large companies alike, though the latter are better equipped to intervene.

Catalyzing change. In order to generate substantial activity around obesity prevention and management in the private sector, it will be crucial to align the interests of the three key stakeholder groups of these programs, namely the employers, the employee, and the health plans. In the public sector, the service provision role adds the residents of the community as another stakeholder.

The issue of who benefits?—and who pays?—is central to this notion of stakeholder alignment. The employers need to be able to clearly identify how they will benefit if they are to make investments in the application of obesity solutions at the worksite, especially in the context of employee turnover and short-term financial program costs. For private sector employers answerable to boards of directors and/or shareholders, this "bottom line" approach is consistent with most business models. For public sectors employers, however, where productivity is harder to measure directly, public dollars directed to "employee benefits" may be politically sensitive, even if management is convinced that substantial return on investment will result. The employee, who enjoys complete portability of the health benefits of program participation (i.e. they experience and keep the health benefit even if they leave the organization), needs to recognize a significant benefit that will exceed the readiness-to-participate threshold and hence be sufficiently persuasive to drive meaningful levels of participation—whether this benefit (or incentive) is financial or not does not matter. Finally, the health plans are stakeholders since they may benefit from healthier members if the interventions are effective, thereby lessening their financial risk exposure when the employer is a fully-insured customer. On the other hand, when the employer is a self-insured customer, identified health plan benefits may include a stronger relationship with the employer customer, a more seamless integration of health programming with insurance benefit products (for example, reduced co-pay or premiums for those who participate in the worksite programs), and a closer connection between worksite-based obesity programs and clinical care—obesity tends to be associated with many diseases and disorders that require regular medical care (e.g., diabetes, hypertension, heart disease, and cancers).

An excellent early step in outlining the benefits for each stakeholder and the approach to take for implementation is the initiation and ongoing maintenance of an open dialogue among these groups. Conducting an employee needs assessment, even a brief survey, may provide a starting point in fostering this communication.

Program/Policy Elements & Cost Considerations

Program design elements may vary widely and may be difficult to prioritize since so many have been utilized and so little data evaluating them, alone or in combination, is available. Many approaches quickly become complex as programs need to consider multiple settings, audiences, behaviors, communication media, and meaningful evaluation and reporting for a variety of customers. However, workplace program design elements are certain to include the identification of the intervention components, the channels through which the program will be implemented, the methods by which the program will be marketed and communicated, the reasons why employees will recognize the benefits of participation (could include the incentives), the methods of evaluating the effectiveness of the initiative, and the financial and budget implications. For example, a workplace obesity initiative may, by design, be multi-component so it will be able to address both prevention and management (treatment). The importance of the program and processes for access may be outlined in company newsletters, table-tents in the cafeteria, e-mail reminders, and memos from the CEO. It may have individual-level coaching and counseling programs for physical activity and healthy eating, presented via a website and online options as well as a phone-based option in order to meet employee preferences and learning styles. In addition, it may implement several organizational-level interventions by adopting a physical activity work break policy that allows employees to use company time for two 10-minute walking breaks throughout the course of the day (while prohibiting this for other behaviors such as smoking) and a policy that allows for all the stairwells to be more fully utilized for physical activity by installing point-of-decision prompts promoting stair walking at all elevators. The initiative will be evaluated for its impact on health-related outcomes through the use of annual health risk appraisals, satisfaction-related outcomes through annual employee surveys, and economic impacts through analyses of obesity-related health care utilization in collaboration with the health plans. This initiative becomes a part of the organizational identity and culture because it is actively supported by the executives of the company and enjoys oversight from an employee advisory committee that is representative of the company's population.

From a program design perspective, focusing on a set of simple rules that directly relate to the realities of implementation in the real-world setting is paramount (Langley, 1996; Wheatley & Kellner-Rogers, 1996). A simple operationally-derived model has been proposed that involves four design steps that effectively combine science and practice, the "4-Ss" of program design (Pronk, 2003). The 4-Ss of program design include size, scope, scalability, and sustainability. Size refers to the degree of impact the program will induce, i.e., effect size. This can be based on a review of all available evidence which subsequently is used in the translation of such evidence into an operationally feasible program solution. Scope refers to the range of program operations and the extent of program activities. Scalability refers to the ability of the program to follow a systematically timed, planned, and graded series of steps that cumulatively account for the increasing reach of a program until a critical mass is attained or the entire target population is engaged. Finally, sustainability refers to the long-term, ongoing support for the program in relation to an accepted value proposition that balances allocated resources (e.g., time, money, people, etc.) against generated revenues or other benefits. Sustainability includes the confirmation of long-term program support through adequate proof of program performance (Pronk, 2003).

The program design steps represented by the 4-Ss include all program marketing, promotions and communications issues. Scalability of programs is directly related to how well a program is marketed and made accessible to employees. Since participation is one of the most important process measures to consider, a variety of strategies should be considered. These strategies include the successful inclusion of union leadership in the program design and planning phases, special outreach to workers of color and lower SES workers, the buy-in of executive leadership, the active support for program implementation of managers, targeted outreach to subgroups identified as key groups to reach based on analyses of available data (for example, groups incurring high health care costs, multiple risk factor groups, among others), and the inclusion of all levels of the company's hierarchy, as well as the ethnic/gender diversity representative(s) of the company in the health promotion or wellness committee (Baun, Horton, Storlie, & Association for Worksite Health Promotion., 1994; Linnan et al., 2005).

Approaches to Evaluation

Evaluation should be an integral part of every worksite health promotion intervention. Appropriate process and outcome assessment will: (1) allow for a data-driven approach to programming; and (2) ensure that continuous (rapid cycle) improvement can take place while generating periodic reporting of program performance (Langley, 1996; Pronk, 2003; Wheatley & Kellner-Rogers, 1996). The evaluation approach needs to recognize that certain aspects of the program are designed to support the individual employee in changing behaviors whereas other aspects are more concerned with the work environment for the employees. Hence, individual (employee)-level as well as organizational-level metrics should be included in the evaluation. In addition, measures should be utilized that are directly related to the goals and objectives of the program and they should be directly applicable to the overarching business needs that are relevant to program performance. Using this approach, evaluation metrics should capture the influence of the program at the level of the employee and the organization, and hence, include measures that reflect health-, weight-, productivity-, and medical cost-related outcomes (Table 15.2).

Table 15.2 Individual- and organizational-level evaluation metrics.

Type of Outcome	Employee-centered variables	Organizationally-focused variables
Weight or lifestyle change program participation and climate	Participation as well as the degree of participation (enrollment, engagement, completion, etc.) must be tracked in order to evaluate the attractiveness of the program options, the degree to which marketing efforts have been effective, and the potential to document whether or not a given employee is eligible for program-related incentives	Changes in company policy, company culture, and the physical environment for employees should be tracked and documented, e.g., the implementation of healthy food options in the cafeteria, the willingness of the CEO to participate in company walks or lead exercise breaks, and the opening of a corporate fitness center
Weight loss or weight maintenance	Weight-related outcomes that reflect how well the program impacts on excess weight (prevention of weight gain and/or weight loss) are central to the evaluation efforts	Performance-related outcomes (e.g., productivity or work performance) (Riedel et al., 2001) are directly applicable to the organization's interest. For example, since presenteeism (the decrement in productivity among workers while they are at work) is estimated to represent over 60% of the total cost of illness for employees (Pronk N. P., 2003) performance while-at-work is recognized as an increasingly important variable in the evaluation of worksite programs
	Health behaviors related to weight	
Health status, health care utilization, and quality of life	Health-related outcomes are required to document the impact on overall employee health, including the prevention or management of diseases and disorders. For example, efforts to optimally manage weight may directly influence the management of chronic diseases in a worker afflicted with diabetes and hypertension	Cost-related outcomes (e.g., workers' compensation, health insurance ratings) are also one of the most important organizational-level metrics to be included in the evaluation
	Other categories of variables to consider for inclusion are medical and pharmacy utilization, and quality of life indicators	

Some evaluation may be done by company personnel. However, this poses a dilemma related to the data, as they represent sensitive information about co-workers. The data gathered should be managed in a way that protects and maintains confidentiality, abiding by rules and regulations outlined by the Health Insurance Portability and Accountability Act (HIPAA) and other applicable state laws. Individual-level data should not be shared with the employer in identifiable format.

Evaluation efforts must also consider the associated costs. The more comprehensive the intervention and the higher the investment made, the greater the need for a rigorous and thorough approach to evaluation. More complicated analyses also call for greater resources.

Guiding Principles

Several important messages can be drawn from this review of workplace approaches to obesity prevention. A summary and synthesis of these messages follows below.

Summary

- Socio-ecological principles suggest that the workplace is a key component in a multilevel approach to behavior change.
- Workplace obesity prevention and control intervention may assist in creating the social norms and political will to drive development, adoption and enforcement of aggressive obesity control legislation, e.g., taxes on obesity-promoting goods and services, subsidies to permit widespread distribution of affordable and high-quality produce, "Good Samaritan" laws to protect individuals and organizations providing time and space for physical activity from litigation. These approaches may also link to childhood obesity prevention, where the greatest traction currently resides in assuming societal responsibility and taking social action to combat obesity, e.g., as the majority of parents are workers, arguments to policymakers and social marketing messages promoting parental modeling of fit lifestyles, stress management benefits enhancing parenting capacity.
- Increased focus is needed in implementing environmental and policy interventions to promote physical activity, particularly engaging underserved populations, and maximizing evaluation conduct and rigor within resource constraints, e.g., through partnerships between academic institutions and public/private sector—simplified evaluation strategies are within resources and expertise of most programs (Glanz & Kristal, 2002).
- The levers to encourage environmental and policy change may differ between private and public sector employers, and this should inform the marketing and promotion of wellness policies/programs. The public sector has greater mission- and cost-related motivation, as they bear responsibility and costs for staff and residents of the communities they serve. The link to health disparities and social inequity issues may also provide momentum for policy change advocacy efforts, e.g., class action litigation to redress the maldistribution of parks and open space.
- All private industries are worksites, including those targeted in public health advocacy, e.g., food industry, TV/film production and distribution,

automobile industry—this may provide leverage for changes in business practices, since obesity-related health care and productivity costs are markedly affecting the bottom line.

- The level of risk reduction needed to offset program costs is probably modest (estimates range from 8 to 42%), with lesser effect sizes likely needed for programs engaging higher proportions of the total employee population (increasing representation of overweight, lower SES and ethnic minority workers, i.e. those with more "room for improvement") (Ozminkowski, Goetzel, Santoro, Saenz, Eley, & Gorsky, 2004).

Future Directions

- Public sector employers should offer wellness incentives to employees, and invest in their evaluation. Cost and productivity data may assist in adoption of models that may be made available to private employers to expand opportunities for their staff. In addition, their considerable purchasing power for various institutional work settings (e.g., schools, prisons, government building cafeterias) may be leveraged to place greater emphasis on nutritional value in the bidding and letting of these contracts (Trust for America's Health., 2005). This, in turn, may enhance the viability of businesses offering healthy food products, presenting the demand to assist the market economy in supplying a greater variety of healthy products at lower cost.
- Legislative action in this arena should be encouraged, e.g., the Healthy Workforce Act, SB 2558 (O'Donnell, 2005). Since liability for injuries incurred is a barrier commonly cited employers to integrating physical activity into workplace routine, legislative policy change addressing this issue may also be appropriate (Backman et al., 2004). Despite the imperfect science, tobacco control efforts should be emulated, in which policy changes were implemented without foreknowledge of their efficacy with rigorous evaluation to permit "mid-course corrections." The cost of waiting for better evidence is excessive, especially for underserved communities.
- Typically, work breaks have been reserved for smoking and coffee (health-compromising or -neutral behaviors), and have been aggressively protected by workers and their unions (Taylor, 2005). Converting or expanding these breaks into opportunities for health-promoting behaviors with similar stress reduction and socializing benefits (i.e. the affective enhancement associated with short bouts of moderate intensity movement) (Bixby, Spalding, & Hatfield, 2001; Ekkekakis et al., 2000; Thayer, 1989; VanLanduyt, Ekkekakis, Hall, & Petruzzello, 2000) may be a way to capitalize on the social and physical infrastructure of the workplace. Given their possible framing as an entitlement (garnering union protection and advocacy), there is great potential for dissemination and institutionalization.

Conclusion

Worksite intervention is central to population-based obesity control. Workplaces provide unparalleled opportunities to engage captive audiences of adults of all ethnic and socioeconomic backgrounds in healthy eating and active living. They also bridge key levels of intervention, i.e. individual (education/information), sociocultural environmental (group experiential learning and social support, role modeling influencing norms) and physical environmental/organizational systems (healthier vending options, stairwell renovation, distant parking incentives, brief exercise bouts during paid work hours). Furthermore, every sector and industry (including those profiting from the sale of tasty nutrient-poor foods and enticing sedentary entertainment and transportation products) are also employers adversely affected by the epidemic, and potential beneficiaries of improvements in population health and fitness status.

Worksites are particularly important settings at this early juncture in our development of policy and environmental approaches to obesity prevention and control. In these settings, decision-making by a single leader can positively influence the health of many people, at little "cost" to the individual, thereby potentiating demand for fitness-promoting goods and services, e.g., walkable neighborhoods and Farmers' Markets. Substantial increases in demand—one clinic, religious institution, corporation, health department, small business, or civic organization at a time—may create the political will to drive the passage of aggressive legislation. Such legislative policy change will reflect and advance the profound societal change required to produce dramatic behavioral change. Thus, the workplace can and should play a critical role in building the social change movement necessary to arrest the obesity pandemic.

References

Algert, S. J., Agrawal, A., & Lewis, D. S. (2006). Disparities in access to fresh produce in low-income neighborhoods in Los Angeles. *American Journal of Preventive Medicine, 30*(5), 365–370.

Andersen, R. E., Franckowiak, S. C., Snyder, J., Bartlett, S. J., & Fontaine, K. R. (1998). Can inexpensive signs encourage the use of stairs? Results from a community intervention. *Annals of Internal Medicine, 129*(5), 363–369.

Anderson, L. H., Martinson, B. C., Crain, A. L., Pronk, N. P., Whitebird, R. R., & O'Connor, P. J., et al. (2005). Health care charges associated with physical inactivity, overweight, and obesity. *Preventing Chronic Disease, 2*(4), A09.

Backman, D. R., Carman, J. S., & Aldana, S. G. (2004). *Fruits and vegetables and physical activity at the worksite: Business leaders and working women speak out on access and environment.* Sacramento, CA: California Department of Health Services.

Bandura, A. (1986). *Social foundations of thought and action: A social cognitive theory.* Englewood Cliffs, N.J.: Prentice-Hall.

Baun, W. B., Horton, W. L., Storlie, J., & Association for Worksite Health Promotion. (1994). *Guidelines for employee health promotion programs.* Champaign, IL: Human Kinetics.

Beresford, S. A., Thompson, B., Feng, Z., Christianson, A., McLerran, D., & Patrick, D. L. (2001). Seattle 5 a Day worksite program to increase fruit and vegetable consumption. *Preventive Medicine, 32*(3), 230–238.

Bixby, W. R., Spalding, T. W., & Hatfield, B. D. (2001). Temporal dynamics and dimensional specificity of the affective response to exercise of varying intensity: Differing pathways to a common outcome. *Journal of Sport & Exercise Psychology, 23*(3), 171–190.

Blair, S. N., Piserchia, P. V., Wilbur, C. S., & Crowder, J. H. (1986). A public health intervention model for work-site health promotion. Impact on exercise and physical fitness in a health promotion plan after 24 months. *Journal of the American Medical Association, 255*(7), 921–926.

Breslow, L. (2001). Why health promotion lags knowledge about healthful behavior. *American Journal of Health Promotion, 15*(5), 388–390.

Caban, A. J., Lee, D. J., Fleming, L. E., Gomez-Marin, O., LeBlanc, W., & Pitman, T. (2005). Obesity in U.S. workers: The national health interview survey, 1986 to 2002. *American Journal of Public Health, 95*(9), 1614–1622.

California Nutrition Network, & California Department of Health Service. (2004). Workplace Nutrition and Physical Activity. *Issue Brief, 1*(1), 1–8.

Campbell, M. K., Tessaro, I., DeVellis, B., Benedict, S., Kelsey, K., & Belton, L., et al. (2002). Effects of a tailored health promotion program for female blue-collar workers: health works for women. *Preventive Medicine, 34*(3), 313–323.

Colditz, G., & Mariani, A. (2000). The cost of obesity and sedentarism in the United States. In C. Bouchard (Ed.), *Physical activity and obesity* (pp. vii, 400). Champaign, IL: Human Kinetics.

Coleman, K. J., & Gonzalez, E. C. (2001). Promoting stair use in a U.S.-Mexico border community. *American Journal of Public Health, 91*(12), 2007–2009.

Crawford, P. B., Gosliner, W., Strode, P., Samuels, S. E., Burnett, C., & Craypo, L., et al. (2004). Walking the talk: Fit WIC wellness programs improve self-efficacy in pediatric obesity prevention counseling. *American Journal of Public Health, 94*(9), 1480–1485.

Daly, J., Licata, M., Gillham, K., & Wiggers, J. (2005). Increasing the health promotion practices of workplaces in Australia with a proactive telephone-based intervention. *American Journal of Health Promotion, 19*(3), 163–166.

Day, K. (2006). Active living and social justice: Planning for physical activity in low-income, black, and Latino communities. *Journal of the American Planning Association, 72*(1), 88–99.

Dishman, R. K., Oldenburg, B., O'Neal, H., & Shephard, R. J. (1998). Worksite physical activity interventions. *American Journal of Preventive Medicine, 15*(4), 344–361.

Donnelly, J. (2005). Physical activity across the curriculum/Take 10! Wichita, KS: Institute of Medicine: Progress in Addressing Childhood Obesity meeting.

Eastman, K. L., Corona, R., Ryan, G. W., Warsofsky, A. L., & Schuster, M. A. (2005). Worksite-based parenting programs to promote healthy adolescent sexual development: A qualitative study of feasibility and potential content. *Perspectives on Sexual and Reproductive Health, 37*(2), 62–69.

Ekkekakis, P., Hall, E. E., VanLanduyt, L. M., & Petruzzello, S. J. (2000). Walking in (affective) circles: Can short walks enhance affect? *Journal of Behavioral Medicine, 23*(3), 245–275.

Elbel, R., Aldana, S., Bloswick, D., & Lyon, J. L. (2003). A pilot study evaluating a peer led and professional led physical activity intervention with blue-collar employees. *Work, 21*(3), 199–210.

Emmons, K. M. (2000). Behavioral and social science contributions to the health of adults in the United States. In B. D. Smedley, S. L. Syme & Institute of Medicine (U.S.). Committee on Capitalizing on Social Science and Behavioral Research to Improve the Public's Health. (Eds.), *Promoting health: intervention strategies from social and behavioral research* (pp. xiv, 493). Washington, DC: National Academy Press.

Emmons, K. M., Linnan, L., Abrams, D., & Lovell, H. J. (1996). Women who work in manufacturing settings: factors influencing their participation in worksite health promotion programs. *Womens Health Issues, 6*(2), 74–81.

Englberger, L. (1999). Prizes for weight loss. *Bull World Health Organ, 77*(1), 50–53.

Estabrooks, P. A., Lee, R. E., & Gyurcsik, N. C. (2003). Resources for physical activity participation: Does availability and accessibility differ by neighborhood socioeconomic status? *Annals of Behavioral Medicine, 25*(2), 100–104.

Ewing, R., Schmid, T., Killingsworth, R., Zlot, A., & Raudenbush, S. (2003). Relationship between urban sprawl and physical activity, obesity, and morbidity. *American Journal of Health Promotion, 18*(1), 47–57.

Finkelstein, E., Fiebelkorn, C., & Wang, G. (2005). The costs of obesity among full-time employees. *American Journal of Health Promotion, 20*(1), 45–51.

Finkelstein, E. A., Fiebelkorn, I. C., & Wang, G. (2003). *National medical spending attributable to overweight and obesity: How much, and who's paying?*: Health Affairs.

Finkelstein, E. A., Fiebelkorn, I. C., & Wang, G. (2004). State-level estimates of annual medical expenditures attributable to obesity. *Obesity Research, 12*(1), 18–24.

Fox, L. D., Rejeski, W. J., & Gauvin, L. (2000). Effects of leadership style and group dynamics on enjoyment of physical activity. *American Journal of Health Promotion, 14*(5), 277–283.

French, S. A., Jeffery, R. W., Story, M., Breitlow, K. K., Baxter, J. S., & Hannan, P., et al. (2001). Pricing and promotion effects on low-fat vending snack purchases: The CHIPS Study. *American Journal of Public Health, 91*(1), 112–117.

Galbally, R. L. (1997). Health-promoting environments: Who will miss out? *Australia and New Zealand Journal of Public Health, 21*(4 Spec No), 429–430.

Giles-Corti, B., & Donovan, R. J. (2002). The relative influence of individual, social and physical environment determinants of physical activity. *Social Science & Medicine, 54*(12), 1793–1812.

Glanz, K., & Kristal, A. R. (2002). Worksite nutrition programs. In M. P. O'Donnell (Ed.), *Health promotion in the workplace* (3rd ed., pp. 274-292). Albany: Delmar Thomson Learning.

Glasgow, R. E., Vogt, T. M., & Boles, S. M. (1999). Evaluating the public health impact of health promotion interventions: The RE-AIM framework. *American Journal of Public Health, 89*(9), 1322–1327.

Goetzel, R. Z., Ozminkowski, R. J., Bruno, J. A., Rutter, K. R., Isaac, F., & Wang, S. (2002). The long-term impact of Johnson & Johnson's Health & Wellness Program on employee health risks. *Journal of Occupation and Environmental Medicine, 44*(5), 417–424.

Golaszewski, T., & Fisher, B. (2002). Heart check: The development and evolution of an organizational heart health assessment. *American Journal of Health Promotion, 17*(2), 132–153.

Hammond, S. L., Leonard, B., & Fridinger, F. (2000). The centers for disease control and prevention director's physical activity challenge: An evaluation of a worksite health promotion intervention. *American Journal of Health Promotion, 15*(1), 17–20, ii.

Hemp, P. (2004). Presenteeism: At work—but out of it. *Harv Bus Rev, 82*(10), 49–58, 155.

Hertz, R. P., Unger, A. N., McDonald, M., Lustik, M. B., & Biddulph-Krentar, J. (2004). The impact of obesity on work limitations and cardiovascular risk factors in the U.S. workforce. *Journal of Occupation and Environmental Medicine, 46*(12), 1196–1203.

Hill, J. O., Thompson, H., & Wyatt, H. (2005). Weight maintenance: What's missing? *Journal of the American Dietetic Association, 105*(5 Suppl 1), S63–S66.

Hill, J. O., & Wyatt, H. R. (2005). Role of physical activity in preventing and treating obesity. *Journal of Applied Physiology, 99*(2), 765–770.

Hunt, M. K., Stoddard, A. M., Barbeau, E., Goldman, R., Wallace, L., & Gutheil, C., et al. (2003). Cancer prevention for working class, multiethnic populations through small businesses: the healthy directions study. *Cancer Causes & Control, 14*(8), 749–760.

Institute of Medicine (U.S.). (2004). *Weight management: State of the science and opportunities for military programs. Available from: http://www.nap.edu/catalog/10783.html*: Subcommittee on Military Weight Management, Committee on Military Nutrition Research.

Institute of Medicine (U.S.). (2006). *Progress in preventing childhood obesity: Focus on industry – Brief summary: Institute of medicine regional symposium*. Washington, DC: National Academies of Sciences.

Institute of Medicine (U.S.). Committee to Assess Worksite Preventive Health Program Needs for NASA Employees. (2005). *Integrating employee health: A model program for NASA*. Washington, DC: National Academies Press.

Jeffery, R. W., & Utter, J. (2003). The changing environment and population obesity in the United States. *Obesity Research, 11*(Suppl. 11), 12S–22S.

Kaplan, G. D., Brinkman-Kaplan, V., & Framer, E. M. (2002). Worksite weight management. In M. P. O'Donnell (Ed.), *Health promotion in the workplace* (3rd ed., pp. xxvi, 614). Albany: Delmar Thomson Learning.

Katz, D. L., O'Connell, M., Yeh, M. C., Nawaz, H., Njike, V., & Anderson, L. M., et al. (2005). Public health strategies for preventing and controlling overweight and obesity in school and worksite settings: A report on recommendations of the task force on community preventive services. *Medicine and Science in Sports and Exercise, 54*(RR-10), 1–12.

Kimm, S. Y., Glynn, N. W., Obarzanek, E., Kriska, A. M., Daniels, S. R., & Barton, B. A., et al. (2005). Relation between the changes in physical activity and body-mass index during adolescence: A multicentre longitudinal study. *Lancet, 366*(9482), 301–307.

Kumanyika, S. (2002). Obesity treatment in minorities. In T. A. Wadden & A. J. Stunkard (Eds.), *Obesity: theory and therapy* (3rd ed., pp. xiii, 377). New York: Guilford Publications, Inc.

Kumanyika, S., & Grier, S. (2006). Targeting interventions for ethnic minority and low-income populations. *Future of Children, 16*(1), 187–207.

Kumanyika, S. K. (2001). Minisymposium on obesity: Overview and some strategic considerations. *Annu Rev Public Health, 22*, 293–308.

Lakdawalla, D. N., Bhattacharya, J., & Goldman, D. P. (2004). Are the young becoming more disabled? *Health Affairs, 23*(1), 168–176.

Lakdawalla, D. N., Goldman, D. P., & Shang, B. (2005). The health and cost consequences of obesity among the future elderly. *Health Affairs*.

Langley, G. J. (1996). *The improvement guide: A practical approach to enhancing organizational performance* (1st ed.). San Francisco: Jossey-Bass Publishers.

Lara, A. (2004, December 6, 2004). *Obesidady diabetes: Participacion de la sociedad civil*. Paper presented at the Public Health Institute Board of Directors Meeting, Puerto Vallarte, Mexico.

Leslie, J., Yancey, A., McCarthy, W., Albert, S., Wert, C., & Miles, O., et al. (1999). Development and implementation of a school-based nutrition and fitness promotion program for ethnically diverse middle-school girls. *Journal of the American Dietetic Association, 99*(8), 967–970.

Linenger, J. M., Chesson, C. V., 2nd, & Nice, D. S. (1991). Physical fitness gains following simple environmental change. *American Journal of Preventive Medicine, 7*(5), 298–310.

Linnan, L., LaMontagne, A. D., Stoddard, A., Emmons, K. M., & Sorensen, G. (2005). Norms and their relationship to behavior in worksite settings: An application of the Jackson return potential model. *American Journal of Health Behavior, 29*(3), 258–268.

Lloyd, L. K., Cook, C. L., & Kohl, H. W. (2005). A pilot study of teachers' acceptance of a classroom-based physical activity curriculum tool: TAKE 10! Texas Association for Health, Physical Education, Recreation, and Dance (TAHPERD) Journal, 73(3), 8–11.

Maibach, E. W. (2003). Recreating communities to support active living: A new role for social marketing. *American Journal of Health Promotion, 18*(1), 114–119.

Marcus, B., Williams, D., Dubbert, P. M., Sallis, J. F., King, A. C., & Yancey, A. K., et al. (2006, December12). Physical activity interventions: What we know and what we need to know. A statement from the Council on Clinical Cardiology (Subcommittee on Exercise, Rehabilitation, and Prevention) and the Council on Nutrition, Physical Activity, and Metabolism (Subcommittee on Physical Activity) of the American Heart Association. *Circulation, 114*(24), 2739–2752. Epub (2006, December 4).

Matson-Koffman, D. M., Brownstein, J. N., Neiner, J. A., & Greaney, M. L. (2005). A site-specific literature review of policy and environmental interventions that promote physical activity and nutrition for cardiovascular health: What works? *American Journal of Health Promotion, 19*(3), 167–193.

Matsudo, S. M., Matsudo, V. R., Araujo, T. L., Andrade, D. R., Andrade, E. L., & de Oliveira, L. C., et al. (2003). The Agita Sao Paulo Program as a model for using physical activity to promote health. *Revista panamericana de salud pública, 14*(4), 265–272.

McKeever, C., Faddis, C., Koroloff, N., & Henn, J. (2004). Wellness within REACH: mind, body, and soul: A no-cost physical activity program for African Americans in Portland, Oregon, to combat cardiovascular disease. *Ethnicity and Disease, 14*(3 Suppl 1), S93–S101.

Metzler, M. W., & Williams, S. (In press, 2007). A classroom-based physical activity and academic content program: more than a "pause that refreshes"? *Journal of Classroom Interaction.*

Mummery, W. K., Schofield, G. M., Steele, R., Eakin, E. G., & Brown, W. J. (2005). Occupational sitting time and overweight and obesity in Australian workers. *American Journal of Preventive Medicine, 29*(2), 91–97.

Naik, G. (2005, November 16). New buildings help people fight flab. *Wall Street Journal,* B1–B2.

Nicoll, G. (2007). Spatial measure associated with stair use. *American Journal of Health Promotion, 21*(4S), 346–352.

O'Donnell, M. P. (1986). Definition of health promotion: Part II: Levels of programs. *American Journal of Health Promotion, 1*(2), 6–9.

O'Donnell, M. P. (2005). The healthy workforce act, S2558. *American Journal of Health Promotion, 19*(3), 9–10.

Oldenburg, B. F., Sallis, J. F., Ffrench, M. L., & Owen, N. (1999). Health promotion research and the diffusion and institutionalization of interventions. *Health Education Research, 14*(1), 121–130.

Ozminkowski, R. J., Goetzel, R. Z., Santoro, J., Saenz, B. J., Eley, C., & Gorsky, B. (2004). Estimating risk reduction required to break even in a health promotion program. *American Journal of Health Promotion, 18*(4), 316–325.

Ozminkowski, R. J., Ling, D., Goetzel, R. Z., Bruno, J. A., Rutter, K. R., & Isaac, F., et al. (2002). Long-term impact of Johnson & Johnson's Health & Wellness Program on health care utilization and expenditures. *Journal of Occupation and Environmental Medicine, 44*(1), 21–29.

Passe, D. H., Horn, M., & Murray, R. (2000). Impact of beverage acceptability on fluid intake during exercise. *Appetite, 35*(3), 219–229.

Peltomaki, P., Johansson, M., Ahrens, W., Sala, M., Wesseling, C., & Brenes, F., et al. (2003). Social context for workplace health promotion: Feasibility considerations in Costa Rica, Finland, Germany, Spain and Sweden. *Health Promotion International, 18*(2), 115–126.

Peterson, M., & Wilson, J. F. (2002). The Culture-Work-Health model and work stress. *American Journal of Health Behavior, 26*(1), 16–24.

Pierce, J. P., White, M. M., & Gilpin, E. A. (2005). Adolescent smoking decline during California's tobacco control programme. *Tobacco Control, 14*(3), 207–212.

Pohjonen, T., & Ranta, R. (2001). Effects of worksite physical exercise intervention on physical fitness, perceived health status, and work ability among home care workers: Five-year follow-up. *Preventive Medicine, 32*(6), 465–475.

Powell, L. M., Slater, S., & Chaloupka, F. J. (2004). The relationship between community physical activity settings and race, ethnicity, and SES. *Evidence-Based Preventive Medicine, 1*(2), 135–144.

Pronk, N. P. (2003). Designing and evaluating health promotion programs: Simple rules for a complex issue. *Disease Management and Health Outcomes, 11*(3), 149–157.

Pronk, N. P., Martinson, B., Kessler, R. C., Beck, A. L., Simon, G. E., & Wang, P. (2004). The association between work performance and physical activity, cardiorespiratory fitness, and obesity. *Journal of Occupation and Environmental Medicine, 46*(1), 19–25.

Pronk, S. J., Pronk, N. P., Sisco, A., Ingalls, D. S., & Ochoa, C. (1995). Impact of a daily 10-minute strength and flexibility program in a manufacturing plant. *American Journal of Health Promotion, 9*(3), 175–178.

Puska, P., Nissinen, A., Tuomilehto, J., Salonen, J. T., Koskela, K., & McAlister, A., et al. (1985). The community-based strategy to prevent coronary heart disease: Conclusions from the ten years of the North Karelia project. *Annu Rev Public Health, 6,* 147–193.

Task Force on Community Preventive Services. (2002). Recommendations to increase physical activity in communities. *American Journal of Preventive Medicine, 22*(Suppl. 4), 67–72.

Riedel, J. E., Lynch, W., Baase, C., Hymel, P., & Peterson, K. W. (2001). The effect of disease prevention and health promotion on workplace productivity: A literature review. *American Journal of Health Promotion, 15*(3), 167–191.

Rogers, E. M. (2003). *Diffusion of innovations* (5th ed.). New York: Free Press.

Seabury, S. A., Lakdawalla, D., & Reville, R. T. (2005). *The Economics of integrating injury and illness prevention and health promotion programs* (No. Working Paper No. WR-243-ICJ. 2005). Santa Monica, CA: RAND Corporation.

Sevick, M. A., Dunn, A. L., Morrow, M. S., Marcus, B. H., Chen, G. J., & Blair, S. N. (2000). Cost-effectiveness of lifestyle and structured exercise interventions in sedentary adults: Results of project ACTIVE. *American Journal of Preventive Medicine, 19*(1), 1–8.

Shephard, R. J. (1992). A critical analysis of work-site fitness programs and their postulated economic benefits. *Medicine and Science in Sports and Exercise, 24*(3), 354–370.

Sorensen, G., Barbeau, E., Stoddard, A. M., Hunt, M. K., Kaphingst, K., & Wallace, L. (2005). Promoting behavior change among working-class, multiethnic workers: Results of the healthy directions—small business study. *American Journal of Public Health, 95*(8), 1389–1395.

Sorensen, G., Hunt, M. K., & Morris, D. H. (1990). Promoting healthy eating patterns in the worksite: The Treatwell intervention model. *Health Education Research, 5,* 505–515.

Sorensen, G., Linnan, L., & Hunt, M. K. (2004). Worksite-based research and initiatives to increase fruit and vegetable consumption. *Preventive Medicine, 39*(Suppl. 2), S94–S100.

Sorensen, G., Stoddard, A., Peterson, K., Cohen, N., Hunt, M. K., & Stein, E., et al. (1999). Increasing fruit and vegetable consumption through worksites and families in the treatwell 5-a-day study. *American Journal of Public Health, 89*(1), 54–60.

Sorensen, G., Stoddard, A. M., LaMontagne, A. D., Emmons, K., Hunt, M. K., & Youngstrom, R., et al. (2002). A comprehensive worksite cancer prevention intervention: Behavior change results from a randomized controlled trial (United States). *Cancer Causes & Control, 13*(6), 493–502.

Stahl, T., Rutten, A., Nutbeam, D., Bauman, A., Kannas, L., & Abel, T., et al. (2001). The importance of the social environment for physically active lifestyle—results from an international study. *Social Science & Medicine, 52*(1), 1–10.

Steckler, A., & Goodman, R. (1989). How to institutionalize health promotion programs. *American Journal of Health Promotion, 3*(4), 34–44.

Steckler, A., Goodman, R. M., McLeroy, K. R., Davis, S., & Koch, G. (1992). Measuring the diffusion of innovative health promotion programs. *American Journal of Health Promotion, 6*(3), 214–224.

Steenhuis, I. H., Van Assema, P., & Glanz, K. (2001). Strengthening environmental and educational nutrition programmes in worksite cafeterias and supermarkets in the Netherlands. *Health Promotion International, 16*(1), 21–33.

Sternfeld, B., Wang, H., Quesenberry, Jr. C. P., Abrams, B., Everson-Rose, S. A., & Greendale, G. A., et al. (2004). Physical activity and changes in weight and waist circumference in midlife women: Findings from the study of women's health across the nation. *Am J Epidemiol, 160*(9), 912–922.

Stewart, J. A., Dennison, D. A., Kohl, H. W., & Doyle, J. A. (2004). Exercise level and energy expenditure in the TAKE 10! in-class physical activity program. *Journal of School Health, 74*(10), 397–400.

Stokols, D., Grzywacz, J. G., McMahan, S., & Phillips, K. (2003). Increasing the health promotive capacity of human environments. *American Journal of Health Promotion, 18*(1), 4–13.

Sturm, R. (2002). The effects of obesity, smoking, and drinking on medical problems and costs. Obesity outranks both smoking and drinking in its deleterious effects on health and health costs. *Health Affairs, 21*(2), 245–253.

Taylor, W. C. (2005). Transforming work breaks to promote health. *American Journal of Preventive Medicine, 29*(5), 461–465.

Thayer, R. E. (1989). *The biopsychology of mood and arousal.* New York: Oxford University Press.

Thompson, D., Edelsberg, J., Kinsey, K. L., & Oster, G. (1998). Estimated economic costs of obesity to U.S. business. *American Journal of Health Promotion, 13*(2), 120–127.

Thorpe, K. E., Florence, C. S., Howard, D. H., & Joski, P. (2004). The impact of obesity on rising medical spending. *Health Affairs, Suppl Web Exclusives*, W4-480–486.

Titze, S., Martin, B. W., Seiler, R., & Marti, B. (2001). A worksite intervention module encouraging the use of stairs: Results and evaluation issues. *Sozial- und Präventivmedizin, 46*(1), 13–19.

Trust for America's Health. (2005). F as in fat: how obesity policies are failing in America. Washington, DC: Trust for America's Health.

United States. Dept. of Health and Human Services. (2003). *Prevention makes common "cents".* Washington, DC: U.S. Dept. of Health and Human Services.

UnumProvident Corporation. (2006). *UnumProvident Obesity-Related Disability Claims Study. Available from:*
http://www.unumprovident.com/newsroom/news/corporate/obesity.aspx.
Chattanooga, TN: UnumProvident Corporation.

VanLanduyt, L. M., Ekkekakis, P., Hall, E. E., & Petruzzello, S. J. (2000). Throwing the mountains into the lakes: On the perils of nomothetic conceptions of the exercise-affect relationship. Journal of Sport & Exercise Psychology. *Journal of Sport & Exercise Psychology, 22*, 208–234.

Vincent, M. L., Clearie, A. F., & Schluchter, M. D. (1987). Reducing adolescent pregnancy through school and community-based education. *Journal of the American Medical Association, 257*(24), 3382–3386.

Walker, D. (2005, October 23). Black colleges aiming to fight obesity. *Associated Press.*

Wang, F., McDonald, T., Champagne, L. J., & Edington, D. W. (2004). Relationship of body mass index and physical activity to health care costs among employees. *Journal of Occupation and Environmental Medicine, 46*(5), 428–436.

Westerterp-Plantenga, M. S., Verwegen, C. R., Ijedema, M. J., Wijckmans, N. E., & Saris, W. H. (1997). Acute effects of exercise or sauna on appetite in obese and nonobese men. *Physiology & Behavior, 62*(6), 1345–1354.

Wheatley, M. J., & Kellner-Rogers, M. (1996). *A simpler way* (1st ed.). San Francisco: Berrett-Koehler Publishers.

Whitt, M. C., DuBose, K. D., Ainsworth, B. E., & Tudor-Locke, C. (2004). Walking patterns in a sample of African American, Native American, and Caucasian women: The cross-cultural activity participation study. *Health Education & Behavior, 31*(Suppl. 4), 45S–56S.

Wilcox, S., Laken, M., Anderson, T., Bopp, M., Bryant, D., & Gethers, O., et al. (In press 2006). The Health-e-AME Faith-Based Physical Activity Initiative: Program Description and Baseline Findings. (2007) *Health Promotion Practice, 8*(1): 69–78.

Wolf, A. M., & Colditz, G. A. (1998). Current estimates of the economic cost of obesity in the United States. *Obesity Research, 6*(2), 97–106.

Yancey, A. K., Jordan, A., Bradford, J., Voas, J., Eller, T., & Buzzard, M., et al. (2003). Engaging high-risk populations in community-level fitness promotion: ROCK! Richmond. *Health Promotion Practice, 4*(2), 180–188.

Yancey, A. K., Lewis, L. B., Guinyard, J. J., Sloane, D. C., Nascimento, L. M., & Galloway-Gilliam, L., et al. (2006). Putting promotion into practice: The African Americans Building a Legacy of Health organizational wellness program. *Health Promotion Practice, 7*(3), 233S–246S.

Yancey, A. K., Lewis, L. B., Sloane, D. C., Guinyard, J. J., Diamant, A. L., & Nascimento, L. M., et al. (2004a). Leading by example: A local health department-community collaboration to incorporate physical activity into organizational practice. *Journal of Public Health Management and Practice, 10*(2), 116–123.

Yancey, A. K., McCarthy, W. J., Harrison, G. G., Wong, W. K., Siegel, J. M., & Leslie, J. (2006). Challenges in improving fitness: Results of a community-based, randomized, controlled lifestyle change intervention. *Journal of Women's Health, 15*(4), 412–429.

Yancey, A. K., McCarthy, W. J., Taylor, W. C., Merlo, A., Gewa, C., & Weber, M. D., et al. (2004b). The Los Angeles Lift Off: A sociocultural environmental change intervention to integrate physical activity into the workplace. *Preventive Medicine, 38*(6), 848–856.

Yancey, A. K., Miles, O., & Jordan, A. (1999). Organizational characteristics facilitating initiation and institutionalization of physical activity programs in a multi-ethnic, urban community. *Journal of Health Education, 30*(2), S44–S51.

Yancey, A. K., Ory, M. G., & Davis, S. M. (2006). Dissemination of physical activity promotion interventions in underserved populations. *American Journal of Preventive Medicine, 31*(4S), 82–91.

Yancey, A. K., Tanjasiri, S. P., Klein, M., & Tunder, J. (1995). Increased cancer screening behavior in women of color by culturally sensitive video exposure. *Preventive Medicine, 24*(2), 142–148.

Yancey, A. K., & Walden, L. (1994). Stimulating cancer screening among Latinas and African-American women. A community case study. *J Cancer Educ, 9*(1), 46–52.

Zernike, K. (2003, Oct 12). Fight against fat shifting to the workplace. *New York Times,* p. A1.

Chapter 16

Obesity Prevention in School and Group Child Care Settings

Eileen G. Ford, Stephanie S. Vander Veur, and Gary D. Foster

Introduction

Childhood obesity rates have tripled over the past few decades. The most recent National Health and Nutrition Examination Surveys (NHANES) data estimate that 17.1% of children aged 2–19 years were obese and 16.5 % of children aged 2–19 were overweight[*]. For the same age group, Mexican American and non-Hispanic black children have higher rates of obesity, at 19% and 20% respectively (Ogden et al., 2006). United States Department of Agriculture (USDA) data indicate that 26% of the 3.8 million preschool children served by the nation's Special Supplement Nutrition for Women, Infants and Children (WIC) programs were overweight (Cole, 2001). Among a recent sample of 1,740 predominantly African American and Latino, eighth graders in school settings, nearly half (49%) were at or above the 85th percentile for BMI (The STOPP-T2D Prevention Study Group, 2006). The need for effective prevention strategies relates to serious health and social consequences that occur during childhood and adolescence as well as the increased likelihood that obese children, especially obese older children, will become obese adults (Guo & Chumlea, 1999; Daniels et al., 2005).

As with adult weight management, treatment options for children are labor intensive and costly and have limited reach. Therefore, interest has shifted to an emphasis on structural changes for primary prevention, achieved through interventions in systems and institutions (described in detail in Chapter 12). The chapter addresses two critical settings for influencing children's environments to foster behaviors conducive to obesity prevention: schools and child care centers. Specifically, we provide: (1) the rationale for intervention in these settings; (2) a conceptual model to facilitate an understanding of how to

---

[*] The Institute of Medicine (IOM) report defines overweight in children as those with a body mass index (BMI) ≥85th percentile and obesity as those with a BMI >95th percentile (Institute of Medicine, 2005) while the Center for Disease Control (CDC) uses the terms at risk of overweight and overweight (Kuczmarski et al. 2000). We will use the terms overweight and obesity for these two cutoffs, respectively in this chapter.

operate within these settings; (3) a literature review of obesity interventions based in school or child care center programs, and their efficacy; (4) insights for planning, implementing, and evaluating interventions in these settings; and (5) recommendations for future directions.

Rationale for Schools and Child Care Centers as Settings for Obesity Prevention

Schools

The school environment presents significant opportunities for obesity prevention. Over 90% of children are enrolled in schools and spend a significant amount of their time there (Baranowski, Cullen, Nicklas, Thompson & Baranowski, 2002). No other institution has as much contact with children (Story, 1999). Children attend school for 13 years (K-12) for 180 plus days spanning 10 months per year. Children who participate in the National School Breakfast (NSB) and National School Lunch Program (NSLP) receive up to two-thirds of their daily caloric requirements from these meals, in addition to calories consumed from after school snacks and in some cases twilight or evening meals. A study from Texas middle schools assessed the potential impact of school food policies that reduced sweetened beverages and high-fat, salty and sweet food portions offered on snack bars (Cullen & Thompson, 2005). Policy changes produced a 47 calorie per day reduction in intake, a modest daily decrease but with the potential to impact long term energy balance. Schools also provide a broad platform for obesity prevention including classroom learning opportunities (health and science); physical education programs; and health services such as nursing and a growing number of health and dental clinics (Story, 1999).

Child Care Centers

Like schools, child care centers serve as an ideal setting to access large groups of young children for obesity prevention (Story, 1999). Relevant child care settings include day care centers, Head Start, maternal and child health clinics, and WIC programs (Daniels et al., 2005). These centers can be a valuable resource to reach children at very young ages and to involve parents to affect the determinants of childhood obesity. Children begin developing behaviors related to diet and activity early in life through a combination of modeling by family members and personal preference, thus making child care centers an ideal place to intervene (Fitzgibbon, Stolley, Dyer, Van Horn, & Kaufer-Christoffel, 2002) (see Chapter 19).

Parents of preschool-aged children play an active role with their child's day care center due to the dependent nature of their children in these settings. Because of this relationship, parents are relatively accessible in preschool settings for promotion of healthy eating and physical activity in their children. As the child progresses in school beyond elementary years, access to parents becomes increasingly limited.

Conceptual Framework

School environments are complex and multi-faceted, and obesity prevention initiatives should be part of coordinated, comprehensive and integrated efforts that address all of the key elements. Drawing on a comprehensive health program model for schools proposed by Allensworth and Kolbe (Allensworth & Kolbe, 1987), Story (1999) identified the components of an integrated comprehensive model for school-based obesity prevention (Figure 16.1). These eight interacting components are briefly summarized below.

The first component is health education. Curriculum for health instruction should outline how to adopt healthy eating behaviors and regular physical activity through material geared towards increasing knowledge, changing attitudes, and developing behavioral skills. Emphasis is placed on both the development and maintenance of these skills while exploring the benefits of the desired behaviors and common practices to achieve them. The curriculum includes discovery learning, group interaction, situational analysis, and goal setting with extensive teacher training and engagement. Thus, the curriculum becomes the backdrop for the behavior changes.

The second and third components are the utilization of school health services and school counseling and psychological services. These services are needed for weight screening, counseling, weight management assessment, treatment, and referral. These services, if available, are typically coordinated by school nurses. Unfortunately, screening and referral policies and procedures are sporadic. With proper staff training on techniques of measurement, interpretation

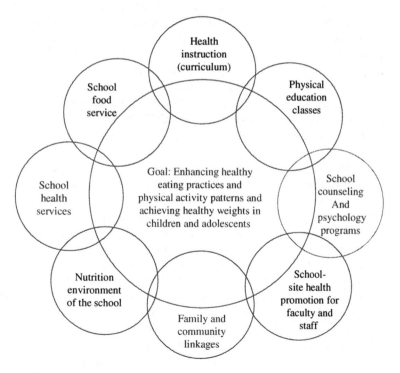

Figure 16.1. Components of an integrated comprehensive model for school-based obesity prevention (from Story, 1999).

of BMI growth charts, counseling skills, and referrals, school health services can become a more integral part of a multi-component prevention strategy.

School food service is the fourth component in the model. Although lunches and breakfasts eligible for federal reimbursement are required to follow the Dietary Guidelines for Americans (U.S. Department of Health and Human Services and U.S. Department of Agriculture, 2005), vending and a la carte options are not yet regulated. Popular high-fat and high-calorie food items are available to the students and profitable to school food service. Extending beyond school food services, the total school nutrition environment is identified as the fifth component of the model. Food is available in various locations within the school such as food stores, through fund-raising, vending outside the cafeteria, school parties, rewards and food advertising. These different venues need to be included when reviewing areas for nutrition improvement or policy change.

The sixth component in the model is physical education. Physical education classes serve the role of increasing energy expenditure and fulfilling at least a part of the daily physical activity. Efforts are needed to increase the duration and intensity of the physical activity while shifting the educational approach from competition and organized sports to lifelong fitness.

School worksite health promotion is the seventh component in the model. Improving the school environment for nutrition and physical activity can also serve the adult population of the schools. Providing opportunities for physical activity and improved nutrition to the school staff embraces the entire school community and can help adults serve as role models for the students. This approach minimizes mixed messages such as those conveyed when vending machines are removed from the school cafeterias while they remain in teacher's lounges. For this to be effective, school commitment and support need to be demonstrated by school administrators at the school and district level. Support is required from the administrators for the staff educational efforts.

The eighth and final component of the model is the degree of integration of the school efforts within the child's community. Aspects of the program need to include peers, teachers, and parents. The reach of the program into the child's life in and outside of school enhance the chances of maintaining the desired behaviors. Support from parents can reinforce all other efforts from all components in the model.

Many different conceptual frameworks have been used to guide school-based obesity prevention research studies. Based on a systematic review of this literature, Summerbell et al. (2005) concluded that approaches that considered structure and environment produced environmental change but not sustainable changes in behavior, and those utilizing a theoretical framework geared at impact on individual behavior produced individual change but did not change the environment. They suggest that environmental approaches may change the environment but must be tied into individual behavior change for sustainable and purposeful results. Story's conceptualization, described above, is an example of dual emphasis on environmental and individual change.

While there have been no formal models developed to guide pre-school and child care center obesity prevention programs, Daniels et al. review the important role of parents and teachers skills in aiding young children to learn and practice healthy behaviors (Daniels et al., 2005). Table 16.1

Table 16.1 Target behaviors for child-care center model.

1. Increasing consumption of fruits and vegetables to the goal of "5-a-day"

2. Increasing consumption of fiber-containing grain products

3. Switching from full-fat to 1% or reduced fat dairy products after age 2

4. Preparing and eating meals at home with the family

5. Increasing physical activity to goal of active play for at least 1 hour per day

6. Limiting daily sedentary time to <2 hours per day

outlines six target behaviors for obesity prevention in pre-school aged children that can be used as endpoints for the development of future prevention programs. It is likely that the same principles and practices described by Story for school settings will be largely applicable to child care settings as well.

Review of Intervention Studies

School-Based Interventions

There are numerous reviews of school based programs to improve nutrition and increase physical activity (Doak, Visscher, Renders, & Seidell, 2006; Kahn et al., 2002; Baranowski et al., 2000; Story, Kaphingst, & French, 2006; Summerbell et al., 2005; Katz et al., 2005). Table 16.2 details the design and findings of school-based research to improve nutrition and increase physical activity. Studies presented do not cover the entire literature, rather these are representative projects showing various approaches, target populations, and findings. The data demonstrate that although it is feasible to conduct interventions related to food service or physical activity, few studies, to date, have been effective in changing targeted weight outcomes such as BMI. Some of the successful studies are highlighted below.

Interventions targeting the total food environment focus on: increasing fruits and vegetables; lowering fat and sodium content; offering dessert and snack items in single serving portions; and eliminating soda and sugar sweetened beverages. The feasibility of these strategies has been demonstrated in terms of implementation and the ability to increase the nutritional quality of the food served (Donnelly et al., 1996; Lytle et al., 1996). These intervention studies typically demonstrate modest effects, such as increases of about a third of a fruit, juice or vegetable serving consumed by the students (Sahota et al., 2001).

Interventions for physical activity focus on increasing the amount of moderate to vigorous physical activity (MVPA) in Physical Education (PE) classes by: adding more classes into the school schedule; lengthening the existing class time for PE; increasing the amount of MVPA in the existing PE period; and increasing physical activity through popular activities. Extensive reviews of these interventions are available elsewhere (IOM, 2005; Kahn et al., 2002). Although many studies have demonstrated increases in physical activity time, MVPA and energy expenditure (Donnelly et al., 1996; McKenzie et al., 1996; Sallis et al., 1997; Simons-Morton, Parcel, Baranowski, Forthofer, & O'Hara, 1991), only one

Table 16.2 Comparison of selected school-based interventions.

Study/Author	Study population and intervention	Key findings
CATCH (McKenzie et al., 1996; Luepker et al., 1996; Nader et al., 1996, 1999; Lytle et al., 1996)	– 3 year intervention – 3rd–5th graders – 96 schools in 4 states Randomized multicomponent intervention to improve diet, physical activity, nonsmoking status	– Increased PE time; – Increased MVPA in class – Implemented 90% of food service goals – Decreased fat content of lunch meal – Decreased self-reported fat intake – No significant changes in body weight, cholesterol or blood pressure
SPARK (McKenzie, 1997)	– 4 year intervention – 4th graders – 7 schools Comparison of 3 physical education conditions (trained classroom teachers, physical education specialists, controls) in two parts: (1) effects of health-related physical education program on quantity and quality of lessons; (2) maintenance effects	– Specialists produced best outcomes – Trained classroom teachers were significantly better than non-trained peers – After termination of intervention, withdrawal of the specialists significantly reduced the quantity and quality of physical education – Trained teachers maintained specialists frequency but had a decline in student activity of 88% of intervention levels
Planet Health (Gortmaker et al., 1999a)	– 2 year intervention – 6–7th graders – 10 schools Intervention to decrease sedentary behavior, increase MVPA, decrease fat intake and increase fruit/vegetable intake	– Decrease prevalence of obesity in girls – Greater remission of obesity among intervention girls – Reduced TV viewing – Increased fruit and vegetable intake
Eat Well and Keep Moving (Gortmaker et al., 1999b)	– 2 year intervention – 4th–5th graders – 14 schools Classroom lessons to decrease high fat foods, increase fruits and vegetables, decrease TV and increase physical activity	– Significant reduction in total energy from fat and saturated fat in intervention group – Significant increase in fruit and vegetable intake in intervention group
Robinson, 1999	– 6 month intervention – 3rd–4th graders – 2 schools Randomized controlled trial to reduce TV, videotape, and video games use.	– Relative decrease in BMI for intervention group – Decreases in TSF, waist and waist-to-hip ratio in intervention group – Decrease TV viewing – Decrease in meals eaten in front of TV – No significant changes in fat intake or MVPA
APPLES (Sahota et al., 2001) (England)	– 1 year intervention – 7–11 year olds – 10 schools	– Increase vegetable consumption in intervention group – No significant changes in BMI

	Teacher training to modify meals and target PE and activity	
Pathways (Caballero et al., 2003)	– 3 year intervention – 3rd–5th grade American Indian Children Intervention to promote changes in diet, increases in physical activity. Delivery via classroom activities on healthy eating and family involvement	– No significant decrease in body fat – Significant reduction in percent calories from fat observed – Total energy intake via 24 hour recalls decreased but inconsistent with observations – No change in physical activity – Significant changes in knowledge and attitudes for intervention group
New Moves (Neumark-Sztainer et al.,2003)	– 16 week intervention – high school girls Multi- component intervention aimed to increase enjoyment and self efficacy of physical activity	– Feasibility indicated by strong satisfaction ratings by schools, subjects, parents and teachers – No significant changes on outcome variables
James et al., 2004	– 1 year intervention – 7–11 year olds – 6 schools Cluster randomized controlled trial to reduce carbonated drinks	– Consumption of carbonated drinks decreased by 0.6 glasses. – Consumption increased by 0.2 glasses in control group. – Increase in the percentage of overweight and obesity in control group – Decrease in percentage of overweight and obesity in the intervention group
Kain et al., 2004	– 1 year intervention – K-8th graders – 5 schools Behavioral program to increase physical activity time and nutrition education for students and parents	– Positive effects on adiposity measures for boys only – Increased physical fitness
TEENS Study (Lytle et al., 2004)	– 2 year intervention – 7th–8th graders – 16 schools 10 sessions of TEENS curriculum and cafeteria changes	– No significant differences in food choices except for score given to making lower fat choices for intervention group
WAY (Wellness, Academics, & You) Program (Spiegel & Foulk, 2006)	– 1 year intervention – 4th–5th graders – 16 schools in 4 states randomized within schools Teachers trained to provide intervention to address health issues in core curriculum as health impacts academic performance and decision making is a learned skill	– Reduction of 2% in the number of students with BMI greater than 85th percentile in intervention group

study reported significant changes in BMI (Manios, Moschandreas, Hatzis & Kafatos, 1999).

Some notable success stories of school based interventions for obesity prevention have been reported. James et al. demonstrated positive effects from an intervention focusing on decreasing soda consumption in six elementary schools in England (James, Thomas, Cavan, & Kerr, 2004). Intervention schools showed significantly greater reductions in soda consumption and obesity prevalence then did the control schools after 1 year. Foster et al. evaluated the effect of a school-based, beverage policy and snack guideline on 4th–6th graders in 10 elementary schools in Philadelphia. The incidence rates of overweight (i.e., crossing the 85th percentile threshold) were halved in the intervention compared to control schools over a two-year period (Foster et al., 2006).

Making It Happen!, a joint project of several federal agencies, outlines school success stories that provide students with healthier food choices (U.S. Department of Agriculture, U.S. Department of Education, U.S. Department of Health and Human Services, CDC, 2005b). The six primary approaches suggested in *Making It Happen!* to change the total food environment include: establishing nutrition standards for competitive food; influencing food and beverage contracts; making more healthful foods and beverages available; adopting marketing techniques to promote healthful choices; limiting student access to competitive foods; and using fundraising activities and rewards that support student health. Table 16.3 provides specific examples of strategies for changing the total school food environment.

In addition to the environmental and policy interventions in food service and physical education, researchers have also promoted curriculum and interventions geared towards decreasing screen time: TV watching, video games and computer use. Most of these programs use a behavioral approach by increasing self awareness through self monitoring, goal setting and setting limits or budgets on actual screen time. Programs of this nature usually involve parental support, as the primary intervention time takes place in the home. Although most programs do not make specific activity recommendations for the child, it is assumed that decreasing screen time will result in the child's choice of an alternative activity, hopefully a physical activity.

Gortmaker et al. studied a multi-component program composed of nutrition changes, PE curriculum and TV viewing with two populations: Eat Well and Keep Moving in Baltimore and Planet Health in Boston (Gortmaker et al., 1999a, 1999b). Planet Health had a positive effect on decreasing TV viewing in the treatment schools. The program resulted in a 24.2% reduction in the prevalence of obesity in girls only, while there was no intervention effect for boys. In addition to the reduction in prevalence, Planet Health observed higher rates of obesity remission in the intervention group. Planet Health also demonstrated a direct relationship between reductions in TV/video time and lower prevalence of obesity.

Robinson reported significant decreases in TV and video time and other sedentary activities associated with participation in a school-based program (Robinson, 1999). Although the children reported less screen time, they did not consistently increase their physical activity time. Nevertheless, the study demonstrated a significant intervention effect on decreasing BMI and skinfold measurements.

Table 16.3 Specific examples of strategies for change in the total school food environment (adapted from *Making it Happen!*).

Specific example in the school
• Establish specifications for healthy foods based on nutrient content and portion size
• Prohibit use of "foods of minimal nutritional value" in schools including fundraising (candy, soda)
• Encourage healthy snacks from home as well, such as fresh fruits and vegetables only
• Internalize vending contracts to increase control – no external companies; let the school food service control vending with healthy choices and receive the revenue
• Limit all vending beverages to water
• Request vendors to price healthier options appropriately and replace food advertisements with picture of physical activity on vending machines
• Include water, milk, yogurt
• Fresh fruits and vegetables
• Vegetables with low fat dip or salsa
• Salads (both fruit and vegetable)
• Air popped popcorn
• Whole grain foods
• Taste test new products
• Information and promotional messages at point of purchase
• Include students in the food selection process
• Develop school wide promotions for healthier food choices
• Price healthier foods at a lower price than unhealthy foods
• Limit snacks available to all students
• Reduce portion size to a prescribed calorie amount (i.e. <200 calories)
• Eliminate vending machines in elementary and middle schools
• Use non food rewards, substitute pizza party with a walk with the Principal
• Sell fruit baskets or gift wrapped fruit for fundraisers
• Sell breakfast cart items instead of candy for fundraisers
• Use placemats or table covers to decorate the cafeteria and make the dining experience rewarding
• Invite guests, celebrities or the Principal to dine with the students focusing on the company rather than the food
• Allow music in the cafeteria as a reward

Child Care Center Interventions

Like school-based studies, multi-component efforts are being attempted to address poor nutrition and lack of physical activity in child care settings by making changes to the food environment, increasing parental involvement, decreasing sedentary time and increasing physical activity. Hip Hop to Health Jr. found smaller increases in BMI at 1 and 2 years among children at Head Start centers receiving an intervention compared with children at control centers. This intervention was conducted in centers serving predominantly African American and Latino children. A subsequent analysis suggested that the effects were in the African American centers (Fitzgibbon et al., 2006). Table 16.4 outlines this intervention and other promising programs that have been developed

Table 16.4 Comparison of preschool-based interventions.

Study/Author	Study population and intervention	Key findings

Hip Hop to Health Jr. (Fitzgibbon et al., 2002)	– 5 year intervention
	– 3–5 year olds
	  • African American and Hispanic
	  • 24 Head Start programs
	
	Intervention had the following aims: decrease dietary fat, increase dietary fiber, decrease physical activity, and inclusion of family and was delivered via 45 min intensive intervention 3 times per week for 14 weeks, parental newsletters. Aerobics classes (2 per week) were offered to parents at intervention sites
		– Intervention had smaller increases in BMI compared with controls at 1 and 2 years
		– Only significant difference: at 1 year in % of kcals from saturated fat, 11.6% vs 12.8%

NAP SACC (Ammerman & Ward, 2003)	– 6 month pilot study
	– 3–5 year olds
	  • 20 childcare centers
	  • 8 counties in NC
	
	Used NAP SACC self assessment instrument to evaluate efficacy of intervention. Intervention consisted of 3 workshops on childhood obesity, healthy eating, and physical activity
		– Insignificant differences between the intervention and control centers at baseline for overall, nutrition and physical activity score
		– Both intervention and control centers improved on their scores at the end of the pilot intervention
		– Intervention centers increased an average of 13 points, control centers improved by an average of 8 points on the NAP-SACC instrument at follow-up

Fit WIC (Crawford et al., 2005)	– 1 year intervention
	– sample varied by intervention site
	  • WIC programs
	  • 5 states
	
	Intervention for obesity prevention focused on 3 key concepts: parental component, staff component, community component (specific intervention programs varied by state)
		– Training, materials and increased time with participants allowed staff to address issues
		– Education should focus on healthy behaviors not weight issues
		– Parents were eager to receive info
		– Physical activity promotion was important to the promotion of healthy eating
		– Staff felt more effective when wellness opportunities were provided at work
		– Stakeholders recognized WIC in the role of leader in obesity prevention

Color Me Healthy (Dunn et al., 2006)	– 1 year program
	– 4–5 year olds
	  • Child care providers
	  • 47 counties in NC
	
	Curriculum used interactive learning tools for physical activity and nutrition. Trained public health professionals to teach health care providers to use the curriculum.
		– 92% of providers indicated that using Color Me Healthy increased physical activity in their children
		– 91.8% indicated that it increased their children's knowledge about movement
		– 93% indicated that CMH increased their children's knowledge about healthy eating

to affect nutrition, physical activity, and BMI in preschool-aged children in child care settings.

Dennison and colleagues were the first to show a decrease in television and video game use following an intervention program in preschool aged children (Dennison, Russo, Burdick, & Jenkins, 2004). Pre-intervention, the intervention and control groups were viewing 11.9 and 14.0 h/wk of television and videos. Post-intervention, the intervention group decreased viewing time by 3.1 h/wk whereas the control group increased their viewing time by 1.6 h/wk. Dennison has also found television watching was significantly higher if the child had a television in his/her bedroom (2002). Even among preschoolers, average mean TV viewing times were high: 14.9, 16.3, 18.4 hours per week for the 2, 3, 4 year old children respectively. As increased opportunity to watch television is a strong marker for an increased risk of being overweight among preschool children, it is an obvious intervention target.

Insights for Planning, Implementation, and Evaluation

Schools and child care centers are political, complex, interactive, evolving environments. In order to intervene, it is important to understand the barriers and challenges. This section will focus on aspects of the school and child care environments for program planning and developing program evaluations.

Planning Interventions

Although there are many opportunities to influence the determinants of obesity in schools, there are also many challenges. Financial constraints exist for many schools and child care centers, particularly low income schools with a limited tax base and a dependence on limited available state support. With the No Child Left Behind legislation, schools must answer the call to increase test scores and Adequate Yearly Progress (AYP) for federal funding of basic programs (*No Child Left Behind Act*, 2002). Although it is important to increase the proficiency of U.S. children in academic areas, No Child Left Behind competes with efforts to influence health change in a school setting.

Child care centers can provide the opportunity to teach proper eating and physical activity habits. Unfortunately, the quality of care provided by many centers is often inadequate making issues related to overall care more important than those related to food and activity behaviors. Lack of training and experience, low pay, and high turnover among child care providers all play a major role in poor quality of child care. On-the-job experience could compensate for lack of formal training, but such experience is hard to find because of high turnover rates. Turnover is a result of deficient compensation and high teacher to student ratios. On average, child care teachers earn just slightly over $14,000 a year and often earn no benefits. The result is an annual turnover rate that reached 27% among child care workers in 1997 and 39% for child care assistants (Friedman, 2006).

Although there is growing support for obesity prevention programs in schools, these same initiatives present a potential burden to administrators with respect to the time needed for planning and supervision in their school; a burden to teachers for training and implementation time; a burden to students from potential time away from academic studies; and, finally, a burden to families related to the potential economic burden or stress of providing healthier food and safe physical activities. Efforts to understand and appreciate the school and center environments and cultures can be helpful in limiting the extent to which programs are burdensome.

Total School Food Environments

The USDA provides federally defined standards based on the Dietary Guidelines for Americans for the breakfast and lunch programs (USDA, 2005b). Failure to comply with standards affects commodity availability and cash reimbursements for the meals. This means that the meals must contain less than 30% of the calories from fat and less than 10% from saturated fat. Lunches must provide one third of the recommended dietary allowance (RDA) for protein, calcium, iron, Vitamin A, Vitamin C and calories. Breakfasts must contain one fourth of the RDAs for the same key nutrients. For many school districts, menus are calculated based on an average for all students' grades 1 through 12. As a result, elementary students may exceed RDA for calories while middle schools may be slightly below. Schools receive reimbursement for the meals based on participation of students in the program. Unfortunately, participation declines with both age and as other food options proliferate. Of note with respect to obesity prevention, efforts to decrease the total calories of federally funded meals are met with resistance because reimbursement will not be possible if the meals fall below their prescribed calorie amount.

The total school food environment has changed over recent years. In addition to the USDA meal programs offered, schools seeking revenue rely on competitive food sales: foods available for purchase from vending, school stores, canteens and snack bars that compete with federally funded meals. By using the 2004 School Health Profiles for public schools, the CDC examined competitive foods sold in 27 states in 11 large urban districts (CDC, 2005a). Results indicated that 89.5% of secondary schools surveyed allowed students to purchase snack food and beverages from vending, school stores, canteen, or snack bars. Although the schools offered both nutritious and non-nutritious food items, 65% offered chocolate and other candies, 74% offered salty snack foods, 92% offered soft drinks, sports drinks, and non-100% fruit juices. As for nutritious offerings, only 44% offered fruits and vegetables, 60% offered low fat-baked snacks, and 84% offered 100% fruit juice. Notably, 94% served bottled water. Snacks were available before school in 60% of the schools surveyed and 22% allowed purchases during any school hours when meals were not served. This analysis demonstrates the need for stronger school food policies to create environments where eating healthy foods is more likely.

Although there are strict guidelines directing the nutritional quality of federally funded breakfast and lunches, minimal guidelines exist for competitive foods. USDA restricts the sale of "foods of minimal value": soda, water ices, chewing gum, candies such as hard candy, jelly beans, marshmallow candies, licorice, spun candy and candy-coated popcorn, but the definition of foods of minimal value has not been updated since originally proposed 30 years ago. In an effort to offset losses in revenues and to make school food services potentially revenue neutral, the sale of competitive foods through vending, snack lines, a la carte and snack bars has become commonplace and accepted. Schools and school food services arrange for companies to sell popular food items directly to students through contracts that provide services to financially stricken schools. None of these food opportunities are regulated.

Thus, while posters may decorate the cafeterias asking students to have "5-A-Day", the schools are serving pizza, subs, and sodas from popular vendors. Contracts often require brand name displayed in prominent places throughout the school environment such as score boards, vending machines, or signage in the cafeteria. Companies not only gain access to young purchasers but also enjoy unfettered access to marketing and brand name exposure throughout the student's day.

If competitive foods were regulated and limited to healthy food choices, such as fresh vegetables and fruits, diet quality would clearly improve. However, it is less clear if these qualitative shifts would affect BMI. In addition, even when policies exist within a school system, there is often a disconnect between the food service directors and the school principals about existence of the policies and how to enforce and regulate the policies (McDonnell, Probart, Weirich, Hartman & Bailey-Davis, 2006). For example, fundraisers and rewards in schools traditionally revolve around foods. These events are permitted to occur during lunches and, therefore, also compete with the federally reimbursed meals. Alternative fundraising events and rewards need to be explored, not only to decrease competition with higher quality foods but also to decrease confusion of school messages or lessons through health classes. Rewards related to physical activity would be beneficial to students, as would fundraisers such as dance-a thons, car washes or sponsored walks.

The Alliance for a Healthier Generation, Clinton Foundation and the American Heart Association along with key industry leaders set forth a school beverage guideline in May, 2006 (Alliance for Healthier Generation, 2006). The guidelines set the beverage criteria for the Healthy Schools Program, with a shift to lower calorie and nutritious beverages for children during school hours and throughout extended day programs. The focus of the guideline is on calories and the educational environment in which those calories are consumed. By adopting these guidelines, the American Beverage Association, PepsiCo, Coca-Cola and Cadbury Schweppes have agreed to specific beverage selections, times of day, implementation goals and reporting.

Beverage selections under the new guidelines are determined by grade category. For elementary schools, choices will now be limited to: water; less than or equal to eight ounce serving of milk or juice; fat free or low fat milk and nutritionally equivalent USDA milk alternatives; fat free or low fat nutritionally equivalent flavored milk with less than 150 calories per eight ounce serving; 100% juice with no added sweeteners with less than 120 calories per eight ounce serving and 10% DV (daily value) for more than 3 micronutrients. Middle schools follow the same guidelines as the elementary schools with the following exceptions: juice and milk meet the same standards but may be available in 10 ounce servings. High School beverage guidelines include: water; no or low calorie beverages with less than 10 calories per eight ounce serving (diet sodas and teas); less than a 12 ounce serving of milk, light juice, juice and sports drinks; fat free or low fat milk and nutritionally equivalent USDA milk alternatives; fat free or low fat nutritionally equivalent flavored milk with less than 150 calories per eight ounce serving; 100% juice with no added sweeteners with less than 120 calories per eight ounce serving and 10% DV (daily value) for more than 3 micronutrients; light juices and sports drinks with less than 66 calories per eight ounce serving; and greater than 50% of the beverages are water and no or low calorie options (less than 10 calories per eight ounces).

When a middle school and high school share a campus, the guidelines suggest following the high school guidelines.

The times of day stipulated by the school beverage policy apply to before school, during school and after-school. After-school events or programs under the control of the school or parties on behalf of the school still require the beverage policy. This includes clubs, band and after-school programs. The policy does not apply to school-related events where parents and other adults comprise a significant portion of the audience such as interscholastic events, school plays or concerts.

The guidelines apply to future contracts but efforts will be made to amend existing contracts within financial fairness. It is the goal of the Alliance to implement the policy for 75% of schools under contract with beverage companies prior to the beginning of the 2008–2009 school year and all schools by 2009–2010 school year.

Finally, the guideline requires reporting beginning in August 2007 with regards to the impact and status of the policy. Reporting will include beverage sales data through vending, a la carte and school stores from both vendors and school fundraising activities.

Broader policy changes may be forthcoming after the Institute of Medicine publishes their report on Nutrition Standards for Foods in Schools (due January 2007). The charge of the committee writing this report is to review the gathered information, including results of public meetings, and make recommendations on nutrition standards in the school environment (IOM, 2006).

Total School Environments for Physical Activity
Current recommendations for physical activity in children are a total of 60 minutes of moderate-to-vigorous physical activity each day (IOM, 2005; DHHS & USDA, 2005). It is estimated that children spend half of their waking day in schools. It is thereby recommended that they complete at least 30 minutes of their recommended 60 minutes per day being physically active in schools (IOM, 2005; Strong, Malina, Bumke, Daniels, Dishman, Gutin, Hergenroeder, Must, Nixon, Pivarnik, Rowland, Trost & Trudeau, 2005). This amount of physical activity is important not only to prevent childhood obesity but improves the cardiovascular system, musculoskeletal system, mental health and emotional well being and is also relevant for chronic disease prevention (IOM, 2005).

Despite very clear objectives set forth in *Healthy People 2010* for physical activity (DHHS, 2000), adolescents are increasingly less likely to participate in physical education classes as they move through the middle school and high school grades (Burgeson, Wechsler, Brener, Young & Spain, 2001). Burgeson found that although 96.4% of the schools require some physical education, the number varied greatly based on grade level, decreasing dramatically from around 50% in grades 1–5, to 25% in grade 8, to only 5% by 12th grade. The study also reported that only 8% of elementary, 6% of middle or junior high schools and 6% of high schools offered daily PE for all students in all grades thus meeting *Healthy People 2010* Objective 22–8. Daily PE classes are supported by many of the national health and education related organizations (AAP, 2000; CDC, 1997; DHHS, 2000; IOM 2005). Although PE and health education are mandated in most states, there are no required guidelines as to the amount or frequency of time needed for either.

As mentioned previously, the No Child Left Behind Act of 2000, while holding schools, teachers and students accountable for academic perform- ances, leaves less and less time available in a school day for non-tested sub- jects including PE. The possibility exists that PE could help to improve academic performance although to date, few studies have demonstrated a clear relationship. Taras reviewed the available research relating physical activity to academic performance (Taras, 2005) and found limited positive effect on short term cognitive benefits. Sallis et al. evaluated academic achievement in Project Spark (Sallis, McKenzie, Kolody, Lewis, Marshall, & Rosengard, 1999) and found that the benefits of physical activity adequately compensated for the time spent away from academic areas (Sallis et al., 1999).

Education about physical activity is available in PE class and health class. Opportunities for actual physical activity are often limited to PE class, recess and after-school activities such as intramural sports and clubs and inter- scholastic sports, if available (Story et al., 2006). After school programs with a wide variety of approaches toward physical activity, whether sports related or ethnic dance or even creative social action fundraising efforts (walk-a thons), increase the likelihood of accessing wide and varied groups of students as participants. Other opportunities for physical activity during the day include teacher or school initiated breaks. These breaks serve as a chance for the students to stretch, move and refocus integrating physical activity into lessons during health or science about the body or take healthy walks exploring neigh- boring environments. Jago and Baronowski reviewed other efforts such as painting playgrounds as ways to increase non-class time physical activity in the school environment (Jago & Baranowski, 2004).

Recess provides unstructured time for students to release energy, serves as stress management, and promotes the development of social skills with peers while negotiating rules for unsupervised games and activities (Story et al., 2006). These skills are valuable for the student in future decision making and for developing a life long appreciation and desire for physical activity. To gain the benefits of recess, it needs to be offered as a stand alone time of impor- tance for social and physical development. Recess is not a substitute for PE but a complement, a chance to use the skills taught in PE (CDC, 1997; IOM, 2005). Not all students have physically active recess opportunities, however. Some schools may use recess time for remediation efforts to improve state mandated test scores.

Child Care Center Environments for Nutrition and Physical Activity
The Child and Adult Care Food Program (CACFP) is a nutrition education and reimbursement program for licensed child care centers, funded by the U.S. Department of Agriculture (USDA) (CACFP, 2006). CACFP provides federal money for meals and snacks served to preschool children in licensed child care centers, Head Start programs, and licensed child care homes (USDA, 2005). In 2004, CACFP served almost 2 million children per day in child care settings and Head Start programs and more than 913,000 in private child care homes. On average, CACFP served more than 2.8 million children in these types of settings (FRAC, 2006). Many centers depend on CACFP to offset expenses. In addition, parents depend on the center and, inadvertently, on the CACFP to provide meals and snacks to their children, which defrays their expenses (Parker, 2000).

Currently, CACFP is not regulated according to the USDA's Dietary Guidelines for Americans, 2005. These guidelines outline how Americans two years of age and older can eat nutritiously to prevent disease and live a healthy life. Requiring CACFP to comply with the Dietary Guidelines could be a way to regulate what children in child care centers are eating, which could dramatically affect what millions of children eat daily.

Similar to the situation with meals, there is a large variation in the quality and amount of physical activity in preschool settings (Pate, Pfeiffer, Trost, Ziegler & Dowda, 2004). Many of the federally funded programs focus on infant and toddler nutrition for health, but few policies and guidelines are available to guide healthcare providers and teachers to direct parents and their children towards increasing physical activity and decreasing sedentary time. Although the 2005 Dietary Guidelines for Americans recommend that children and adolescents are active for at least 60 minutes on most days of the week (DHHS & USDA, 2005), limited curriculum is available for implementing these recommendations in child care centers.

Child care settings cater to large numbers of children within different developmental stages. Infants and toddlers vary greatly in social, cognitive and nutritional needs. This creates a barrier to implementation of a single effort towards obesity prevention and may be one of the reasons why efforts to increase physical activity and improve food quality in child care settings are not more common.

Implementing and Evaluating Interventions

Implementing obesity prevention interventions in schools and childcare settings requires an assessment of where things are initially and a plan of action that includes benchmarks against which to judge progress. The new requirement for schools that participate in federally-funded school meal programs to develop and to implement wellness policies creates a mandate to develop such a plan of action. This requirement was included in the Child Nutrition and WIC Reauthorization Act of 2004 (USDA, 2004). Policies must address both nutrition and physical activity and be in place by the start of the 2006–2007 school year. The National Alliance for Nutrition and Activity has worked with a variety of relevant organizations to create a set of model policies for local school districts (NANA, 2006). From a process perspective, implementation activities should involve both internal and external influences and stakeholders, that is, people who have authority over or vested interests in both developing a plan and seeing that it is implemented and effective. This includes involving the students themselves, wherever feasible.

School Needs Assessment: School Health Index

The Centers for Disease Control and Prevention (CDC) School Health Index (SHI) is a self-assessment and planning guide designed to help schools identify the strengths and weaknesses of their nutrition and physical activity programs and policies. While the CDC specifies schools, this tool can easily be tailored to child care centers. The SHI helps schools to identify the policies and practices most likely to be effective in improving youth health risk behaviors. It is structured around CDC's eight-component model of a coordinated school health program. These components include:

1. School Health and Safety Policies and Environment
2. Health Education
3. Physical Education and Other Physical Activity Programs
4. Nutrition Services
5. Health Services
6. Counseling, Psychological, and Social Services
7. Health Promotion for Staff
8. Family and Community Involvement

The SHI allows a school or school district to assess the extent to which they have implemented the types of policies and practices recommended by CDC to promote healthy eating, physical activity and other health related practices (U.S. DHHS, 1996). Schools start by developing School Health Councils comprising teachers, food service personnel, parents, school administrators and students. These teams are charged with completing the 8 module self-assessment process, identifying recommended actions and prioritizing these recommendations, which serve as the basis for completion of the School Health Improvement Plan. A school's Improvement Plan lists steps in implementing recommended actions and develops a process for monitoring progress and reviewing recommendations for change (CDC, 2005b).

Engaging School Stakeholders

School and pre-school based obesity prevention programs need to effect change in the school culture. School culture is set by all stakeholders: students, families, teachers, administration and school staff; as well as the location and surrounding areas, external political influences and mandates and local school board mission. In order to both assess and address prevention interventions in a school, it is important to understand all of the stakeholders involved and the interrelated roles that they play. School stakeholders can be divided into four categories (see Table 16.5): external influences; structural/administrative levels; internal school layers; and the local school community.

External Influences: External influences include local, state and federal political leaders and initiatives. Due to financial needs and the state and federal Department of Education mandates, schools must answer to issues sensitive to political influence. The No Child Left Behind legislation is a current example. For full federal funding, schools must implement these initiatives, which may be incompatible, or perceived as incompatible with PE and health education needs.

Structural/Administrative Levels: All school districts have their own structure, and the administrative organizational structure is unique from one district to the next. Determining who the key decision makers are for the district is critical for program development and success. Understanding the roles of each department at the central level as well as the layers of administration from the central district will foster program acceptance and decrease potential competition among programs in the district. In order to better understand and work with the school district, first develop

Table 16.5 Summary of essential school stakeholders.

Stakeholder group	Stakeholder members
External influences	• Political leaders (local, state, federal initiatives and mandates) • Health Department • Nonprofit health promotion groups or coalitions • Externally funded health education grants

Structural or administrative levels	• School Board or Council
	• CEO or Superintendent
	• Area or Regional Superintendent
	  • Categorical or regional
	• Specific departments:
	  • Department of Student Services
	  • Wellness programs
	  • Nursing
	  • School Food Services
	  • Department of Health & Physical Education
	  • Academic Office, Curriculum
	• District Parent Association

Internal school layers	• Principal • Assistant Principal or Deans • School Health Council • Teachers • Parent Association • Food Service Manager & Workers • Students
Local school community	• Parents • Recreation centers • After-school programs

partnerships with key identified decision makers. Ideally these key decision makers include: the School District Superintendent or Chief Executive Officer and Chief Academic Officer, but accessibility to these individuals may be limited if available at all. Therefore, program introduction needs to take place in both the middle levels with the Director of the Office of Research, Director of Student Services, Director of Special Services (those who oversee nurses and health educators), Director of Food Service, and Director of PE and with individual school Principals. These insiders will help to navigate the structure and keep the program politically afloat. Identifying school board directors who have voiced concern of student health issues as well as forming alliances with the head of key departments will keep obesity prevention programs and interventions on the administrative agenda. A multi-prong approach increases the possibility of program acceptance and approval.

Internal School Layers: Once a program or intervention has district-wide approval or acceptance, it is important to work within the internal school layers. Although the Principal is necessary and responsible for all school activities, buy-in with the teachers and staff is essential. Meetings and information sessions as well as advisory boards will assist in keeping all stakeholders informed and serve as a feedback mechanism. If the school already has a School Health Council, plans should be made to work with that group. As many programs focus on dietary change, all food service employees need to be included in planning and implementing any proposed changes. The Food Service Director makes the decisions, but the food service employees interact at the point of service or purchase with the students on a daily basis and can exhibit influence.

Focus groups or informal meetings with students will provide an opportunity for direct constituent involvement and increase the likelihood of student acceptance of the program. Identifying decisions in which students can have a voice will facilitate program ownership for this critical audience, e.g., involving students in the selection of music, incentives or other aspects of school wide events. Allowing the students to name the program or a component of the program locally also helps them to identify with the effort. In order to effectively utilize student input, program staff should have conducted preliminary research and present the students with top choices for names or incentives, as students cannot be expected to undertake the initial stages of the process.

Local School Community: If the total school environment is to change, it will need to include efforts provided at home, in the community, or by parent volunteers. School stores and parties are usually organized and staffed by parents; therefore including these parent groups from the beginning will enhance engagement and decrease competitive messages. Finally, after school programs either at the school or local recreation centers need to be coordinated as well.

The intervention or program cannot appear to sweep into the school without regard for the existing programs and demands of the stakeholders. Careful relationship building with all of these groups is paramount to success. Again, utilizing the CDC SHI is a recommended starting point. Developing lasting partnerships with all groups is an active and ongoing process.

Engaging Child Care Center Stakeholders

Since the majority of child care centers are for-profit entities, due to the primary function of day care, their stakeholders differ from schools. Forty percent of children aged 3 to 4 years whose mothers are working full-time spend more than 35 hours per week in non-parental care (Capizzano & Adams, 2000) with the largest percent of the child's care coming from center-based care (Casper, 1996). The stakeholders in child care settings are outlined in Table 16.6.

External Stakeholders: External stakeholders include outside influences from local, federal and state initiatives. Additionally, many local and state health departments are involved with policy and initiatives in state funded and supported child care centers. Health education grant funding is also an area of external influence that could prove to be beneficial to child care centers and could help to offer more programs specifically for preschool aged children.

Table 16.6 Summary of essential child care center stakeholders.

Stakeholder group	Stakeholder members
External influences	• Political leaders (local, state, federal initiatives and mandates)
	• Health Department
	• Nonprofit health promotion groups or coalitions
	• Externally funded health education grants
Structural or administrative levels	• CEO
	• Management group
Internal layers	• School or Center Director
	• Teachers
	• Teaching Assistants
	• Students
Local community	• Parents

Structural/Administrative Level: At a structural or administrative level, a preschool CEO or management company that is involved with privately funded or state funded day care centers can play a role in decision making processes and the overall structure of a child care setting. These administrative figures sometime view the financial needs of the center as a first priority and choose less expensive, less healthy foods to replace more expensive, better quality foods. Like schools, child care centers might see the day when competitive foods are necessary to augment financial stability.

Internal School Layers: At the internal level, center directors, like school principals, handle day-to-day operational needs and quality control within the center. Their role is to oversee the care that children receive from teachers and assistants employed by the centers. Children's care and safety are the main concern of every child care center director, and children's nutritional and physical needs may be of much lower concern or priority. The ability to provide nutrition and physical activity programs would improve if structured nutrition and activity programs or guidelines were readily available to encourage provision of a healthy environment for the children. Head Start may provide such a model. It is designed to meet the needs of low income children but the principles and guidelines for nutrition and activity could be much more widely applied. Because one Head Start objective is to provide an ongoing source of healthcare to children, heights and weights are being collected, BMI's calculated and parents are given guidelines on nutrition and physical activity for their children. Although it is unclear how these data are being used and distributed to families, Head Start provides a good model for privately funded programs to adapt and implement based on their individual needs (Story, Kaphingst, & French, 2006).

Teachers and teaching assistants serve the role of instructing and providing safe care for children at their centers. Unfortunately, overcrowding and large ratios of children per teacher may make their jobs extremely difficult. With the demand of caring for so many children at one time, teachers and their assistants have little time for program development and implementation. Teachers roles in providing healthcare to children could become easier with the support of a program similar to Head Start. With the support and guidance of a developed program, the burden of providing this additional care to children could diminish.

Local Community: Children at preschool age are usually more dependent on parents than school-aged children. In particular, they are dependent on them to provide nutrition, transportation, assistance with basic decision-making and even simple hygienic needs. This dependency could make parents more accessible to their children's child care centers for programs and interventions. Involving parents in a nutrition and physical activity component of preschool could be provided through weekly newsletters or homework assignments that mirror that of what their children are being taught as nutrition or physical activity lessons weekly at their center. Fitzgibbon found that 61% of parents of intervention children in Hip Hop to Health Jr. completed at least one of three homework assignments per week and 88% reported reading the weekly newsletter. Fitzgibbon's study (2002) was limited to Head Start programs, but could be adapted to work with privately funded child care centers.

Evaluation

Outcome measures for program evaluation should include: BMI measurements; measurements of intervention goals such foods served or physical activity offered and MVPA; and measures of dietary intake, physical activity and sedentary activity. To fully evaluate the program's effect on the school culture additional measures should include: academic performance, such as standardized test scores, absenteeism and disciplinary action school; environmental influences; and economic costs and benefits. Outcome evaluations are only one type of evaluation needed, in part because a long time may be needed to influence outcomes. Interim measures of process and intermediate variables can indicate whether the efforts are on track and sufficiently comprehensive and integrated. Principles of action for obesity prevention have been identified, applicable to diverse settings (Kumanyika, Jeffrey, Morabia, Ritenbaugh, & Antipatis, 2002). These principles were used by Doak et al. (2006) to form 12 specific questions used to evaluate intervention programs for childhood obesity. Although these questions were utilized for a literature review, they serve as useful criteria for any school based intervention or evaluation. Table 16.7 lists the 12 question criteria for evaluating interventions drawing on criteria by Kumanyika et al. (2002).

Recommendations

This section provides recommendations for both school-based and child care center prevention programs. Schools and child care centers differ greatly in structure but both offer opportunities to make changes to physical activity and eating habits among children and adolescents. While the literature and the environment vary for schools and child care centers, the planning and implementation steps necessary to guide primary prevention efforts remain remarkably similar. Future programs in both types of settings should follow parallel paths.

Table 16.7 Criteria for evaluating interventions in school and child care settings (adapted from Doak et al., 2006; Kumanyika et al., 2002).

1. Does the intervention address dietary habits, physical activity patterns and television viewing of children?

2. For interventions that include physical activity intervention, does the intervention include activities inside and outside school?

3. Does the intervention seek to change behaviors by changing the physical, economic, or sociocultural environment within the school and/or child care setting?

4. Is the program sustainable over time at the structural and institutional level with minimal additional inputs?

5. What is the level of involvement from the participants, parents, teachers and/or broader community?

6. Is the intervention a primary prevention program tailored to the needs of the local community, schools and/or families that are included in the target population?

7. To what extent does the intervention address family and individual factors and the interaction of these with school and/or child care factors?

8. If effective, does the intervention have external validity to national, regional, or community levels?

9. Does the intervention build links between sectors by involving multiple organizations/groups that may otherwise be viewed as independent?

10. Does the intervention reach all children in the community?

11. Is there potential for integrating the program into existing initiatives? Did the program tap into existing initiatives or preexisting programs?

12. Did the program build on existing theory and evidence?

Robinson and Sirard suggest that while there is increasing interest in applying environmental and policy approaches for preventing childhood obesity, the research to inform policy change is lagging (Robinson & Sirard, 2005). Research has historically followed a problem-oriented model designed to identify causality of disease states, or in this case, determinants of childhood obesity. The authors strongly promote a change in paradigm towards solution-oriented research for school based environmental research and programs for primary prevention of childhood obesity. The obvious difference in these approaches is that the solution-oriented research paradigm leads to research questions with direct relevance to policy and practice. Examples of solution-oriented research paradigm questions include: without waiting for proof that soda sales in schools causes obesity, the question posed would be: will eliminating soda in schools affect childhood obesity? This type of question results in answers to both association and effect of soda removal.

Despite the number of research articles published on school-based interventions, relatively few studies exist with consistent designs and findings with which to compare and make evidence-based recommendations and determine the most cost effective and health promoting strategies to achieve healthy weights in youth (Summerbell et al., 2005). The Cochrane Collaboration Report suggests that future research should be undertaken with evaluation designs sufficiently powered to determine what works and what does not. In addition, interventions with sufficient sustainability and parental involvement are suggested. Other research areas recommended by the Cochrane group include designing methods of following participants for long term evaluation; reporting of BMI as well as other measures of adiposity; evaluating sustainability and cost effectiveness, and the inclusion of process evaluation measures.

Table 16.8 IOM recommendations for schools (IOM, 2005).

USDA, state, and local authorities, and schools should:

• Develop and implement nutritional standards for all competitive foods and beverages sold or served in schools

• Ensure that all school meals meet the Dietary Guidelines for Americans

• Develop, implement and evaluate pilot programs to extend school meal funding in schools with a large percentage of children at risk of obesity

State and local educational authorities and schools should:

• Ensure that all children and youth participate in a minimum of 30 min of moderate to vigorous physical activity during the school day

• Expand opportunities for physical activity through physical education classes; intramural and interscholastic sports programs and other physical activity clubs, programs, and lesson; after-school use of facilities, use of schools as community centers; and walking- and biking-to-school programs

• Enhance health curricula to devote adequate attention to nutrition, physical activity, reducing sedentary behaviors, and energy balance, and to include a behavioral skills focus

• Develop, implement, and enforce school policies to create schools that are advertising-free to the greatest extent possible

• Involve school health services in obesity prevention efforts

• Conduct annual assessments of each student's weight, height, and gender- and age-specific BMI percentile and make this information available to parents

• Perform periodic assessments of each school's policies and practices related to nutrition, physical activity, and obesity prevention

Federal and state departments of education and health professional organizations should:

• Develop, implement, and evaluate pilot programs to explore innovative approaches to both staffing and teaching about wellness, healthful choices, nutrition, physical activity, and reducing sedentary behaviors. Innovative approaches to recruiting and training appropriate teachers are also needed

As discussed earlier in this chapter, the vast majority of children and youth are in school and child care for extended periods of time, affording opportunities for them to not only learn about the desired health behaviors but providing a safe place for them to practice these behaviors. Schools can influence this process by teaching, providing, demonstrating and modeling and reinforcing examples of healthy behaviors likely to influence obesity. The IOM recommends, "Schools should provide a consistent environment that is conducive to healthful eating behaviors and regular physical activity" (IOM, 2005). Table 16.8 lists and describes the recommendations for improving school environments to facilitate obesity prevention. Some of these recommendations are directed to federal agencies, but many can be implemented by state and local authorities.

Summary

The prevalence and consequences of childhood overweight and obesity are staggering. Schools and child-care centers provide an opportunity to systematically improve eating and activity habits through both environmental change and education. This opportunity has not yet been realized however. Significant barriers exist, the most prominent of which is the perceived and/or real competition of nutrition and physical activity programs with the core mission of academic achievement or of providing safe and nurturing but cost effective child care.

Many interventions have been attempted in school settings. With some notable exceptions, most interventions have not affected BMI. The reasons for this are unclear but may include insufficient dose, programs that were too broad, focused more on individual behavior than on policy change, were not sufficiently comprehensive (related to dose), or had inadequate evaluation. Given the stakes, we suggest that intervention and evaluation efforts continue in schools and child care centers as described in this chapter. While top-down, protocol driven efforts are useful for proof-of-concept in laboratory settings or efficacy studies, schools and child care centers may also be well-served by policy-driven approaches that have their roots in the local school culture. The importance of continued evaluation cannot be overstated, particularly evaluations that can provide clues to why programs are effective or not effective. Ultimately, if BMI or similar summative outcomes remain largely unaffected by a new generation of studies, it may be time to conclude that child-care center and school-based interventions are necessary but not sufficient to affect BMI among children.

References

Allensworth, D. D., & Kolbe, L. J. (1987). The comprehensive school health program. Exploring an expanded concept. *Journal of School Health, 57*, 409–412.

Alliance for a Healthier Generation. (2006, May 3). *Memorandum of understanding*. Retrieved November 16, 2006, from http://www.healthiergeneration.org/engine/renderpage.asp?pid=s017

American Academy of Pediatrics (AAP). (2000). Physical fitness and activity in schools. *Pediatrics, 105*(5), 1156–1157.

American Diabetes Association. (2006). Presence of diabetes risk factors in a large U.S. eighth-grade cohort. *Diabetes Care, 29*(2), 212–217.

Baranowski, T., Mendlein, J., Resnicow, K., Frank, E., Cullen, K., & Baronowski, J. (2000). Physical activity and nutrition in children and youth: An overview of obesity prevention. *Preventive Medicine, 31*, S1–S10.

Baranowski, T., Cullen, K. W., Nicklas, T., Thompson, D., & Baranowski, J. (2002). School based obesity prevention: A blueprint for taming the epidemic. *American Journal of Health Behavior, 26*(6), 486–493.

Burgeson, C. R., Wechsler, H., Brener, N. D., Young, J. C., & Spain, C. G. (2001). Physical education and activity: Results from the School Health Policies and Programs Study 2000. *Journal of School Health, 71*(7), 279–293.

Caballero, B., Clay, T., Davis, S. M., Ethelbah, B., Rock, B. H., Lohman, T., et al. (2003). Pathways: A school-based, randomized controlled trial for the prevention of obesity in American Indian schoolchildren. *American Journal of Clinical Nutrition, 78*(5), 1030–1038.

Capizzano, J., & Adams, G. (2000). The hours that children under five spend in child care: variations across states. *Urban Institute, B-8*, 1–11.

Casper, L. M. (1996). Who's minding our preschoolers? *United States Bureau of the Census: Current Population Reports, P70-53*, 1–7.

Centers for Disease Control and Prevention. (1997). Guidelines for school and community programs to promote lifelong physical activity among young people. *Morbidity and Mortality Weekly Report, 46*, 1–36.

Centers for Disease Control and Prevention. (2005a). Competitive foods and beverages available for purchase in secondary schools—selected sites, United States, 2004. *Morbidity and Mortality Weekly Report, 54*(37), 917–921.

Centers for Disease Control and Prevention. (2005b). *School health index: A self assessment and planning guide*. Atlanta. Retrieved July 11, 2005, from http://www.cdc.gov/healthyyouth/shi

Child and Adult Care Food Program (CACFP). (1999). Retrieved May 26, 2006 from http://www.cacfp.org/index.html

Child Nutrition and WIC Reauthorization Act of 2004. S.2507. Section 204. Local Wellness Policy. Retrieved December 2, 2006, from http://www.schoolwellnesspolicies.org/resources/Section204LocalWellnessPolicies.pdf,

Cole, N. (2001). *The prevalence of overweight among WIC children*. Alexandria, VA: U.S. Department of Agriculture, Food, and Nutrition Service.

Cullen, K. W., & Thompson, D. I. (2005). Texas school food policy change related to middle school a la carte/ snack bar foods: potential savings in kilocalories. *Journal of the American Dietetic Association, 105*(12), 1952–1954.

Daniels, S. R., Arnett, D. K., Eckel, R. H., Gidding, S. S., Hayman, L. L., Kumanyika, S., et al. (2005). Overweight in children and adolescents: Pathophysiology, consequences, prevention and treatment. *Circulation, 111*, 1999–2012.

Dennison, B. A., Erb, T. A., & Jenkins, P. L. (2002). Television viewing and television in bedroom associated with overweight risk among low-income preschool children. *Pediatrics, 109*, 1028–1035.

Dennison, B. A., Russo, T. J., Burdick, P. A., & Jenkins, P. L. (2004). An intervention to reduce television viewing by preschool children. *Archives of Pediatric and Adolescent Medicine., 158*(2), 170–176.

Doak, C. M., Visscher, T. L. S., Renders, C. M., & Seidell, J. C. (2006). The prevention of overweight and obesity in children and adolescents: A review of interventions and programmes. *Obesity Reviews, 7*, 111–136.

Donnelly, J. E., Jacobsen, D. J., Whatley, J. E., Hill, J. O., Swift, L. L., Cherrington, A., et al. (1996). Nutrition and physical activity program to attenuate obesity and promote physical and metabolic fitness in elementary school children. *Obesity Research, 4*, 229–243.

Dunn, C., Thomas, C., Ward, D., Pegram, L., Webber, K., & Cullitan, C. (2006). Design and implementation of a nutrition and physical activity curriculum for child care settings. *Preventing Chronic Disease, 3*(2), 1–8.

Fitzgibbon, M. L., Stolley, M. R., Dyer, A. R., Van Horn, L., & Kaufer-Christoffel, K. (2002). A community-based obesity prevention program for minority children: Rationale and study design for hip-hop to health jr. *Preventive Medicine, 34*, 289–297.

Fitzgibbon, M. L., Stolley, M. R., Schiffer, L., Van Horn, L., KauferChristoffel, K., & Dyer, A. (2006). Hip-Hop to Health Jr. for Latino preschool children. *Obesity, 14*(9), 1616–1625.

Foster, G. D., Sherman, S., Grundy, K., Sargent, S., Shults, J., Kumanyika, S. K., et al. (2006). A randomized trial of a school-based obesity prevention program. *Obesity, 14*(9) Abstract Supplement: A49.

The Food Research and Action Center (FRAC), "Child Nutrition Fact Sheet: Child and Adult Car Food Program (CACFP)". (2006). Retrieved May 31, 2006, from http://www.frac.org/pdf/cncacfp.PDF

Friedman, M. (2006). *Child care. Coalition of human needs*.Retrieved May 31, 2006from http://www.policyalmanac.org/social_welfare/child care.shtml

Gortmaker, S. L., Peterson, K., Wiecha, J., Sobol, A. M., Dixit, S., Fox, M. K.et al. (1999a). Reducing obesity via a school-based interdisciplinary intervention among youth: Planet Health. *Archives of Pediatric and Adolescent Medicine, 153*(4), 409–418.

Gortmaker, S. L., Cheung, L. W., Peterson, K. E., Chomitz, G., Cradle, J. H., Dart, H., et al. (1999b). Impact of a school-based interdisciplinary intervention on diet and physical activity among urban primary school children: Eat well and keep moving. *Archives of Pediatric and Adolescent Medicine, 153*(9), 975–983.

Guo, S. S., & Chumlea, W. C. (1999). Tracking of body mass index in children in relation to overweight in adulthood. *American Journal of Clinical Nutrition, 70*, 145S–148S.

Institute of Medicine (IOM). (2005). J. P. Koplan, C. T. Liverman, & V. I. Kraak (Eds.), *Preventing childhood obesity, health in the balance.* Washington, DC: National Academies Press.

Institute of Medicine (IOM). (2006, October 12). *Nutrition standards for foods in schools.* Retrieved November 16, 2006, from http://www.iom.edu/CMS/3788/30181.aspx.

Jago, R., & Baranowski, T. (2004). Non-curricular approaches for increasing physical activity in youth: A review. *Preventive Medicine, 39*, 157–163.

James, J., Thomas, P., Cavan, D., & Kerr, D. (2004). Preventing childhood obesity by reducing consumption of carbonated drinks: Cluster randomized controlled trial. *British Medical Journal, 328*(7450), 1236.

Kahn, E. B., Ramsey, L. T., Brownson, R. C., Heath, G. W., Howze, E. H., Powell, K. E., et al. (2002). The effectiveness of interventions to increase physical activity: A systematic review. *American Journal of Preventive Medicine, 22*(4S), 73–107.

Kain, J., Uauy Albala, R., Vio, F., Cerda, R., & Leyton, B. (2004). School-based obesity prevention in Chilean primary school children: Methodology and evaluation of a controlled study. *International Journal of Obesity, 28*, 483–493.

Katz, D. L., O'Connell, M., et al. (2005). Public health strategies for preventing and controlling overweight and obesity in school and worksite settings: A report on recommendations of the Task Force on Community Preventive Services. *Morbidity and Mortality Weekly Report. Recommendations & Reports., 54*(RR-10), 1–12.

Kuczmarski, R. J., Ogden, C. L., Grummer-Strawn, L. M., Flegal, K. M., Guo, S. S., Wei, R., et al. (2000). CDC growth charts: United States. *Advance Data, 8*(314), 1–27.

Kumanyika, S., Jeffrey, R. W., Morabia, A., Ritenbaugh, C., & Antipatis, V. J. (2002). Obesity prevention: The case for action. *International Journal of Obesity and related metabolic disorders, 26*, 425–436.

Luepker, R. V., Rastam, L., Hannan, P. J., Murray, D. M., Gray, C., Baker, W. L.,et al. (1996). Community education for cardiovascular disease prevention. Morbidity and Mortality results from the Minnesota Heart Health Program. *American Journal of Epidemiology, 144*, 351–362.

Lytle, L. A., Stone, E. J., Nichaman, M. Z., Perry, C. L., Montgomery, D. H., Nicklas, T. A., et al. (1996). Changes in nutrient intakes of elementary school children following a school-based intervention: Results from the CATCH study. *Preventive Medicine, 25*, 465–477.

Lytle, L. A., Murray, D. M., Perry, C. L., Story, M., Birnbaum, A. S., Kubik, M. Y.,et al. (2004). School-based approaches to affect adolescents' diets: Results from the TEENS study. *Health Education & Behavior, 31*(2), 270–287.

Manios, Y., Moschandreas, J., Hatzis, C., & Kafatos, A. (1999). Evaluation of a health and nutrition education program in primary school children of Crete over a three-year period. *Preventive Medicine, 28*, 149–159.

McDonnell, E., Probart, C., Weirich, E., Hartman, T., & Bailey-Davis, L. (2006). School competitive food policies: Perceptions of Pennsylvania public high school foodservice directors and principals. *Journal of the American Dietetic Association, 106*(2), 271–276.

McKenzie, T. L., Nader, P. R., Strikmiller, P. K., Yang, M., Stone, E. J., Perry, C. L., et al. (1996). School physical education: Effect of the Child and Adolescent Trial for Cardiovascular Health. *Preventive Medicine, 25*, 423–431.

McKenzie, T. L., Sallis, J. F., Kolody, B., & Faucette, F. N. (1997). Long-term effects of a physical education curriculum and staff development program: SPARK. *Res Q Exerc Sport, 68*(4), 280–291.

Nader, P. R., Sellers, D. E., Johnson, C. C., Perry, C. L., Stone, E. J., Cook, K. C., et al. (1996). The effect of adult participation in a school-based family intervention to improve children's diet and physical activity: The child and adolescent trial for cardiovascular health. *Preventive Medicine, 25*, 455–464.

National Alliance for Nutrition and Activity (NANA). (2006). *Model school wellness policies*. Retrieved December 2, 2006, from http://www.cspinet.org/nutritionpolicy/nana.html

Neumark-Sztainer, D., Story, M., Hannan, P. J., & Rex, J. (2003). New moves: A school-based obesity prevention program for adolescent girls. *Preventive Medicine, 37*(1), 41–51.

No Child Left Behind Act 200. (U.S.C) Public Law 107-110.115 STAT. 1425. (2002).

Ogden, C. L., Carroll, M. D., Curtin, L. R., McDowell, M. A., Tabak, C. J., & Flegal, K. M. (2006). Prevalence of overweight and obesity in the United States, 1999–2004. *Journal of the American Medical Association, 295*, 1549–1555.

Parker, L. (2000). The federal nutrition programs: A safety net for very young children. *Zero to Three, 21*(1), 29–36.

Pate, R. R., Pfeiffer, K. A., Trost, S. G., Ziegler, P., & Dowda M. (2004). Physical activity among children attending preschools. *Pediatrics, 114*(5), 1258–1263.

Robinson, T. N. (1999). Reducing children's television viewing to prevent obesity: A randomized controlled trial. *Journal of the American Medical Association, 282*, 1561–1567.

Robinson, T. N., & Sirard, J. R. (2005). Preventing childhood obesity: A solution-oriented research paradigm. *American Journal of Preventive Medicine, 28*(2 Suppl. 2), 194–201.

Sahota, P., Rudolf, M. C., Dixey, R., Hill, A. J., Barth, J. H., & Cade, J. (2001). Evaluation of implementation and effect of primary school based intervention to reduce risk factors for obesity. *British Medical Journal, 323*(7320), 1027–1029.

Sallis, J. F., McKenzie, T. L., Alcaraz, J. E., Kolody, B., Faucette, N., & Hovell, M. F. (1997). The effects of a 2-year physical education program (SPARK) on physical activity and fitness in elementary school students. Sports, Play and Active Recreation for Kids. *American Journal of Public Health, 87*, 1328–1334.

Sallis, J. F., McKenzie, T. L., Kolody, B., Lewis, M., Marshall, S. & Rosengard, P. (1999). Effects of health-related physical education on academic achievement: Project SPARK. *Research Quarterly for Exercise and Sport, 70*(2), 127–134.

Simons-Morton, B. G., Parcel, G. S., Baranowski, T., Forthofer, R., & O'Hara, N. M. (1991). Promoting physical activity and a healthful diet among children: Results of a school-based intervention study. *American Journal of Public Health, 81*, 986–991.

Spiegel, S. A., & Foulk, D.(2006). Reducing overweight through a multidisciplinary school-based intervention. *Obesity, 14(1)*, 88–96.

The STOPP-T2D Prevention Study Group, Kaufman, F. R., Baranowski, T., Cooper, D. M., Harrell, J., Hirst, K., Goran, M., & Resnicow, K. (2006). Presence of diabetes risk factors in a large U.S. eighth-grade cohort. *Diabetes Care, 29*(2), 212–217.

Story, M. (1999). School-based approaches for preventing and treating obesity. *International Journal of Obesity and related metabolic disorders, 23*(Suppl. 2), S43–S51.

Story, M., Kaphingst, K. M., & French, S. (2006). The role of child care settings in obesity prevention. *Childhood Obesity, 16*(1), 143–168.

Strong, W. B., Malina, R. M., Bumke, C. J. R., Daniels, S. R., Dishman, R. K., Gutin, B., et al. (2005). Evidence based physical activity for school-age youth. *J Pediatrics, 146*, 732–737.

Summerbell, C. D., Waters, E., Edmunds, L. D., Kelly, S., Brown, T., & Campbell, K. J. (2005). Interventions for preventing obesity in children (Review). *Cochrane Database Syst Rev, 3*, CD001871.

Taras, H. (2005). Physical activity and student performance at school. *Journal of School Health, 75*(6), 214–218.

U.S. Department of Agriculture (USDA). (2004). The Child Nutrition and WIC Reauthorization Act of 2004. Public Law 108–265. Section 204. *Local school wellness policies.* http://www.fns.usda.gov/cnd/Governance/Legislation/Historical/PL_108-265.pdf

U.S. Department of Agriculture (USDA). (2005). Fit WIC: Programs to Prevent Childhood Overweight in Your Community. Alexandria, VA: U.S. Department of Agriculture, Food and Nutrition Service. http://www.fns.usda.gov/oane.

U.S. Department of Agriculture, U.S. Department of Education, U.S. Department of Health and Human Services, CDC. Making it happen! School Nutrition success stories. Alexandria (September 7, 2005);
http://www.cdc.gov/healthyyouth/nutrition/making-it=happen/index.htm

U.S. Department of Health and Human Services. (1996). Physical activity and health: A report of the Surgeon General. Atlanta, Georgia: U.S. Department of Health and Human Services, Public Health Service, CDC, National Center for Chronic Disease Prevention and Health Promotion.

U.S. Department of Health and Human Services, U.S. Department of Education. (2000). Promoting better health for young people through physical activity and sports: A report to the president from the secretary of health and human services and the secretary of education. Atlanta, Georgia: U.S. Department of Health and Human Services.

U.S. Department of Health and Human Services and U.S. Department of Agriculture. (2005). *Dietary Guidelines for Americans* (6th ed.). Government Printing Office.

Chapter 17

Individual Behavior Change

Myles S. Faith and Eva Epstein

Introduction

All obesity prevention and treatment strategies ultimately depend on individual behavior change related to caloric intake and expenditure. What differentiates approaches is whether they engage individuals through direct interpersonal contact or attempt to influence their behavior indirectly, e.g., through information dissemination or environmental manipulations, and the unit of intervention, i.e., single individuals, groups of individuals, or whole communities. Much of the potentially relevant knowledge about individual behavior change is drawn from studies that were designed to produce weight loss (treatment) rather than to prevent weight gain. As discussed in Chapter 5, although the types of behaviors targeted are similar, obesity prevention may require conceptual frameworks and approaches that differ from those for obesity treatment (Kumanyika & Obarzanek, 2003). The specific program goals and populations addressed will also influence the extent to which obesity treatment evidence and models apply. For example, individual or group based obesity treatment approaches that involve intensive personal counseling may be quite applicable for a program to prevent obese children from becoming obese adults or to stabilize weight in overweight children or adults during periods that pose a high risk of rapid weight gain (e.g., during pubertal or perimenopausal transitions; immediately postpartum, during smoking cessation, or when medications that tend to cause weight gain are prescribed (Arenz, Ruckerl, Koletzko, & von Kries, 2004; Copeland, Martin, Geiselman, Rash, & Kendzor, 2006; Littrell, Hilligoss, Kirshner, Petty, & Johnson, 2003; Menza et al., 2004). For normal weight children and adults in the general population, broadly based social marketing strategies to motivate permanent adoption of specific but modest changes in routine eating and physical activity patterns may be appropriate, perhaps combined with some direct, individual-level advice.

The purpose of this chapter is to describe overall principles and concepts related to changing individual behavior that apply across life stages, intervention approaches, and settings. This 'primer' provides background for Chapters 18 through 21 in particular. These chapters, respectively, review concepts and evidence related to obesity prevention during gestation and infancy, preschool and school age years, pre-adolescence and adolescence,

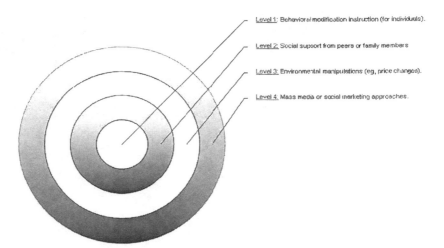

Level 1: Behavioral modification instruction (for individuals).

Level 2: Social support from peers or family members

Level 3: Environmental manipulations (eg, price changes).

Level 4. Mass media or social marketing approaches.

Figure 17.1 Concentric circles representing the four levels of behavior change that emanate from an ecological model.

and adulthood. In the present chapter, we describe and highlight evidence on behavior change approaches at four complementary levels that emanate from an ecological model (see Figure 17.1): (1) *behavioral modification* instruction, e.g., personalized counseling in techniques geared to changing eating or physical activity behaviors; (2) *social support* from peers or family members for making behavior changes; (3) *environmental manipulations* such as pricing structure changes at food purchase locations; and (4) *mass media or social marketing* approaches for information dissemination. Theories that support these different approaches are referenced. Two additional, cross cutting issues are also discussed: tailoring, i.e., adaptation of interventions to improve relevance for specific ethnic, gender, or socioeconomic subgroups, and motivation, i.e., the extent to which individuals or groups perceive obesity as a paramount problem in their lives and are ready to make changes. We have provided a selective review of the literature to highlight key issues; more extensive reviews of specific interventions are available elsewhere (Brug & van Lenthe, 2005; *Committee on Prevention of Obesity in Children and Youth. Preventing Childhood Obesity. Health in Balance*, 2004; Doak, Visscher, Renders, & Seidell, 2006; Kahn et al., 2002; Matson-Koffman, Brownstein, Neiner, & Greaney, 2005; Summerbell et al., 2005).

Behavior Change Theories and Frameworks

Many theoretical models have been developed to account for pathways to behavior change. This section summarizes several of the most prominent theoretical models that have been developed and tested over the years: Learning theory/operant conditioning, Social learning theory, Behavioral economics, Transtheoretical model, Social ecological model, and Diffusion theory. Most of these are testable theory-based models, although some are planning frameworks that may incorporate theory (e.g., the socioecological model). Although these frameworks did not evolve specifically to address nutrition and obesity prevention per se, they have been applied to these issues.

Learning theory/operant conditioning. This theoretical model describes how behaviors are initiated and maintained as a function of their consequences (Ferster & Skinner, 1957). Thus, behaviors that are followed by positive consequences tend to be sustained whereas behaviors that are followed by negative consequences are less likely to occur. For example, the theory predicts that children will be more likely to eat fruits and vegetables if they are repeatedly praised for these choices by parents compared to children whose parents do not praise or otherwise reinforce such choices. Classical behavioral treatment studies for obese adults, conducted by Stuart (1967), were based on learning theory.

Social learning theory. This theoretical model describes how behaviors are initiated and maintained by social learning and role modeling, in addition to the direct consequences outlined by traditional learning theory. This model, also called social cognitive theory (Bandura, 1977, 1986), underscores the role of observational learning. For example, the theory predicts that children will be more likely to eat chips and pretzels as snacks if their own caregivers eat those same snacks themselves, compared to children whose caregivers role model healthier snack choices. Social learning principles are relevant for understanding why social support enhances weight control efforts among family members (discussed below).

Behavioral economics theory. This theoretical model describes how behavioral choices are critically dependent upon cost as well as other choices that are concurrently available. The model incorporates many concepts from economic theory and is also influenced by basic animal studies (Bickel, Madden, & Petry, 1998; Bickel & Vuchinich, 2000). Behavioral economic studies have been applied to many laboratory-based food choice studies with obese and nonobese adults and children (Epstein & Saelens, 2000). These studies show how the decision to eat healthier foods can be increased by either reducing access to, or increasing the cost of, less healthy foods.

Transtheoretical model. This theoretical model describes the different levels of readiness to change that people experience when contemplating behavior change. The framework posits that behavior change progresses or cycles through six stages of change: precontemplation, contemplation, preparation, action, maintenance, and determination (Prochaska & Velicer, 1997). The framework recognizes that not all members of a group or community recognize a disorder or are prepared to make changes, and emphasizes the importance of assessing an individual's readiness to make behavior changes. The framework has been applied to the topics of diet (Di Noia, Schinke, Prochaska, & Contento, 2006; Horwath, 1999) and exercise interventions (Marcus & Simkin, 1994).

Social ecological model. This theoretical model describes the importance of studying how children or adults interact with others over prolonged periods of time, in the natural environment, for understanding the development of human behavior (Bronfenbrenner, 1979). The model underscores that behavioral choices are not made in a vacuum or in isolation of the broader social environment; the roles of family, community, and broader society are critical to this theory. The social ecological model is pertinent to current interests in the "toxic environment"–factors that may be saturating the environment with inexpensive and low nutrient foods and thereby contributing to rising obesity rates (Battle & Brownell, 1996; Brownell & Horgen, 2004).

Diffusion theory. This theoretical model describes the manner in which new technological ideas or techniques migrate from creation to use on a larger social level (Rogers, 1995). The theory posits that technological innovations are communicated through different channels, over time, as they become incorporated into the larger social system. Interpersonal channels are important aspects of model, which describes various stages of technological innovation including *knowledge, persuasion, decision, implementation,* and *confirmation.* This model is pertinent to many current technological innovations related to weight control behavior change, including Internet-based approaches (Womble et al., 2004).

Behavior Modification

The "nuts and bolts" of lasting behavior change are framed at the individual level. Many of the specific strategies for individual behavior change come from the obesity treatment literature, although these principles have been applied in obesity prevention studies conducted in clinics (Epstein et al., 2001) and schools (Robinson, 1999). These strategies generally strive to: (1) *enhance awareness* of targeted behavior; (2) *modify* the antecedent situations and/or consequences, associated with the targeted behavior; and (3) *reinforce* changes in the targeted behavior. As summarized below, these aims are achieved through a series of processes that stem from operant conditioning and social learning theories (described previously). These processes include self-monitoring, a "functional analysis of behavior," goal setting, feedback, stimulus control, and reinforcement procedures (Wadden, Crerand, & Brock, 2005). Each process is explained below.

Self-monitoring. A critical step for initiating, and ultimately maintaining, individual behavior change is *self-monitoring* (Foreyt & Goodrick, 1991). The main utility of self-monitoring is to provide feedback on the frequency with which the target behavior typically occurs, something that individuals can be notoriously poor at estimating. When adults are challenged to estimate how much television they watch during a typical week, or how many servings of fruits and vegetables they consume each day, estimates are often inaccurate despite the best of intentions. Self-monitoring addresses this problem, by requiring one to record each time a targeted behavior occurs during an observation period (Korotitsch & Nelson-Gray, 1999). The situation in which the target behavior occurs can also be monitored, to raise awareness of the contextual cues that relate to the target behavior and for a functional analysis of behavior (see below). A variety of target behaviors can be monitored, including the intake of specific foods (e.g., fruits and vegetables, energy-dense foods), total food intake, minutes of physical activity, and television or screen viewing time. Therefore, precisely defining the target behavior is a key part of self-monitoring.

There are a variety of diaries, forms, logs, and formats that can be used for self-monitoring. In addition, the mere action of tracking one's behavior can promote behavior change and, therefore, can be an effective intervention (Kazdin, 2001). The frequency with which individuals self-monitor is a reliable predictor of weight loss in obese children and adults (Berkowitz, Wadden, Tershakovec, & Cronquist, 2003; Wadden et al., 2005) and is associated with long-term weight loss maintenance (Wing & Hill, 2001). At the same time, successful weight loss, increased feelings of control, and enhanced weight control are often powerful reinforcements that can enhance the act of monitoring. Finally, self-monitoring can provide an "objective" benchmark against which goal setting (see below) can be determined and behavior change can be evaluated.

Functional analysis of behavior. Understanding the functions that behaviors serve can facilitate behavior change. To this end, a functional analysis of behavior (FAB) can be used to determine the situational circumstances that promote a target behavior and the consequences that sustain it. Self-monitoring strategies can raise awareness of these relations and allow for a FAB. Specifically, FAB involves a detailed analysis of the *antecedents* of the target behavior (i.e., What factors or contexts precede behavior change?), the target *behavior* itself, and the *consequences* of the behavior (e.g., What reactions does the behavior elicit from others that might sustain behavior change?). When successfully implemented, a FAB can highlight environmental changes that might be helpful in facilitating behavior changes among individuals who are exposed to the environments in question.

Goal setting. Goal setting is a well-established individual behavior change strategy. Based on the learning principle of *successive approximation*, individuals are encouraged to set small attainable goals that build up to a larger goal. Smaller goals are more likely to be attained, thereby providing a sense of mastery that can support additional behavior change (Wadden & Foster, 2000). Reappraisal of goals, a common strategy for behavior change, involves setting new goals if initial goals were not achieved, and revisiting or revising goals that have not yet been achieved. An important consideration is establishing achievable goals. It is well documented, for example, that many obese adults hold weight loss goals that are unlikely to be achieved even with superior behavior modification programs (Foster, Wadden, Vogt, & Brewer, 1997; Wadden et al., 2003). This may lead to frustration and hinder behavior change.

Stimulus control. Increasing the frequency of more healthy behaviors (e.g., fruit and vegetable intake) is easier when cues for less healthy behaviors are removed or limited from the environment (Heatherton & Nichols, 1994), a concept known as *stimulus control*. Examples of stimulus control for reducing intake of undesirable foods include restricting the location where eating takes place (e.g., limiting eating at home to the kitchen and/or dining room), the people with whom social eating occurs (e.g., friends who regularly go for ice cream), the activities associated with undesirable food choices (e.g., television viewing), or the times when eating occurs out of the home (i.e., on the way home from work) (Wadden & Foster, 2000). As another example, Robinson (1999) demonstrated that altering the home environment to limit television access was associated with increased physical activity and weight gain prevention in children.

Television watching may influence both physical activity, or inactivity, and eating behavior (Robinson, 2001).

Stimulus control not only involves the removal of cues that prompt undesirable behaviors, but it also includes the provision or amplification of cues that prompt desirable behaviors. A case in point is the literature on food provisions in the context of weight loss interventions for adult obesity. Behavioral interventions that provided obese patients with healthier foods to take home generally achieved greater weight loss success than comparable behavioral interventions that did not incorporate food provisions (Jeffery, 1995; Wing et al., 1996).

Feedback. Feedback is a critical component to behavior change and is typically achieved through careful self-monitoring of behavior. Feedback on weight control can also be achieved by regularly weighing oneself (e.g., weekly), which appears to be important for longer term maintenance of weight loss (Wing & Hill, 2001).

Positive Reinforcement Strategies. Positive reinforcement is an important component to individual behavior change, especially when it can help offset the discomfort of giving up less healthy behaviors (Wadden et al., 2005). Praise and recognition can be among the strongest strategies, which may explain why weight loss is enhanced when peers and family members are supportive. This is especially true for childhood obesity prevention and treatment strategies (Epstein, Myers, Raynor, & Saelens, 1998). Individual behavior change can be facilitated by self-reinforcement strategies in which people identify ways to reward their own behavior change without the use of foods (e.g., buying a special gift for oneself for reaching key goals).

An interesting concept related to positive reinforcement is that of *displacement* or *substitution*. There is some evidence that reinforcing, and thereby increasing, fruit and vegetable intake can lead to the "natural" displacement of energy-dense foods (Epstein et al., 2001; Goldfield & Epstein, 2002). This has been documented in at least one randomized clinical trial of children who were at-risk for obesity, whose parents were trained either to reward increased fruit and vegetable intake or reduced energy-dense food intake by their children (Epstein et al., 2001). Results indicated that both groups showed comparable reductions in percent overweight, suggesting that increasing fruit and vegetable intake may have displaced fat or sugar intake. However, there is considerable debate on this topic (Rolls, Ello-Martin, & Tohill, 2004). This issue is also relevant to other "levels" of intervention addressed in this chapter, most notably whether subsidization of healthier foods in vending machines will necessarily displace the purchase and intake of energy-dense foods.

Social Support

Social learning theory, summarized previously in this chapter, underscores the importance of social support for facilitating individual behavior change. Indeed, studies do indicate that peers and family members can play pivotal roles in facilitating individual behavior change for weight control. The best evidence for the role of *peer support* comes from randomized weight loss interventions that manipulated the extent to which additional patient or provider contact was provided to obese patients. Renjilian et al. (Renjilian et al., 2001) used a 2 (individual vs. group treatment) $\times$ 2 (preferred vs. non-preferred treatment modality) design to evaluate whether weight loss differed as a function of individual vs. group treatment, and whether the patient received his/her preferred treatment modality (i.e., preferred individual treatment vs. preferred group treatment). Results indicated that weight loss was significantly greater for individuals receiving group as opposed to individual treatment (mean weight losses = 11.0 kg vs. 9.0 kg, respectively). Whether or not patients received their preferred treatment modality did not influence weight loss.

A series of randomized weight loss trials by Perri and colleagues indicate that enhancing interpersonal contacts after weight loss treatment ends can improve maintenance of weight loss (Perri, 1992). Across studies, they found that weight loss maintenance was generally enhanced when adults were trained to form their own self-help or "buddy groups" after treatment ended, by providing post-treatment mail and phone contact with the weight loss counselor and by participating in a "social influence" program that included strategies for providing peer support by phone and group meetings.

One of the more illustrative examples of "enforced" peer support in a real world setting is the Trevose Behavior Modification Program, which is administered and directed by lay individuals, staffed by volunteers, and is free of charge to participants. Like conventional behavior modification programs, there are weekly 1-hour group sessions that teach behavior modification techniques (described previously). However, this program places strict attention to regular attendance and attaining behavior goals (i.e., they must reduce at least 15% of their initial body weight). Failure to achieve regular attendance and/or certain weight loss goals can result in dismissal from the group. In an uncontrolled study, Latner et al. (2000) reported that, among 171 obese individuals who entered the Trevose program between 1992 and 1993, the group's mean weight loss (even after assuming no benefit for those who dropped out) was 12.8 kg, or 13.7% of their initial body weight. Members who completed two years of treatment lost 19.3% of their initial body weight. The extent to which these impressive outcomes can be attributed specifically to enhanced social support per se needs to be evaluated.

Verheijden et al. (2005) provide a critical conceptual review on the role of social support in weight loss. They distinguish "structural" as opposed to "functional" social support for weight control, with the former referring to the availability of *actual* support givers (e.g., the number of friends in a self-help group), whereas the latter refers to *perceived* support givers. Their review of the literature concludes that few intervention studies had clear conceptual definitions or measures of social support. They recommend that future studies more precisely conceptualize and measure social support constructs.

With respect to *family support*, Brownell et al. (1978) conducted one of the first studies to document the role of family support for enhancing weight control. They studied the 8-month weight loss of obese adults assigned to one of three behavioral weight loss treatment conditions: (1) cooperative spouse-couples training, in which both the obese patient and his/her spouse attended all training sessions; (2) cooperative spouse-subject alone training, in which only the obese patient received treatment despite having a spouse who was willing to attend treatment; and (3) non-cooperative spouse training, in which the obese patient received treatment alone because his/her spouse was unwilling to attend. Participants and their spouses were randomized to the first two conditions, but not to the third condition. The behavioral training program was consistent for all patients. Results indicated that weight loss was significantly greater among subjects in the first group (13.6 kg) than for subjects in the second or third groups (8.8 kg and 6.8 kg, respectively). Similar to Brownell et al.'s (1978) results, other studies also found that weight loss is enhanced when spouses are included in treatment (Pearce, LeBow, & Orchard, 1981); however, not all studies found that including spouses in treatment improved weight loss for the target obese patient (Wing, Marcus, Epstein, & Kupfer, 1983).

More consistent evidence for the role of family support comes from family-based intervention studies for pediatric obesity. Reviews of this literature are provided elsewhere (Epstein et al., 1998); however, there is compelling evidence that obese children lose more weight when their parents are actively involved in treatment compared to when they are not. Epstein et al. (1994) provided 10-year follow up data on obese children and their parents who were randomly assigned to one of three family-based behavioral weight loss interventions: (1) an intervention that targeted the parent and child together; (2) an intervention that just targeted the child; or (3) a non-specific intervention that reinforced the families for attendance. Parents in the first group were trained actively in the behavioral change strategies (see next section) that could be applied to their children to help them achieve better lifestyle changes. Results indicated that 43% of the children in this first group reduced their percent overweight by at least 20% (a relatively large treatment effect), in comparison to only 22% of the children in the second group and 29% of the children in the third group.

Golan et al. (1998) compared the effects of a behavioral weight control intervention for obese children ages 6–11 years that targeted either the parent or the obese child as the active "agent" of behavior change. Both interventions used the same behavior change principles, including self-monitoring, stimulus control, and reinforcement (see below). After one year, reduction in child percent overweight was significantly greater among the intervention targeting parents (mean reduction = 14.6%) compared to the intervention targeting children (mean reduction = 8.1%). After seven years, the superior outcome of the parent intervention group remained significant (mean reductions = 29% vs. 20.2% in the two groups, respectively, $p < 0.05$) (Golan & Crow, 2004).

Taken together, these studies underscore the importance of peer and family support to individual weight control. These studies primarily come from randomized weight loss trials of overweight or obese adults, rather than prevention studies per se. However, the findings are pertinent to the topic of prevention and suggest that interpersonal support systems may be important variables for predicting outcomes. Additional research is needed to address this question.

Environmental and Policy Changes

The social ecological model, summarized previously in this chapter, emphasizes the role of broader community and societal influences on individual behavior. The model describes how people can choose only from options that are available in the environment and, therefore, provides a framework for showing how the positive or negative consequences for choices established in society (e.g., through the price and availability of foods) influence individual behavior. Guided by this model, several community-based interventions have attempted to promote healthier diets through providing incentives ("*incentivization*", i.e., reinforcement) of more nutritious foods. Incentivization refers to rewarding the purchase of healthier foods, which is achieved by reducing their prices. By contrast, others have discussed *taxation* (punishment) as a social ecological strategy to discourage unhealthier food choices. A series of articles by Brownell and colleagues, which advocate for public policy and legislation approaches to the prevention of obesity, have addressed this issue extensively (Brownell & Horgen, 2004; Horgen & Brownell, 2003; Jacobson & Brownell, 2000). These approaches are also covered in Chapter 13, 15, and 16 as they apply, respectively to communities, worksites, and schools.

With respect to incentivization, a series of experimental studies has demonstrated that reducing the price of healthier foods in school and worksite vending machines (French et al., 2001), school cafeterias (French, Story et al., 1997), and restaurants (Horgen & Brownell, 2002) will reliably lead to increases in the purchase of those foods. For example, in a 10-week intervention, French et al. (1997) manipulated the price of low-fat snacks at nine vending machines in a university setting. When the prices of low-fat snacks (i.e., ≤3 grams of fat per package) were experimentally reduced by 50%, the sales of low-fat foods increased by almost 150%. Interestingly, the sales of regular (i.e., not low-fat) snacks declined by approximately 20% during this period even though they were not targeted. This suggests that another behavioral principle, *displacement* or *substitution*, may occur as a secondary effect of incentivization. The concept stems from behavioral economics theory, described above, and occurs when the reinforcement of a desired behavior leads to the concurrent reduction of an undesirable behavior.

In another study, French et al. (2001) added low-fat snacks to 55 vending machines in 12 secondary schools and 12 worksites and experimentally manipulated the price of these items relative to existing snack foods (i.e., equal price, 10% reduction, 25% reduction, 50% reduction) as well the signs at the vending machines (i.e., no signs, low-fat items labeled, low-fat items labeled plus promotional signs for low-fat items). Sales of low-fat vending snacks were measured continuously for 12 months. Results indicated that reducing the price of low-fat snack foods by 10%, 25%, and 50%, respectively, was associated with 9%, 39%, and 93% increases in those items, respectively (see Figure 17.2). Promotional signage (i.e., an information based strategy) was only weakly associated with increases in low-fat snack sales.

The effectiveness of strategies that rely on negative reinforcement, or punishment, e.g., taxation or price increases on unhealthy foods, is less well studied and also more controversial or at least less popular than approaches based on positive reinforcement. Despite the lack of data, the notion of

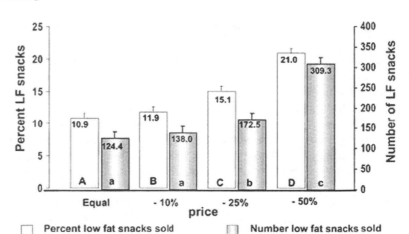

Figure 17.2 Changes in low-fat snack food purchases as a function of price reduction of those items in the "CHIPS" study (from French et al., 2001).

"fat taxes" has received much attention in the popular press. In a provocative paper, Jacobson and Brownell (2000) proposed that a small sales tax (e.g., 1¢) be imposed on the sales of foods of low nutritional value (e.g., soft drinks, candy, chewing gum, or snack foods). Although the proposed taxes likely would be too small to reduce purchases of those foods by individuals, Jacobson and Brownell propose that the generated revenues could be directed towards health promotion programs for obesity prevention. At least one population-based survey found relatively low public support for regulatory or taxation-based strategies for childhood obesity prevention initiatives (Evans, Finkelstein, Kamerow, & Renaud, 2005). The percent of respondents supporting various environmental interventions for childhood obesity prevention is summarized in Table 17.1. Respondents placed the majority of

Table 17.1 Support for childhood obesity intervention strategies as reported in a population-based survey (from Evans et al., 2005).

Intervention	Percent in favor
School vending machines	
Increasing promotion and marketing of healthy foods and drinks in school vending machines	85.4%
Restricting the availability of less healthy foods and drinks in school vending machines	73.6%
Allowing only the sale of healthy foods and drinks in school vending machines	70.9%
Increasing cost of less healthy foods and drinks in school vending machines	45.3%
Removing all vending machines from schools	35.9%
Still favor change in current vending practices in schools if it meant less money available to schools for other school activities	58.9%
School cafeterias	
Restricting the availability of less healthy foods and drinks in school cafeterias	74.5%
Allowing only the sale of healthy foods and drinks in school cafeterias	67.4%

Removing all fast food and other less healthy foods and drinks from school cafeterias	61.4%
Increasing the cost of less healthy foods and drinks in school cafeterias	44.0%
Still favor changes in school cafeterias if it meant a loss of money available to schools	67.8%
School curriculum	
Requiring schools to teach students healthy eating and exercise habits	93.9%
Requiring more physical education classes in school	82.3%
Requiring more recess and supervised intramural activities in school	68.9%
Still favor changes in school curriculum if it meant less time for traditional academic courses such as math, science, English, and history	34.1%
Evaluating children's weight in schools	
Providing students who are obese with weight loss and exercise programs in school	72.9%
Sending parents a health report card of their children's weight on a regular basis	57.1%
Recording students' weight on a regular basis	49.5%
Still favor evaluation of students' health if it meant some students would be embarrassed by the results	49.0%
Promotion of fast food and other less healthy food marketed to children	
Restricting the amount of fast food and less healthy food advertisements during children's television programs	75.3%
Prohibiting the advertising and promotion of fast food and less healthy foods marketed to children	47.9%
Increasing the tax on fast food and less healthy foods marketed to children	39.1%
Still favor restrictions on fast food and less healthy foods if it meant the government would have more control on what foods are available to children	43.9%
Still favor the above or other actions if it meant an increase of $25 a year in income taxes that you owe	70.9%
Still favor the above or other actions if it meant an increase of $100 a year in income taxes that you owe	49.8%

responsibility for childhood obesity prevention on parents rather than the government. See Chapter 6 for additional discussion of consumer perspectives and "personal responsibility" issues.

In sum, there is mounting experimental support for the notion that incentivizing healthier foods by lowering their prices will cause a greater number of individuals to purchase those foods. It is unclear, however, if incentivization strategies necessarily will lead to increased consumption of those foods and/or prevention of weight gain over time, and there are no strong data addressing the effects of taxing less healthy foods on the purchase or ultimate consumption of those foods. These are important questions for future research.

Mass Media and Social Marketing

Mass media and social marketing strategies for obesity prevention have traditionally targeted individual behavior change through population-based *information dissemination*. These interventions can reach a large number of individuals in communities or worksites, providing information on behavior modification strategies for weight control and for other health behaviors (e.g., smoking cessation). Taylor and Stunkard (Taylor & Stunkard, 1993) reviewed classic studies of this type, two of which were the pioneering Stanford Three-Community Study (Farquhar et al., 1977) and the Stanford Five-City Study (Farquhar et al., 1985; Taylor et al., 1991). These community interventions primarily attempted to reduce coronary risk factors rather than prevent weight gain per se, although the strategies are pertinent to weight gain prevention. Compared to citizens in the control communities in these studies, citizens in the intervention communities that received intensive media campaigns showed only modest prevention of weight gain. In the Three Community study, experimental communities did not gain weight, while control communities gained 0.45 kg on average. In the Five Community Study, experimental communities gained 0.54 kg on average vs. 1.25 kg in the control communities. As concluded by an Institute of Medicine committee that reviewed results of weight control studies (IOM, 1995), "Obesity turned out to be far harder to control than the other coronary risk factors" (p. 158).

Following up on the initial Stanford reports, a series of studies conducted by investigators at the University of Minnesota specifically tested community-based weight gain prevention and cardiovascular disease reduction programs. The Minnesota Heart Health Program (MHHP), a 13-year research project involving 6 communities, evaluated whether a multi-component education campaign could reduce population-wide risk factors for cardiovascular disease. Intervention communities received risk factor screenings, mass media education, adult education classes, worksite interventions, home correspondence programs, school-based programs, restaurant programs, and point-of-purchase education in supermarkets over 7 years. Weight gain prevention was emphasized for all adults, and weight loss was encouraged among those who were obese. Results of the intervention were deemed to be "disappointing," with strong upward weight trends observed in both control and intervention communities (Jeffery, 1995).

The "Healthy Worker Project" tested the effects of worksite health promotion programs for weight loss and smoking cessation among 16 intervention and 16 control worksites in the Minneapolis/St. Paul metropolitan area between 1987 and 1990 (Lando, Jeffery, McGovern, Forster, & Baxter, 1993). The intervention was a combination of on-site educational classes addressing weight loss and cigarette cessation, in conjunction with a financial incentive system involving payroll reduction. Specifically, participants committed to reduce their weekly payroll by a given amount (at least $5) which they could regain by achieving their target weight loss goals. There were 2,041 workers who enrolled in the weight loss program across sites. Weight loss goals were determined by participants and were structured as to not exceed 1% of body weight per week. Results indicated no significant differences between intervention and control worksites in the 2-year BMI changes (Jeffery, Forster et al., 1993).

In the "Pound of Prevention" (POP) study, 228 men and 998 women were randomly assigned to one of three intervention groups: (1) no-contact control, (2) monthly educational newsletters, and (3) monthly educational newsletters plus incentives for participation (Jeffery & French, 1999). The educational newsletters emphasized the themes of weighing oneself weekly, eating at least two servings of fruit each day, eating at least three servings of vegetables each day, reducing high-fat food intake, and increasing regular exercise. Compared to the control group, participants in both intervention groups significantly increased the frequency of healthy dieting practices and self-weighing over three years. However, weight gain during this period did not significantly differ between the three groups (i.e., the mean 3-year estimated weight gains were 0.6 kg, 0.6 kg, and 0.5 kg for the three groups, respectively).

In sum, in spite of the intuitive sense that mass media and social marketing strategies to dissemination information should work, the balance of studies that used mass media and social marketing approaches as the primary strategy to change behavior and improve weight control appeared to have little effect on weight gain prevention. This finding is noteworthy, as many of the current "obesity prevention" initiatives in the United States apparently continue to be based on information dissemination, for example, the Department of Health and Human Services' "Small Steps" campaign (http://www.smallstep.gov/sm_steps/sm_steps_index.html). The theoretical reasons why information dissemination alone is not effective were described earlier. Recognition that improvements in knowledge alone do not generally result in substantive behavior modification, many investigators are now focusing on environmental manipulations and policy changes that will present individuals with a set of behavior options that are more conducive to obesity prevention (French et al., 2001).

Tailoring to Participant Characteristics

There is growing interest in the topic of "tailoring" interventions in order to enhance individual behavior change efforts. Tailoring can be defined as "Any combination of information or change strategies *intended to reach one specific person*, based on characteristics that are unique to that person, related to the outcome of interest, and have been *derived from an individual assessment*" [italics in original] (Kreuter & Skinner, 2000) (p. 1). Key to this formulation are the distinct but related concepts of *cultural targeting* and *cultural tailoring*. According to Kreuter and colleagues (Kreuter, Lukwago, Bucholtz, Clark, & Sanders-Thompson, 2003), cultural targeting refers to development of a single intervention for a single subgroup that takes into account shared characteristics of that subgroup. Such targeting efforts are consistent with many public health frameworks in that they attempt to address the most affected individuals within a population, rather than the whole population, and by making the materials more relevant to the subgroup being targeted. Five types of strategies have been used to enhance the cultural appropriateness of intervention materials and have been labeled *peripheral, evidential, linguistic, constituent-involving,* and *sociocultural strategies* (Kreuter et al., 2003):

Peripheral strategies. This refers to the appearance of intervention materials, to make them more appealing or relevant to a given subgroup. This may be achieved through the selection of certain colors, images, fonts, or pictures, or titles used in the materials. This strategy enhances cultural relevance through "peripheral" means of information processing (Petty & Cacioppo, 1981).

Evidential strategies. This refers to efforts to enhance the relevance of the health issue by presenting evidence of impact for the subgroup. Such evidence can come for epidemiological studies showing, for example, that a given disorder or disease is more common in that subgroup compared to the general population.

Linguistic strategies. This refers to efforts to make intervention materials more accessible by providing them through the dominant or native language of the subgroup.

Constituent-involving strategies. This refers to efforts to involve members of the subgroup in the intervention process in order to draw directly on their experiences. Examples include training paraprofessionals or students from targeted community as interventionists, and enlisting active involvement from community stakeholders in decision-making aspects of the intervention.

Sociocultural strategies. This refers to efforts to discuss health-related issues in the broader context of social and/or cultural values of the subgroup. Unlike peripheral strategies previously mentioned, sociocultural strategies attempt to enhance cultural relevance through a more central pathway, or "deep structure," of information processing (Resnicow, Baranowski, Ahluwalia, & Braithwaite, 1999).

The concept of cultural *tailoring* recognizes that there is considerable diversity and individual differences even within subgroups. That is, "although culture is shared, individuals within a given culture can have varying levels of certain cultural beliefs" (Kreuter et al., 2003) (p. 137). Cultural tailoring, therefore, is a process for assessing the extent to which a given member of the subgroup endorses a purported cultural belief or attitude and, if so, how the intervention will be individualized for that person. Kreuter et al. (2003) provide a useful example of how tailoring was conducted in the "Cultural Tailoring for Cancer Prevention in Black Women" study. Specifically, questionnaires were used to assess the importance for individuals of four identified cultural characteristics: religiosity, collectivism, racial pride, and perception of time. Health education messages subsequently were tailored for each of the four cultural characteristics and, depending on the importance of each domain, different messages were provided to different participants.

Rakowski (1999) also provides a thoughtful discussion on tailoring program messages or interventions, emphasizing the role of broader contextual factors that impact on behavior. His model emphasizes the combination of behavior, population, and setting when considering the "focal points" for tailoring interventions. To illustrate this framework, one could consider a prevention study that is tailored to increase fruit and vegetable intake (behavioral focus), among urban dwelling families (population focus), enrolled in a church-based intervention (setting focus). Rakowski also identifies a number of culturally relevant variables for tailoring behavioral interventions that are presented in Table 17.2. Kumanyika (2004) provides additional discussion of this topic.

With respect to obesity prevention per se, individual behavior change may be better achieved when prevention initiatives are tailored to participant characteristics. However, there has been limited research into this important area. As reviewed by Kumanyika (2002), the potential importance of tailoring interventions for weight loss was recognized by the NHLBI Obesity Education Initiative Expert Plan (NHLBI, 1998). Based on limited but supportive evidence, the expert panel concluded that "the possibility that a standard approach to weight loss will work differently in diverse patient populations must be considered when setting expectations about treatment outcomes."

Table 17.2 Culturally relevant variables important for tailoring behavioral interventions (from S. Kumanyika, 2004 as adapted from Rakowski, 1999).

Client or population characteristics:

- Age, race/ethnicity, gender and socioeconomic variables
- Risk perception/perceived threat of illness
- Readiness for change; stage of change
- Self-efficacy perceptions
- Attitudes about the health practice or illness
- Information processing style
- Attribution of causality for illness
- Availability of family/friend support; social support systems
- Reliance on medical professionals to determine one's health actions
- Tendency to avoid or approach the health care system
- Level of acculturation to mainstream

Required psychosocial resources and performance

- Demands
- Holding a positive self-image
- Social support to assist the change process
- Optimism/long-range time perspective
- Sense of timing/scheduling
- Tolerance of discomfort

Several studies tailored behavioral interventions for weight loss and/or weight gain prevention have been conducted with African Americans. One set of examples was in Phase 1 of the Girls Health Enrichment Multi-Site Studies (GEMS), an overview of which is provided by Kumanyika et al. (Kumanyika, Obarzanek, Robinson & Beech, 2003; Kumanyika, Story et al., 2003). The aim of GEMS Phase 1 was to develop and pilot test a series of culturally appropriate weight gain prevention interventions for African American preadolescent girls. Critical to this research program, four sites (Baylor University, University of Memphis, University of Minnesota, and Stanford University) began with a formative assessment in which the interventions were developed, evaluated for cultural appropriateness, and reviewed for acceptability by key stakeholders (e.g., adolescents, parents, treatment providers). A key lesson was that the establishment of trust and strong working relations among community leaders, as well as investigators, is critical for facilitating individual behavior change (Kumanyika, Obarzanek et al., 2003). Following the formative assessments, all four sites pilot tested the resulting intervention approaches. The two approaches that were found to be sufficiently feasible and effective to warrant further testing in full scale studies (at Stanford University and the University of Memphis) are described below. Outcomes of the full scale two year trials will be forthcoming.

Robinson et al. (2003) randomized 61 girls, 8 to 10 years old, to an after-school dance class and television (TV) reduction intervention or a health education control intervention. For the active treatment, "GEMS Jewels" dance classes were offered after school 5 days per week at three community centers. These sessions included provision of a healthful snack and an hour long homework period, followed by 45–60 minutes of moderate-to-vigorous physical activity. Dance lessons were taught by African American college students, who taught traditional African dance, hip-hop, and step dances. The TV reduction component of the intervention consisted of five home visit lessons for parents and children, providing behavioral strategies to reduce television viewing. The control group received health-related newsletters and lectures. After the 3-month pilot study period, trends were in the expected direction (i.e., improvements in the treatment group relative to controls) for BMI, waist circumference, after school physical activity, screen time (TV, videotape and video game use), and school grades. Statistically significant reductions in household television viewing and eating dinners while watching TV in the treatment vs. the control group children were also found.

Beech et al. (2003) randomized 60 African American girls, 8–10 years old, to one of three intervention groups: child-targeted family intervention, parent-targeted family intervention, or self-esteem enhancement comparison group. The first two intervention groups were culturally tailored family-based interventions targeting enhanced nutrition and physical activity, with the primary difference being the family member who was actively treated (i.e., child vs. parent). The specific intervention content of the 12 respective sessions were derived from extensive focus group research with children and parents, a summary of which is provided in Table 17.3. Table 17.4 summarizes the 12 session topics for the two respective groups, which also included some discussion of body image appraisal and acceptance. The self-esteem enhancement group (controls) participated in arts and crafts activities, "friendship building," and games. Compared to the self-esteem intervention, girls receiving the active interventions (combining the child-targeted and parent-targeted groups) showed smaller 3-month gains in BMI and waist circumference, reduced consumption of sweetened beverage consumption, increased water intake, and increased physical activity.

Gans et al. (2003) described the development of *SisterTalk*, a community-based and culturally tailored weight control intervention for black women delivered via cable television. The intervention applied the conceptual framework of Kumanyika (Kumanyika, Morssink, & Agurs, 1992) for relating cultural influences to weight management programs and, in doing so, considered a variety of factors such as how the educational materials would be processed by the target audience, the packaging of information, and the use of language and imagery. The intervention also made explicit use of Social Action Theory, which attends to a range of contextual, social interaction, motivation, generative capabilities, and problem solving considerations (see Figure 17.3). This study illustrates the utility of a clear theoretical framework for culturally tailoring interventions to individuals within communities.

There have been other efforts to tailor established weight loss programs for African American adults who were treated in clinical or community settings. As reviewed by Kumanyika (Kumanyika, 2002), the greatest weight losses were approximately 0.4 kg/week over 11–14 weeks (McNabb, Quinn, Kerver, Cook, & Karrison, 1997; Pleas, 1988) with other studies reporting weight losses of 0.30–0.35 kg/week over 8–10 weeks (Kanders et al., 1994; S. K. Kumanyika & Charleston, 1992) or smaller weight losses.

Table 17.3 Select child and parent focus group findings and their associated intervention activities in the Memphis GEMS weight gain prevention study in African American preadolescent girls (from Beech et al., 2003).

Child intervention		Parent intervention	
Child focus group findings	Related intervention activities	Parent focus group findings	Related intervention activities
Physical activity		**Physical activity**	
Strong dislike of traditionally structured P.E. classes (e.g., push up, sit ups, running laps, etc.)	Included "fun" activities for movement Encouraged girls to take "ownership" of the program and suggest new activities	Parents enjoy dancing with friends and family members, not seen as a direct form of exercise	Physical activity component included different forms of dance ("dancing to oldies" and new "line" dancing to popular music)
Girls enjoy movement in the form of dance	Incorporation of hip-hop aerobics into the main active component Encouragement of girls to dance/move during commercials when watching TV	Typical family activities and outings do not include physical activity	Information presented in the didactic portion of the physical activity component regarding ways to increase family activity (e.g., washing cars, cleaning house to music, walking after dinner, etc.)
Younger girls (8–10) expressed an interest in a variety of physical activities (e.g., soccer, basketball, kickball, bike riding, etc.)	Spotlight/brief discussion of activity alternatives discussed each week Challenge sheets (reward for trying different activities)	Continuous feedback and information regarding lifestyle changes provides support and is instrumental in creating new healthy habits	Goal setting cards were used for parents to select weekly family activities and record their progress
Nutrition		**Nutrition**	
Girls assist their families with meal preparation and often perform microwave cooking alone	Inclusion of weekly food preparation activities with child-friendly recipes Food "art" and taste-testing activities to encourage a broad exposure to different fruits and vegetables	Parents are very knowledgeable about nutrition, but lacked information about how to implement this knowledge into their daily practices	Provision of "tips" on how to include healthy snacks for kids and modify traditional recipes to make them healthier Nutrition games provided fun ways to learn new strategies (e.g., Who Wants to be Healthy?)
Importance of Sunday family dinners	Messages regarding food moderation were given for times when traditional heavy meals are likely to be consumed	The relationships between weight and health was seen as primarily genetic; lack of acceptance of the connection between behavioral practices and body size	Emphasis on healthy lifestyles, rather than on weight Focus on increased physical activity to promote and maintain health; disease prevention approach
Existence of neighborhood "candy ladies"	Recognition of an environmental immutable exposure; message regarding frequency of visitation and quantity of candy purchased were presented	Time constraints impacted the preparation of health meals Desire to prepare healthier foods that their families would enjoy	Healthy, easy-to-prepare recipes were distributed at every session Hands-on food preparation of kids-friendly recipes were included

Table 17. 4 Session-by-session intervention themes in the University of Memphis' GEMS weight gain prevention study in African American pre-adolescent girls (from Beech et al., 2003).

Session	Child targeted intervention		Parent targeted intervention:	
	Nutrition	Physical Activity	Nutrition	Physical Activity
1	• Hip-hop aerobics • Encourage a variety of physical activities	• Increasing vegetable consumption • Make a vegetable salad and stamped napkins	• Introduction to the "Old School" dance	• Importance of water and F&V consumption
2	• Hip-hop aerobics • Decrease sedentary activities • Encourage walking	• Decreasing sweetened beverages • Vegetable tray • Low sugar drinks/ water • Blind taste test	• Stretching • "Old School" dance • Importance of walking	• Cooking activity; importance of breakfast consumption • Decrease sweetened beverages
3	• Hip-hop aerobics • Exercise with a partner • Active games	• Increase fruit consumption • Fruit platter/dip • GEMS heart	• Stretching • "Old School" dance	• Nutrition game • Low fat lunch options
4	• Hip-hop aerobics • Using the "talk" test when exercising • Encourage jogging	• Increase fruits as snacks • "Snack attack" bags • Fruit/vegetable art	• Stretching • "Old School" dance	• Cooking activity-decrease salt intake and increase use of seasonings
5	• Hip-hop aerobics • Exercise when bored or angry • Encourage jump roping	• Eat a variety of healthy foods • "Ants on a log" • Triscuit pyramid	• Stretching • Line dancing	• Nutrition game • Increase water consumption • Low fat snacks
6	• Hip-hop aerobics • Encourage playing sports	• Recognize fullness/ satiety • Satiety demo • Bountiful burritos	• Stretching • Line dancing • Cleaning to music	• Cooking activity • Label reading
7	• Hip-hop aerobics • Ways to overcome barriers to exercise • Encourage stairs	• Eating a healthful breakfast • Make fruit roll-ups • GEMS oven mitts	• Stretching • Line dancing • Low-cost/no cost family	• Nutrition game • Making healthier fast food choices
8	• Hip-hop aerobics • Encourage use of community resources to increase activity • Encourage bike riding	• Eating a healthy lunch • Drink more water • Turkey roll-up	• Stretching • Line dancing	• Cooking activity • Importance of the family dinner • "Drink less sugar"
9	• Hip-hop aerobics • Decrease sedentary activities • Encourage swimming	• Eating a healthy dinner • Pita pocket pile up • Soup basket mix	• Stretching • Dance • Importance of daily exercise	• Nutrition game • Veggies and kids • Eating while watching TV
10	• Hip-hop aerobics • Decrease sedentary activities • Encourage roller	• Smart snacks • Teddy fruit toss • Memo book	• Stretching • Dance	• Cooking activity • Low-fat eating • Increase water consumption
11	• Hip-hop aerobics • Ways to keep moving	• Healthy fast food choices • Create a better burger	• Stretching • Dance • Importance of parental role modeling	• Nutrition game • Portion control
12	• Hip-hop aerobics	• Nutrition Twister • Vegetable and fruit tray • Turkey roll-ups	• Stretching • Dance	• Healthy snacks • Certification/awards

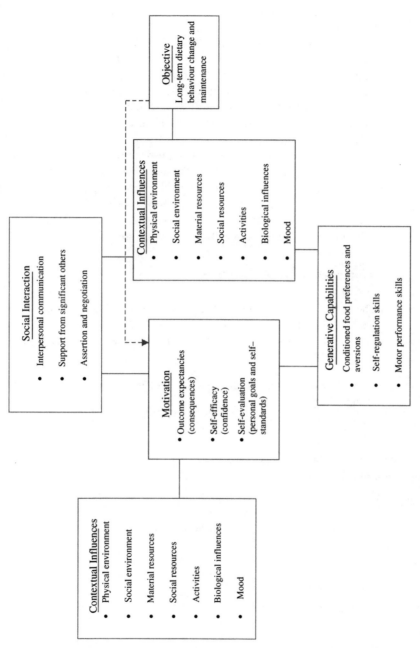

Figure 17.3 Social action theory framework as applied in the *SisterTalk* weight control intervention (from Gans et al., 2003).

Interventions also may be tailored by gender and stage of life. For example, the Women's Healthy Lifestyle Project was a 5-year dietary and physical activity intervention program that targeted prevention of weight gain during menopause, with the participants being 535 healthy pre-menopausal women aged 44–50 years at study enrollment. Participants were assigned either to an assessment only control group or to a comprehensive lifestyle intervention. The lifestyle intervention had behavioral goals of limiting food intake to 1,300 kcal/day and increasing physical activity expenditure to 1,000–1,500 kcal/week. They were also given a weight loss goal of 2.3–6.8 kg by the end of the trial (Simkin-Silverman, Wing, Boraz, & Kuller, 2003). After 4.5 years of treatment, 55% of the intervention participants were at or below their baseline weights compared to 26% of the controls ($p < 0.001$). Reduction in waist circumference was also significantly greater among intervention than control participants (means $= -2.9$ cm vs. -0.5 cm, $p < 0.05$).

In sum, the tailoring of existing interventions for enhancing individual behavior change arguably is one of the more pressing needs in obesity prevention research. The studies reviewed in this section suggest the promise of such approaches, with GEMS serving as a richly informative example. While additional studies are undertaken, Table 17.5 provides a useful set of guidelines for tailoring interventions to specific cultural groups (Kumanyika, 2002).

Motivation for Prevention

The perception that obesity is an important problem, or potential impeding medical problem, for oneself or one's family may be a critical determinant of individual behavior change. Some individuals who are obese or who have

Table 17.5 Recommended guidelines for adapting weight loss programs for effectiveness in diverse populations (from Kumanyika, 2002)

1. Provide a setting or treatment venue that:
   • Is physically acceptable to participants
   • Incorporates features likely to be familiar to participants
   • Is free of negative psychosocial connotations
   • Is free of factors that create a large social distance among participants or between participants and counselors
   • Promotes active participant involvement and high participant self-esteem and self efficacy

2. Involve staff who are:
   • Culturally self-aware
   • Culturally competent in working with diverse audiences

3. Use educational and counseling approaches that anticipate a suitable diversity and range in participants':
   • Preexisting knowledge base
   • Day-to-day routine and discretionary time
   • Financial resources and living situation
   • Cultural preferences for food and activity

4. Facilitate integration of weight management advice with other aspects of health care and self-care

5. Expect and allow for program modifications based on patient feedback and preferences

obese children, in fact, may not perceive there to be a problem and therefore may not be inclined to make changes. Evidence to support this comes primarily from focus group studies with parents from low income families, who were enrolled in the federal Supplemental Program for Women Infants and Children (WIC) (Baughcum, Chamberlin, Deeks, Powers, & Whitaker, 2000). For example, Baughcum et al. (1998) conducted focus groups with over 600 low-income mothers of young children to assess their attitudes concerning child feeding. Results indicated three major themes: (1) parent beliefs that a heavy child is a healthy child, (2) parent concerns that a child is not getting enough to eat, and (3) parent use of food to influence children's behavior.

Similarly, Jain et al. (2001) reported that mothers of children who were overweight and at risk for overweight did not use the definition of child overweight based on the standard growth charts. Instead, these mothers related their children's weight status to weight-related teasing and their ability to partake in physical activity. Finally, in a survey study of 277 mothers whose perceptions about childhood obesity were assessed, 33% of the mothers of overweight or obese children reported that their child's weight was "about right" (Jeffery, Voss, Metcalf, Alba, & Wilkin, 2005).

Most clinic-based weight control interventions have studied motivated individuals or family members who were willing to undergo time-intensive treatments. These individuals perceived obesity as a problem and were motivated to make individual behavior changes. However, this may not be the case for all overweight or obese individuals in the broader population. Some people who are generally motivated to lose weight may have limited readiness to undertake the specific behavior changes required for weight loss. Or, other pressing life responsibilities and commitments may take priority. How these issues are negotiated on an individual-by-individual, or community-by-community, basis warrants additional research to empower individual behavior change.

Conclusion

This chapter summarizes the principles underlying individual behavior change, with implications for obesity or weight gain prevention initiatives that can be implemented across a range of social settings. Theories, principles and specific strategies were reviewed ranging from those that engage individuals directly to those implemented at a community or whole population level. Much of the existing evidence comes from the obesity treatment literature. Conceptual frameworks for obesity prevention should bridge the fields of basic science, health promotion, and risk reduction.

References

Arenz, S., Ruckerl, R., Koletzko, B., & von Kries, R. (2004). Breast-feeding and childhood obesity-a systematic review. *International Journal of Obesity*, 28(10), 1247–1256.

Bandura, A. (1977). *Social learning theory*. New Jersey: Prentice-Hall.

Bandura, A. (1986). *Social foundations of thought and action: A social cognitive theory*. Englewood Cliffs, NJ: Prentice-Hall.

Battle, E. K., & Brownell, K. D. (1996). Confronting a rising tide of eating disorders and obesity: Treatment vs. prevention and policy. *Addictive Behaviors*, 21(6), 755–765.

Baughcum, A. E., Burklow, K. A., Deeks, C. M., Powers, S. W., & Whitaker, R. C. (1998). Maternal feeding practices and childhood obesity: A focus group study of low-income mothers. *Archives of Pediatrics & Adolescent Medicine, 152*(10), 1010–1014.

Baughcum, A. E., Chamberlin, L. A., Deeks, C. M., Powers, S. W., & Whitaker, R. C. (2000). Maternal perceptions of overweight preschool children. *Pediatrics, 106*(6), 1380–1386.

Beech, B. M., Klesges, R. C., Kumanyika, S. K., Murray, D. M., Klesges, L., McClanahan, B., et al. (2003). Child- and parent-targeted interventions: The Memphis GEMS pilot study. *Ethnicity and Disease, 13*(1 Suppl. 1), S40–S53.

Berkowitz, R. I., Wadden, T. A., Tershakovec, A. M., & Cronquist, J. L. (2003). Behavior therapy and sibutramine for the treatment of adolescent obesity: A randomized controlled trial. *Journal of the American Medical Association, 289*(14), 1805–1812.

Bickel, W. K., Madden, G. J., & Petry, N. M. (1998). The price of change: The behavioral economics of drug dependence. *Behavior Therapy, 29*, 545–565.

Bickel, W. K., & Vuchinich, R. E. (2000). *Reframing Health Behavior Change with Behavioral Economics.* Mahwah, NJ: Lawrence Erlbaum.

Bronfenbrenner, U. (1979). *The Ecology of Human Development.* Cambridge, MA: Harvard University Press.

Brownell, K. D., Heckerman, C. L., Westlake, R. J., Hayes, S. C., & Monti, P. M. (1978). The effect of couples training and partner co-operativeness in the behavioral treatment of obesity. *Behavior Research and Therapy, 16*(5), 323–333.

Brownell, K. D., & Horgen, K. B. (2004). *Food Fight.* New York: Contemporary Books.

Brug, J., & van Lenthe, F. (2005). *Environmental determinants and interventions for physical activity, nutrition, and smoking: A review.* Rotterdam: Ikenweij.

Clinical Guidelines on the Identification, Evaluation, and Treatment of Overweight and Obesity in Adults—The Evidence Report. National Institutes of Health. Obes Res. 1998 Sep;6 Suppl 2:51S–209S. Review. No abstract available. Erratum in: Obes Res 1998 Nov; 6(6): 464.

Committee on Prevention of Obesity in Children and Youth. (2004). *Preventing childhood obesity. Health in balance.* Washington, DC: National Academies Press.

Copeland, A. L., Martin, P. D., Geiselman, P. J., Rash, C. J., & Kendzor, D. E. (2006). Smoking cessation for weight-concerned women: Group vs. individually tailored, dietary, and weight-control follow-up sessions. *Addictive Behaviors, 31*(1), 115–127.

Di Noia, J., Schinke, S. P., Prochaska, J. O., & Contento, I. R. (2006). Application of the transtheoretical model to fruit and vegetable consumption among economically disadvantaged African-American adolescents: Preliminary findings. *American Journal of Health Promotion, 20*(5), 342–348.

Doak, C. M., Visscher, T. L., Renders, C. M., & Seidell, J. C. (2006). The prevention of overweight and obesity in children and adolescents: A review of interventions and programmes. *Obesity Reviews, 7*(1), 111–136.

Epstein, L. H., Gordy, C. C., Raynor, H. A., Beddome, M., Kilanowski, C. K., & Paluch, R. (2001). Increasing fruit and vegetable intake and decreasing fat and sugar intake in families at risk for childhood obesity. *Obesity Research, 9*(3), 171–178.

Epstein, L. H., Myers, M. D., Raynor, H. A., & Saelens, B. E. (1998). Treatment of pediatric obesity. *Pediatrics, 101*(3, Pt. 2), 554–570.

Epstein, L. H., & Saelens, B. E. (2000). Behavioral economics of obesity: Food intake and energy expenditure. In W. K. V. Bickel, R.E. (Ed.), *Reframing health behavior change with behavioral economics* (pp. 293-311). Mahwah, NJ: Lawrence Erlbaum.

Epstein, L. H., Valoski, A., Wing, R. R., & McCurley, J. (1994). Ten-year outcomes of behavioral family-based treatment for childhood obesity. *Health Psychology, 13*(5), 373–383.

Evans, W. D., Finkelstein, E. A., Kamerow, D. B., & Renaud, J. M. (2005). Public perceptions of childhood obesity. *American Journal of Preventive Medicine, 28*(1), 26–32.

Farquhar, J. W., Fortmann, S. P., Maccoby, N., Haskell, W. L., Williams, P. T., Flora, J. A., et al. (1985). The Stanford Five-City Project: Design and methods. *American Journal of Epidemiology*, *122*(2), 323–334.

Farquhar, J. W., Maccoby, N., Wood, P. D., Alexander, J. K., Breitrose, H., Brown, B. W., Jr. et al. (1977). Community education for cardiovascular health. *Lancet*, *1*(8023), 1192–1195.

Ferster, C., & Skinner, B. (1957). *Schedules of reinforcement*. New York: Appleton-Century-Crofts.

Foreyt, J. P., & Goodrick, G. K. (1991). Factors common to successful therapy for the obese patient. *Medicine Science Sports and Exercise*, *23*(3), 292–297.

Foster, G. D., Wadden, T. A., Vogt, R. A., & Brewer, G. (1997). What is a reasonable weight loss? Patients' expectations and evaluations of obesity treatment outcomes. *Journal of Consulting and Clinical Psychology*, *65*(1), 79–85.

French, S. A., Jeffery, R. W., Story, M., Breitlow, K. K., Baxter, J. S., Hannan, P., et al. (2001). Pricing and promotion effects on low-fat vending snack purchases: The CHIPS Study. *American Journal of Public Health*, *91*(1), 112–117.

French, S. A., Jeffery, R. W., Story, M., Hannan, P., & Snyder, M. P. (1997). A pricing strategy to promote low-fat snack choices through vending machines. *American Journal of Public Health*, *87*(5), 849–851.

French, S. A., Story, M., Jeffery, R. W., Snyder, P., Eisenberg, M., Sidebottom, A., et al. (1997). Pricing strategy to promote fruit and vegetable purchase in high school cafeterias. *Journal of the American Dietetic Association*, *97*(9), 1008–1010.

Gans, K. M., Kumanyika, S. K., Lovell, H. J., Risica, P. M., Goldman, R., Odoms-Young, A., et al. (2003). The development of SisterTalk: A cable TV-delivered weight control program for black women. *Preventive Medicine*, *37*(6, Pt. 1), 654–667.

Golan, M., & Crow, S. (2004). Targeting parents exclusively in the treatment of childhood obesity: Long-term results. *Obesity Research*, *12*(2), 357–361.

Golan, M., Weizman, A., Apter, A., & Fainaru, M. (1998). Parents as the exclusive agents of change in the treatment of childhood obesity. *American Journal of Clinical Nutrition*, *67*(6), 1130–1135.

Goldfield, G. S., & Epstein, L. H. (2002). Can fruits and vegetables and activities substitute for snack foods? *Health Psychology*, *21*(3), 299–303.

Heatherton, T. F., & Nichols, P. A. (1994). Personal accounts of successful versus failed attempts at life change. *Personality and Social Psychology Bulletin*, *20*, 664–675.

Horgen, K. B., & Brownell, K. D. (2002). Comparison of price change and health message interventions in promoting healthy food choices. *Health Psychology*, *21*(5), 505–512.

Horgen, K. B., & Brownell, K. D. (2003). Confronting the toxic environment: Environmental and public health actions in a world crisis. In T. A. Wadden & A. J. Stunkard (Eds.), *Handbook of obesity treatment* (pp. 95–106). New York, NY: Guilford Press.

Horwath, C. (1999). Applying the transtheoretical model to eating behaviour change: Challenges and opportunities. *Nutrition Research Reviews*, *12*(2), 281–317.

IOM. (1995). *Weight the options: Criteria for evaluating weight-management programs*. Washington, DC: National Academy of Sciences.

Jacobson, M. F., & Brownell, K. D. (2000). Small taxes on soft drinks and snack foods to promote health. *American Journal of Public Health*, *90*(6), 854–857.

Jain, A., Sherman, S. N., Chamberlin, L. A., Carter, Y., Powers, S. W., & Whitaker, R. C. (2001). Why don't low-income mothers worry about their preschoolers being overweight? [see comment]. *Pediatrics*, *107*(5), 1138–1146.

Jeffery, A. N., Voss, L. D., Metcalf, B. S., Alba, S., & Wilkin, T. J. (2005). Parents' awareness of overweight in themselves and their children: Cross sectional study within a Cohort (EarlyBird 21). *British Medical Journal*, *330*, 23–24.

Jeffery, R. W. (1995). Community programs for obesity prevention: The Minnesota Heart Health Program. *Obesity Research*, *3*, 283s–288s.

Jeffery, R. W., Forster, J. L., French, S. A., Kelder, S. H., Lando, H. A., McGovern, P. G., et al. (1993). The healthy worker project: A work-site intervention for weight control and smoking cessation. *American Journal of Public Health*, *83*(3), 395–401.

Kahn, E. B., Ramsey, L. T., Brownson, R. C., Heath, G. W., Howze, E. H., Powell, K. E., et al. (2002). The effectiveness of interventions to increase physical activity. A systematic review. *American Journal of Preventive Medicine*, *22*(Suppl. 4), 73–107.

Kanders, B. S., Ullmann-Joy, P., Foreyt, J. P., Heymsfield, S. B., Heber, D., Elashoff, R. M., et al. (1994). The black American lifestyle intervention (BALI): The design of a weight loss program for working-class African-American women. *J Am Diet Assoc*, *94*(3), 310–312.

Kazdin, A. (2001). *Behavior modification in applied settings* (6th ed.). Belmont, CA: Wadsworth/Thomson Learning.

Korotitsch, W. J., & Nelson-Gray, R. O. (1999). An overview of self-monitoring research in assessment and treatment. *Psychological Assessment*, *11*, 415–425.

Kreuter, M. W., Lukwago, S. N., Bucholtz, D. C., Clark, E. M., & Sanders-Thompson, V. (2003). Achieving cultural appropriateness in health promotions programs: Targeted and tailored approaches. *Health Education Behavior*, *30*, 133–146.

Kreuter, M. W., & Skinner, C. S. (2000). Tailoring: What's in a name? *Health Education Research*, *15*(1), 1–4.

Kumanyika, S. (2004). Cultural differences in treatment. In G. A. Bray, & C. Bouchard (Eds.), *Handbook of obesity* (2nd ed., pp. 45–67). New York: Marcel Dekker.

Kumanyika, S. K. (2002). Obesity treatment in minorities. In T. A. Wadden, & A. J. Stunkard (Eds.), *Handbook of obesity treatment* (3rd ed., pp. 416–446). New York: Guilford Publications, Inc.

Kumanyika, S. K., & Charleston, J. B. (1992). Lose weight and win: A church-based weight loss program for blood pressure control among black women. *Patient Education Counseling*, *19*(1), 19–32.

Kumanyika, S. K., Morssink, C., & Agurs, T. (1992). Models for dietary and weight change in African-American women: Identifying cultural components. *Ethnicity and Disease*, *2*(2), 166–175.

Kumanyika, S. K., & Obarzanek, E. (2003). Pathways to obesity prevention: Report of a National Institutes of Health workshop. *Obesity Research*, *11*(10), 1263–1274.

Kumanyika, S. K., Obarzanek, E., Robinson, T. N., & Beech, B. M. (2003). Phase 1 of the Girls health Enrichment Multi-site Studies (GEMS): Conclusion. *Ethnicity and Disease*, *13*(1 Suppl. 1), S88–S91.

Kumanyika, S. K., Story, M., Beech, B. M., Sherwood, N. E., Baranowski, J. C., Powell, T. M., et al. (2003). Collaborative planning for formative assessment and cultural appropriateness in the Girls health Enrichment Multi-site Studies (GEMS): A retrospection. *Ethnicity and Disease*, *13*(1 Suppl. 1), S15–S29.

Lando, H. A., Jeffery, R. W., McGovern, P. G., Forster, J. L., & Baxter, J. E. (1993). Factors influencing participation in worksite smoking cessation and weight loss programs: The Healthy Worker Project. *American Journal of Health Promotion*, *8*(1), 22–24.

Latner, J. D., Stunkard, A. J., Wilson, G. T., Jackson, M. L., Zelitch, D. S., & Labouvie, E. (2000). Effective long-term treatment of obesity: A continuing care model. *International Journal of Obesity*, *24*(7), 893–898.

Littrell, K. H., Hilligoss, N. M., Kirshner, C. D., Petty, R. G., & Johnson, C. G. (2003). The effects of an educational intervention on antipsychotic-induced weight gain. *Journal of Nursing Scholarship*, *35*(3), 237–241.

Marcus, B. H., & Simkin, L. R. (1994). The transtheoretical model: Applications to exercise behavior. *Medicine Science Sports and Exercise*, *26*(11), 1400–1404.

Matson-Koffman, D. M., Brownstein, J. N., Neiner, J. A., & Greaney, M. L. (2005). A site-specific literature review of policy and environmental interventions that promote physical activity and nutrition for cardiovascular health: What works? *American Journal of Health Promotion*, *19*(3), 167–193.

McNabb, W., Quinn, M., Kerver, J., Cook, S., & Karrison, T. (1997). The PATHWAYS church-based weight loss program for urban African-American women at risk for diabetes. *Diabetes Care*, *20*(10), 1518–1523.

Menza, M., Vreeland, B., Minsky, S., Gara, M., Radler, D. R., & Sakowitz, M. (2004). Managing atypical antipsychotic-associated weight gain: 12-month data on a multi-modal weight control program. *Journal of Clinical Psychiatry*, *65*(4), 471–477.

Pearce, J. W., LeBow, M. D., & Orchard, J. (1981). Role of spouse involvement in the behavioral treatment of overweight women. *Journal of Consulting and Clinical Psychology*, *49*(2), 236–244.

Perri, M. G. (1992). Improving maintenance of weight loss following treatment by diet and lifestyle modification. In T. A. Wadden & T. B. VanItallie (Eds.), *Treatment of the seriously obese patient* (pp. 456–477). New York: Guilford.

Petty, R., & Cacioppo, J. (1981). *Attitudes and persuasion: Classic and contemporary approaches*. Dubuque, IA: W.C. Brown.

Pleas, J. (1988). Long-term effects of a lifestyle-change obesity treatment program with minorities. *Journal of the National Medical Association*, *80*(7), 747–752.

Prochaska, J. O., & Velicer, W. F. (1997). The transtheoretical model of health behavior change. *American Journal of Health Promotion*, *12*(1), 38–48.

Rakowski, W. (1999). The potential variances of tailoring in health behavior interventions. *Annals of Behavioral Medicine*, *21*(4), 284–289.

Renjilian, D. A., Perri, M. G., Nezu, A. M., McKelvey, W. F., Shermer, R. L., & Anton, S. D. (2001). Individual versus group therapy for obesity: Effects of matching participants to their treatment preferences. *Journal of Consulting and Clinical Psychology*, *69*(4), 717–721.

Resnicow, K., Baranowski, T., Ahluwalia, J. S., & Braithwaite, R. L. (1999). Cultural sensitivity in public health: Defined and demystified. *Ethnicity and Disease*, *9*(1), 10–21.

Robinson, T. N. (1999). Reducing children's television viewing to prevent obesity: A randomized controlled trial. *Journal of the American Medical Association*, *282*(16), 1561–1567.

Robinson, T. N. (2001). Television viewing and childhood obesity. *Pediatric Clinics of North America*, *48*(4), 1017–1025.

Robinson, T. N., Killen, J. D., Kraemer, H. C., Wilson, D. M., Matheson, D. M., Haskell, W. L., et al. (2003). Dance and reducing television viewing to prevent weight gain in African-American girls: The Stanford GEMS pilot study. *Ethnicity and Disease*, *13*(1 Suppl. 1), S65–S77.

Rogers, E. M. (1995). *Diffusion of innovations* (4th ed.). New York: The Free Press.

Rolls, B. J., Ello-Martin, J. A., & Tohill, B. C. (2004). What can intervention studies tell us about the relationship between fruit and vegetable consumption and weight management? *Nutrition Reviews*, *62*(1), 1–17.

Simkin-Silverman, L. R., Wing, R. R., Boraz, M. A., & Kuller, L. H. (2003). Lifestyle intervention can prevent weight gain during menopause: Results from a 5-year randomized clinical trial. *Annals of Behavioral Medicine*, *26*(3), 212–220.

Stuart, R. (1967). Behavioral control of overeating. *Behavior Research Therapy*, *5*, 357.

Summerbell, C. D., Waters, E., Edmunds, L. D., Kelly, S., Brown, T., & Campbell, K. J. (2005). Interventions for preventing obesity in children. *Cochrane Database System Review*, *3*, CD001871.

Taylor, C. B., Fortmann, S. P., Flora, J., Kayman, S., Barrett, D. C., Jatulis, D., et al. (1991). Effect of long-term community health education on body mass index. The Stanford Five-City Project. *American Journal of Epidemiology*, *134*(3), 235–249.

Taylor, C. B., & Stunkard, A. J. (1993). Public health approaches to weight control. In A. J. Stunkard & T. A. Wadden (Eds.), *Obesity: Theory and Therapy* (2nd ed., pp. 335–353). New York: Raven Press.

Verheijden, M. W., Bakx, J. C., van Weel, C., Koelen, M. A., & van Staveren, W. A. (2005). Role of social support in lifestyle-focused weight management interventions. *European Journal of Clinical Nutrition, 59*(Suppl. 1), S179–S186.

Wadden, T. A., Crerand, C. E., & Brock, J. (2005). Behavioral treatment of obesity. *Psychiatric Clinics of North America, 28*(1), 151–170, ix.

Wadden, T. A., & Foster, G. D. (2000). Behavioral treatment of obesity. *Medical Clinics of North America, 84*(2), 441–461, vii.

Wadden, T. A., Womble, L. G., Sarwer, D. B., Berkowitz, R. I., Clark, V. L., & Foster, G. D. (2003). Great expectations: "I'm losing 25% of my weight no matter what you say". *Journal of Consulting and Clinical Psychology, 71*(6), 1084–1089.

Wing, R. R., & Hill, J. O. (2001). Successful weight loss maintenance. *Annual Review of Nutrition, 21*, 323–341.

Wing, R. R., Jeffery, R. W., Burton, L. R., Thorson, C., Nissinoff, K. S., & Baxter, J. E. (1996). Food provision vs structured meal plans in the behavioral treatment of obesity. *International Journal of Obesity, 20*(1), 56–62.

Womble, L. G., Wadden, T. A., McGuckin, B. G., Sargent, S. L., Rothman, R. A., & Krauthamer-Ewing, E. S. (2004). A randomized controlled trial of a commercial internet weight loss program. *Obesity Research, 12*(6), 1011–1018.

Chapter 18

Obesity Risk Factors and Prevention in Early Life: Pre-Gestation through Infancy

Nicolas Stettler

Introduction

As with other age-groups in the U.S. population, the prevalence of overweight has increased among children 6 to 24 months of age: from 7.2% in 1976–1980 to 11.6% in 1999–2000 in a nationally representative sample (Ogden, Flegal, Carroll, & Johnson, 2002). Nutritional surveillance data for low-income children show similar trends (Mei et al., 1998). Although the increase in the prevalence of overweight has been less rapid in this age group compared to older children and adolescents (Ogden et al., 2002), these trends suggest that the obesity epidemic may begin in infancy. This justifies a closer look at the possibility of initiating childhood obesity prevention very early in life.

Although the evidence in this area is not definitive, early life risk factors for obesity development in the offspring may include, for pregnant women, obesity, excessive weight gain, or diabetes during pregnancy, and, for the infant, high infant birth weight, not being breastfed or for only a short period, and rapid infancy weight gain. Maternal obesity is one of the strongest predictors for obesity in the offspring (Whitaker, Wright, Pepe, Seidel, & Dietz, 1997). Public health concern about this potential obesity risk factor for the offspring has increased markedly with the increase in obesity among U.S. women. In adolescent females, the prevalence of overweight, defined as a body mass index (BMI) at or above age and gender specific 95th percentile of the relevant Centers for Disease Control standard (see Chapter 2), has increased from 5.3% in 1976–1980 to 16.4% in 2003–2004 (Ogden et al., 2006; Ogden et al., 2002). During the same period, the prevalence of obesity, defined as a BMI of 30 kg/m^2 or more, in women ages 20 to 39 years increased from 12.3% to 28.9% (Flegal, Carroll, Ogden, & Johnson, 2002; Ogden et al., 2006).

Some potential risk factors for early obesity development are more common in ethnic minority and low socioeconomic status groups. For example, obesity prevalence is notably higher in Black American, Mexican American, and Native American women, compared to White women and is also generally higher in women living below or near the poverty line (Bolen, Rhodes, Powell-Griner, Bland, & Holtzman, 2000; Ogden et al., 2006; Zhang & Wang, 2004), Diabetes is also more prevalent in these population groups (Harris et al., 1998; United States

Dept. of Health and Human Services, 2001). As obesity and diabetes are more frequent in Black than in White women, and as these conditions are associated with high birth weight, it would be expected that the prevalence of low birth weight should be lower in Black than in White women. However, the opposite is observed (United States Dept. of Health and Human Services, 2001). These smilingly paradoxical observations may be explained by the fact that obesity is also a risk factor for hypertension, which is a major risk factor for low birth weight, or by other factors associated with low birth weight that are more frequent among Black women. Breastfeeding is less frequent among Black mothers and among those with lower educational levels (United States Dept. of Health and Human Services, 2001).

Overweight status in infancy is only a modest predictor of adulthood obesity and its complications. Although overweight toddlers are at higher risk for adulthood obesity, only one in four children who are overweight in the second year of life is likely to become an obese adult (Whitaker et al., 1997). Nevertheless, as will be discussed, the longer term benefits of preventive interventions begun very early in life are not necessarily mediated through the prevention of overweight during infancy. Early interventions could, therefore, also lead to a decrease in obesity much later in life, after a latency period and without impact on infancy overweight status.

As the first of several chapters discussing the potential for obesity prevention during different stages of life, this chapter focuses on fetal life and infancy. See the Box for explanations and definitions of several key concepts and terms used in the chapter. In the following narrative, the lifecourse perspective on obesity epidemiology and prevention (Gillman, 2004), which serves as the conceptual framework for this chapter, is first explained, after which other key aspects of the developmental context for obesity prevention during fetal life and infancy and the associated risks of intervening during these periods are highlighted. A review of evidence for maternal and infant factors that may increase the risk for obesity development follows, together with potential pre- and post-natal opportunities for prevention, identified in the contexts of existing nutrition and weight gain guidelines for pregnant women and infants and settings that offer natural access.

Box 18.1. Definitions and Key Concepts

Infancy
Infancy is the period between birth and first birthday. The first four weeks of life are called the **neonatal period** and the infant is called a **newborn**.

Gestational Age at Birth
Gestational age at birth is the duration, usually measured in weeks, between the first day of the last normal menstruation of the pregnant woman and the day of delivery. This definition assumes a regular 28-day cycle and that ovulation occurred 14 days after the first day of menstruation. Normal pregnancy duration and gestational age at birth (but really the period with no menstruation) are 37.0 to 41.9 weeks or 259 to 293 days.

Gestational age can be determined by history of the last menstruation, but this method is often unreliable, as blood discharges sometimes happen in early pregnancy and can be mistaken for menstruation. Preferred methods of gestational age determination are prenatal ultrasounds or assessment of physical and neurological development of the newborn after birth. Infants born before 37 weeks are called **preterm or premature newborns**, while those born at or after 42 weeks are called **post-term newborns**. Risk factors for premature birth can be maternal, including cervix insufficiency, infection, pre-eclampsia, and smoking, or can be fetal, including malformation and fetal distress.

Premature Infants

Infants born before 37 weeks are called **preterm or premature newborns**. The physical and neurological developments of premature infants are expected first to continue as they would in utero and only then to follow the development of an infant born at full term gestation. Preterm infants are, therefore, often characterized by their **corrected age** in addition to chronological age. Corrected age is calculated by subtracting the difference between gestational age and 40 weeks from the chronological age. For example, an infant with a chronological age of eight months born at 32 weeks of gestation is considered about two months premature and its corrected age would then be six months.

Birth Weight

Birth weight is the weight of the newborn measured shortly after birth and before feeding. Duration of gestation is the main determinant of birth weight. Other important determinants are maternal health, maternal smoking, race, parity, and season of birth. Birth weight is considered normal between 2,500 and 4,000 g. Infants born with a weight below 2,500 g are called **"low birth weight" (LBW)** and those above 4,000 g **"high birth weight" or macrosomic**, regardless of the duration of the gestation. Thus, LBW may be due to short gestation or slow growth during fetal life. Infants born with a birth weight below 1,500 g are called **"very low birth weight" (VLBW)** and those born below 1,000 g **"extremely low birth weight" (ELBW)**.

Birth Weight Relative to Gestational Age

Because birth weight varies with gestational age, sets of reference percentiles of birth weight for gestational age have been established (Battaglia & Lubchenco, 1967). Newborns are called **small-for-gestational age (SGA)** if their weight is below the 10th percentile, **large-for-gestational age (LGA)** if their weight is above the 90th percentile, and **appropriate-for-gestational age (AGA)** otherwise. Infants with a birth weight below the 3rd percentile are sometimes referred as **severely SGA**. As weight for gestational age accounts for the duration of gestation, it is a better indicator of intrauterine growth than birth weight. A newborn with LBW can be AGA and have had normal intrauterine growth before a premature birth. As some determinants and consequences of premature birth and **intrauterine growth retardation (IUGR)** are different, this distinction is important from a lifecourse perspective. However, birth weight for gestational age does not necessarily reflect the dynamic process of fetal growth or the body proportions of the newborn. Two infants may present with the same birth weight for gestational age, but may have experienced growth retardation at different stage of fetal life or may have different body proportions, such as a preservation of the brain growth at the expense of other organs, resulting in disproportional fetal growth patters. These distinctions are also important from a lifecourse perspective as the causes and consequences of these growth patterns may be different.

Overweight in Infancy

There is no universally recognized definition of overweight in the first year of life. A frequently used definition is a weight for length at or above the 95th percentile of the reference population (Kuczmarski et al., 2000). BMI is typically not used during infancy, but some have used the ponderal index (weight in kg divided by length in m at the power three) to describe weight relative to length in infants.

Developmental Context

Lifecourse Perspective

The lifecourse approach posits that susceptibility to adult disease is determined by a dynamic process that occurs over the lifespan (Ben-Shlomo & Kuh, 2002; Kuh & Ben-Shlomo, 1997). Perturbations or insults determining adult health may occur at any time from pre-conception to embryonic, fetal, infant, childhood, adolescent, and adult life. These insults can affect both somatic growth and maturation of metabolic systems, and they include a range of societal, lifestyle, and biological determinants, which act in concert with each other (Figure 18.1). Under the lifecourse approach, one possibility is that health determinants work through a critical period model, in

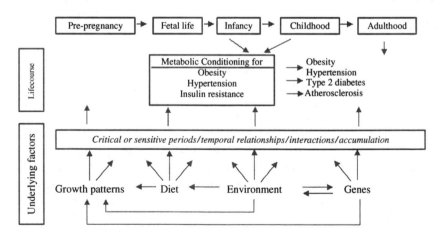

Figure 18.1 A conceptual framework of the lifecourse approach to obesity epidemiology and prevention. Susceptibility to obesity is determined by a dynamic process that occurs over the lifespan, with societal, lifestyle, and biological determinants acting during critical or sensitive periods on the development of obesity and its complications.

which an insult during a specific period of development has lasting effects on the structure or function of organs, tissues and body systems (Gillman, 2004). Some prefer to call these periods sensitive rather than critical if the insult is not completely deterministic. For example, the association of stroke mortality with low social class is stronger for social class measured in childhood than in adulthood (Smith, Hart, Blane, & Hole, 1998); therefore, childhood can be considered a sensitive period for this association. Other lifecourse models are also possible, such as the accumulation of risk models (Gillman, 2004). The concept of critical periods can also include latency before the development of the outcome. That is, exposure during a sensitive or critical period can be associated with the development of a condition such as obesity after a delay in which excessive adiposity is not apparent. Thus, this concept differs from "tracking" of risk factors from early life to adulthood.

Prevention models based on a lifecourse perspective would argue that interventions targeted to critical or sensitive periods confer long-term benefits potentially greater than interventions occurring during less sensitive periods. Identifying and intervening upon modifiable factors that occur during such short critical or sensitive periods could be particularly effective at preventing the development of obesity. In fact, the lifecourse approach may be especially well suited to the prevention of obesity as, unlike other chronic diseases of adulthood, obesity has a significant occurrence during childhood, with complications evident in young adulthood and even childhood.

Fetal Life and Infancy

Fetal life and infancy represent the periods of the life cycle with the largest number and magnitude of biological, developmental, behavioral, environmental, and nutritional changes. It is thus natural to hypothesize that these two periods may be critical for the long-term development of health and disease, including obesity.

Growth and Metabolism

During a normal gestation, the human fetus grows from a microscopic single-cell organism to a highly complex organism of about 3,200 g. In the first year of life, body weight increases threefold and body composition changes noticeably. Fat mass increases from approximately 500 g at birth (14% of body weight) to more than 2,000 g at 12 months of age (23% of body weight). In the first year of life, energy requirements increase from about 500 to 750 kcal/day, a slower increase than the increase in body weight. Thus, relative to body weight, energy requirements decrease from about 110 to 80 kcal/kg/day. Energy use also changes dramatically during this period. Energy deposition for growth accounts for about 40% of the energy requirements in the first month of life but only for about 2 to 3% at 12 months. The remaining energy requirements are divided between energy for activity and basal metabolic rate. Brain metabolic rate accounts for 87% of the basal metabolic rate in the newborn, but only 53% in the 12-month-old infant.

Important changes in the hormonal control of growth and metabolism also happen during fetal life and infancy. While fetal growth is mainly under the control of insulin, thyroid hormone and insulin-like growth factors, infant growth is mainly controlled by pituitary growth hormones (Fowden & Forhead, 2004). Perhaps more important for understanding the developmental determinants of obesity, leptin, a hormone produced in the adipose tissue that regulates food intake and body weight (Friedman, 2000), has been shown to be produced both by the human fetus and placenta in the third trimester of pregnancy. At birth, leptin levels are high and remain high for the first six hours of life but plunge rapidly to low levels by 12 to 16 hours of life. A gradual increase takes place during the following weeks and months (Himms-Hagen, 1999).

In humans, brain size increases considerably during the last three months of fetal life and the first three years of post-natal life. The peak velocity in brain growth occurs around birth, when the brain size already reaches 30% of adult size. At 18 months, the brain has reached 60% and at three years more than 80% of adult size. The complex microscopic structure of the brain is achieved by neuronal migration, a process during which neurons arrange themselves in the brain by migrating to the places where they are supposed to be located to fulfill their individual function. Neuronal migration reaches its height at the end of the first trimester of pregnancy. Neurogenesis, the process by which new neurons are created, and myelinization, the process by which nerve fibers are isolated to facilitate communication between brain cells, begin in mid-gestation and continue in the first two years of life. Programmed neuron cell death, which starts at the end of fetal life, further contributes to the plasticity and maturation of the brain.

Gross Motor Development and Feeding Patterns

The anatomic changes of the brain during early life correlate with remarkable developmental and behavioral changes (Behrman, Kliegman, & Jenson, 2004). Gross motor development, which is critical for later physical activity, starts at eight weeks of fetal life, when the first muscle contractions can be observed. At full-term birth, muscle tone is sufficient to partially hold the newborn's head. In the first six months of life, the infant starts to learn voluntary muscle contractions that generate predictable tactile and visual stimuli and lead to the progressive development of voluntary movements (Behrman et al., 2004). On average, infants are able to sit without support around six months of life and to walk around one year of life. These developmental milestones set the stage for increased independence and socialization. As soon as the child is able to walk independently, he or she increases control of his/her environment and the range of available food and activity choices.

To paraphrase Behrman et al., (2004) in the first year of life, parenting progresses from care of a near-sighted newborn with mainly uncontrolled movements, urgent, unclear and often exhausting needs to a relationship with an increasingly independent child who clearly communicates non-verbally, explores his/her environment, feeds him/herself, makes choices, and is suspicious of strangers. The first year of life is also a time when food intake behaviors, appetite, and energy regulation mechanisms are organized; it is also a time of significant changes in nutritional patterns and diet. In fetal life, nutrients are passively supplied to the fetus through the placenta. However, some evidence suggests that the fetus is already exposed, through the amniotic fluid, to tastes that vary with the diet of the pregnant woman and may influence later choices (Mennella, Jagnow, & Beauchamp, 2001).

Minutes after birth, the newborn is placed at the breast and for the first time experiences feeding, hunger, and satiety. The highly complex and redundant systems that will regulate the finely tuned energy balance for the rest of the individual's life are first put into use and possibly set at that time. Initially, the discomfort of hunger leads to tension and crying that, in turn, leads the caring parent to provide food and, for the newborn, results in feeding, pleasant tactile and visual stimulation, and the relief of hunger (Behrman et al., 2004). Progressively, the infant adapts to more regular feeding schedules and by the end of the first year to an adult pattern of three main meals with snacks. The infant's diet also changes drastically in the first year of life. While there is evidence that the taste of breast milk varies with maternal diet (Mennella et al., 2001), the formula-fed infant experiences months of a remarkably monotonous diet, constant in taste. In the first year of life, the diet changes from 100% breast milk or formula to the progressive introduction of complementary foods, exposure to new textures and tastes, and, by 12 months, a diet that resembles the family diet.

Long Term Impact of the Early Life Environment

The remarkable biological and behavioral developments during fetal life and the first year of human life are, at least in part, influenced by environmental factors. Thus, interventions during this period have the potential to have long-term beneficial or harmful health consequences. The field of developmental biology provides many examples from animal models of the long-term impact of the early life environment, usually referred to as imprinting or programming. Among the many mechanisms that underlie these influences, variations in the expression of existing genes, a process studied by the emerging field of epigenetics, has received increasing attention. In humans, several historical examples of harmful programming are well known. Exposure of the human fetus to diethylstilbestrol, a synthetic estrogen prescribed to pregnant women to prevent miscarriages, leads to the development of a particular cancer of the vagina and cervix in female offspring decades later. The malformations associated with fetal exposure to thalidomide and the neurodevelopmental consequence of fetal exposure to high levels of methyl-mercury in Minamata, Japan, provide other striking and extreme examples. The consequences of more subtle environmental manipulations in early life are of increasing interest and the potential of early life interventions for chronic disease prevention, particularly obesity, has opened an exciting, hopeful field of new research. The flipside of this exciting potential is that the possibility for imprinting and programming in early life also highlights the high vulnerability of the fetus and infant and the risk for long-term unwanted health consequences. Thus, any intervention during this period should be carefully thought through and observed over the long term.

The concept of prevention of early life causation of adult chronic diseases was popular in the 19th century but was largely forgotten by the second half of the 20th. In 1976, however, Ravelli, Stein and Susser (Ravelli, Stein, & Susser, 1976) published a study of young Dutch men who had been exposed during various stages of fetal life and infancy at the end of World War II to a short period of famine. This study suggested that exposure to famine at the beginning of fetal life was associated with an increased risk for adult obesity, while exposure at the end of fetal life and early infancy was associated with a decreased risk. In the following years, David Barker, in the United Kingdom, published a series of studies demonstrating the association of low birth weight first with ischemic heart disease mortality, then with ischemic heart diseases, elevated blood pressure, and insulin resistance. In his 1998 book, Barker further refined his "fetal origin hypothesis." During the same period, renewed interest in early life determinants of chronic diseases, including determinants in early post-natal life, led to several epidemiological studies and to the conceptualization of the lifecourse approach to chronic disease epidemiology by Kuh and Ben-Shlomo (1997).

Risk Factors and Opportunities for Obesity Prevention

The Prenatal Period: Pregnant Women

Weight Status of Pregnant Women
Maternal overweight status has been associated with overweight in the offspring at various ages and in many populations (Parsons, Power, Logan, & Summerbell, 1999; Whitaker et al., 1997). Furthermore, there seems to be a continuous association between maternal and offspring weight status along the continuum of maternal weight (Stettler et al., 2000). The most obvious hypothetical contributing factor for this association is a genetic predisposition to obesity shared by mother and child, as has been demonstrated in studies of children adopted at birth (Stunkard et al., 1986). The environment that mother and child share also likely contributes to this association in weight status, which could be mediated through several factors. Overweight women tend to have infants with higher birth weight, which is associated with later obesity. Overweight women are also less likely to breastfeed successfully, and breastfeeding has been associated with a protective effect for obesity development in the offspring.

When examining the association between maternal and offspring weight status, several important confounding factors need to be considered, including paternal weight status, race/ethnicity, socioeconomic status, maternal age, and parity. Because no intervention studies have examined this question and because the association between maternal and offspring weight status could be entirely explained by non-modifiable factors, it is unclear if a better control of weight status in women of child-bearing age would result in obesity prevention in the offspring. But, at a minimum, the strong association between maternal and offspring weight status is informative for prevention, to help identify children at risk for developing obesity. The prevention of obesity in female adolescents and women of child-bearing age is addressed in Chapters 21 and 22.

Weight Gain and Nutrition during Pregnancy
Weight gain during pregnancy is recommended to fall within 11.5 to 16.0 kg in non-obese women, 7.0 to 11.5 kg in overweight women, and 12.5 to 18.0 kg in underweight women (Institute of Medicine (U.S.) Subcommittee on Nutritional Status and Weight Gain during Pregnancy & Institute of Medicine (U.S.) Subcommittee on Dietary Intake and Nutrient Supplements during Pregnancy, 1990). These ranges are associated with optimal pregnancy, fetal, and neonatal outcomes. Excessive weight gain during pregnancy is associated

with higher birth weight, which, in turn, is associated with overweight in childhood and adulthood. Data from the Dutch Famine study provide indirect evidence that poor weight gain in late pregnancy may be associated with a decreased risk for obesity in the adult offspring (Ravelli et al., 1976). However, observational studies directly addressing this question are sparse. Two published observational studies did not demonstrate a link between weight gain during pregnancy and obesity in the offspring during childhood (Fisch, Bilek, & Ulstrom, 1975; Whitaker, 2004), but two preliminary reports suggest a positive association (Oken, Taveras, Kleinman, Rich-Edwards, & Gillman, 2005; Seidman, Laor, Shemer, Gale, & Stevenson, 1996). The nature of the association between weight gain during pregnancy and overweight in the offspring is unclear, but could be mediated through high birth weight, fetal glucocorticoid exposure, and/or metabolic programming, or explained by confounding factors, such as socioeconomic factors, shared environment, or genetic determinants.

No intervention studies have specifically addressed the hypothesis that preventing excessive weight gain during pregnancy could prevent obesity in offspring later in life. Interventions to prevent excessive weight gain during pregnancy for reasons other than prevention of obesity in offspring have, however, been systematically reviewed and found to be possible (Kramer & Kakuma, 2003), although the number of studies (three) and total number of subjects was relatively small and the impact on birth weight inconsistent. More recent studies confirm the feasibility and effectiveness of excessive weight gain prevention during pregnancy (Olson, Strawderman, & Reed, 2004; Polley, Wing, & Sims, 2002), but the long-term impact on offspring overweight status is unknown.

Another important question is whether a woman's diet or intake of specific nutrients during pregnancy may have an impact on the risk for overweight in the offspring. This possibility is suggested by animal studies. Although the impact of a woman's diet during pregnancy on several outcomes, mostly neonatal outcomes, has been extensively studied in humans, the association of diet during pregnancy with the development of overweight in the offspring remains understudied. One of the potential mechanisms for this association may be through prenatal exposure to tastes in the amniotic fluid impacting taste preference and food choices later in life (Mennella et al., 2001). Once again, when studying the association of the diet of pregnant women with overweight in the offspring, important confounding factors should be kept in mind but are often difficult to measure. Thus, only intervention studies will provide sufficient justification for modifying pregnant women's diets as a public health tool for the prevention of obesity in the offspring.

Diabetes During Pregnancy

Diabetes during pregnancy is associated with increased birth weight and other obstetrical, fetal, or neonatal complications that can be, at least in part, prevented by optimized diabetes control during pregnancy (Metzger & Coustan, 1998). The goal of diabetes control during pregnancy is to maintain a fasting glucose at or below 5.3 mmol/l (95 mg/dl) and a two-hour postprandial glucose at or below 6.7 mmol/l (120 mg/dl) through dietary and physical activity interventions and insulin injections when needed (Metzger & Coustan, 1998). Pregnant women can have three types of diabetes. Type 1 diabetes is caused by a destruction of insulin-producing pancreatic cells during childhood or early adulthood and usually precedes pregnancy. Women with type 1 diabetes always require insulin; therefore, this type of diabetes is often called "insulin-dependent diabetes." This nomenclature may be misleading, though, as the other types of diabetes may also require insulin treatment. With the increase in obesity in the U.S. population, more and more women of childbearing age and adolescents have type 2 diabetes, once known as adult-onset diabetes or non-insulin-dependent diabetes. Type 2 diabetes is usually caused by obesity-related insulin resistance and the progressive failure by the pancreas to meet the increased requirements for insulin to overcome this tissue resistance. Type 2 diabetes is treated by weight loss, insulin-sensitizing oral medications, or insulin. Because pregnancy is a contraindication to insulin-sensitizing oral medications, many pregnant women with type 2 diabetes are treated with insulin injections to optimize diabetes control. Furthermore, pregnancy is a physiological state of insulin resistance. In predisposed women, about 2 to 3% of women of childbearing age, this pregnancy-induced insulin resistance may become more significant and result in gestational diabetes (Kuhl, 1998). Often gestational diabetes is reversible and resolves after delivery, but in some women, it can remain present as type 2 diabetes after pregnancy (Kuhl, 1998). Many women do not meet the criteria of gestational diabetes, but nonetheless present some degree of insulin resistance and glucose intolerance during pregnancy.

Regardless of the type of diabetes, the fetus of a diabetic woman with poor diabetes control is exposed to high blood sugar and consequently increases its own insulin production. As insulin is one of the main growth factors during fetal life, offspring of women with poor diabetes control during pregnancy are born LGA or macrosomic (see Box 18.1 for definitions). This neonatal macrosomia is the main cause of obstetrical and neonatal complications. In addition, diabetes during pregnancy is a risk factor for premature birth and fetal malformations. Diabetes during pregnancy has also been associated with obesity in the offspring during adolescence (Gillman, Rifas-Shiman, Berkey, Field, & Colditz, 2003; Silverman, Rizzo, Cho, & Metzger, 1998). However, most studies of pregnancy diabetes and offspring obesity are unable to separate the effect of the intrauterine environment from a genetic predisposition to obesity and diabetes. One study, though, suggests that the intrauterine environment itself may predispose the offspring to obesity. Pima Indians in Arizona have high prevalence of obesity and type 2 diabetes. In a study of Pima Indians, Pettitt, Nelson, Saad, Bennett, & Knowler (1993) compared siblings born before and after their mother developed diabetes, thus partially controlling for their familial predisposition. The sibling born after being exposed to pregnancy diabetes in utero was more likely to become an obese child or adolescent than the sibling born before development of diabetes in the mother, suggesting a direct effect of the intrauterine environment on the risk for obesity in the offspring.

The association between diabetes during pregnancy and obesity in the offspring could be explained by high birth weight, fetal exposure to high blood sugar, high fetal blood insulin, and metabolic programming. However, another intriguing observation suggests a different possible mechanism. Comparing children of diabetic mothers who were breastfed by their mother or fed banked breast milk from non-diabetic women, Plagemann, Harder, Kerstin, & Kohlhoff

(Plagemann, Harder, Kerstin, & Kohlhoff, 2002) showed an increased risk for obesity in the children fed the milk of their diabetic mothers, suggesting an effect of breast milk of mothers who are diabetic. An area of great interest but uncertainty is the impact on the offspring's weight status of glucose intolerance in women who do not meet the criteria for gestational diabetes. As the cutoff points for the definition of gestational diabetes are relatively arbitrary, one could speculate that glucose intolerance during pregnancy is a milder form of gestational diabetes with similar but milder effects on the risk for obesity in the offspring.

No intervention study to prevent or control diabetes during pregnancy has investigated a possible impact on the offspring's weight status after the neonatal period. Thus, evidence is currently insufficient to recommend such intervention for the prevention of obesity in the offspring. A limited number of intervention studies to optimize diabetes control or to improve glucose tolerance during pregnancy have shown improved glycemic control and, for some, a reduction in high birth weight through caloric restriction, other dietary manipulations or physical activity (Bevier, Fischer, & Jovanovic, 1999; Jovanovic-Peterson, Bevier, & Peterson, 1997; Jovanovic-Peterson, Durak, & Peterson, 1989; Knopp, Magee, Raisys, Benedetti, & Bonet, 1991). However, a systematic review deemed existing data insufficient for reaching reliable conclusions on the effectiveness of such interventions (Tuffnell, West, & Walkinshaw, 2003).

Smoking During Pregnancy

Recently, several observational studies have suggested that smoking during pregnancy may be associated with an increased risk for obesity in the offspring (von Kries, Toschke, Koletzko, & Slikker, 2002; Whitaker, 2004) and that a dose-response association may be present (Wideroe, Vik, Jacobsen, & Bakketeig, 2003). The mechanism for this association is unclear and most likely not mediated through fetal growth, as infants of smoking women usually have a lower birth weight than those of non-smokers. As for several other potential targets for intervention described in this chapter, the association between smoking during pregnancy and obesity in the offspring is subject to important potential confounding variables that are difficult to measure, particularly the elusive concept of "health consciousness." The lack of intervention studies with long-term follow-up of the offspring weight status limits the ability to draw conclusions about causality or to estimate the potential of smoking cessation to prevent obesity in the offspring. In fact, one would expect smoking cessation to be associated with an increased body weight in the pregnant woman and an increased birth weight, of which both are associated with an increased risk for obesity in the offspring. Interventions to promote smoking cessation during pregnancy have, however, been tested for the other health benefits. A systematic review found that these interventions are effective in decreasing the proportion of women who continue to smoke (Lumley, Oliver, Chamberlain, & Oakley, 2004).

Birth Weight and Gestational Age

The direct association between birth weight and weight status later in life is consistent between populations, across a wide range of age of the offspring and across various methods of weight status measurements (Gillman, 2004;

Parsons et al., 1999). These studies have demonstrated associations between birth weight status and later weight status both using continuous or dichotomous variables of weight status. Among studies that adjust for gestational age or maternal weight status, birth weight remained independently associated with weight status later in life. Although this association, as such, is not a subject of debate, no intervention studies have demonstrated a cause-effect relationship. Being born LGA and being obese later in life could be due to common genetic or environmental predispositions or to other unmeasured confounding factors. However, a study of monozygotic twins suggests that the association of birth and adolescent weight status is not entirely explained by genetic or common environmental factors and that fetal growth may have a long-term impact on weight status (Pietilainen, Kaprio, Rasanen, Rissanen, & Rose, 2002).

In most studies, being born SGA has been associated with a decreased risk for obesity later in life, regardless of whether the birth is full- or pre-term. Some studies, however, suggest a U-shaped curve between birth weight and later weight status, that is, both low birth weight and high birth weight may predispose to later obesity (Curhan et al., 1996). However, an association between low birth weight for gestational age and later obesity has not been clearly demonstrated in humans, despite evidence from animal models.

When individuals born SGA do become obese, they tend to have a more central fat distribution (Barker, Robinson, Osmond, & Barker, 1997), a risk factor for insulin resistance and cardiovascular diseases. This increased risk for central obesity in individuals born SGA is compatible with Barker's fetal origin of adult disease hypothesis (Barker, 1998). Restricted fetal growth has been most clearly associated with cardiovascular disease and with risk factors other than generalized obesity. No intervention studies have been conducted to test the hypothesis that preventing SGA birth weight could impact fat distribution.

In studying possible associations of premature birth with obesity later in life, birth weight for gestational age needs to be carefully taken into account. This is a frequent problem, because some of the determinants of premature birth are the same as the determinants of intrauterine growth retardation, and many premature infants also are SGA. Being born before term gestation, per se, does not appear to be associated with increased BMI later in life (Johansson et al., 2005) and may actually be associated with decreased adult BMI if fetal growth retardation is also present. For example, male (but not female) subjects born premature with a VLBW had a lower BMI at age 20 years than subjects born at full term (Hack et al., 2003). This observation could be explained by fetal growth retardation, as the subjects born with a VLBW were, on average, also SGA at birth. Another study suggests that the lower BMI of adolescents born premature is due to lower fat mass (Fewtrell, Lucas, Cole, & Wells, 2004). These results were, however, not adjusted for birth weight for gestational age status and may have also been confounded by intrauterine growth retardation.

Challenges of Prenatal Interventions in Pregnant Women
Several prenatal interventions with the potential to decrease the risk for obesity in offspring are already recommended or standard practices for other health reasons. The prevention of overweight and obesity in adolescent girls and women of childbearing age is a public health priority, as in other population groups (U.S. Department of Health and Human Services, 2001; 2001a),

and is discussed elsewhere in this book. The prevention of excessive weight gain during pregnancy is standard practice to prevent obstetrical and neonatal complications (Institute of Medicine (U.S.) Subcommittee on Nutritional Status and Weight Gain during Pregnancy & Institute of Medicine (U.S.) Subcommittee on Dietary Intake and Nutrient Supplements during Pregnancy, 1990). In diabetic women and women with glucose intolerance, glycemic control is also recommended to decrease obstetrical and neonatal complications (Metzger & Coustan, 1998). Reduction of smoking exposure during pregnancy has well-established benefits for the pregnant woman and the fetus and represents one of the goals of Healthy People 2010 (United States Dept. of Health and Human Services, 2001).

Although these interventions already are recommended and thought to have public health benefits, their impact on the prevention of obesity in the offspring is unknown. Thus, long-term follow-up of the offspring should be encouraged to measure the impact of any of these prevention strategies on obesity prevention. There is, however, an ethical challenge to designing studies of prenatal interventions that are already recommended for other reasons in order to test their impact on the long-term health of the offspring. As these interventions already are established, randomized controlled trials would require less than optimal care for the control group and, in most cases, would be unethical. Thus, more creative research designs such as quasi-experiments or offspring follow-up of historical clinical trials may be needed.

When interventions are appropriate, they require changes in well-established behaviors or habits. Therefore, it is unlikely that health education alone would be successful and, most likely, behavior modification interventions will be required to achieve the desired changes. Such behavior modification could be formatted for individual or group interventions. Some prenatal interventions may be associated with potential risks. For example, insufficient weight gain could be an unintended adverse effect of overzealous attempts to prevent excessive weight gain during pregnancy, with impaired nutrition and consequent damage to the fetus. Thus, such interventions should take place under close medical supervision.

The Postnatal Period: Infants

Breastfeeding

Early observational studies did not support the hypothesis that breastfeeding could decrease the risk of developing obesity in offspring (Butte, 2001). More recently, however, several studies and meta-analyses of observational studies have suggested a dose-dependent protective effect of breastfeeding against obesity development (Arenz, Ruckerl, Koletzko, & von Kries, 2004; Owen, Martin, Whincup, Smith, & Cook, 2005). Several mechanisms have been hypothesized. Breastfed infants tend to gain weight more slowly than formula-fed infants (Dewey, 1998), thus the association of formula feeding with later obesity may be mediated by rapid infancy weight gain. Breast milk itself contains biological factors not contained in formula that may decrease the long-term risk of developing obesity. Another possible mechanism is through the establishment during the neonatal period of infant feeding self-regulation or of feeding interactions between parent and child. Infants who feed at the breast self-regulate their energy intake by their sucking behavior. Breast milk production is directly dependent on the infant sucking, and overfeeding is unlikely to happen with breastfeeding. In contrast, bottle-fed infants may be subject to overfeeding if parents think that the infant should finish the bottle or adhere to rigid feeding guidelines. Parental control of dietary intake has been associated with overweight in older children (Faith, Scanlon, Birch, Francis, & Sherry, 2004) and may be more prevalent in children who have been bottle-fed (Taveras et al., 2004).

The main weakness of the evidence for a protective effect of breastfeeding against obesity development is that these observational studies are subject to confounding factors that are difficult to measure, particularly the "health consciousness" of families that may be more likely to breastfeed and less likely to engage in behaviors associated with later obesity. In an attempt to control for these family factors, Nelson, Gordon-Larsen, & Adair (2005) conducted an observational study of siblings discordant for breastfeeding status and found no association of breastfeeding with obesity in adolescence, after adjustment for sibling status. A more definite answer to this controversial question will likely come from follow-up data from randomized controlled trials of breastfeeding promotion, but, to date, no such data have been published that address obesity prevention in the offspring. Promising data are currently being collected in nearly 14,000 six-and-a-half-year-old children of mothers who were subjects of the Promotion of Breastfeeding Intervention Trial (PROBIT) study (Kramer et al., 2001). Using the model developed for the World Health Organization Baby Friendly Hospital Initiative, hospitals in Belarus were randomized to the intervention or usual care and included about 17,000 mother-infant pairs. At three months of age, 43.3% of the intervention infants were exclusively breastfed, compared to 6.4% of control infants, and at six months of age, 7.9% compared to 0.6%. The effect of the intervention persisted at twelve months when 19.7% of intervention infants still received some breastfeeding compared to 11.4% of infants in the control group. However, some may not be swayed by results of such trials because breastfeeding promotion interventions do not lead to a 100% successful breastfeeding rate. Intention-to-treat analyses of randomized trials do not allow an accounting for the achieved breastfeeding rate. Furthermore, breastfeeding may be more or less protective against obesity at different times of the lifecycle and longer follow-up will be necessary to assess the long-term consequences of breastfeeding in the PROBIT and other breastfeeding promotion trials.

Breastfeeding promotion is already recommended for public health benefits other than obesity prevention (American Academy of Pediatrics. Committee on Nutrition & Kleinman, 2004; "Breastfeeding and the use of human milk. American Academy of Pediatrics. Work Group on Breastfeeding," 1997) and, considering the low potential for risks, is one of the strategies recommended by the Surgeon General (U.S. Department of Health and Human Services & Health Service, 2001) and the Institute of Medicine (Institute of Medicine (U.S.) Committee on Prevention of Obesity in Children and Youth, 2005) to prevent childhood obesity, based on observational evidence only. Currently, exclusive breastfeeding is recommended for the first six months of life, with progressive introduction of complementary foods thereafter. Some breastfeeding for at least the first twelve months of life is also recommended, in addition to the complementary foods. For mothers unwilling or unable to breastfeed, infant formulas are considered acceptable substitutes for breast milk. In the United States, rates of breastfeeding initiation and maintenance remain low (Fox, Pac, Devaney, & Jankowski, 2004), and breastfeeding promotion could be one of the strategies to prevent obesity.

Several studies have successfully promoted breastfeeding initiation and maintenance, particularly in low-income countries, but also in the United States (Dyson, McCormick, & Renfrew, 2005; Sikorski, Renfrew, Pindoria, & Wade, 2002). The PROBIT study may be one of the largest and most relevant to the U.S. context (Kramer et al., 2001) and achieved significant increase in breastfeeding rates, as described above. Thus, breastfeeding promotion is possible and effective, but its potential to prevent obesity in offspring is unknown.

Complementary Foods

Optimizing complementary food introduction to adhere to the American Academy of Pediatric (AAP) guidelines is another intervention already recommended (American Academy of Pediatrics. Committee on Nutrition. & Kleinman, 2004; "Breastfeeding and the use of human milk. American Academy of Pediatrics. Work Group on Breastfeeding," 1997). Despite these recommendations, complementary foods are often introduced before six months of age (Fox et al., 2004). For example, according to the 2002 Feeding Infants and Toddlers study (Fox et al., 2004), among infants ages four to six months, 66% consume grain or grain products, 14% meat, and 10% desserts at least once a day. Between the ages of nine and eleven months, 9% of infants consume French fries or other fried potatoes, 6% salty snacks, and 11% sweetened beverages at least once a day. Thus, there is much room for improvement of adherence to the AAP breastfeeding and nutrition recommendations for infants.

The association between early introduction of complementary food and obesity development remains controversial. Observational studies provide contradictory results (Agras, Kraemer, Berkowitz, & Hammer, 1990; Burdette, Whitaker, Hall, & Daniels, 2006; Kramer, 1981; Wilson et al., 1998). These studies, however, are also subject to confounding factors that are difficult to measure and the lack of positive results may be explained by reversed causality, i.e., infants who grow more slowly may be more likely to receive complementary feeding to improve growth. In addition to the timing of complementary food introduction, the type of complementary food may be associated with later risk for obesity. Experimental data suggest that taste preference may be established during infancy (Birch, 1999; Mennella et al., 2001). For example, infants who develop early preferences for high fat and high sugar foods may continue to prefer these foods as they grow older, and it has been suggested that childhood diet quality may be associated with obesity (Lee, Mitchell, Smiciklas-Wright, & Birch, 2001). However, data to support a direct association between the type of complementary food introduced during infancy and obesity later in life are lacking. One interventional study aimed at decreasing cardiovascular risk factors other than obesity may provide useful information, though. This large randomized controlled trial of cardiovascular prevention conducted in Finland, the Special Turku Coronary Risk Factor Intervention Project for Babies (STRIP) study (Niinikoski et al., 1996), compared usual care to a low saturated fat and low cholesterol diet starting at age seven months and continuing during childhood, together with physical activity promotion. The prevalence of overweight at age 10 years was lower among girls in the intervention group than in the control group, but no effect was observed among boys (Hakanen et al., 2006). In this study, it is difficult to attribute the difference in the prevalence of obesity to the type of complementary food introduced in infancy, as the intervention continued during childhood and included many other recommendations regarding nutrition and physical activity. This study, however, demonstrates the feasibility and safety of a diet low in saturated fat in infants as young as age seven months (Niinikoski et al., 1997; Rask-Nissila et al., 2000).

Motor Development and Activity Patterns

Little is known about a possible association between gross motor development, spontaneous physical activity or sedentary activities during infancy with later development of obesity in healthy individuals born at full-term gestation. Children with severe impairment of gross motor development often have long-term disabilities and it has recently been shown that children with limitations in physical activity are more likely to be overweight than other children (Bandini, Curtin, Hamad, Tybor, & Must, 2005). However, the pertinence of these findings to other children is unknown. Although about 60% of children under age two years watch television on a typical day, the long-term consequences of these early sedentary activities on obesity development are unknown. Interventions to promote physical activity or decrease sedentary activities in healthy infants during the first year of life have not been conducted.

Infancy Weight Gain

Several observational studies suggest a positive association between the rate of weight gain during the first year, first few months, and even first week of life with weight status and obesity in childhood and adulthood (Baird et al., 2005; Monteiro & Victora, 2005; Stettler et al., 2005). These results are, however, very dependent on the statistical method used to analyze the data. The best method to identify a sensitive or critical period of weight gain for the development of obesity remains controversial. One method developed by Cole (2004) to identify sensitive periods of weight gain is known as the lifecourse plot. However, using different analytical methods, other studies have concluded that infancy is not a critical period for the development of obesity (Kinra, Baumer, & Davey Smith, 2005). The association between early infancy weight gain and later obesity appears to be independent and to have no interaction with birth weight (Stettler, Zemel, Kumanyika, & Stallings, 2002).

Animal models support the imprinting of obesity in early postnatal life and have suggested potential mechanisms, including programming of the appetite regulation centers of the brain (Plagemann et al., 1999) and of insulin metabolism (Waterland & Garza, 2002). Another mechanism for an association between early infancy weight gain and later obesity could be through behaviors established in early life. Stunkard, Berkowitz, Schoeller, Maislin, & Stallings (2004) showed that the sucking behavior at age three months was predictive of weight status at age two years, confirming previous observations (Agras et al., 1990). Observational studies investigating the association between early infancy weight gain and later obesity are subject to many confounding factors, including common genetic and environmental determinants of rapid infancy weight gain and later obesity.

Preliminary results from a sibling study, however, suggest that this association is not entirely explained by common genetic background and environment (Stettler & Faith, 2004).

Convincing evidence for early infancy nutrition programming of metabolism is also provided by a series of reports by Singhal et al. (Singhal, Cole, Fewtrell, Deanfield, & Lucas, 2004; Singhal, Cole, & Lucas, 2001; Singhal et al., 2002; Singhal, Fewtrell, Cole, & Lucas, 2003) from a randomized controlled trial of preterm infant nutrition. Usual or enriched formulas were randomly assigned to a group of preterm infants from birth to hospital discharge for a median duration of four weeks. The infants randomized to the usual formula grew more slowly than those randomized to the enriched formula. A sub-sample of these subjects was located and studied during adolescence. Subjects randomized to the enriched formula during this short postnatal period had more insulin resistance (Singhal et al., 2003), higher blood pressure (Singhal et al., 2001), and early signs of cardiovascular disease (Singhal et al., 2004). Although they were not more likely to be obese, they did show signs of leptin resistance, which is one of the hypothesized mechanisms for obesity (Friedman, 2000; Singhal et al., 2002). These randomized controlled trial results suggest that early infant nutrition may have long-term metabolic consequences independent of confounding factors. The main limitations of these studies are the low follow-up rate (only about one in four eligible subjects were examined in adolescence) and the uncertainly of generalizing data from premature infants to the general population of infants.

Little effort has been dedicated to preventing rapid weight gain in infancy as, so far, the emphasis has been on preventing under-nutrition, particularly in SGA infants and infants from low-income countries. The benefits of preventing under-nutrition during the first year of life on neurological development, infection prevention, optimal statural growth, and overall morbidity and mortality have been well established ("The State of the World's Children 1998: a UNICEF report. Malnutrition: causes, consequences, and solutions," 1998). Furthermore, catch-up growth in LBW infants has shown some short- and long-term benefits both in low- and high-income countries (Henderson, Fahey, & McGuire, 2005; Luo, Albertsson-Wikland, & Karlberg, 1998; Victora, Barros, Horta, & Martorell, 2001). Thus, it is unknown if prevention of excessive weight gain during infancy is safe and possible, and, if so, if it is effective in preventing the development of later obesity.

The potential approaches to preventing excessive weight gain during infancy include breastfeeding promotion and starting complementary food only after age six months, of which both are recommended for other reasons. Other potential strategies to prevent excessive weight gain that have not been evaluated for safety or efficacy include restricting breast milk or formula intake, restricting the quantity of complementary foods, or altering complementary food options. Since during the first year of life dietary intake is much under the control of the caregivers, such interventions would probably have the format of health education, but may require intensive reassurance and support to address the concerns of caregivers and extended family about perceived insufficient weight gain.

Challenges of Postnatal Interventions in Infants
As discussed above for prenatal interventions, to design interventions to promote breastfeeding and optimize complementary feeding in the first year of

life, one has to balance ethical and scientific considerations. Long-term follow-up is important to establish the balance between benefits, costs, and risks of these interventions. Educational approaches most likely need to be complemented by behavioral and/or support strategies, in order to change traditional or cultural practices of infant feeding that are no longer recommended. When designing interventions to promote breastfeeding and to optimize infant nutrition, in addition to targeting mothers, researchers and public health officials should consider targeting fathers, members of the extended family, and other elements of the maternal support system and environment, particularly the work environment.

Intervention Settings

A natural setting for pre- and post-natal interventions is the health care setting, including prenatal care clinics, obstetrician, pediatrician, or family practice offices. The prenatal period and infancy are times when women and their children have frequent encounters with health professionals, thus offering numerous opportunities for obesity prevention. Women of childbearing age are recommended to get PAP smear screening at least every three years and 79% of them comply with this recommendation (United States. Dept. of Health and Human Services, 2001). During pregnancy, early and frequent prenatal care visits are recommended and more than 95% of U.S. women receive at least some prenatal care (Martin et al., 2005). Obstetricians can play a particularly important role in breastfeeding promotion, as most women decide if they will breastfeed long before delivery. Infants also frequently interact with the health system. The AAP recommends a minimum of eight preventive health care visits during the first year of life (Committee on Practice and Ambulatory Medicine, 2000). At age 19–35 months, more than 95% of children have completed at least three injections against diphtheria, tetanus, and pertussis, clearly having seen a health care provider at least three times, most likely during infancy ("National, state, and urban area vaccination coverage among children aged 19–35 months—United States, 2004," 2005). These frequent interactions with health professionals provide a unique window of opportunity for obesity prevention to be integrated into other preventive care encounters. Additionally, pregnancy and infancy may be periods when many families are particularly receptive to recommendations from health professionals to optimize the health of their offspring.

Other community-based settings may also be suitable. For nutrition interventions, these include governmental programs that support women and their infants. A large number of pregnant, postpartum and breastfeeding women and infants take part in the U.S. Government Special Supplemental Nutrition Program for Women, Infant, and Child (WIC), which provides nutrition supplementation and consultation to lower income families (Martin et al., 2005; U.S. Department of Agriculture Food and Nutrition Service Office of Analysis Nutrition and Evaluation, 2003). As part of WIC benefits, participants receive nutrition education and counseling at WIC clinics by experienced nutrition professionals, thus offering significant opportunities for obesity prevention. WIC is an especially appropriate setting, as nutrition education by professional nutritionists is closely integrated with other benefits of the program. Recent recommendations by the Institute of Medicine to change WIC food packages hold great promise for obesity prevention early in life (Institute of Medicine (U.S.) Committee to Review the WIC Food Packages, 2005). Daycare centers also represent another possible setting for infant feeding interventions.

Research Directions

As for other public health nutrition interventions, the safety and effectiveness of new interventions, i.e., those that are not otherwise recommended, for obesity prevention from pre-gestation through infancy must be clearly demonstrated before these interventions are translated into recommendations. As can be seen in this chapter, many research questions are unanswered and evidence-based obesity prevention strategies in this period of the life cycle may take decades to be defined. Many intervention studies aimed at outcomes other than obesity prevention have not yet reported data on obesity. As noted previously, although most prenatal interventions have already been studied for health benefits other than obesity prevention in the offspring, much research is needed to assess if these interventions may have a long term impact on the development of obesity in the offspring. Additionally, there are several scientific questions for which observational studies are needed before conducting intervention studies.

To establish effectiveness requires an explicit theoretical framework and rigorous research methods, particularly when harm is possible. For example, the optimal rate of weight gain during infancy for optimal long-term health is not clearly established and evidence for a positive association between infancy weight gain and later obesity has challenged the paradigm that, for infant weight gain, "more is better." As optimal infancy weight gain is not defined, the condition of uncertainly (i.e., the best option is not known) required for randomized control trials is met and this type of design would be the strongest to test excessive weight gain prevention interventions.

Interventions to optimize gross motor development and physical activity and/or to decrease sedentary activities, including exposure to television also require evaluation. There is a dearth of literature available to inform researchers and public health officials on potential approaches for such interventions. These types of interventions are unlikely to be associated with significant risk, but should nonetheless be implemented in a well controlled research setting with long-term follow-up for safety and efficacy.

The potential of a lifecourse approach to obesity prevention, starting before conception, is so substantial that this research agenda needs to be addressed urgently. Furthermore, if short interventions during critical periods can have long-term public health benefits, such strategies could be particularly cost effective. An important guiding principle for interventions aimed at growing, developing, and vulnerable individuals, is to plan, from initiation of the intervention, long-term safety and efficacy evaluations. This principle is challenging, however, as research and public health funding typically are for short periods relative to possible lifelong benefits or risks. Thus, funding agencies may need to consider the specific case of a lifecourse approach to chronic disease prevention and create original funding strategies to advance this promising field of prevention.

Summary and Implications

At this juncture, the interventions that can be recommended for obesity prevention during the vulnerable prenatal and postnatal periods are those that are recommended for other indications and that might also have the benefit of preventing the conditions that lead to obesity in the offspring in short or long term. These interventions include the prevention of overweight and excessive weight gain in pregnant women, optimal management of diabetes during gestation, smoking prevention during pregnancy, promotion of breastfeeding, and adherence to the AAP recommendations for the introduction of complementary feeding.

Otherwise, strategies that are not currently advised and that have not been deemed safe or beneficial should only be implemented in a rigorous research setting, with close monitoring of adverse events and long-term follow-up of the various critical outcomes that could be negatively affected. For example, the potential risks of limiting infant growth through dietary restriction include decreased statural growth, increased risk for infection, and, more importantly, sub-optimal neurological development. As discussed above, the first year of life is an important period for the development of the human brain and any dietary restriction during this period has the potential for negative long-term consequences. Furthermore, the nutritional needs for normal brain development during the first year of life have not been clearly defined. Such concerns have been the main reason that, for example, cardiovascular disease prevention by reducing fat and cholesterol intake has not been recommended before age two years. Some reassurance about these concerns can be derived from the results of the STRIP study described above, where the children who had been randomized to a low saturated fat, low cholesterol diet at age seven months had the same neurological development at age five years as the children of the control group (Rask-Nissila et al., 2000). These children, however, did not have a restricted infancy weight gain.

In conclusion, the prevention of obesity from pre-conception through infancy today remains only a promising theoretical concept, but, if supported by scientific evidence of safety and efficacy, may, in the future, play a critical role in comprehensive public health strategies for obesity prevention.

References

Agras, W. S., Kraemer, H. C., Berkowitz, R. I., & Hammer, L. D. (1990). Influence of early feeding style on adiposity at 6 years of age. *Journal of Pediatrics, 116*(5), 805–809.

American Academy of Pediatrics, Committee on Nutrition. (2004). InKleinman, R. E.. *Pediatric nutrition handbook* (5th ed.). Elk Grove Village, IL: American Academy of Pediatrics.

American Academy of Pediatrics, Work Group on Breastfeeding. Breastfeeding and the use of human milk. (1997). *Pediatrics, 100*(6), 1035–1039.

Arenz, S., Ruckerl, R., Koletzko, B., & von Kries, R. (2004). Breast-feeding and childhood obesity—a systematic review. *International Journal of Obesity, 28*(10), 1247–1256.

Baird, J., Fisher, D., Lucas, P., Kleijnen, J., Roberts, H., & Law, C. (2005). Being big or growing fast: Systematic review of size and growth in infancy and later obesity. *British Medical Journal, 331*(7522), 929.

Bandini, L. G., Curtin, C., Hamad, C., Tybor, D. J., & Must, A. (2005). Prevalence of overweight in children with developmental disorders in the continuous national health and nutrition examination survey (NHANES) 1999-2002. *Journal of Pediatrics, 146*(6), 738–743.

Barker, M. (1998). *Mothers, babies and health in later life*. Edinburgh: Harcourt Brace & Co, Ltd.

Barker, M., Robinson, S., Osmond, C., & Barker, D. J. (1997). Birth weight and body fat distribution in adolescent girls. *Archives of Disease in Childhood, 77*(5), 381–383.

Battaglia, F. C., & Lubchenco, L. O. (1967). A practical classification of newborn infants by weight and gestational age. *Journal of Pediatrics, 71*(2), 159–163.

Behrman, R. E., Kliegman, R., & Jenson, H. B. (2004). *Nelson textbook of pediatrics* (17th ed.). Philadelphia, PA: Saunders.

Ben-Shlomo, Y., & Kuh, D. (2002). A life course approach to chronic disease epidemiology: Conceptual models, empirical challenges and interdisciplinary perspectives. *International Journal of Epidemiology, 31*(2), 285–293.

Bevier, W. C., Fischer, R., & Jovanovic, L. (1999). Treatment of women with an abnormal glucose challenge test (but a normal oral glucose tolerance test) decreases the prevalence of macrosomia. *American Journal of Perinatology, 16*(6), 269–275.

Birch, L. L. (1999). Development of food preferences. *Annual Review of Nutrition, 19*, 41–62.

Bolen, J. C., Rhodes, L., Powell-Griner, E. E., Bland, S. D., & Holtzman, D. (2000). State-specific prevalence of selected health behaviors, by race and ethnicity—Behavioral Risk Factor Surveillance System, 1997. *Morbidity and Mortality Weekly Report. CDC Surveillance Summaries, 49*(2), 1–60.

Burdette, H. L., Whitaker, R. C., Hall, W. C., & Daniels, S. R. (2006). Breastfeeding, introduction of complementary foods, and adiposity at 5 y of age. *American Journal of Clinical Nutrition, 83*(3), 550–558.

Butte, N. F. (2001). The role of breastfeeding in obesity. *Pediatric Clinics of North America, 48*(1), 189–198.

Cole, T. J. (2004). Modeling postnatal exposures and their interactions with birth size. *Journal of Nutrition, 134*, 201–204.

Committee on Practice and Ambulatory Medicine. (2000). Recommendations for preventive pediatric health care. *Pediatrics, 105*(3), 645–646.

Curhan, G. C., Chertow, G. M., Willett, W. C., Spiegelman, D., Colditz, G. A., Manson, J. E., et al. (1996). Birth weight and adult hypertension and obesity in women. *Circulation, 94*(6), 1310–1315.

Dewey, K. G. (1998). Growth characteristics of breast-fed compared to formula-fed infants. *Biology of the Neonate, 74*(2), 94–105.

Dyson, L., McCormick, F., & Renfrew, M. J. (2005). Interventions for promoting the initiation of breastfeeding. *Cochrane Database System Review, 2*, CD001688.

Faith, M. S., Scanlon, K. S., Birch, L. L., Francis, L. A., & Sherry, B. (2004). Parent-child feeding strategies and their relationships to child eating and weight status. *Obesity Research, 12*(11), 1711–1722.

Fewtrell, M. S., Lucas, A., Cole, T. J., & Wells, J. C. (2004). Prematurity and reduced body fatness at 8-12 y of age. *American Journal of Clinical Nutrition, 80*(2), 436–440.

Fisch, R. O., Bilek, M. K., & Ulstrom, R. (1975). Obesity and leanness at birth and their relationship to body habitus in later childhood. *Pediatrics, 56*(4), 521–528.

Flegal, K. M., Carroll, M. D., Ogden, C. L., & Johnson, C. L. (2002). Prevalence and trends in obesity among US adults, 1999-2000. *Journal of the American Medical Association, 288*(14), 1723–1727.

Fowden, A. L., & Forhead, A. J. (2004). Endocrine mechanisms of intrauterine programming. *Reproduction, 127*(5), 515–526.

Fox, M. K., Pac, S., Devaney, B., & Jankowski, L. (2004). Feeding infants and toddlers study: What foods are infants and toddlers eating? *Journal of the American Dietetic Assocation*, *104*(1 Suppl. 1), s22–s30.

Friedman, J. M. (2000). Obesity in the new millennium. *Nature*, *404*(6778), 632–634.

Gillman, M. W. (2004). Lifecourse approach to obesity. In D. Kuh & Y. Ben-Shlomo (Eds.), *A life course approach to chronic disease epidemiology*. New York: Oxford University Press.

Gillman, M. W., Rifas-Shiman, S., Berkey, C. S., Field, A. E., & Colditz, G. A. (2003). Maternal gestational diabetes, birth weight, and adolescent obesity. *Pediatrics*, *111*(3), e221–e226.

Hack, M., Schluchter, M., Cartar, L., Rahman, M., Cuttler, L., & Borawski, E. (2003). Growth of very low birth weight infants to age 20 years. *Pediatrics*, *112*(1, Pt. 1), e30–e38.

Hakanen, M., Lagstrom, H., Kaitosaari, T., Niinikoski, H., Nanto-Salonen, K., Jokinen, E., et al. (2006). Development of overweight in an atherosclerosis prevention trial starting in early childhood. The STRIP study. *International Journal of Obesity*, *30*(4), 618–626.

Harris, M. I., Flegal, K. M., Cowie, C. C., Eberhardt, M. S., Goldstein, D. E., Little, R. R., et al. (1998). Prevalence of diabetes, impaired fasting glucose, and impaired glucose tolerance in U.S. adults. The Third National Health and Nutrition Examination Survey, 1988-1994. *Diabetes Care*, *21*(4), 518–524.

Henderson, G., Fahey, T., & McGuire, W. (2005). Calorie and protein-enriched formula versus standard term formula for improving growth and development in preterm or low birth weight infants following hospital discharge. *Cochrane Database System Review*, *2*, CD004696.

Himms-Hagen, J. (1999). Physiological roles of the leptin endocrine system: Differences between mice and humans. *Critical Reviews in Clinical Laboratory Science*, *36*(6), 575–655.

Institute of Medicine (U.S.) Committee on Prevention of Obesity in Children and Youth., Koplan, J., Liverman, C. T., Kraak, V. I., Institute of Medicine (U.S.). Food and Nutrition Board, & Institute of Medicine (U.S.). Board on Health Promotion and Disease Prevention. (2005). *Preventing childhood obesity: Health in the balance*. Washington, DC: National Academies Press.

Institute of Medicine (U.S.) Committee to Review the WIC Food Packages. (2005). *WIC food packages: Time for a change*. Washington, DC: National Academies Press.

Institute of Medicine (U.S.) Subcommittee on Nutritional Status and Weight Gain during Pregnancy & Institute of Medicine (U.S.). Subcommittee on Dietary Intake and Nutrient Supplements during Pregnancy. (1990). *Nutrition during pregnancy: Part I, weight gain; Part II, nutrient supplements*. Washington, DC: National Academy Press.

Johansson, S., Iliadou, A., Bergvall, N., Tuvemo, T., Norman, M., & Cnattingius, S. (2005). Risk of high blood pressure among young men increases with the degree of immaturity at birth. *Circulation*, *112*(22), 3430–3436.

Jovanovic-Peterson, L., Bevier, W., & Peterson, C. M. (1997). The Santa Barbara County Health Care Services program: Birth weight change concomitant with screening for and treatment of glucose-intolerance of pregnancy: A potential cost-effective intervention? *American Journal of Perinatology*, *14*(4), 221–228.

Jovanovic-Peterson, L., Durak, E. P., & Peterson, C. M. (1989). Randomized trial of diet versus diet plus cardiovascular conditioning on glucose levels in gestational diabetes. *American Journal of Obstetrics and Gynecology*, *161*(2), 415–419.

Kinra, S., Baumer, J. H., & Davey Smith, G. (2005). Early growth and childhood obesity: A historical cohort study. *Archives of Disease in Childhood*, *90*(11), 1122–1127.

Knopp, R. H., Magee, M. S., Raisys, V., Benedetti, T., & Bonet, B. (1991). Hypocaloric diets and ketogenesis in the management of obese gestational diabetic women. *Journal of the American College of Nutrition*, *10*(6), 649–667.

Kramer, M. S. (1981). Do breast-feeding and delayed introduction of solid foods protect against subsequent obesity? *Journal of Pediatrics, 98*(6), 883–887.

Kramer, M. S., Chalmers, B., Hodnett, E. D., Sevkovskaya, Z., Dzikovich, I., Shapiro, S., et al. (2001). Promotion of Breastfeeding Intervention Trial (PROBIT): A randomized trial in the Republic of Belarus. *Journal of the American Medical Association, 285*(4), 413–420.

Kramer, M. S., & Kakuma, R. (2003). Energy and protein intake in pregnancy. *Cochrane Database Syst Rev*(4), CD000032.

Kuczmarski, R. J., Ogden, C. L., Grummer-Strawn, L. M., Flegal, K. M., Guo, S. S., Wei, R., et al. (2000). CDC growth charts: United States. *Adv Data, 8*(314), 1–27.

Kuh, D., & Ben-Shlomo, Y. (1997). *A life course approach to chronic disease epidemiology*. Oxford, England: Oxford University Press.

Kuhl, C. (1998). Etiology and pathogenesis of gestational diabetes. *Diabetes Care, 21*(Suppl. 2), B19-B26.

Lee, Y., Mitchell, D. C., Smiciklas-Wright, H., & Birch, L. L. (2001). Diet quality, nutrient intake, weight status, and feeding environments of girls meeting or exceeding recommendations for total dietary fat of the American Academy of Pediatrics. *Pediatrics, 107*(6), E95.

Lumley, J., Oliver, S. S., Chamberlain, C., & Oakley, L. (2004). Interventions for promoting smoking cessation during pregnancy. *Cochrane Database System Review, 4,* CD001055.

Luo, Z. C., Albertsson-Wikland, K., & Karlberg, J. (1998). Length and body mass index at birth and target height influences on patterns of postnatal growth in children born small for gestational age. *Pediatrics, 102*(6), E72.

Martin, J. A., Hamilton, B. E., Sutton, P. D., Ventura, S. J., Menacker, F., & Munson, M. L. (2005). Births: Final data for 2003. *National Vital Statistics Report, 54*(2), 1–116.

Mei, Z., Scanlon, K. S., Grummer-Strawn, L. M., Freedman, D. S., Yip, R., & Trowbridge, F. L. (1998). Increasing prevalence of overweight among US low-income preschool children: The Centers for Disease Control and Prevention pediatric nutrition surveillance, 1983 to 1995. *Pediatrics, 101*(1), E12.

Mennella, J. A., Jagnow, C. P., & Beauchamp, G. K. (2001). Prenatal and postnatal flavor learning by human infants. *Pediatrics, 107*(6), E88.

Metzger, B. E., & Coustan, D. R. (1998). Summary and recommendations of the Fourth International Workshop-Conference on Gestational Diabetes Mellitus. The Organizing Committee. *Diabetes Care, 21*(Suppl. 2), B161–B167.

Monteiro, P. O., & Victora, C. G. (2005). Rapid growth in infancy and childhood and obesity in later life—a systematic review. *Obesity Review, 6*(2), 143–154.

National, state, and urban area vaccination coverage among children aged 19-35 months—United States, 2004. (2005). *Morbidity and Mortality Weekly Report, 54*(29), 717–721.

Nelson, M. C., Gordon-Larsen, P., & Adair, L. S. (2005). Are adolescents who were breast-fed less likely to be overweight? Analyses of sibling pairs to reduce confounding. *Epidemiology, 16*(2), 247–253.

Niinikoski, H., Lapinleimu, H., Viikari, J., Ronnemaa, T., Jokinen, E., Seppanen, R., et al. (1997). Growth until 3 years of age in a prospective, randomized trial of a diet with reduced saturated fat and cholesterol. *Pediatrics, 99*(5), 687–694.

Niinikoski, H., Viikari, J., Ronnemaa, T., Lapinleimu, H., Jokinen, E., Salo, P., et al. (1996). Prospective randomized trial of low-saturated-fat, low-cholesterol diet during the first 3 years of life. The STRIP baby project. *Circulation, 94*(6), 1386–1393.

Ogden, C. L., Carroll, M. D., Curtin, L. R., McDowell, M. A., Tabak, C. J., & Flegal, K. M. (2006). Prevalence of overweight and obesity in the United States, 1999-2004. *Journal of the American Medical Association, 295*(13), 1549–1555.

Ogden, C. L., Flegal, K. M., Carroll, M. D., & Johnson, C. L. (2002). Prevalence and trends in overweight among US children and adolescents, 1999-2000. *Journal of the American Medical Association, 288*(14), 1728–1732.

Oken, E., Taveras, E. M., Kleinman, K. P., Rich-Edwards, J. W., & Gillman, M. W. (2005). Maternal weight gain during pregnancy and child adiposity at age 3 years. *Pediatric Research, 58*(5), 1127 (Abstract).

Olson, C. M., Strawderman, M. S., & Reed, R. G. (2004). Efficacy of an intervention to prevent excessive gestational weight gain. *American Journal of Obstetrics and Gynecology, 191*(2), 530–536.

Owen, C. G., Martin, R. M., Whincup, P. H., Smith, G. D., & Cook, D. G. (2005). Effect of infant feeding on the risk of obesity across the life course: A quantitative review of published evidence. *Pediatrics, 115*(5), 1367–1377.

Parsons, T. J., Power, C., Logan, S., & Summerbell, C. D. (1999). Childhood predictors of adult obesity: A systematic review. *International Journal of Obesity, 23*(Suppl. 8), S1–S107.

Pettitt, D. J., Nelson, R. G., Saad, M. F., Bennett, P. H., & Knowler, W. C. (1993). Diabetes and obesity in the offspring of Pima Indian women with diabetes during pregnancy. *Diabetes Care, 16*(1), 310–314.

Pietilainen, K. H., Kaprio, J., Rasanen, M., Rissanen, A., & Rose, R. J. (2002). Genetic and environmental influences on the tracking of body size from birth to early adulthood. *Obesity Research, 10*(9), 875–884.

Plagemann, A., Harder, T., Kerstin, F., & Kohlhoff, R. (2002). Long-term impact of neonatal breast-feeding on body weight and glucose tolerance in children of diabetic mothers. *Diabetes Care, 25*(1), 16–22.

Plagemann, A., Harder, T., Rake, A., Waas, T., Melchior, K., Ziska, T., et al. (1999). Observations on the orexigenic hypothalamic neuropeptide Y-system in neonatally overfed weanling rats. *Journal of Neuroendocrinology, 11*(7), 541–546.

Polley, B. A., Wing, R. R., & Sims, C. J. (2002). Randomized controlled trial to prevent excessive weight gain in pregnant women. *International Journal of Obesity, 26*(11), 1494–1502.

Rask-Nissila, L., Jokinen, E., Terho, P., Tammi, A., Lapinleimu, H., Ronnemaa, T., et al. (2000). Neurological development of 5-year-old children receiving a low-saturated fat, low-cholesterol diet since infancy: A randomized controlled trial. *Journal of the American Medical Association, 284*(8), 993–1000.

Ravelli, G. P., Stein, Z. A., & Susser, M. W. (1976). Obesity in young men after famine exposure in utero and early infancy. *New England Journal of Medicine, 295*(7), 349–353.

Seidman, D. S., Laor, A., Shemer, J., Gale, R., & Stevenson, D. K. (1996). Excessive maternal weight gain during pregnancy and being overweight at 17 years of age. *Pediatric Research, 39*(4), 656 (Abstract).

Sikorski, J., Renfrew, M. J., Pindoria, S., & Wade, A. (2002). Support for breastfeeding mothers. *Cochrane Database System Review, 1*, CD001141.

Silverman, B. L., Rizzo, T. A., Cho, N. H., & Metzger, B. E. (1998). Long-term effects of the intrauterine environment. The Northwestern University Diabetes in Pregnancy Center. *Diabetes Care, 21*(Suppl. 2), B142–B149.

Singhal, A., Cole, T. J., Fewtrell, M., Deanfield, J., & Lucas, A. (2004). Is slower early growth beneficial for long-term cardiovascular health? *Circulation, 109*(9), 1108–1113.

Singhal, A., Cole, T. J., & Lucas, A. (2001). Early nutrition in preterm infants and later blood pressure: Two cohorts after randomised trials. *Lancet, 357*(9254), 413–419.

Singhal, A., Farooqi, I. S., O'Rahilly, S., Cole, T. J., Fewtrell, M., & Lucas, A. (2002). Early nutrition and leptin concentrations in later life. *American Journal of Clinical Nutrition, 75*(6), 993–999.

Singhal, A., Fewtrell, M., Cole, T. J., & Lucas, A. (2003). Low nutrient intake and early growth for later insulin resistance in adolescents born preterm. *Lancet, 361*(9363), 1089–1097.

Smith, G. D., Hart, C., Blane, D., & Hole, D. (1998). Adverse socioeconomic conditions in childhood and cause specific adult mortality: Prospective observational study. *British Medical Journal*, *316*(7145), 1631–1635.

The State of the World's Children 1998: A UNICEF report. Malnutrition: Causes, consequences, and solutions (1998). *Nutrition Review*, *56*(4, Pt. 1), 115–123.

Stettler, N., & Faith, M. S. (2004). A sibling analysis of the association between early infancy weight gain and childhood obesity. *Circulation*, *109*, e71 (Abstract).

Stettler, N., Stallings, V. A., Troxel, A. B., Zhao, J., Schinnar, R., Nelson, S. E., et al. (2005). Weight gain in the first week of life and overweight in adulthood: A cohort study of European American subjects fed infant formula. *Circulation*, 111(15), 1897–1903.

Stettler, N., Tershakovec, A. M., Zemel, B. S., Leonard, M. B., Boston, R. C., Katz, S. H., et al. (2000). Early risk factors for increased adiposity: A cohort study of African American subjects followed from birth to young adulthood. *American Journal of Clinical Nutrition*, *72*(2), 378–383.

Stettler, N., Zemel, B. S., Kumanyika, S., & Stallings, V. A. (2002). Infant weight gain and childhood overweight status in a multicenter, cohort study. *Pediatrics*, *109*(2), 194–199.

Stunkard, A. J., Berkowitz, R. I., Schoeller, D., Maislin, G., & Stallings, V. A. (2004). Predictors of body size in the first 2 y of life: A high-risk study of human obesity. *International Journal of Obesity*, *28*(4), 503–513.

Stunkard, A. J., Sorensen, T. I., Hanis, C., Teasdale, T. W., Chakraborty, R., Schull, W. J., et al. (1986). An adoption study of human obesity. *New England Journal of Medicine*, *314*(4), 193–198.

Taveras, E. M., Scanlon, K. S., Birch, L., Rifas-Shiman, S. L., Rich-Edwards, J. W., & Gillman, M. W. (2004). Association of breastfeeding with maternal control of infant feeding at age 1 year. *Pediatrics*, *114*(5), e577–e583.

Tuffnell, D. J., West, J., & Walkinshaw, S. A. (2003). Treatments for gestational diabetes and impaired glucose tolerance in pregnancy. *Cochrane Database System Review*, *3*, CD003395.

U.S. Department of Agriculture Food and Nutrition Service Office of Analysis Nutrition and Evaluation. (2003). *WIC Participant and Program Characteristics 2002*. Alexandria, VA.

U.S. Department of Health and Human Services (2001). *The Surgeon General's call to action to prevent and decrease overweight and obesity*. Rockville, MD: U.S. Department of Health and Human Services.

U.S. Department of Health and Human Services. (2001a). *Healthy People 2010: Understanding and improving health* (Rev. ed.). Boston: Jones and Bartlett Publishers.

Victora, C. G., Barros, F. C., Horta, B. L., & Martorell, R. (2001). Short-term benefits of catch-up growth for small-for-gestational-age infants. *International Journal of Epidemiology*, *30*(6), 1325–1330.

von Kries, R., Toschke, A. M., Koletzko, B., & Slikker, W., Jr. (2002). Maternal smoking during pregnancy and childhood obesity. *American Journal of Epidemiology*, *156*(10), 954–961.

Waterland, R. A., & Garza, C. (2002). Early postnatal nutrition determines adult pancreatic glucose - responsive insulin secretion and islet gene expression in rats. *Journal of Nutrition*, *132*(3), 357–364.

Whitaker, R. C. (2004). Predicting preschooler obesity at birth: The role of maternal obesity in early pregnancy. *Pediatrics*, *114*(1), e29–e36.

Whitaker, R. C., Wright, J. A., Pepe, M. S., Seidel, K. D., & Dietz, W. H. (1997). Predicting obesity in young adulthood from childhood and parental obesity. *New England Journal of Medicine*, *337*(13), 869–873.

Wideroe, M., Vik, T., Jacobsen, G., & Bakketeig, L. S. (2003). Does maternal smoking during pregnancy cause childhood overweight? *Pediatric and Perinatal Epidemiology*, *17*, 171–179.

Wilson, A. C., Forsyth, J. S., Greene, S. A., Irvine, L., Hau, C., & Howie, P. W. (1998). Relation of infant diet to childhood health: Seven year follow up of cohort of children in Dundee infant feeding study. *British Medical Journal, 316*(7124), 21–25.

Zhang, Q., & Wang, Y. (2004). Socioeconomic inequality of obesity in the United States: Do gender, age, and ethnicity matter? *Social Science and Medicine, 58*(6), 1171–1180.

Chapter 19

Obesity Prevention During Preschool and Elementary School-Age Years

Marilyn S. Nanney

Introduction

Overweight and obesity are defined as the accumulation of excess fat (adipose tissue). Definitions for children are more complex than for adults due to the variations by age and gender. For this chapter, which focuses on preschool and early childhood years, overweight status is defined using sex- and age-specific growth charts developed by the Centers for Disease Control and Prevention (CDC), with at risk of overweight as a BMI ≥85th percentile and <95th percentile, and overweight as ≥95th percentile. For children, these CDC designations apply the term overweight instead of obesity (which is the term used in adults) to the highest weight category and "at risk of overweight" to the category that is termed "overweight" in adults. However, for clarity, the terms overweight and obesity are used in this chapter. The sex specific BMI for age growth charts are based on national data from 1963 to 1994 (Kuczmarski et al., 2002). As explained in Chapter 2, this method of defining childhood obesity is limited in determining excess fatness as such. However, for a variety of reasons, the BMI for age cutpoints are currently the preferred measure for use in children for public health as well as clinical purposes (Whitlock et al., 2005).

The proportion of children who are overweight or obese has increased dramatically in the past 25 years. Even with substantial progress it seems highly unlikely that the national "Healthy People 2010" goal of reducing the prevalence of obesity (95th percentile cutoff) in children to 5% (Healthy People 2010, 2006) can be met. Among 2- to 5- year-olds, overweight doubled from 5% in the early 1970's to >10% in 2000 (Ogden et al., 2002). When overweight children (85th percentile cutoff) are included, one in every four preschoolers is affected in the general U.S. population (Hedley et al., 2004). Obesity is even more pronounced among low-income preschool children (Sherry et al., 2004). Among 6- to 11- year-olds, obesity has tripled during the same timeframe. Between 1963 and 2000, average weights increased eleven pounds among both 10-year-old girls (from 77 to 88 pounds) and boys (from 74 to 85 pounds) (Ogden et al., 2004).

Although recent increases in the prevalence of overweight and obesity among children are not limited to one location, age, gender, or ethnic group,

429

the impact is greater in certain demographic subgroups (Crawford et al., 2001). Obesity is especially prevalent among African American, Hispanic, and American Indian children (Flegal & Troiano, 2000; Ogden et al., 2002) (see Chapter 3). Among whites, obesity prevalence is especially high among low-income families whereas the effects of socioeconomic status (SES) on youth obesity are less clear in other ethnic groups (Koplan et al 2005; Troiano et al., 1995; Ogden et al 2003). In addition, although parental SES is associated inversely with childhood obesity among whites, higher SES does not seem to protect African American and Hispanic children against overweight (Crawford et al., 2001). Reasons for the excess obesity risk in minority and low-income individuals may involve less favorable access to healthful foods and fewer options for physical activity, as well as familial and sociocultural influences (Kumanyika & Grier, 2006). Living in a rural setting also seems to be associated with excess risk of obesity in young children (Tai-Seale & Chandler, 2003). For example, McMurray and colleagues (1999) reported significantly increased risk (by a ratio of about 1.6:1) of obesity among rural compared with urban third- and fourth- grade children after controlling for race, gender and SES.

Being an obese preschooler indicates a 25% chance of becoming an obese adult, while that figure jumps to 41% and 75% if obesity is maintained at age seven and twelve, respectively (Perry, 1997).

Because of poor treatment outcomes and the likelihood of obesity tracking from childhood into adolescence and then adulthood, prevention options are best. It also makes sense to focus efforts on the younger generations, when health education, environmental and policy change can shape a lifetime of healthy lifestyle practices and prevent excess weight gain (Caballero, 2004; Koplan et al., 2005); and because the consequences of obesity do not wait for adulthood to emerge. The best approach to this problem in young children is prevention of abnormal weight gain (Daniels et al., 2005) using a health-centered, rather than a weight-centered, approach that focuses on the whole child (Berg et al., 2003).

This chapter reviews the rationale and developmental context for obesity prevention during childhood years from about age 2 through 11 or 12. Obesity prevention before preschool years is discussed in Chapter 18 and for the preadolescent and adolescent years in Chapter 20. We review evidence in relation to a range of potential risk factors for obesity development that can be considered as intervention targets, and describe selected interventions that have been reported for children in preschool and school age years. This chapter complements the discussion of childhood obesity prevention approaches conducted in schools, child care, and community settings in Chapters 13 and 16. In addition, detailed reviews on many of the issues covered in this chapter have been published, related to both individually oriented and policy and environmental approaches (Summerbell et al., 2005; Brug & VanLenthe, 2005; Doak et al., 2006; Story et al, 2006a; Story et al, 2006b; Lindsay et al, 2006).

Consequences of Childhood Overweight and Obesity

Obesity has adverse effects on physical health and maturation, psychosocial adjustment, and academic performance during childhood in addition to the potential longer term consequences when obesity tracks into adulthood.

Adverse health outcomes of obesity include type 2 diabetes, obstructive sleep apnea, high blood pressure, high cholesterol, and the metabolic syndrome (Daniels et al., 2005; Ogden et al., 2003). The evidence supporting prevention of childhood obesity to prevent adverse obesity-related outcomes in adulthood is compelling, based on longitudinal studies affirming that adult obesity frequently originates during childhood (Dietz, 1994; Troiano et al., 1995; Whitaker et al., 1998). For individuals born in the United States in 2000, assuming that current obesity levels do not change, the lifetime risk of being diagnosed with diabetes at some point in their lives is estimated at 30% for boys and 40% for girls (Narayan et al., 2003). This estimated lifetime risk is even higher among certain ethnic minority groups.

Approximately one-third of overweight preschool children and one-half of overweight school aged children grow up to be obese adults (Serdula et al., 1993; Whitaker et al., 1998). In the Bogalusa Heart Study data, based on periodic BMI and triceps skin fold thickness measurements between 1973 and 1996 in 2,610 children initially ages 2–17 years, the magnitude of these associations increased with childhood age. BMI levels of even the youngest (2–5 years) children were moderately ($r = 0.33-0.41$) associated with adult adiposity with increased associations at 6–8 years ($r = 0.41-48$) and 9–11 years ($r = 0.51-0.56$). Overweight 2–5 year olds were more than 4 times as likely to become obese adults (Freedman et al., 2005).

In a population based sample, approximately 60% of obese children aged 5–10 years had at least one physiological cardiovascular disease risk factor such as elevated total cholesterol, triglycerides, insulin, or blood pressure levels, and 25% had two or more risk factors (Freedman et al., 1999). Overweight children also tend to mature earlier than non overweight children (Frisch & Revelle, 1971), and advanced sexual maturation has been associated with insulin resistance (Dimartino-Nardi, 1999), higher serum levels of insulin-like growth factors (Bideci et al., 1997), exaggerated adrenal response and polycystic ovary syndrome (Lazar et al., 1995) either during or after childhood. Increasing lifetime exposure to estrogen, partially due to early menarche, may increase the risk for both breast and ovarian cancers (Key, 1995). Additionally, excess body weight during puberty is linked to increased bone mineral density (Hasanoglu et al., 2000), advanced bone ages (De Simone et al., 1995), and orthopedic complications due to the effect of increased weight on the hip growth plate (Wilcox & Leighley, 1988).

Childhood obesity not only has physical effects but also has serious psychosocial effects. Many studies show that children who are overweight have lower self-esteem (Hill & Pallin, 1998) and report poorer quality-of-life (Schwimmer et al., 2003). A cross-sectional study of 106 five- to eighteen-year-olds who were severely obese (mean BMI of 34.7) had a similar quality-of-life as those diagnosed with cancer compared with healthy children and adolescents (Schwimmer et al., 2003). As noted above, overweight children have advanced maturation; that children who mature early tend to have lower self-esteem has been documented for some time (Brooks-Gunn, 1988). One study demonstrated significantly decreased levels of global self-esteem and consequent higher rates of sadness, loneliness, and nervousness in obese versus non-obese Hispanic and white females (Strauss, 2000). In addition, these obese children who had decreasing levels of self-esteem over a four-year period were more likely to engage in unhealthy behaviors such as cigarette and alcohol consumption. The effect of how adults treat children with excess weight has not been well studied. However, one can imagine that since overweight children tend to be taller than their non-overweight peers, they most likely are viewed as older than their chronological age and expected to behave accordingly. This expectation may cause frustration and a "turning inward" by the overweight child (Dietz, 1998).

Physically active children exhibit higher self-esteem and lower levels of anxiety and stress—all linked to better academic performance (Symons et al., 1997). A meta-analysis of 200 studies showed that physical activity supports learning (Etnler et al., 1997). A large-scale study done by the California Department of Education matched Fitnessgram data with SAT scores and found a strong correlation between academic achievement and fitness (Action for Healthy Kids, 2004). The connection between weight and academic performance has been less studied. Many potential confounding factors must be controlled for in observational studies on overweight children and academic success, including socioeconomic status, parents' level of education, poor nutrition and/or inadequate physical education. No randomized controlled trials (of academic outcomes before and after receiving or not receiving effective obesity treatment) are published that provide definitive answers on the link between academic performance and child weight-gain. However, one recent observational study conducted among kindergarteners supports the hypothesis that being overweight is causally linked to poorer academic outcomes during childhood. An analysis of more than 11,000 children in the Early Childhood Longitudinal Study data set indicated that test scores in both reading and math were lower for overweight kindergarteners compared to their non-overweight classmates and that these lower test scores among the overweight kids persisted into first grade (Datar et al., 2004). Overweight kindergarten boys had significantly lower math and reading test scores that could not be explained by other factors such as socioeconomic status, race/ethnicity, parent-child interaction, birth weight, physical activity, and television watching. A subsequent wave of data collection found that moving from not-overweight to overweight between kindergarten entry and end of third grade was significantly associated with reductions in math and reading test scores among girls and more absenteeism for boys (Datar & Sturm, 2006). One mechanism for the effect of overweight on school performance may be through absenteeism, which is directly linked to academic performance. Children who are overweight tend to miss more school due to health-related concerns. For example, Schwimmer et al. (2003) reported that severely overweight students were absent up to four times more often than normal weight students. Although reasons for absenteeism were not investigated in that study, increased school absenteeism has been documented in children with other chronic diseases including diabetes and asthma (Vetiska et al., 2000; Diette et al., 2000).

Developmental Context

During childhood and adolescence, growth is expected, and thus, weight and body size are constantly changing. However, there may be vulnerable periods for excess weight gain during childhood that offer opportunities for prevention of overweight (Daniels et al., 2005). Dietz (1994) has suggested that there are three critical periods for the development of overweight in children and youth: (1) the intrauterine environment and early infancy (discussed in Chapter 18); (2) between the ages of 3–7 years (also called "adiposity rebound" period), and (3) adolescence (discussed in Chapter 20). Although the mechanisms remain unclear, obesity that begins at these periods appears to increase the risk of persistent obesity and its complications (Dietz, 1994).

Adiposity rebound refers to the rise in BMI that occurs between ages 3 and 7 years (also see Chapter 2). Several studies have found that an early post-infancy rise in the body mass index increases the risk for overweight in adolescence and adulthood (Flynn et al., 2006; Freedman et al., 2001) and may account for about 30% of adult obesity (Dietz, 2000; Whitaker et al., 1998). If a child experiences adiposity rebound early, there is an increased likelihood that the child will be overweight during adolescence and adulthood. Therefore, understanding the determinants of excess body fat in young children may be particularly critical for preventing adult obesity.

Compared to infancy, the preschool years are characterized by a decreased rate of physical growth, and a child's interest in eating may diminish during this period. However, the preschool years are a period of rapid social, intellectual and emotional growth and are important in the development of positive attitudes toward food and learning to make food choices. Often the preschool period is characterized by "food jags" during which the child may eat only a few foods or may want the same food meal after meal. Parents are often concerned when a preschooler shows decreased interest in eating and refuses some favorite foods (Mitchell, 1994). During the early school years the velocity of growth slows but remains relatively steady until the preadolescent growth spurt at about 10 years of age in girls and 12 in boys. Most food-related behavior problems of the preschool years have been resolved by school age. Older children develop more autonomy with eating and take the initiative in making changes, usually accepting a wider variety of foods. Food preferences are increasingly influenced by peers and other factors outside the home as children mature.

For physical activity, the period between 5 and 8 years of age appears to be one of transition in the development of strength and motor performance with considerable variation among children (Malina, et al., 2004). Movement skills developed in the early years are building blocks for more complex movement tasks that later enable children to participate in physical activity successfully and with enjoyment (e.g., being able to jump, throw, skip, hop, catch, and kick). Even though overall physical growth is decelerating, motor skills are being fine-tuned. Developmental learning opportunities gained through group physical activities include problem solving, self-expression, socialization, and conflict resolution skills (National Association for Sport and Physical Education, 2001).

Overall, childhood is a period of slow, steady growth, the rate of which is determined by genetic and environmental factors. In the short-term, growth is characterized by spurts and latent periods. Children's energy and nutrient needs are determined by body size, body composition, rate of growth and level of activity. Because of day-to-day variation in the rate of growth, energy needs of children will vary and the child's appetite is an indicator of daily caloric needs. Resources are available to provide guidance to child-feeding during this phase of development. For example, in 2005, *MyPyramid for Kids* was released to reach children ages 6–11 years with targeted messages about the importance of making healthful eating and physical activity choices and an interactive computer game to apply these messages (USDA, 2005). With respect to physical activity, emphasis during the preschool and elementary school years is on developing basic motor skills that allow participation in a variety of physical activities and on developing an appreciation and under-standing of the important wellness and fitness concepts that are the foundation for being physically active for a lifetime. In 1999, The Youth Sport Council and The National Association for Sport and Physical Education developed a resource entitled *Choosing the Right Sport & Physical Activity Program for Your Child* (Youth Sport Council and The National Association for Sport and Physical Education, 1999) outlining considerations by child specific character-istics (skill level, maturity, interests, special needs), safety considerations (nec-essary safety equipment, play area free of obstacles and hazards, first aid supplies accessible, ratio of coaches/staff 1:10, warm-up and conditioning activities to prevent injuries), child's readiness to participate (skill level match, emotional and social maturity matches activity, group or team, cultural and gender diversity are encouraged) and administration & organization of the pro-gram (philosophy: fun versus winning, training of coaches, development of fair play, teamwork and sportsmanship, number and length of practices).

Risk Factors for Obesity Development

Obesity can be defined as a set of complex interactions among genetic, envi-ronmental, and behavioral factors, all acting on energy balance, and approaches for prevention of childhood obesity can be just as complex. At the population level the factors contributing to obesity in U.S. adults and children have been well-described: declining levels of physical activity and increased levels of inactivity (French et al., 2003; Jeffery & Utler, 2003; Brownson et al., 2005; Koplan et al., 2005). Overall, food consumption patterns have probably changed more dramatically than physical activity levels, suggesting to some observers that increases in youth obesity are primarily related to changes in diet (Sturm, 2005). However, decreases in physical activity and increases in inactivity in children have also been substantial. For example, Sturm noted a major decline in children's walking to school from 20.2% in 1997 to only 12.5% in 2001. The precise magnitudes of temporal effects are difficult to esti-mate due to poor historical data. The availability and quality of school physi-cal education have declined and the popularity of sedentary leisure time pursuits has increased. Elementary schools (grades 1 through 5) requiring physical education is around 50% (Story, 2006a). Time actually spent being physically active has been estimated at far less than the national recommenda-tions of moderate to vigorous physical activity at least 50% of class time (Simons-Morton, 1994).

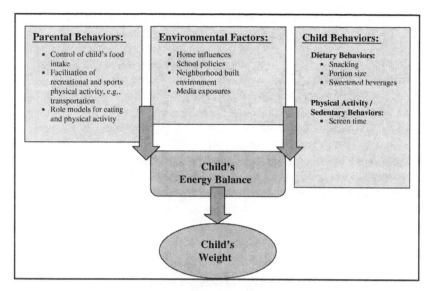

Figure 19.1 Factors Determining Childhood Weight.

(Source: Parrott & Myers, 2005).

Taken as a whole, the best available evidence identifies three types of factors influencing the energy balance, and therefore weight, of preschool and younger children: (1) environmental and policy factors, (2) child behaviors, and 3) parental behaviors. Specific potential influences within each of these categories are listed in the Figure 19.1 (Parrott & Myers, 2005) and reviewed in the following sections. Some of these determinants have been relatively well studied in attempts to discover possible preventive strategies for childhood obesity, while the role of others is still speculative.

Environmental Factors

Contextual influences such as the home environment, school policies, the neighborhood built environment, and media advertising that have changed dramatically in recent years tend to encourage increased energy intake and decreased energy output and have widespread impact on child behaviors (Sallis & Glanz, 2006). The nature of these influences is highlighted below and discussed in detail in several other chapters in this book, which are cross-referenced. Schools as settings for obesity prevention interventions are addressed in Chapter 16. Neighborhood design is discussed in Chapter 8, and media and marketing issues are addressed in Chapter 10. These environmental factors can be targeted through policy-oriented interventions, to complement interventions directed to individual children or families.

Home Influences

As discussed earlier, parents indirectly influence children's eating and activity through parental modeling. In addition, parents directly influence the development of these patterns through the home environment. Children are more likely to eat foods that are available and easily accessible (Patrick & Nicklas, 2005). Of the determinants of children's fruit and vegetable intake that have been studied, availability, accessibility, and taste preferences are the most consistently and positively related determinants to consumption (Blanchette & Brug, 2005; Cullen et al., 2003). Presence of a television set in the child's bedroom appears to be a good indicator of the prevalence of overweight among children even after adjustment for potential confounders (age, gender, viewing hours, mother's BMI, education and race/ethnicity). In cross-sectional data from the Supplemental Nutrition Program for Women, Infants, and Children (WIC) programs in 49 New York agencies (n = 2,761 mothers of 1– 5 year old children), children with a TV set in their room were 1.3 times more likely to be overweight than those without a bedroom TV (Dennison, 2002). A TV in the child's bedroom is an even stronger marker for increased risk of being overweight than viewing times per week. In this study, children with a TV in their bedrooms (40%) spent an additional 4.6 hours per week watching television or videos.

School Policies

There is widespread consensus among governmental agencies, professional associations of dietitians and pediatricians, and other experts that improving the overall school environment is critical in addressing the obesity epidemic among children (Koplan et al., 2005; Nicklas & Johnson, 2004; American Academy of Pediatrics, 2004). Healthy People 2010 objectives indicate that schools should provide an opportunity for preventing overweight and obesity by promoting physical activity and healthy eating habits. The National Association for Sport and Physical Education recommends that elementary schools offer 225 minutes of physical education per week. As reported in a 2004 Research Brief by the National Institute for Health Care Management (NIHCM, 2004) kindergarteners on average receive only 57 minutes of physical education per week while first graders receive only 65 minutes per week. The CDC estimates that just 8% of elementary schools provide daily physical education.

The decrease in physical education (PE) programs can be partly attributed to the need for various curricular areas and programs that compete for the limited resources available to schools. In addition, there is also competition for time in the school day and some of the decline in PE classes has been attributed to the need or interest of schools to replace PE with other subjects in order to increase standardized test scores (Action for Healthy Kids, 2004). This is in spite of evidence that adding physical activity time may support improved academic performance (National Association for Sport and Physical Education, 2001; Sallis et al., 1999; Shephard, 1997). Physical education can not only improve test scores but also has health benefits which may indirectly improve academic performance by reducing absenteeism (Action for Healthy Kids, 2004; National Institute for Health Care Management, 2004).

The 2004 NIHCM Research Brief reported that a one hour increase in PE instruction per week was associated with lower BMI levels (.31) among overweight and at-risk-of-overweight girls in 1st grade (Datar, 2004). Adding to the body of evidence, overweight children in this study had more absences (National Institute for Health Care Management, 2004). There has also been speculation that increased homework loads have also been blamed for contributing to the childhood obesity epidemic. However, on average, American students at all grade levels apparently spend less than one hour studying on any given day, a figure which has not changed much in the past twenty years (Sturm, 2005). This makes it unlikely that homework is a key factor.

The importance of school foods in a child's diet appears to be highest among children aged six to eleven years (Lin et al., 1999). In a survey of changes in energy consumption from elementary school foods between 1991–92 and 1998–99, a 3% increase in energy content of lunch consumed at school was reported, while energy from breakfast decreased by 4% (Sturm, 2005). The contribution of federally funded meals to this change could not be determined. School environment influences on children's food intake are not limited to the federally funded breakfast and lunch programs, however. They include other foods sold in the school lunchroom, foods sold for fundraisers (e.g., candy sales) or brought to school as special treats on occasions such as children's birthdays, and nutrition education provided in regular or health oriented classes. National estimates (2003–2004) indicate that 83% of elementary schools have one or more competitive food sources (e.g., ala carte line, vending machines, school stores) (Government Accountability Office, 2005). See Chapter 16 for a discussion of policies and programs that can potentially influence these aspects of the school environment. Guidelines for the healthfulness of all foods available to children in schools are currently under development (Committee of the Institute of Medicine, Nutrition standards for foods in schools, 2006). Positive steps taken recently concerning the food industry include the negotiated agreement between the Alliance for a Healthier Generation and five major snack food manufacturers to adhere to nutrition standards in school foods (http://www.clintonfoundation.org/index.htm).

Neighborhood Built Environment
The rapid rise in childhood overweight in a relatively short time period emphasizes the importance of environmental factors on this issue (Ebbeling et al., 2002). The way the built environment is developed affects daily eating and activity decisions (Chapter 8). Preschool children are more active when there are more places available nearby to spend time and play. A handful of studies have shown that children with access to recreational facilities and programs, usually near their homes, are more active than those without such access (Sallis et al., 2000). A few studies among preschool children have found that the more time spent outdoors, the higher their activity levels (Lindsay et al., 2006). More children walk to school in neighborhoods with sidewalks (Ewing et al., 2004). Unfortunately, there has been a major decline in children's walking to school from 20.2% in 1997 to only 12.5% in 2001. Parental concerns over safety (crime and traffic) may make playing outdoors and walking to school more difficult. A California Safe Routes to School program found a 64% increase in walking and a 114% increase in bicycling to school when promotional activities combined with improved street crossings and more sidewalks were implemented (Staunton et al., 2003).

Data on the influence of the built environment on weight levels of preschool children are inconsistent. A cross-sectional study of 7,020 low-income children 3–5 years of age living in Cincinnati, Ohio found no association between overweight prevalence in preschoolers and the proximity of the children's residences to playgrounds or fast food restaurants or to the safety of the children's neighborhoods, where the neighborhood characteristics were measured objectively (Burdette et al., 2004). Contrary findings that suggest an association are based on parental reports of the perceived safety of the neighborhood (Lumeng, 2006). Cross-sectional analysis among 768 urban and rural parents of first graders from 10 sites across the U.S. showed that parents of children who were overweight perceived their neighborhoods as significantly less safe than parents of children who were not overweight.

Research on the role of the neighborhood food environment and overweight in older children is more limited than that for the physical activity environment. However, the Early Childhood Longitudinal Study, which followed a nationally representative sample of kindergarten children over 4 years into elementary school grades, permitted a prospective examination of the association of neighborhood food prices and food outlet density with changes in BMI among elementary school children over time. Lower neighborhood prices for vegetables and fruits were found to predict a significantly lower gain in BMI between kindergarten and third grade, whereas lower meat prices had the opposite effect (Sturm & Datar, 2005).

Media and Advertising

The media environment is a major influence on children's eating and physical activity patterns. Electronic media (e.g., television, the internet, video games, wireless telephones) today more than ever, plays a central role in the socialization of young children and commercial marketing is a substantial component of this influence (McGinnis et al., 2006). This is critically important because children do not understand the persuasive intent and lack the defense skills to discern marketing content until about age 8 (American Academy of Pediatrics, 1995). The Institute of Medicine Committee on Food Marketing and the Diets of Children and Youth (2006) makes a strong case that exposure to television advertising is associated with adiposity in children ages 2 to 11 (McGinnis et al., 2006).

Watching television is a sedentary activity, but the potential influence of television on weight is not simply a matter of decreased physical activity. Television also communicates powerful messages about diets, food products, and social norms. Furthermore, television creates an appealing, and often 'nurturing' environment exposing the vast majority of American children to a steady 'diet' of commercials for energy-dense food products. Based on a review of the commercials aired during the top-ranked prime-time network shows for the 2-to 11-year-old age category, 40% of the food advertisements were for fast-food products, of which, french fries represented 80% of the vegetables advertised (Parrott & Myers, 2005). Moreover, commercials increase a child's preference for advertised products. This presumably contributes to the finding that children who are heavy television viewers are more likely to have an unhealthy perceptions about nutrition than children less frequently exposed to television (Borzekowski & Robinson, 2001).

Traditional television, radio, print, and billboard food and beverage marketing accounted for only 20% of exposures in 2004 (McGinnis et al., 2006). An unprecedented shift in marketing has occurred through product placement, character licensing, sponsoring school activities, and adventure games. The contribution of these other channels for advertising to the obesity epidemic in children has not yet been ascertained (Koplan et al, 2005).

Child Behaviors

Dietary Behaviors

The methodological limitations on both dietary and physical activity assessment as well as the difficulty of assessing energy balance of individuals complicate the ability to show an association between dietary composition and the prevalence of obesity as such. Although fat eaten in excess leads to a positive energy balance and obesity, there is no strong evidence that fat intake is the chief reason for the ascending trend of childhood obesity. Limiting fat intake is, therefore, not a common childhood obesity preventive strategy. In fact, the National Health and Nutrition Examination Survey (NHANES) data show a decline in fat consumption of American children over the last three decades, at the same time that obesity levels have increased (Dehghan et al., 2005). This is indirect evidence that changes in dietary fat intake are not the major cause of the increase in obesity in children.

As discussed in the following section, changes in specific eating behaviors that may be associated with excess energy intake (e.g., snacking, portion sizes) may help to explain the increase in obesity rates. Diet trends in a nationally representative sample of preschool children ages 3 to 5 between 1977 and 1998 indicated an increase in added-sugars and excess juice consumption as well as total calories (Kranz et al., 2004). No significant increased trends in energy intake were observed in children aged 6–11 years during the same time period, although children in this age group eat fewer vegetables, drink less than half the amount of milk and exceed recommendations for added sugars by 6–12 teaspoons than in 1977. On a typical day, approximately 25% of children aged 4–8 years old and 26% of 9–13 years old eat fast food (Bowman et al., 2004).

Snacking. The research on snacking is complicated by the unclear definition of what constitutes a snack or snack food. The United States Department of Agriculture Food and Nutrition Service defines snacks as mini-meals that help provide nutrients and food energy children need to grow, play, and learn (USDA, 2003). Snacks fill in the gaps between regular meals and are an important part of a child's daily nutritional intake, since children can not get enough nutrition in three meals. By all definitions snacks tend to be higher in energy density and fat content than meals, and high snack consumption has been associated with high intakes of fat, sugar and calories. Snacking frequency appears to have increased along with the prevalence of overweight. Enns et al., who analyzed data from the Continuing Survey of Food Intakes by Individuals (CSFII) 1989–91, 1994–96 and 1998 and the Nationwide Food Consumption Survey 1977–78, found two significant trends in snacking patterns among 6–11 year olds: (1) the intake of chips/crackers/popcorn/pretzels roughly tripled from the mid-1970s to the mid-1990s and (2) the intake of soft drinks roughly doubled during the same period. Percentage of 6–11 year old salty snack consumers increased from 16–34% for boys and 18–37% among girls. More specifically, the intake of chips, crackers, popcorn and pretzels increased by about one-third of a cup from 1977–78 to 1994–96 and 1998 per day for girls and boys. For the same time periods, consumers of soft drinks rose from 31–47% for boys and 30–45% for girls. Soft drink consumption increased by about 3 ounces per day for girls and 4 ounces per day for boys. (Sturm, 2005).

Portion size. Food portion sizes affect total energy intakes in children (Rolls et al., 2000; Smiciklas-Wright et al., 2003). In the United States, portion sizes of many foods have been increasing since the 1970s. This trend has been observed in a variety of settings including restaurants, supermarkets, and in the home. Increases in portion size have occurred in parallel with the rise in the prevalence of obesity, which suggests that large portion sizes could play a role in the increase in body weight among children. This impression is supported by a comparison of food service portion sizes from 1957 to 1997. The typical fast-food outlet hamburger in 1957 contained a little more than one ounce of cooked meat, compared to a burger weighing up to six ounces in 1997. The average theatre serving of popcorn consisted of three cups in 1957, compared with 16 cups in 1997. A typical muffin weighed less than 1.5 ounces in 1957, compared with five to eight ounces in 1997. These observations, which are based on food supply data, cannot be linked directly to individual-level food consumption or body weight. However, based on analyses of national survey data, portion sizes were positively related to both energy intake and body weight in 2–5 year old children (McConahy et al., 2004). Among children 6–11 years, comparing 1989 to 1999 and 1994 to 1996 intake data, ready-to-eat cereal and toasted oat rings were reported as larger portion sizes among the 107 foods examined (Smiciklas-Wright et al., 2003). Several recent studies, including controlled experiments in children, suggest that increased portion sizes promote excessive intake at meals (Fisher et al., 2003; McConahy et al., 2002; Rolls et al., 2000). Children 3 to 5 years of age consumed 25% more of an entrée and 15% more total energy at lunch when presented with portions that were double an age-appropriate standard size (Fisher et al., 2003).

Sweetened beverages. Consumption of sugar-added beverages, particularly soft drinks, has increased dramatically among preschoolers and school-age children (French et al., 2003). Intake of carbonated soft drinks (regular and low calorie) increases as children grow older, with a dramatic rise occurring when they are around 8 years old (Rampersaud et al., 2003). According to a national survey (CSFII data), soft drinks were the sixth leading food source of energy among children, constituting over 50% of total beverage consumption. These same data indicated that 12% of preschoolers (n = 810) and 32% of school-aged children (n = 557) consumed 9 oz a day or more of carbonated soft drinks (regular and low calorie) in 1994 (Harnack et al., 1999). Two- to five-year-old children drinking 9 or more ounces of soft drinks per day consumed significantly more calories than nonconsumers (1,448 versus 1,704 average calories). Similar trends are seen for 6- to 12- year-olds (1,830 versus 2,018 average calories).

Some studies demonstrate that the quantities of 100% fruit juice, fruit drinks, milk, regular and diet soda are associated with total energy intake but are not significantly correlated with increasing BMI among preschool aged children (Skinner & Carruth, 2001; O'Connor et al., 2006). However, researchers speculate that because adiposity rebound, on average, doesn't occur until about 5 to 6 years of age (Whitaker et al., 1998), it is possible that if preschool children were followed through their adiposity rebound, the increased energy intake would translate into an increased BMI after age 6 (O'Connor et al., 2006). One retrospective cohort study found an association between sweetened beverage consumption and overweight among 2- and 3-year-olds during a one year follow-up (Welsh et al., 2005). Among children who were at risk for overweight at baseline, those that consumed 1 to 2 drinks per day were twice as likely to become overweight as those drinking less than one daily sweetened beverage. Similar findings are reported among those children who were overweight at baseline adjusting for age, gender, race, birth weight, intake of high fat and sweet foods, and total calorie.

A few mechanisms have been suggested as to how sugar-sweetened drink consumption increases the prevalence of overweight. First, these drinks are high in calories and contribute to an overall higher caloric intake. Another possibility is that children do not compensate, behaviorally, at meals for the calories they have consumed in sweet drinks. Evidence also suggests that it may be physiologically more difficult to compensate for energy consumed as a liquid than as a solid food, and that consumption of sugar-sweetened beverages, therefore, results in increased energy intake (Parrott & Myers, 2005). Whether the critical factor is the sugar, the calories, or behaviors related to beverage consumption is unknown.

Physical Activity/Sedentary Behaviors

Energy expenditure through physical activity is a key component of energy balance, and it has been suggested that a steady decline in physical activity among all age groups has contributed heavily to rising rates of obesity in children. Trend data for children are limited but suggest that time spent being physically active has declined and imply an association with the rise in overweight and obesity. In 2002, the Youth Media Campaign Longitudinal Survey among a representative sample of children aged 9 to 13 years revealed that 62% did not participate in any organized physical activity during their nonschool hours and 23% did not engage in any free-time physical activity (Centers for Disease Control, 2003). Analyses of available data on youth discretionary time suggests a decline in free time for 3- to 12- year-olds by six hours per week from 1981 to 1997 (Hoefferth & Sandberg, 2001). Unstructured playtime has decreased to make room for organized activities; participation in organized activities (including sports) has increased by 73 minutes per week. Given that time in structured settings away from home has increased (i.e., school and day care), so does the importance of physical activity in those settings. An increase in structured time offers opportunities for interventions that may be more successful at expanding the number of youth who meet minimum-guideline criteria for strenuous physical activity than interventions targeted at diverse and unstructured home environments (Sturm, 2005).

Time spent in sedentary activities is also an important variable to consider. Numerous studies have shown that sedentary behaviors like television viewing and playing computer games are associated with increased prevalence of obesity in children (Marshall et al., 2004). Thus, physical activity and/or reducing sedentary behaviors are usually core components of prevention interventions. Increasing physical activity to achieve energy balance and prevent obesity potentially offers several physiologic and metabolic advantages with respect to body composition. Physical activity helps build and maintain healthy bones, muscles, and joints; builds endurance and muscular strength; maintains weight; lowers risk factors for many chronic diseases; helps control blood pressure; promotes psychological well-being and self-esteem; and reduces feelings of depression and anxiety. The National Association for Sport and Physical Education guidelines recommend that preschoolers have at least 2 hours of activity each day, half in structured activity and the other half unstructured or as active play (National Association for Sports and Physical

Education, 2001). Children ages five to twelve should have at least 60 minutes of daily activity. However, studies on the effects of physical activity on body composition are limited by the inability to determine cause and effect and control for other confounders (such as maturation, genetics and ethnicity).

Most research examining inactivity focuses on television. Because of the concerns about the adverse health effects of television, the Committee on Public Education of the American Academy of Pediatrics has cautioned parents to limit children's exposure to television and other media to a maximum of 2 hours per day. For children younger than 2 years, they completely discourage television viewing (Robinson, 1999). The impact of computers and video games on sedentary behavior is probably not very large, especially when compared with television, as they together comprise only about 10% of the average daily media budget of children aged 2 to 18 (Sturm, 2005). There are, however, large differences in viewing patterns by age and gender. Children younger than 8 years spent a negligible amount of time on video games or computers in 1998, but boys aged 8 to 13 averaged 47 minutes per day playing video games. In a longitudinal analysis of the Framingham Children's Study, data on 106 children followed from 4 to 11 years of age, demonstrated that TV viewing was an independent predictor of change in BMI (Proctor et al., 2003). By 11 years of age, children who watched 3 or more hours of daily TV had a higher BMI, on average, compared to those who watched TV less than 1.75 hours per day after controlling for age, gender, baseline BMI, and activity levels (BMI 20.8 versus 18.7). However, recently an analysis of 52 studies examining the relationship between TV viewing or video game use and obesity among 3–18 year olds found a small but significant effect of TV viewing on obesity, although it is likely to be too small to be of substantial clinical importance (Marshall et al., 2004). Several possible mechanisms have been suggested for TV viewing to cause obesity (Dietz & Gortmaker, 1985). These include: (1) using time that could be spent in physical play, thus reducing energy expenditure; (2) selecting food choices of high energy density promoted though advertising on television; and (3) increasing energy intake by eating during viewing time.

Parental Behaviors

Several studies highlight the centrality of the family in the etiology of childhood overweight (Davison & Birch, 2002). Parents shape their children's dietary practices, physical activity and ultimately their weight status in many ways (Lindsay et al., 2006). Specific parent behaviors that have been identified as influential in the development of lifelong habits during the preschool and preadolescent years include parental control of the child's food intake, encouragement for physical activities and modeling of personal healthy habits.

Control of Child's Food Intake

Parental concern about their child's weight status may be associated with higher risk or prevalence of overweight among children. Parental restriction of highly palatable foods may promote children's desire for such "forbidden foods", interfering with regulation of caloric intake and promoting the development of overweight. The association of parental food restriction with increased body weight in children is supported by a review of studies examining parent to child feeding strategies and their relationships to child eating and weight status (Faith et al., 2004). Nineteen of the twenty-two studies examined (86%) reported at least one significant association between parent feeding style and child weight outcome. Child energy intake or body weight was more likely to be positively associated with feeding restriction rather than general feeding control. Gender appears to be a moderator. Several large scale studies report associations between feeding restrictions and weight in 5–7 year old girls but not in boys especially in mother–daughter relationships (Fisher & Birch, 2002). Even though childhood obesity experts discourage dieting, parents who feel the need to control a child's weight commonly encourage dieting (Lindsay et al., 2006). In addition, when parents assume control of meal size or coerce children to eat rather than allowing them to focus on their internal cues of hunger and satiety, children's ability to regulate meal size in response to energy density is diminished (Johnson & Birch, 1994).

Parental Facilitation of Children's Recreational and Sports Physical Activity

Parents who are supportive of physical activity have physically active children (Davison et al., 2003). Instrumental support (e.g., providing a ride to practice) for children's sports participation is associated with greater levels of physical activity (Davison et al., 2003). One study among 370 boys and 362 girls in 4th and 5th grades identified that frequency of parents transporting children to activity locations explained significant proportions of the activity levels for those children (Sallis et al., 1997). Transporting a child to a location where he or she could be active was more effective than encouraging or even playing with the child (Sallis et al., 1992). In young children, physical activity is mostly informal "active play" and not usually costly, although certain activities for older children can be costly. No or low cost options such as walking or biking as a means of "active transportation" could potentially be a means of increased energy expenditure. Unfortunately, in 2001 average use of active transportation among U.S. children was only eight minutes per day, equating to no more than the energy equivalent of a half can of soda (Sturm, 2005).

Role Models for Eating and Physical Activity

Parents' physical activity and dietary intake patterns can be used to predict children's risk of obesity (Davison & Birch, 2002). At an early age children will eat what their parents eat. For example, parent intake is consistently and positively associated with fruit and vegetable intake among children (Cullen et al., 2003; Nicklas & Johnson, 2004; Fisher et al, 2003). This parent–child correspondence is especially true for mothers and daughters with comparable milk consumption patterns, degree of portion control, and restrained eating (Koplan et al., 2005). The evidence relating parental modeling to child activity behaviors is less substantial than that for eating. Parents often engage in different types of physical activity than children and in different settings, decreasing the opportunity for direct observational learning by their children of these activities. Nevertheless, the Framingham Children's Study among four to seven year old children and their parents found that the children of active mothers were twice as likely to be active as children of inactive mothers. When both parents were active, these children were 5.8 times more likely to be active than the children of two sedentary parents (Hood et al., 2000).

In summary, evidence for an association between each determinant and overweight varies in magnitude and volume. When viewed as a whole, the current evidence does not point to any one specific determinant, but rather to a combination of influences collectively. As a result, a combined approach, addressing multiple determining factors will be required for comprehensive obesity prevention.

Recommendations for Parents

Although the causes of overweight and obesity among young children are many, prevention strategies within the immediate environment of the child include the home, school, neighborhood, and media contexts. Most important, family and home environmental variables are potentially modifiable by the parent for their preschool and early school-aged children. Ways for parents to positively influence child dietary and physical/sedentary activity behaviors within the family and home contexts are summarized here. Recommendations for intervening in the school and neighborhood environments are discussed in Chapters 13 and 16.

Parents can influence their children's eating and physical activity a number of ways. Most notably in the home, the availability and accessibility of healthy foods, parental role modeling of healthy eating and activity behaviors, and parent-to-child interaction around foods can positively influence development of the child's dietary and activity patterns (Haire-Joshu & Nanney, 2002). Around preschool age, when children particularly dislike new foods, it is important for parents to provide early exposure to nutritious foods like fruits and vegetables to increase their preference for them. Therefore, the home physical environment, along with parental role modeling, is critical to exposure to healthy foods and establishing taste preferences. Parents can also reduce opportunities for unhealthful choices by their selection of options when eating away from home. However, as noted previously, excessive restriction of high calorie foods and beverages when they are available may be counterproductive. Advice about controlling the child's food intake emphasizes the division of parental and child responsibility. Satter (Satter, 1986) states that parents are responsible for presenting a variety of healthful foods to children and deciding the manner in which these foods are presented and that children are responsible for whether and how much they eat (Nicklas & Johnson, 2004).

Observational learning through parental modeling between parents and young children has been seen as an effective strategy for improving dietary intakes and activity patterns among children (Haire-Joshu & Nanney, 2002). When parents adopt a healthier lifestyle, those habits contribute to the development of healthful behaviors and patterns in their children. There is concern that portion sizes have become excessively large in recent years, particularly for foods consumed outside of the home. Parents should be helped to identify and make available age-appropriate portion sizes for their children. In general, an appropriate portion size is a tablespoon for every year of the child's age (Mitchell, 1994) Based on the current evidence, the message to parents regarding sweetened beverages is that limiting the child's consumption of soft drinks may help reduce the risk and prevent excessive weight gain that can lead to obesity (American Academy of Pediatrics, 2004). Recommendations for limiting sedentary activity include removing a television from the child's bedroom, if present, limiting overall TV and videogame watching to less than 2 hours per day and offering alternative, more active activities that children find entertaining and enjoyable (Koplan et al., 2005). Specific recommendations for parents are highlighted in Table 19.1.

Table 19.1 What a parent can do to promote healthful eating and physical activity in children (Source: Sothern, 2004; Ritchie et al., 2005).

- Encourage the child to select more healthful snacks, and never give food as a reward

- Serve children an appropriate portion of each food prepared. Teach children that it is okay to leave food on their plate so they will learn to self-regulate and not overeat

- Keep within reach nutritious foods naturally low in fat and sugar. Reduce children's access to high calorie, nutrient poor beverages and foods, both at home and when eating away

- Reduce children's television and video game time by removing the machine from the child's bedroom and limit viewing hours to less than 2 hours per day

- Require that all foods and drinks be consumed in a designated area (kitchen, snack bar), not in front of the television

- Work to find ways to increase exposure to a variety of age and skill appropriate physical activities that are fun and achievable

- Model healthful eating and physical activity practices for children

Interventions During Preschool and Childhood Years and At-Risk Children

Based upon an international review by Summerbell for the Cochrane Collaboration, Caballero (2004) summarized childhood obesity prevention studies for the United States and concluded that most of the successful prevention programs include at least one of the following components: dietary changes, physical activity, behavior and social modifications, and family participation. However, the current evidence suggests that many diet and physical activity interventions to prevent obesity in children are often not effective in preventing weight gain, although they can be effective in influencing positive dietary changes and increased physical activity levels (Summerbell et al., 2005). The majority of interventions in this age group have been in schools or group care settings, which are also discussed in Chapter 16.

Preschool Children

Sixty percent (13 million) of the nation's preschool children spend most of their day in a child care facility (National Center for Educational Statistics, 1996). Day care settings offer a unique opportunity to incorporate strategies that promote healthy weights among preschoolers. These facilities are widely state regulated in some respects but with generally weak standards governing nutrition and physical activity (Story et al., 2006b).

Dennison and colleagues describe a preschool-based intervention that led to reductions in young children's television and video viewing (Dennison et al., 2004). The study, a randomized controlled trial among 16 day care centers in rural upstate New York for 2- to 6-year-olds, provided a 7-session intervention to reduce children's TV viewing, with supporting materials for the day care provider, child, and parents. The adult materials focused on positive aspects of alternative activities to television viewing like the enhanced social skills gained from eating meals together. The child focused materials encouraged activities such as generating a list of activities that they enjoyed other than watching television and making "no television" signs and stickers. Parent reports of the child's frequency of TV/video viewing indicated significant reductions in viewing time in the intervention group (decreased viewing by 3.1 hours/day) compared to the control group (increased viewing by 1.6 hours/day). After the intervention, the percentage of children watching more than 2 hours/day of television/videos was significantly lowered among the intervention group compared to the control group (19% versus 41%). The change in the children's viewing did not differ by child gender, parent education, or the number of hours per week the child attended day care or preschool. Although BMI decreased in the intervention group and increased among the control group, none of the changes in growth measurements (BMI, triceps skin-fold) between the 2 groups were significantly different during the study period.

To date the only reported intervention targeting preschoolers that has been effective in reducing increases in BMI is *Hip-Hop to Health Jr.,* evaluated in a randomized controlled trial of African American and Latino children in 24 Head Start preschools in Chicago, IL (Fitzgibbon et al., 2005). This 14-week dietary/physical activity intervention was developed with input from early childhood educators, nutrition and activity experts, community health advocates, minority health experts and focus groups. The intervention consisted of three, forty minute weekly sessions often incorporating hand-held puppets to present healthy eating and activity concepts and lead them through adventures; and engaging the children in physical activity such as "trips to the zoo" where children pretended to be zoo animals. In addition to the child curriculum, parents in the intervention group received weekly newsletters with information supporting the children's curriculum. At the end of the study period, intervention African American children had significantly smaller increase in BMI (and BMI z-score) compared with control children at 1-year and 2-year follow-up. Differences in BMI between the groups with adjustments for baseline age and BMI were -0.53 kg/m2 (.06 versus .59 mean BMI increase) at year 1 and -0.54 kg/m2 (.54 versus 1.08 mean BMI increase) at year 2. Relative effects of the intervention were similar for boys and girls, for children below and above the median age at baseline, and for children below and above the 85th percentile at baseline. However, the study is not informative as to the types of changes responsible for the BMI difference. Percent calories from saturated fat (11.6% versus 12.8%, respectively ($p = .002$)) was the only food intake or physical activity variable that differed between African American intervention and control children (Fitzgibbon et al., 2005). A subsequent report from this study noted that effectiveness was limited to the six predominantly African American Head Start Centers. No effectiveness was observed in the six predominantly Latino centers, although the program was well received (Fitzgibbon et al, 2006). The authors offer the following possible reasons for the lack of effectiveness among in the Latino preschool children: parent intervention not intensive enough, intervention not targeting ethnic foods and cultural aspects of eating and activity, and a higher BMI (and BMI z-score) at baseline.

Overall, there is a critical shortage of programs aimed at the preschool years which represents an important stage of growth and development (Summerbell et al., 2005). Furthermore, variability among preschool-setting policies and practices offer an important opportunity to influence overall activity levels and dietary intakes of the children the preschools serve. Experts in the field cite the federal preschool program, Head Start, as a model for nutrition standards for other child care programs to look to for guidance (Story et al., 2006b).

Elementary School-Aged Children

The combination of one-to-one mentoring, child-focused computer based tailoring, and parent support holds promise as an obesity prevention approach among elementary school-aged children (Haire-Joshu, 2005). *Partners of All Ages Reading About Diet and Exercise* (PARADE) was incorporated into national mentoring programs delivered as an adjunct to school-based learning, and designed to promote positive diet and activity patterns. PARADE consisted of 8 lesson plans delivered by mentors, addressing key concepts related to diet and activity; 8 child-focused computer-tailored storybooks with messages targeting that child's diet and activity patterns; 8 parent-action newsletters, which highlighted content in each storybook. Schools (n = 121) and children (N = 780; females = 71%; African American = 66%; average age = 8.6 yrs.) were randomized to intervention or control sites. PARADE children maintained their relative weight position as measured by BMI z-score and controls increased BMI z-score (p < .06). Within-group results revealed PARADE children maintained their caloric intake in contrast to controls who reported increases in total calories (p < .06), total % fat calories (p < .04) and saturated fat intake (<.06). There was no significant difference in time spent in activity between groups.

The Medical College of Georgia *FitKid Project* (MCG FitKid) was developed to increase moderate to vigorous physical activity (MVPA) in elementary school children during the 2-hour block of time after school (Yin et al., 2005). Children in nine intervention schools were compared with children in nine control schools. Sixty-eight percent were eligible for free or reduced price lunch. The after school intervention activities included 40 minutes of homework assistance, a healthy snack, and an 80-minute period of activity. The age appropriate activities consisted of 20 minutes of warm-up, 40 minutes of MVPA (i.e., tag and ball game), and 10 minutes of calisthenics and cool-down. The FitKid after school program incorporated a monthly theme and emphasized enjoyment and fun. Children who had greater than 40% attendance decreased in percent body fat, whereas the control participants gained slightly at the end of one school year. The intervention effects were not related to baseline weight status.

In a study involving nearly 1,400 ethnically diverse children at 4 elementary schools in Massachusetts, an individualized *Health Report Card* was associated with increased parental awareness of their child's weight status among overweight children (Chomitz et al., 2003). Families were randomly assigned to a personalized weight and fitness health card intervention, a general information intervention or a control group. The personalized health intervention group received a health report card of their children's height, weight and weight status, fitness test results, and interpretive information. For those children outside of the healthy weight range, the materials referred parents to follow-up with their primary health care provider or the school nurse. Within one to six weeks after the after the *Health Report Card* was sent to homes, a telephone interview was conducted to assess the efficacy of the intervention materials. First, parent awareness of child's weight status was assessed by correctness of classifications (overweight, at risk for overweight, healthy weight, or underweight). Second, parent concern about their child's weight was determined (very, somewhat, slightly, not at all). Third, the planning of weight control activities from a list categorized as medical services (see a pediatrician or school nurse), diet-related activities (put child on diet, skip meals or snacks), physical activities (sign up for sports or exercise class, increase exercise or physical activity). Prior to the mailings and phone interviews, physical education teachers were trained to collect height, weight, and physical fitness data using newly installed stadiometers and scales at each school. Among overweight students, the personalized health report card intervention parents were 3 times more likely to know their child's weight status compared to the control group. Compared to the control group, parents of overweight children were more likely to be concerned about their child's weight status (48% versus 33%). After receiving the personalized *Health Report Card*, the intervention parents were more likely to report initiating or intending to initiate intervention activities compared to the other two groups.

Interactive Multimedia for Promoting Physical Activity in Children (IMPACT) (Goran & Reynolds, 2005) is an 8 week multimedia intervention (interactive CD-Rom, 4 classroom and 4 homework assignments developed using Social Cognitive Theory constructs for 209 4th graders, ages 8 to 11 from four schools). The interactive animated computer game is supplemented by classroom and homework assignments for improving physical activity. The game theme is one of a group of children traveling around the world in search of magic ingredients to concoct an antidote to the elixir generated by an evil doer who wants everybody to hate being physically active. Despite the seeming incongruity of using inactive intervention methods to promote physical activity, *IMPACT* reports significant improvements in light physical activity and reductions in BMI z-score by 1.4% (net difference from control) in girls but not boys, after controlling for baseline age and BMI z-score. The increase in light activity translates to about 20 minutes more per day. The findings of this study suggest the use of technology as an effective intervention strategy that appeals to youth.

Ethnic Minorities and Low-Income Children

Ethnic diversity is increasing in the United States. Recent census bureau estimates place the minority population at about one-third of the U.S. population overall and 45% of U.S. children under age 5 (Population Reference Bureau, 2006). As discussed in Chapter 3, a higher prevalence of obesity has been identified among several minority populations, which indicates susceptibility and a need for programs that specifically target these groups. Ethnic differences in obesity-related risk factors begin as early as 6 to 9 years of age (Winkleby et al., 1999).

In addition to the previously described *Hip Hop for Health* program targeting minority children, one intervention targeting Hispanic preadolescents, *El Paso Catch*, was conducted among 3rd graders (n = 896) representing 8 schools in El Paso, Texas (Coleman et al., 2005). *El Paso Catch* is the translation of a school health curriculum tested with a national clinical research trial (Child and Adolescent Trial for Cardiovascular Health-CATCH), in a community low-income school setting. The intervention program consists of both physical education (PE) and cafeteria components and included a PE training guidebook, activities and curriculum materials and an Eat Smart manual. Training emphasized adapting the national materials to the ethnic and regional variations and school-specific environments of El Paso schools. The translation of an already effective program (CATCH) to low-income schools with Hispanic students successfully slowed the increase in risk of overweight among both boys and girls. *El Paso CATCH* schools reported significant reduction in the rate of increase in risk for overweight among girls (2% versus 13% rate of increase) and boys (1% versus 9% rate of increase). Specifically for girls, the percentage of at risk for overweight or overweight from third grade to fifth grade was higher among control schools (26% to 39% at risk for or overweight) compared to *El Paso Catch* schools (30% to 32% at risk for or overweight). A similar pattern was seen for boys, with a rate of increase for *El Paso Catch* schools (40%–41% at risk for or overweight) that was significantly less than for the control schools (40%–49% at risk for or overweight).

The health and nutritional status of American-Indian children has changed dramatically over the past three to four decades from a problem of under weight and under nutrition to one of excessive body weight (Story et al., 2003). Even as early as 5- to 6-years of age, overweight is more than twice as prevalent in American-Indian children compared to U.S. youth in general, and obesity is more than three times as prevalent (Yu, 1991). As a result, obesity has emerged as one of the most serious public health problems facing American-Indian children and there is an urgent need for effective prevention strategies. To date, the *Pathways* study is the largest and most comprehensive prevention study of American-Indian children. *Pathways* was a multisite school-based curriculum and family intervention for 1704 third–fifth grade American Indian children. The study was designed to promote healthful eating and increasing physical activity and was evaluated in a randomized field trial including 41 schools in seven American Indian communities (Davis et al., 2003). The 21 intervention schools received four components: a classroom curriculum, food service, physical activity, and family modules. The curriculum and family components were based on Social Learning Theory and American Indian concepts. *Pathways* resulted in positive changes in knowledge, identity, a healthful eating and physical activity and environmental change in school food service and documented significant reductions in total energy intake and percent calories from fat. However, it did not reduce the percent body fat or BMI in intervention schools compared to controls. Reasons for this may be that the intervention was not long enough, weight gain that occurred during the 3 months of summer recess when no intervention program was conducted, or compensation for calories reduced in meals at school by consuming more calories at home (Caballero, 2004).

Overall, the number of obesity prevention interventions focusing on minority or other at-risk populations remains inadequate given the higher than average risks of obesity among children in minority populations. Best practices identified among programs targeting minority populations report strong stakeholder involvement in program planning and evaluation (Flynn et al., 2006) and involving parents and other family members as active participants in the intervention (Teufel et al., 1999). Almost nonexistent are interventions addressing special needs of immigrant children who may be especially vulnerable to the obesogenic environment during their transition from home country to the United States (Summerbell et al., 2005). However, programs targeting minority populations may have some applicability to immigrant groups (Flynn et al., 2006).

While weight-gain, prevention interventions for preschool and preadolescent children are clearly in their formative years, encouraging progress has been made with lessons to be learned. Strategies that are shown to be effective among youth of diverse backgrounds are especially needed. Finally, the long-term effectiveness of these interventions should be explored.

Summary and Implications

Prevention of excess weight gain is necessary to reverse one of our most critical public health problems, childhood overweight and obesity. During childhood, growth is expected and weight and body size are constantly changing. Obesity prevention programs for preschool and early preadolescent children should aim to decrease adiposity without weight loss by means of maintenance or stabilization of weight over time. As children grow taller, maintenance of weight can result in a reduction of BMI percentile. Children with excess weight experience physical, psychological and adverse learning effects. Fortunately, clinically-based weight management programs among children and adolescents have demonstrated that a modest decrease in BMI percentile is associated with significant improvements in insulin and lipid levels (Kirk et al., 2005).

A main reason for encouraging healthy eating and activity patterns early on is to create a foundation of healthy lifestyles as children move to adulthood, contributing to a life-long protection from chronic disease risks, like obesity. However, the current environmental experience of young children includes few opportunities for physical activity and an overabundance of high calorie foods (Sothern, 2004). Strategies must be developed that involve parents and incorporate a standard of practice in early childhood settings that establishes positive lifestyle behaviors. Specifically, creating more programs to improve parental behaviors relevant to childhood overweight and targeting child-specific settings for policy interventions are highly promising strategies. An emphasis on energy balance instead of weight is preferred. The Weight Realities Division of the Society for Nutrition Education developed guidelines for childhood obesity prevention programs that encourage a health-centered, rather than a weight-centered, approach that focuses on the whole child, physically, mentally, and socially. The guidelines emphasize living actively, eating in normal and healthful ways, and creating a supportive environment (Berg et al., 2003). Promotion of efforts to reduce excess caloric intake along with efforts to increase energy expenditure should receive paramount attention in the design of interventions targeting our most vulnerable individuals, our children. Most likely, any real influence on the weight status among individual children will be the result of cumulative effects with an emphasis on policy changes targeting influences that dominate their away-from-home environments.

Acknowledgements. The authors recognize the contributions of Darrin Cottle Karen Schliep and Pamela Kosti in the preparation of this chapter.

References

Action for Healthy Kids. (2004). The Learning Connection: The Value of Improving Nutrition and Physical Activity in Our Schools. At: www.ActionForHealthyKids.org. Accessed October 2, 2006.

Alliance for a Healthier Generation. At: www.clintonfoundation.org. Accessed October 24, 2006.

American Academy of Pediatrics. (2004). Soft drinks in schools.. *Pediatrics*, 113, 152–154.

American Academy of Pediatrics. Committee on Communications (1995). Children, adolescents, and advertising. *Pediatrics*, 95(2), 295–297.

Berg, F., Buechner, J., & Parham, E. (2003). Guidelines for childhood obesity prevention programs: Promoting healthy weight in children. *Journal of Nutrition Education and Behavior*, 35(1), 1–4.

Bideci, A., Cinaz, P., Hasanoglu, A., & Elberg, S. (1997). Serum levels of insulin-like growth factor-I and insulin-like growth factor binding protein-3 in obese children. *Journal of Pediatric Endocronology & Metabolism*, 10(3), 295–299.

Blanchette, L., & Brug, J. (2005). Determinants of fruit and vegetable consumption among 6-12 year old children and effective interventions to increase consumption. *Journal of Human Nutrition and Dietetics*, 18(6), 431–443.

Borzekowski, D., & Robinson, T. (2001). The 30-second effect: An experiment revealing the impact of television commercials on food preferences of preschoolers. *Journal of the American Dietetic Association*, 101(1), 42–46.

Bowman, S. A., Gormaker, S. L., Ebbeling, C. B., Pereira, M. A., & Ludwig, D. S. (2004). Effects of fast-food consumption on energy intake and diet quality among children in a National Household Survey. *Pediatrics*, 113(1), 112–118.

Brooks-Gunn, J. (1988). Antecedents and consequences of variations in girls' maturational timing. *Journal of Adolescent Health Care*, 9, 365–373.

Brownson, R. C., Boehmer, T. K., & Luke, D. A. (2005). Declining rates of physical activity in the United States: What are the contributors? *Annual Review of Public Health*, 26, 421–443.

Brug, J., & van Lenthe, F. (2005). Environmental determinants and interventions for physical activity, nutrition and smoking: A review., 31–202.

Burdette, H., Whitaker, R., & Daniels, S. (2004). Parental report of outdoor playtime as a measure of physical activity in preschool-aged children. *Archives of Pediatric and Adolescent Medicine*, 158(4), 353–357.

Caballero, B. (2004). Obesity prevention in children: Opportunities and challenges. *International Journal of Obesity*, 28, S90–S95.

Centers for Disease Control and Prevention. (2003). Physical activity levels among children aged 9-13 years-United States, 2002. *Morbidity and Mortality Weekly Report*. 52(33), 785–788.

Chomitz, V., Collins, J., Kim, J., Kramer, E., & McGowan, R. (2003). Promoting healthy weight among elementary school children via a health report card approach. *Archives of Pediatric and Adolescent Medicine*, 157(8), 765–772.

Coleman, K., Tiller, C., Sanchez, J., Heath, E., Sy, O., Milliken, G., et al. (2005). Prevention of the epidemic increase in child risk of overweight in low-income schools: The El Paso coordinated approach to child health. *Archives of Pediatric and Adolescent Medicine*, 159(3), 217–224.

Committee of the Institute of Medicine. Nutrition standards for foods in schools. Food and Nutrition Board. http://www.nationalacademies.org. Accessed 8/14/06.

Crawford, P., Story, M., Wang, M., Ritchie, L. D., & Sabry, Z. (2001). Ethnic issues in the epidemiology of childhood obesity. *Pediatric Clinics of North America*, 48(4), 855–878.

Cullen, K., Baranowski, T., Owens, E., Marsh, T., Rittenberry, L., & de Moor, C. (2003). Availability, accessibility, and preferences for fruit, 100% fruit juice, and vegetable influence children's dietary behaviors. *Health Education and Behavior*, *30*(5), 615–626.

Daniels, S., Arnett, D., Eckel, R., Gidding, S., Hayman, L., Kumanyika, S., et al. (2005). Overweight children and adolescents: Pathophysiology, consequences, prevention and treatment. *Circulation*, *111*(15), 1866–1868.

Datar, A., & Sturm, R. (2006). Childhood overweight and elementary school outcomes. International Journal of Obesity advance online publication, March 14, 2006; doi:10.1038/sj.ijo.0803311.

Datar, A., Sturm, R., & Magnabosco, J. (2004). Childhood overweight and academic performance: National study of kindergarteners and first-graders. *Obesity Research*, *12*(1), 58–68.

Davis, S., Clay, T., Smyth, M., Gittelsohn, J., Arviso, V., Flint-Wagner, H., et al. (2003). Pathways curriculum and family interventions to promote healthful eating and physical activity in American Indian schoolchildren. *Preventive Medicine*, *37*(1), 24–34.

Davison, K., & Birch, L. (2002). Obesigenic families: Parents' physical activity and dietary intake patterns predict girls' risk of overweight. *International Journal of Obesity and Related Metabolic Disorders*, *26*(9), 1186–1193.

Davison, K., Cutting, T., & Birch, L. (2003). Parents' activity-related parenting practices predict girls' physical activity. *Medicine and Science of Sports and Exercise*, *35*(9), 1589–1595.

Dehghan, M., Akhtar-Danesh, N., & Merchant, A. (2005). Childhood obesity, prevalence and prevention. *Nutrition Journal*, 4, 24. Retrieved on April 9, 2007, from http://www.nutritionj.com/content/4/1/24.

De Simone, M., Farello, G., Palumbo, M., Gentile, T., Ciuffreda, M., Olioso, P., et al. (1995). Growth charts, growth velocity and bone development in childhood obesity. *International Journal of Obesity and Related Metabolic Disorders*, *19*(12), 851–857.

Dennison, B., Erb, T., & Jenkins, P. (2002). Television viewing and television in bedroom associated with overweight risk among low-income preschool children. *Pediatrics*, 109(6), 1028–1035.

Dennison, B., Russo, T., Burdick, P., & Jenkins, P. (2004). An intervention to reduce television viewing by preschool children. *Archives of Pediatric and Adolescent Medicine, 158*(2), 170–176.

Diette, G., Markson, L., Skinner, E. A., Nguyen, T., Algratt-Bergstrom, P., & Wu, A. (2000). Nocturnal asthma in children affects school attendance, school performance, and parents' work attendance. *Archives of Pediatric and Adolescent Medicine, 154*(9), 923–928.

Dietz, W. (1994). Critical periods in childhood for the development of obesity. *American Journal of Clinical Nutrition*, 59(5):955–959.

Dietz, W. (1998). Health consequences of obesity in youth: Childhood predictors of adult disease. *Pediatrics*, 101(Suppl. 3), 518–525.

Dietz, W. (2000). "Adiposity rebound": Reality or epiphenomenon? *Lancet*, *356*(9247), 2027–2028.

Dietz, W., & Gortmaker, S. (1985). "Do we fatten our children at the television set? Obesity and television viewing in children and adolescents." *Pediatrics*, *75*(5), 807–812.

Dimartino-Nardi, J. (1999). Premature adrenarche: Findings in prepubertal African-American and Caribbean-Hispanic girls. *Acta Paediatrica, Supplementum, 88*(433), 67–72.

Doak, C. M., Visscher, T. L. S., Render, C. M., & Seidell, J. C. (2006). The prevention of overweight and obesity in children and adolescents: A review of interventions and programmes. *Obesity Reviews*, *7*, 111–136.

Ebbeling, C., Pawlak, D., & Ludwig, D. (2002). Childhood obesity: Public-health crisis, common sense cure. *Lancet*, *360*(9331), 473–482.

Enns, C., Mickle, S., & Goldman, J. (2002). Trends in food and nutrient intakes by children in the United States. *Family Economics and Nutrient Review*, *14*(2), 56–68.

Etnler, J., Salazaw, W., Landers, D., Petruzzello, S., Han, M., & Nowell, P. (1997). The influence of physical fitness and exercise upon cognitive functioning: A meta-analysis. *Journal of Sports and Exercise Physiology*, *19*(3), 249–277.

Ewing, R., Schroeer, W., & Greene, W. (2004). School location and student travel: Analysis of factors affecting mode choice. *Transportation Research Record*, 55–63.

Faith, M., Scanlon, K., Birch, L., Francis, L., & Sherry, B. (2004). Parent-child feeding strategies and their relationships to child cating and weight status. *Obesity Research*, *12*(11), 1711–1722.

Fisher, J., & Birch, L. (2002). Eating in the absence of hunger and overweight in girls from 5 to 7 y of age. *American Journal of Clinical Nutrition*, *76*(1), 226–231.

Fisher, J., Rolls, B., & Birch, L. (2003). Large portion sizes affect children's intake relative to age-appropriate and self-selected portions. *American Journal of Clinical Nutrition*, *77*, 1164-1170.

Fitzgibbon, M., Stolley, M., Schiffer, L., Van Horn, L., KauferChristoffel, K., & Dyer, A. (2005). Two-year follow-up results for hip-hop to health Jr.: A randomized controlled trial for overweight prevention in preschool minority children. *Journal of Pediatrics*, *146*(5), 618–625.

Fitzgibbon, M., Stolley, M., Schiffer, L., Van Horn, L., KauferChristoffel, K., & Dyer, A. (2006). Hip-hop to health jr. for Latino preschool children. *Obesity (Silver Spring)*, *14*(9), 1616–1625.

Flegal, K., & Troiano, R. (2000). Chages in the distribution of body mass index of adults and children in the U.S. population. *International Journal of Obesity and Related Metabolic Disorders*, *24*, 807–818.

Flynn, M., McNeil, D., Maloff, B., Mutasingwa, D., Wu, M., Ford, C., & Tough, S. (2006). Reducing obesity and related chronic disease risk in children and youth: A synthesis of evidence with 'best practice' recommendations. *Obesity Research*, *7*(Suppl. 1), 7–66.

Freedman, D., Dietz, W., Srinivasan, S., & Berenson, G. (1999). The relation of overweight to cardiovascular risk factors among children and adolescents: The Bogalusa heart study. *Pediatrics*, *103*(6, Pt. 1), 1175–1182.

Freedman, D., Kettel Khan, L., Serdula, M., Srinivasan, S., & Berenson, G. (2001). BMI rebound, childhood height and obesity among adults: The Bogalusa heart study. *International Journal of Obesity and Related Metabolic Disorders*, *25*(4), 543–549.

Freedman, D., Khan, L., Serdula, M., Dietz, W., Srinivasan, S., & Berenson, G. (2005). The relation of childhood BMI to adult adiposity: The Bogalusa heart study. *Pediatrics*, *115*(1), 22–27.

French, S., Lin, B., & Guthrie, J. (2003). National trends in soft drink consumption among children and adolescents age 6 to 17 years: Prevalence, amounts, and sources, 1977-1978 to 1994-1998. *Journal of the American Dietetic Association*, *103*, 1326–1331.

Frisch, R., & Revelle, R. (1971). Heights and weight at menarche and a hypothesis of menarche. *Archives of Disease in Childhood*, *46*, 695–701.

Goran, M., & Reynolds, K. (2005). Interactive multimedia for promoting physical activity (impact) in children. *Obesity Research*, *13*(4), 762–771.

Government Accountability Office. (2005, August). *School meal programs: Competitive foods are widely available and generate substantial revenues for schools.* Washington, DC. 6AD-05-SU3. Retrieved on April 9, 2007, from http://www.gao.gov/new.tnns/dossu3.pdf

Haire-Joshu, D. (2005). *Partners of all ages reading about diet and exercise (PARADE) National Institute of Infant Progress Report.* St. Louis, MO: Saint Louis University School of Public Health.

Haire-Joshu, D., & Nanney, M. (2002). Prevention of overweight and obesity in children: Influences on the food environment. *The Diabetes Educator*, *28*(3), 415–422.

Harnack, L., Stang, J., & Story, M. (1999). Soft drink consumption among US children and adolescents: Nutritional consequences. *Journal of the American Dietetic Association, 99*(4), 436–441.

Hasanoglu, A., Bideci, A., Cinaz, P., Turner, L., & Unal, S. (2000). Bone mineral density in childhood obesity. *Journal of Pediatric Endocronology & Metabolism, 13,* 307–311.

Healthy People 2010. "Reduce the proportion of children and adolescents who are overweight or obese." http://www.healthypeople.gov/document/html/objectives/19-03. htm. Accessed 8/14/06.

Hedley, A., Ogden, C., Johnson, C., Carroll, M., Curtin, L., & Flegal, K. (2004). Prevalence of overweight and obesity among U.S. children, adolescents, and adults, 1999-2002. *Journal of the American Medical Association, 291*(23), 2847–2850.

Hill, A. J., & Pallin, V. (1998). Dieting awareness and low self-worth: Related issues in 8-year-old girls. *International Journal of Eating Disorders, 24,* 405–413.

Hofferth, S. L., & Sandberg, J. F. (2001). Changes in American children's time, 1981-1997. In T. Owens, S. Hofferth, (Eds.), *Children at the millennium: Where have we come from, Where are we going? Advances in life course research.* New York: Elsevier Science.

Hood, M., Moore, L., Sundarajan-Ramamurti, A., Singer, M., Cupples, L., & Ellison, R. (2000). Parental eating attitudes and the development of obesity in children. The Framingham children's study. *International Journal of Obesity, 24*(10), 1319-1325.

Jeffery, R, & Utter, J. 2003. The changing environment and population obesity in the United States. *Obesity Research, 11,* 12S–22S.

Johnson, S., & Birch, L. (1994). Parents' and children's adiposity and eating style. *Pediatrics, 94*(5), 653–661.

Key, T. J. (1995). Hormones and cancer in humans. *Mutation Research, 333*(1-2), 59–67.

Kirk, S., Zeller, M., Claytor, R., Santangelo, M., Khoury, P., & Daniels, S. (2005). The relationship of health outcomes to improvement in BMI in children and adolescents. *Obesity Research, 13*(5), 876–882.

Koplan, J., Liverman, C., & Kraak, V. (2005). *Preventing Childhood Obesity Health in the Balance.* Washington DC: Institute of Medicine National Academy of Sciences.

Kranz, S., Siega-Riz, A. M., & Herring, A. (2004). Changes in diet quality of American preschoolers between 1977 and 1998. *American Journal of Public Health, 94*(9), 1525–1530.

Kuczmarski, R., Ogden, C., Guo, S., Grummer-Strawn, L., Flegal, K., Mei, Z., et al. (2002). 2000 CDC growth charts for the United States: Methods and development. *Vital Health Statistics 11,* 246, 1–190.

Kumanyika, S., & Grier, S. (2006). Targeting interventions for ethnic minority and low-income populations. *The Future of Children, 16*(1), 187–207.

Lazar, L., Kauli, R., Bruchis, C., Nordenberg, J., Galatzer, A., & Perzelan, A. (1995). Early polycystic ovary-like syndrome in girls with central precocious puberty and exaggerated adrenal response. *European Journal of Endocrinology, 133,* 403–406.

Lin, B., Guthrie, J., & Frazao, E. (1999, January-April). Quality of children's diets at and away from home: 1994-6. *Food Review, 22*(1), 2–10.

Lindsay, A., Sussner, K., Kim, J., & Gortmaker, S. (2006). The role of parents in preventing childhood obesity. *Future of Children, 16*(1), 169–186.

Lumeng, J. C., Appugliese, D., Cabral, H. J., Bradley, R. H., & Zuckerman, B. (2006). Neighborhood safety and overweight status in children. *Archives of Pediatric and Adolescent Medicine, 160,* 25–31.

Malina, R. M., Bouchard, C., & Bar-Or, O. (2004). *Growth, maturation, and physical activity* (2nd ed.). Champaign, IL: Human Kinetics.

Marshall, S. J., Biddle, S. J., Gorely, T., Cameron, N., & Murdey, I. (2004). Relationships between media use, body fatness and physical activity in children and youth: A meta-analysis. *International Journal of Obesity and Related Metabolic Disorders, 28*(10), 1238–1246.

McConahy, K., Smiciklas-Wright, H., Birch, L., Mitchell, D., & Picciano, M. (2002). Food portions are positively related to energy intake and body weight in early childhood. *Journal of Pediatrics*, (140), 340–347.

McConahy, K., Smiciklas-Wright, H., Mitchell, D., & Picciano, M. (2004). Portion size of common foods predicts energy intake among preschool-aged children. *Journal of the American Dietetic Association*, (104), 975–979.

McGinnis, J., Gootman, J., & Kraak, V. (2006). *Food marketing to children and youth*: *Threat or opportunity?* Washington DC: Institutes of Medicine of the National Academies.

McMurray, R., Harrell, J., Bangdivala, S., & Deng, S. (1999). Cardiovascular disease risk factors and obesity of rural and urban elementary school children. *Journal of Rural Health*, *15*(4), 365–374.

Mitchell, M. K. (1994). Nutrition during growth: Preschool and school years. In: *Nutrition across the life span* (pp. 127-158). Philadelphia, PA: W.B. Saunders Company.

Narayan, K., Boyle, J., Thompson, T., Sorensen, S., & Williamson, D. (2003). Lifetime risk for diabetes mellitus in the United States. *Journal of the American Medical Association*, *290*(14), 1884–1890.

National Association for Sport and Physical Education (2001). Physical education is critical to a complete education. A position paper from the National Association for Sports and Physical Education. http://www.aahperd.org/NASPE/pdf_files/pos_papers/pe_critical.pdf. Accessed October 14, 2006.

National Center for Educational Statistics. (1996). Child care and early education program participation of infants, toddlers, and preschoolers. In United States Department of Education. (NCCS 95-824) http:// nccs: ed.gov/pubs 95/web 95824.asp. Accessed on April 9, 2007.

National Institute for Health Care Management (2004). Obesity in Young Children: Impact and Intervention. http://www.nihcm.org/finalweb/pg_publications_obesity.htm. Accessed October 2, 2006.

Nicklas, T., & Johnson, R. (2004). Dietary guidance for healthy children aged 2 to 11 years. *Journal of the American Dietetic Association*, *104*, 660–677.

O'Connor, T. M., Yang, S. J., Nicklas, T. A. (2006). Beverage intake among preschool children and its effect on weight status. *Pediatrics*, *118*:1010–1018.

Ogden, C., Carroll, M., & Flegal, K. (2003). Epidemiologic trends in overweight and obesity. *Endocrinology and Metabolism Clinics of North America*, *32*(4), 741–760.

Ogden, C., Flegal, K., Carrol, M., & Johnson, C. (2002). Prevalence and trends in overweight among us children and adolescents, 1999-2000. *Journal of the American Medical Association*, *288*, 1728–1732.

Ogden, C., Fryar, C., Carroll, M., & Flegal, K. (2004). Mean body weight, height, and body mass index, United States 1960–2002. 2004 Oct 27; *Advance Data*, (347): 1–17.

Parrott, J., & Myers, E. (2005). American Dietetic Association evidence-based analysis library. Factors associated with childhood overweight. http://www.adaevidencelibrary.com/topicfm>cnt = 27928. Accessed April 9, 2007.

Patrick, H., & Nicklas, T. (2005). A review of family and social determinants of children's eating patterns and diet quality. *Journal of the American College of Nutrition*, *24*(2), 83–92.

Perry, C. (1997). Preadolescent and adolescent influences on health. In B. D. Smedley, & L. Syme (Eds.), *Promoting health intervention strategies for social and behavioral research*. Washington DC: National Academy Press.

Population Reference Bureau. (2006). *In the news: U.S. population is now one-third minority*. Retrieved October 23, 2006, from http://www.prb.org/Articles/2006/IntheNewsUSPopulationIsNowOneThirdMinority.aspx

Proctor, M. H., Moore, L. L., Gao, D., Cupples, L. A., Bradlee, M. L., Hood, M. Y., & Ellison, R.C. (2003). Television viewing and change in body fat from preschool to early adolescence: The Framingham Children's Study. *International Journal of Obesity and Related Metabolic Disorders, 27*, 827–833.

Rampersaud, G. C., Bailey, L. B., & Kauwell, G. P. (2003). National survey beverage consumption data for children and adolescents indicate the need to encourage a shift toward more nutritive beverages. *Journal of the American Dietetic Association, 103*(1), 97–100.

Ritchie, L., Welk, G., Styne, D., Gerstein, D., & Crawford, P. (2005). Family environment and pediatric overweight: What is a parent to do? *Journal of the American Dietetic Association,* (105), S70–S79.

Robinson, T. (1999). Reducing children's television viewing to prevent obesity: A randomized controlled trial. *Journal of the American Medical Association, 282,* 1561–1567.

Rolls, B., Engell, D., & Birch, L. (2000). Serving portion size influences 5-year-old but not 3-year-old children's food intakes. *Journal of the American Dietetic Association, 100*(2), 232–234.

Sallis, J., & Glanz, K. (2006). The role of built environments in physical activity, eating, and obesity in childhood. *Future of Children, 16*(1), 89–109.

Sallis, J., Alcaraz, J., McKenzie, T., Hovell, M., Kolody, B., & Nader, P. (1992). Parent behavior in relation to physical activity and fitness in 9-year olds. *American Journal of Diseases in Children, 146,* 1383–1388.

Sallis, J., Alcaraz, J., McKenzie T., & Howell, M. (1997). Predictors of change in children's physical activity over 20 months: Variations by gender and level of adiposity. *American Journal of Preventive Medicine, 16,* 222–229.

Sallis, J., McKenzie, T., Kolody, B., Lewis, M., Marshal, S., & Rosengard, P. (1999). Effects of health-related physical education on academic achievement; project spark. *Research Quarterly for Exercise and Sport, 70*(2), 127–134.

Sallis, J., Prochaska, J., & Taylor, W. C. (2000). A review of correlates of physical activity of children and adolescents. *Medicine and Science in Sports and Exercise, 32,* 963–975.

Satter, E. (1986). *Child of mine.* Palto Alto, CA: Bull Publishing.

Schwimmer, J., Burwinkle, T., & Varni, J. (2003). Health-related quality of life of severely obese children and adolescents. *Journal of the American Medical Association, 289*(14), 1818.

Serdula, M., Ivery, D., Coates, R., Freedman, D., Williamson, D., & Byers, T. (1993). Do obese children become obese adults? A review of the literature. *Preventive Medicine, 22*(2), 167–177.

Shephard, R. (1997). Curricular physical activity and academic performance. *Pediatric Exercise Science, 9,* 113–126.

Sherry, B., Mei, Z., Scanlon, K., Mokdad, A., & Grummer-Strawn, L. (2004). Trends in state-specific prevalence of overweight and underweight in 2- through 4-year-old children from low-income families from1989 through 2000. *Archives of Pediatric and Adolescent Medicine, 158*(12), 1116–1124.

Simons-Morton, B., Taylor, W., Snider, S., Huang, I., & Fulton J. (1994). Observed levels of elementary and middle school children's physical activity during physical education classes. *Preventive Medicine, 23*(4), 437–441.

Skinner, J. D., & Carruth, B. R. (2001). A longitudinal study of children's juice intake and growth: The juice controversy revisited. *Journal of the American Dietetic Association, 101*(4), 432–437.

Smiciklas-Wright, H., Mitchell, D., Mickle, S., Goldman, J., & Cook, A. (2003). Foods commonly eaten in the United States, 1989-1991 and 1994-1996; Are portion sizes changing? *Journal of the American Dietetic Association, 103*(1), 41–47.

Sothern, M. (2004). Obesity prevention in children: Physical activity and nutrition. *Nutrition Journal, 20,* 704–708.

Staunton, C., Hubsmith, D., & Kallins, W. (2003). Promoting safe walking and biking to school: The Marin County success story. *American Journal of Public Health, 93,* 1431–1434.

Story, M., Kaphingst, K., & French, S. A. (2006a). The role of schools in obesity prevention. *Future of Children, 16*(1): 109–142.

Story, M., Kaphingst, K., & French, S. A. (2006b). The role of child care settings in obesity prevention. *Future of Children, 16*(1), 143–168.

Story, M., Stevens, J., Himes, J., Stone, E., Rock, B., Ethelbah, B., et al. (2003). Obesity in American-Indian children: Prevalence, consequences, and prevention. *Preventive Medicine,* (37), S3–S12.

Strauss, R. (2000). Childhood obesity and self esteem. *Pediatrics, 105*(1), 15.

Sturm, R. (2005). Childhood obesity-what we can learn from existing data on societal trends, part 1. *Preventing Chronic Disease, 2*(1), 1–9.

Sturm, R., & Datar, A. (2005). Body mass index in elementary school children, metropolitan area food prices and food outlet density. *Public Health, 119*(12), 1059–1068.

Summerbell, C., Waters, E., Edmunds, L., Brown, K., & Campbell, K. (2005). Interventions for preventing obesity in children. (Review). *The Cochrane Database of Systematic Reviews,* CD001871.

Symons, C., Cinelli, B., James, T., & Groff, P. (1997). Bridging student health risks and academic achievement through comprehensive school health programs. *Journal of School Health, 67*(6), 220–227.

Tai-Seale, T., & Chandler, C. (2003). Nutrition and overweight concerns in rural areas. In *Rural healthy people* 2010: *A companion document to healthy people 2010* (Vol. 1). College Station, TX: The Texas A&M University System Health Science Center, School of Rural Public Health, Southwest Rural Health Research Center.

Teufel, N., Perry, C., Story, M., Flint-Wagner, H., Levin, S, Clay, T., et al. (1999). Pathways family intervention for third-grade American Indian children. *American Journal of Clinical Nutrition, 69*(Suppl. 4), 803S–809S.

Troiano, R., Flegal, K., Kuczmarski, R., Campbell, S., & Johnson, C. (1995). Overweight prevalence and trends for children and adolescents: The national health and nutrition examination surveys 1963-1991. *Archives of Pediatric and Adolescent Medicine, 149,* 1085–1091.

United States Department of Agriculture. (2005). *MyPyramid: Steps to a Healthier You.* [Online]. Available: http://www.mypyramid.gov/ [accessed October 4, 2006].

United States Department of Agriculture. Food and Nutrition Service. (2003, March). Nibbles for Health: Nutrition Newsletters for Parents of Young Children. *Why Snacks?* [Online]. Available: http://www.fns.usda.gov/tn/Resources/nibbles.html [accessed October 4, 2006].

Vetiska, J., Glabb, L., Perlman, K., & Daneman, D. (2000). School attendance of children with type 1 diabetes. *Diabetes Care, 23,* 1706–1707.

Welsh, J. A., Cogswell, M. E., Rogers, S., Rockett, H., Mei, Z., & Grummer-Strawn L. (2005). Overweight among low-income preschool children associated with the consumption of sweet drinks: Missouri, 1999-2002. *Pediatrics, 115*(2), 223–229.

Whitaker, R., Pepe, M., & Wright, J. S., Seidel, K. D., Dietz, WH. (1998). Early adiposity rebound and the risk of adult obesity. *Pediatrics, 101*(3), E5.

Whitlock, E., Williams, S., Gold, R., Smith, P., & Shipman, S. (2005). Screening and interventions for childhood overweight: A summary of evidence for the US preventive services task force. *Pediatrics, 116*(1): e125–144.

Wilcox, P. W., Weiner, D. S., & Leighley, B. (1988). Maturation factors in slipped capital femoral epiphysis. *Journal of Pediatric Orthopedics, 8,* 196–200.

Winkleby, M., Robinson, T., Sundquist, J., & Kraemer, H. (1999). Ethnic variation in cardiovascular disease risk factors among children and young adults: Findings from the third national health and nutrition examination survey, 1988-1994. *Journal of the American Medical Association, 281,* 1006–1013.

Yin, Z., Gutin, B., Johnson, M., Hanes, J., Moore, J., Cavnar M., et al. (2005). An environmental approach to obesity prevention in children: Medical college of Georgia FitKid project 1 year results. *Obesity Research*, *13*(12), 2153–2161.

Youth Sport Council and The National Association for Sport and Physical Education. (1999). *Choosing the right sport & physical activity program for your child*. At: http://www.aahperd.org/naspe. Accessed October 13, 2006.

Yu, P. (1991). Heart disease in Asians and Pacific-Islanders, Hispanics, and Native Americans. *Circulation*, *83*, 1475–1477.

Chapter 20

Obesity Prevention During Preadolescence and Adolescence

Alison E. Field

Introduction

Pediatric obesity is a serious public health problem in the United States. According to the 2003–2004 National Health and Nutrition Examination Survey (NHANES), approximately 37% of children and 34% adolescents are overweight or at risk for overweight (i.e., body mass index (BMI) ≥ national 85th percentile for age and sex) (see Chapter 3) (Ogden et al., 2006). The prevalence of overweight is particularly high among African Americans and Hispanics. However, these estimates may underestimate the true prevalence among preadolescents and adolescents due to relying on the pediatric BMI standards from the Centers for Disease Control and Prevention (CDC) (Centers for Disease Control (CDC),2002). The CDC suggests that children and adolescents at or above the 95th percentile of BMI for age and gender be classified as overweight, but at age 13.5 years for boys and age 12 for girls, some children with a BMI greater than 25 kg/m^2, the adult cut-off for over-weight, will not be classified as overweight since that is below the 95th age and gender-specific percentile for BMI (see Chapter 2). This problem is much less of an issue when a BMI ≥85th percentile for age and gender is used to define overweight in youth. In that case, the inconsistent classification does not occur until 17.5 years for the boys and 17 years for girls. Thus the reported prevalence of obesity among adolescents in the United States likely underesti-mates the true prevalence (Gordon-Larsen, Adair, Nelson, & Popkin, 2004).

As discussed in Chapters 18 and 19, obesity prevention in children and youth can be a focus prior to preadolescence and adolescence, but this matu-rational transition period may be particularly important in the prevention of overweight and obesity. The prevalence of adolescent overweight has increased almost three-fold since the late 1980s (Ogden et al., 2006; Ogden, Flegal, Carroll, & Johnson, 2002), suggesting an urgent need to identify and address the causes of this relatively recent, population-wide phenomenon. Weight status during preadolescence and adolescence is a good predictor of adult weight status. For example, Whitaker et al. (Whitaker, Wright, Pepe, Seidel, & Dietz, 1997) observed that the odds of being an obese adult were 28 times higher for an obese 10–14 year old child compared to a non-obese child of the same age. Moreover, obese children are not the only ones who become overweight or obese adults. Those not yet overweight can also benefit from preventive efforts. In a study of 269 children who were initially 8 to 15 years of age, few very lean children became overweight over the following 10 years. However, independent of age and length of follow-up, girls and boys whose BMI was between the 50th and 84th percentile (i.e., in the "healthy weight" range) were approximately four to five times more likely than their leaner peers of becoming overweight or obese as young adults (Field, Cook, & Gillman, 2005). In addition, preadolescence and adolescence correspond to the ages when young people begin to make more of their own decisions. Preventive interventions can target this transitional period in order to foster decision-making that is favorable to the achievement and maintenance of healthy weight.

The objective of the chapter is to foster an understanding of preadolescence and adolescence from developmental and behavioral perspectives and to consider how various factors may influence lifestyles choices among preadolescents and adolescents. Youth are highly influenced by social pressures, media images and marketing, and the beliefs and behavior of their friends and family. These influences are important to consider when planning interventions to prevent obesity. Because they may undermine or overwhelm the impact of knowledge gained from obesity prevention interventions. In reviewing the literature on potential modifiable determinants of obesity or weight gain, results from randomized clinical trials are reported whenever possible and given somewhat greater weight than those from observational and quasi-experimental studies. Clinical trials are less subject to misinterpretation due to selection bias and confounding variables and can be more clearly interpreted with respect to changes resulting from *modifying a risk factor.* However, clinical trials have only evaluated a subset of all the possible modifiable influences on weight gain: dietary intake, physical activity, and screen time. Moreover, many questions about the complex pathways that determine obesity cannot be feasibly answered by clinical trials in which only a few factors are modified (Swinburn, Gill, & Kumanyika, 2005). Among the observational studies, greater weight has been given to longitudinal studies, but in some cases potential insights from cross-sectional have been included. Detailed systematic reviews of obesity determinants and interventions that include studies of children in the preadolescent and adolescent age range (Brug & van Lenthe, 2005; Flynn et al., 2006) may provide a useful complement to this chapter, in addition to the several other chapters in this book related to obesity prevention contexts and settings.

Developmental Context

Maturational Issues

In this chapter preadolescence refers to ages 8 to 12 years and adolescence refers to ages 13 to 20. Among girls, pubertal development normally occurs within preadolescence (Rico et al., 1993). In a nationally representative sample of 4,263 youth, 8 to 19 years of age, in the United States, the median age of onset for breast development among females was 10.4 years among non-Hispanic whites, 9.8 for Mexican Americans, and 9.5 years among non-Hispanic black girls (Sun et al., 2002). For the white and Mexican-

American girls, pubic hair development, which is caused by increased andro-gen secretion, started slightly later. The onset of menses usually occurs approximately two years after the onset breast development. Girls who are overweight are more likely to have an early age at menarche, whereas those who are highly active or have a low body weight are more likely to have a delayed age at menarche. Boys develop later than girls and may extend beyond the preadolescent age range. Among males it was estimated that the median was 12.0 years among non-Hispanic whites, 12.3 years for Mexican Americans, and 11.2 years among non-Hispanic black boys (Sun et al., 2002). Genital development started approximately two years earlier.

During puberty, most females experience a growth spurt and an increase in body fat, as well as lean mass. Among males, the growth spurt occurs later, during adolescence, and is associated with increases in lean mass, but decreases in fat mass. (Rico et al., 1993). However, although some weight change is a normal and healthy part of preadolescence and adolescence, for an increasing number of youth excessive amounts of body weight and body fat are accrued during this period. Moreover, as noted above, overweight youth enter puberty at younger ages. Thus overweight girls start to increase their fat mass at younger ages than their peers and early age of menarche is associated with shorter achieved stature. The combination of having higher fat mass accrual and shorter achieved stature is one reason overweight preadolescent girls are likely to become overweight adults.

Cognitive Changes

Not only do physical changes distinguish children from preadolescents and adolescents, but also the cognitive processes used in these two periods are very different from one another. By the time children have become preadolescents, they should have acquired the ability to think abstractly instead of being con-crete thinkers. Being able to think abstractly markedly changes the ability of children to understand global concepts in nutrition and healthy lifestyle behav-ior choices, which are components of most school-based obesity prevention interventions. Pertinent to the ability to evaluate preventive interventions, the ability to think abstractly is necessary to complete self-report assessments of dietary intake, physical activity, inactivity, and other potential modifiable determinants of obesity. For example, younger children, who are concrete thinkers, are able to report on discrete events, such as lunch on that particular day, but do not have the cognitive skills to report on average lunch intake dur-ing an extended period. Older children are able to report on behaviors they usually engage in over an extended period of time, such as week, month, sea-son, or year. Some preadolescents have not yet reached the development stage of being abstract thinkers and it is, therefore, not surprising that validity of self-report assessments tends to be higher among adolescents than preadoles-cents (Field, Peterson et al., 1999; Himes & Faricy, 2001).

Appetite and Activity

One of the many noticeable changes that occur during the transition from childhood to adolescence is that among males, appetite increases tremen-dously. Because many young males remain active during adolescence and are still growing, the minority of young males becomes overweight. However, for some adolescents, the caloric needs of growing are less than the discrepancy between calories consumed and calories expended through activity; thus, they gain excessive amounts of weight. Although females also grow during preadolescence and adolescence, they do not appear to have the same large increase in appetite, which is fortunate since energy expenditure tends to decrease during this period (Kimm, Glynn et al., 2002).

Another developmental change that occurs around puberty is the beginning of attraction to members of the opposite (or same) sex. Among preadolescents and adolescents, weight concerns and body dissatisfaction are greater among heterosexual than lesbian girls; whereas, among boys, heterosexuals have lower levels of body dissatisfaction than their peers with same sex attractions (S. B. Austin et al., 2004). Among post-pubertal females, who have developed androgen-related changes such as body hair and body odor, one consequence of becoming attracted to members of the opposite sex, is that they are less likely to engage in activities that they worry make them physically unattractive Thus, just as they have begun to increase their fat mass due hormonal changes associated with pubertal development, they are reducing their energy expenditure, which should make them particularly vulnerable to excessive weight gain. One approach to counteracting the decline in activity among adolescent girls is to design separate activity classes for girls so they will not feel self-conscious about their physical appearance (Neumark-Sztainer, Story, Hannan, & Rex, 2003).

Behavioral Determinants of Excess Weight Gain

Eating Patterns and Dietary Composition

Identifying behavioral determinants of obesity development during preadolescence and adolescence is challenging in that, when considering outcomes, one must try to separate determinants of normal and healthy weight gain from those related to excessive weight gain. This is particularly difficult in observational studies and may be one of the reasons that few behavioral factors have consistently been definitively identified as predictors of weight gain during preadolescence and adolescence. In addition to the changes due to physical development, preadolescence and adolescence are also periods when parents have increasingly less control over what their children eat. Youths in this age range may be purchasing more food outside of the home, including fast food, sugar-sweetened beverages, and other convenience foods with high caloric content but otherwise questionable nutritional value that may make them more likely to gain excessive amounts of weight. Moreover, as girls enter puberty they may become very focused on their weight and shape and may adopt unhealthy weight control behaviors, such as skipping breakfast or using diets pills or laxatives to control their weight.

Food Purchased away from Home
Recently there has been a shift towards studying eating patterns instead of intake of specific macro- or micronutrients as predictors of weight gain. One pattern is purchasing food away from home. Guthrie et al. (2002) found that between 1977–1978 and 1994–1996, consumption of foods prepared away from home increased by 14% to 32% of total calories (Guthrie, Lin, & Frazao,

2002). Portion sizes, and thus caloric content, of foods purchased away from home tend to be larger than when the same foods are prepared at home (Briefel & Johnson, 2004; Guthrie, Lin, & Frazao, 2002; Young & Nestle, 2003). Moreover, these foods tend to be higher in fat, particularly unhealthy fats such as saturated fat and trans fat. Thus, eating meals prepared away from home appears to promote intake of excessive calories in a pattern that increases risks for chronic disease development.

There are many places where one can purchase food outside the home, including grocery stores, specialty food stores, food courts, and fast food restaurants. Cross sectional studies have observed that children and adolescents who eat at fast food restaurants have worse diets than their peers who do not eat fast food. Bowman and colleagues (Bowman, Gortmaker, Ebbeling, Pereira, & Ludwig, 2004) studied 6,212 children and adolescents who were 4 to 19 years of age and observed that on any given day, approximately 30% of the participants consumed fast food. Adolescents, males, those with higher household income, and non-Hispanic blacks were most likely to consume fast food. After taking into account the demographic differences, children and adolescents who ate fast food consumed significantly greater calories, more soda, fewer fruits and non-starchy vegetables, and significantly less milk. Similar findings were observed by French et al. in a study of 4,746 students in 7th through 12th grade (French, Story, Neumark-Sztainer, Fulkerson, & Hannan, 2001). They observed that not only was consumption of fast food associated with more calories, more soda, and other unhealthy dietary patterns, it was also associated with greater time watching television, greater availability in the home of unhealthy foods, and the perception of fewer concerns by mother or peers about healthy eating. Despite being associated with known and suspected risk factors for obesity, in this cross-sectional analysis, fast food consumption was not associated with being overweight, which highlights the fact that one should be cautious in interpreting associations of risk factors and outcomes in cross-sectional analyses.

However, in longitudinal studies, the consumption of fried foods and other fast foods has been found to prospectively predict greater weight gain among preadolescents, adolescents, and young adults. Among 101 girls who were 8 to 12 years of age at baseline and followed for approximately six years, frequency of eating foods from quick service restaurants, which included fast food restaurants, sandwich shops, and street vendors, was associated with greater weight gain (Thompson et al., 2004). Others have studied slightly different types of patterns of eating food away from home in relationship to weight gain. In the Growing Up Today Study(GUTS), Taveras et al. (Taveras, Berkey et al., 2005) found that at baseline there was a positive association with the frequency of eating fried foods away from home and intake of calories, trans fat, and sugar-sweetened beverage. In prospective analyses, children who increased their consumption of foods fried away from home from less than weekly to 4 to 7 times a week over the one year of follow-up had larger increases in BMI than their peers. Stronger associations were seen by Pereira and colleagues in a 15-year follow-up of young African-American and White adults ages 18 to 30 at enrollment in the Coronary Artery Risk Development in Young Adults (CARDIA) cohort (Pereira et al., 2003). They observed that both baseline frequency of eating fast food and change in frequency of consuming fast food were independently associated with changes in weight among African Americans and whites; the association was stronger among whites.

Although fast food restaurants have been making efforts to offer some healthier food options, many of the food choices and the 'meals' that are promoted are high in caloric content thus, it is not surprising that fast food intake is predictive of greater gains in BMI.

Snack Food and Soda Consumption

There are a variety of reasons that intake of snack foods might promote weight gain, one of which is that snack foods may be consumed in addition to, not instead of, regular meals. However, despite an ecological association between increasing prevalence of pediatric obesity and intake of snack foods over the past two decades (Jahns, Siega-Riz, & Popkin, 2001; Ogden, Flegal, Carroll, & Johnson, 2002) the relation between snack food intake and weight change is not well understood. Francis et al. (Francis, Lee, & Birch, 2003) followed 173 Caucasian girls from age 5 to 9 years. They observed no relationship between intake of snacks and weight gain among children with lean parents; however, among the girls with at least one overweight parent, snack food intake was associated with greater weight gain. Though, in two other longitudinal studies of preadolescents and adolescents no meaningful association between intake of snack food and change in BMI was observed (Field et al., 2004; Phillips et al., 2004). Unlike Francis et al. (Francis, Lee, & Birch, 2003) Field et al. (Field et al., 2004) observed that offspring of overweight mothers gained more weight than their peers, but that there was not an association between snack food intake and weight change among children of lean mothers or overweight mothers. One limitation of all of these studies is that they did not assess snacking patterns, including snacking on items other than "snack foods," such as cereal, smoothies, sandwiches, breakfast foods, or main dishes that contain at least as many calories as many snack food items.

Several recent prospective studies have observed that weight gain was associated with greater intake of sugar-sweetened beverages (Berkey, Rockett, Field, Gillman, & Colditz, 2004; Ebbeling et al., 2006; Ludwig, Peterson, & Gortmaker, 2001; Phillips et al., 2004; Schulze et al., 2004). However, in two of the studies the effect was relatively small (Berkey, Rockett, Field, Gillman, & Colditz, 2004; Phillips et al., 2004). However, even a small effect over time can translate into a meaningful difference, a point that is often forgotten. The lack of strong association between snack food and soda with subsequent weight gain has been misinterpreted by some to mean that these foods and beverages, which are of low nutritional value but may be high in calories, do not need to be targeted as part of obesity prevention efforts. However, overall, total caloric intake is a predictor of weight gain and overconsumption of any type of food or beverage would, therefore, contribute to weight gain. Since there are a variety of healthy food and beverage options that contain more nutrients and minerals for the same or fewer calories per serving, it is prudent to recommend reducing foods and beverages that contain empty calories, such as snack foods and sugar-sweetened beverages, in an effort to reduce total caloric intake and prevent the development of obesity.

Skipping Breakfast

Researchers have begun to investigate whether skipping breakfast is independently associated with obesity. It is estimated that between 12% and 34%

of children and adolescents skip breakfast (Rampersaud, Pereira, Girard, Adams, & Metzl, 2005). Breakfast skipping is more prevalent among adolescents and females, particularly adolescent females and African American females. There are a variety of reasons that people skip breakfast, including lack or time and dieting to lose weight. Breakfast consumption has been associated with better ability to concentrate, higher test grades, and memory but is less well studied in terms of weight gain (Rampersaud, Pereira, Girard, Adams, & Metzl, 2005). In cross-sectional studies it is usually found that children and adolescents who skip breakfast are heavier than their peers; however, due to the cross-sectional nature of these studies it is unclear whether the association is because skipping breakfast leads to gaining more weight or because children who are heavy are skipping breakfast in an effort to lose weight. There are two prospective investigations that have observed that adolescents and young adults who skip breakfast have larger subsequent gains in BMI. In the GUTS, Berkey et al. (2004) observed that among the overweight participants, those who skipped breakfast experienced larger gains in BMI over the following two 1-year periods. In the CARDIA study, a prospective cohort study of African Americans and Whites who were 18–30 when the study began, independent of baseline BMI, white young adults who skipped breakfast were significantly more likely than their peers to become overweight. The relationship was weaker and not significant among the African Americans. In the National Heart, Lung, and Blood National Growth and Health Study (NGHS), a 10-year prospective study of African American and white girls who were enrolled at ages 9–10, as the girls aged, the frequency of eating breakfast declined over time. Independent of BMI, girls who ate breakfast had lower BMIs, but the association was attenuated and no longer significant after parental education, energy intake, and physical activity were adjusted for in the statistical model (Barton et al., 2005). It is unclear whether the results in the NGHS study varied by weight status as was seen in GUTS. At a minimum, it appears that consuming breakfast is associated with better dietary patterns and may protect against excessive weight gain in some sub-groups.

Dietary Composition

Weight gain is a function of energy intake exceeding energy expenditure, thus total caloric intake is a predictor of obesity. However, the role of specific macronutrients, food groups, and specific foods in the development of obesity is controversial. Although obesity prevention interventions have included efforts to increase servings per day of fruits and vegetables (Gortmaker, Cheung et al., 1999; Gortmaker, Peterson et al., 1999) decrease intake of dietary fat (Baranowski et al., 2003; Beech et al., 2003; Gortmaker, Cheung et al., 1999; Himes et al., 2003; Nader et al., 1999; Robinson et al., 2003; Rochon et al., 2003; Story et al., 2003) and decrease soda intake (Baranowski et al., 2003; Beech et al., 2003; Rochon et al., 2003; Story et al., 2003) it is not clear whether these diet changes are effective at preventing weight gain.

Fiber, Fruits, and Vegetables
Diets rich in fiber or fruits and vegetables are associated with a decreased risk of many chronic diseases (Rimm et al., 1996; Willett, 1994). The association

of fiber, fruit, and vegetable intake to weight gain is not well understood. Despite a lack of data, several obesity-prevention interventions have included efforts to increase the consumption of fruits and vegetables in the hope that these foods will replace more energy dense food choices popular among children and adolescents (Baranowski et al., 2003; Beech et al., 2003; Gortmaker, Cheung et al., 1999; Gortmaker, Peterson et al., 1999; Story et al., 2003) but the interventions were either too small (Baranowski et al., 2003; Beech et al., 2003; Story et al., 2003) or contained a variety of lifestyle modifications (Gortmaker, Cheung et al., 1999; Gortmaker, Peterson et al., 1999). Thus, they were unable to identify a beneficial impact on body weight of increasing fruit and vegetable intake. Many fruits and vegetables are high in dietary fiber, which among adults is associated with less weight gain (Howarth, Huang, Roberts, & McCrory, 2005; Koh-Banerjee et al., 2004; Liu et al., 2003) but the results in children are equivocal. Among the 6,149 girls and 4,620 boys in GUTS, no association was observed between fiber intake and weight gain (Berkey et al., 2000) In the CARDIA study, fiber intake was protective against weight gain among the African American and white young adults and adults (Ludwig, Pereira et al., 1999). It is possible that the discrepancy in results reflects the much larger BMI gains in CARDIA than those seen in GUTS (Berkey et al., 2000; Lewis et al., 2000). Alternatively, the older age of the CARDIA participants means that it is easier to distinguish excessive weight gain from weight gain due to physical development, which should be close to zero among the 18–30 year old participants, thus associations between dietary intake and weight gain should be easier to observe in CARDIA than GUTS. More research is needed to better understand whether increasing fiber intake protects against excessive weight gain.

Among children and adolescents, fruit juice may account for a non-trivial proportion of total fruit intake. Although consumption of fruits and vegetables has been promoted at all ages, there has been a concern that high intake of fruit juice could promote the development of obesity; however, the results have not been consistent across studies (Dennison, Rockwell, & Baker, 1997; Skinner, Carruth, Moran, Houck, & Coletta, 1999). In a three year follow-up of 8,203 girls and 6,715 boys in the Growing Up Today Study, vegetable intake had a weak inverse association with changes in BMI z-score among the boys, but there was no association among the girls (Field, Gillman, Rosner, Rockett, & Colditz, 2003). The lack of a strong effect could be due children and adolescents consuming fruits and vegetables in addition to rather than instead of unhealthy snack foods or other calorie dense foods. Although several randomized trials have included a component focusing on increasing fruit and vegetable consumption, they have also included a variety of other lifestyle changes. It is, therefore, impossible to isolate a specific association between fruit and vegetable intake and weight change. Also, only one of these interventions (Gortmaker, Peterson et al., 1999) found a significant effect on weight at follow-up. Taken together the available evidence suggests that promoting fruits and vegetables specifically for obesity prevention may not be effective unless clearly adopted as a *substitute* for more energy dense foods.

Dietary Fat

The role of dietary fat in weight gain has been widely studied, but remains highly controversial (Pirozzo, Summerbell, Cameron, & Glasziou, 2003;

Willett & Leibel, 2002). On one hand, dietary fat intake has been targeted as a possible cause of obesity because it is more energy-dense per gram than protein or carbohydrate. Moreover, foods that are high in fat tend to be very palatable, and therefore people may consume them in large quantities, thus ingesting a large number of calories. Nevertheless, the results are far from conclusive. In the CARDIA study of young adults dietary fat intake predicted greater weight gain (Lewis et al., 1997); whereas, in the Growing Up Today Study, dietary fat was not related to weight gain (Berkey et al., 2000).

Calcium

The role of calcium intake in weight regulation is also controversial. Neither Philips (Phillips et al., 2003) in a small prospective study nor Berkey (Berkey, Rockett, Willett, & Colditz, 2005) in a large prospective cohort observed an association between dairy food or calcium intake and weight gain. Moreover, among 59 girls in a dietary calcium intervention, Lappe et al. (Lappe, Rafferty, Davies, & Lypaczewski, 2004) did not observe a difference in weight or body fat gain between the high-calcium diet group and the usual diet group. Similarly, in a one-year dietary calcium intervention among 155 young adult women, there were no differences in change in fat mass between controls, medium (to achieve 1,000–1,100 mg/day), and high dairy (to achieve 1,300–1,400 mg/day) groups (Gunther et al., 2005). However, Skinner et al. (Skinner, Bounds, Carruth, & Ziegler, 2003) prospectively studied 52 8-year old white children and their mothers and found that dietary calcium was inversely related to percent of body fat, as measured by DEXA. In other prospective studies of pre-school students (Carruth & Skinner, 2001) and young adult women (Lin et al., 2000) calcium was also observed to have an inverse association with change in body fat. It is unclear why the results are so inconsistent. Until the relationship is better understood it would be prudent to continue promoting calcium for bone health, but not necessarily as an obesity prevention method.

Glycemic Index

Another highly debated area is the role of glycemic index or glycemic load in weight gain. Glycemic index is a property of carbohydrate-containing food that describes the increase in blood glucose after a meal. Foods that are digested and absorbed rapidly, such as potatoes and refined grains, have a high glycemic index (Foster-Powell & Miller, 1995; Wolever, Jenkins, Jenkins, & Josse, 1991). In controlled studies oral administration of glucose or foods with a high glycemic index produce rapid elevations in blood glucose and insulin levels, which are followed in many individuals by a period of reactive hypoglycemia with continued modest elevation in insulin levels. This situation results in hunger and increased food intake (Campfield, Smith, Rosenbaum, & Hirsch, 1996) possibly leading to cycles of hypoglycemia and hyperphagia. Results of a cross-over feeding study of 12 obese teenage boys are consistent with the idea that intake of high glycemic foods may promote hunger and increase food intake, which could lead to greater weight gain (Ludwig, Majzoub et al., 1999). Moreover, Ebbeling and colleagues reported that a low glycemic load diet was more effective than an energy-restricted lowfat diet in treating 14 obese youth in a randomized trial. However, in a more recent trial of 23 young adults in a 12-month intervention (Ebbeling et al., 2005) patients in the low glycemic load arm lost a similar amount of weight (8.4%) as those in the energy-restricted lowfat diet arm (7.8%) and both groups remained below their baseline weight when followed one year later. No association was seen between glycemic index or load and weight change among the 6,149 female and 4,620 male preadolescents and adolescents in the Growing Up Today Study (Berkey et al., 2000).

There may not be enough studies on this topic among preadolescents and adolescents to reach any firm conclusions. However, there are at least several possible explanations for the discrepancies in results across studies. It is possible that a reduced glycemic load diet is more important for weight loss and weight loss maintenance than prevention of weight gain and the development of obesity. Alternatively, it may be that the benefit can only be seen among heavier participants, particularly overweight participants who adhere strictly to the diet. It is also possible that the beneficial effect of a low glycemic is relatively small and thus in studies that use food frequency questionnaires, the measurement error in the diet assessment obscures the true association. More studies are needed to better understand the role of glycemic index and load in relation to weight gain and the development of obesity.

The conclusions that can be supported by the available data on how these potentially modifiable variables relate to obesity prevention are summarized in Table 20.1. These conclusions are specific for obesity prevention, however, and should not necessarily be applied to questions of whether modifications in these variables should be targeted to improve other health or social outcomes.

Table 20.1 Summary of associations of dietary behaviors and nutrient intakes with obesity prevention during pre-adolescence and adolescence.

	Obesity prevention	Other health effects
Food purchased away from home, particularly fried foods	Associated with poor diet quality and greater weight gain in one cohort study, but not another	
Snack foods and soda	Add empty and perhaps excessive calories, but the results are inconsistent as to whether they make a preadolescent or adolescent gain more weight	Associated with increase risk of diabetes among adults
Skipping breakfast	Associated with weight gain	May be a marker for unhealthy weight concerns and weight control behaviors
Fiber, fruit, and vegetable intake	Results of fiber being protective against weight gain are inconclusive. Fruit and vegetable intake not strongly associated with weight change	Decreased risk of certain cancers among adults
Dietary fat intake	Results of dietary fat promoting weightgain are inconclusive.	Trans and saturated fat increase risk for cardiovascular disease (CVD) among adults; monounsaturated fats have CVD benefits
Calcium intake	No association	Possible benefit on bone health
Glycemic index	Inconsistent findings related to prevention, although decreases in consumption of high glycemic index foods have been associated with more weight loss	Inversely associated with diabetes in adults

Body Dissatisfaction and Dieting

Although the prevalence of overweight and obesity are increasing, the desire to be thin or to have well defined or toned muscles is still very wide spread. Weight concerns and dieting are less common among males than females (Field, Colditz, & Peterson, 1997; French, Story, Downes, Resnick, & Blum, 1995); however, recent data suggest that these concerns are becoming more prevalent (Braun, Sunday, Huang, & Halmi, 1999). Body shape concerns of males may be slightly different from those of females. Among females, weight dissatisfaction increases with relative weight, but among males the relationship is more complicated (Neumark-Sztainer, Story, Hannan, Perry, & Irving, 2002). For both males and females it is undesirable to be overweight, but for males it is also undesirable to be too lean or not sufficiently muscular (Labre, 2002; Neumark-Sztainer et al., 2002).

Most of the research on body dissatisfaction has focused on a desire to be thin and the unhealthy methods people, mainly females, use to achieve that goal. (Boutelle, Neumark-Sztainer, Story, & Resnick, 2002; Field, Camargo, Taylor, Berkey, Frazier et al., 1999). The prevalence of a desire to be more muscular and correlates of using unhealthy methods to increase muscle mass or definition are less well studied (McCabe & Ricciardelli, 2001). Data on the association of using protein powder, creatine, dehydroepiandrosterone (DHEA), steroids, or other supplements and pro-hormones with dietary intake and weight change are not readily available.

Among preadolescents and adolescents, those who are dieting or using other methods to lose weight report engaging in more physical activity (Field, Austin et al., 2003; Lowry, Galuska, Fulton, Wechsler, & Kann, 2002) and smoking (Lowry et al., 2002). The association of weight control efforts and dietary intake appears to depend on whether the weight control method is healthy or unhealthy. In the Growing Up Today Study, dieters reported consuming fewer snack foods, a lower percentage of energy from fat, a higher percentage of energy from carbohydrate and more caffeine (Field, Austin et al., 2003). However, among the 4,144 middle and high school students in Project Eat, Neumark-Sztainer et al. observed that adolescent girls who engaged in unhealthy weight control strategies had lower intakes of fruits, vegetables, and calcium than their peers who were not using healthy or unhealthy weight control behaviors (Neumark-Sztainer, Hannan, Story, & Perry, 2004). Unhealthy weight control behaviors do not appear to protect against weight gain among adult women (Field, Manson, Taylor, Willett, & Colditz, 2004).

Paradoxically, dieting has been observed to predict greater subsequent BMI increases among preadolescent and adolescent girls and boys (Field, Austin et al., 2003; Stice, Cameron, Killen, Hayward, & Taylor, 1999). The concept of dieting implies a relatively short-term change in dietary intake versus a more permanent lifestyle change. Since drastic changes in dietary intake are rarely sustainable, it is not surprising that self-described dieting does not protect against weight gain. It is likely that some dieters may alternate between periods of restrictive eating and periods of overeating that more than negate any positive effect of the periods of reduced intake. In other words, people—including preadolescents and adolescents who are unhappy with their weight may be willing and able to make at least short term changes in dietary intake, but either they are self-selecting ineffective diets and/or are unable to make long-term beneficial changes in dietary intake.

Physical Activity and Inactivity

By definition, activity is related to weight gain since change in weight reflects energy intake not being in equilibrium with energy output. However, demonstrating this association in a way that provides guidance for obesity prevention is difficult. The literature on the association between physical activity and weight change is equivocal. Some studies have found an inverse association between activity level and subsequent weight change (Kimm et al., 2005; Schmitz, Jacobs, Leon, Schreiner, & Sternfeld, 2000) while others have not (Nader et al., 1999; Story et al., 2003). Some studies have found that activity is protective against weight gain only among females (Berkey et al., 2000; Kettaneh et al., 2005) while other studies have seen the protective effect only among males (Gordon-Larsen, Adair, & Popkin, 2002). There is some evidence that increasing activity is associated with decreased adiposity among overweight children but is less effective in preventing weight gain among leaner children and adolescents (Strong et al., 2005). Some of the discrepancies in the literature may be due to error in activity assessments or measurement error in the outcome. It is also possible that failure to control for *inactivity*, (i.e., extent of sedentary behavior), in some studies may contribute to the discrepancies in the findings.

Most studies of the relationship between activity and weight or fatness use BMI as the outcome measure; however, one cross-sectional population study of 2,714 12-year old students in France, Klein-Platat et al. (2005) used waist circumference instead of BMI as their measure of fatness. They observed that independent of BMI, structured activity was inversely related to waist circumference in both males and females. However, causality cannot be inferred due to the cross-sectional design. Gordon-Larsen and colleagues (Gordon-Larsen et al., 2002) conducted a quasi-prospective study using the National Longitudinal Study of Adolescent Health (Add Health). They assessed whether baseline activity levels and change in activity levels predicted overweight status at follow-up, but did not control for baseline BMI or weight status; hence it is unclear whether the association was due to baseline weight or changes in overweight status. They found that among the 12,759 adolescent girls and boys, the level of moderate to vigorous activity at baseline was protective against obesity at follow-up and that among the boys, but not the girls, increases in moderate to vigorous activity also decreased the odds of being obese at follow-up.

The results from prospective studies are more consistent for females than males. In the NGHS, a prospective cohort study of 1,152 black and 1,135 white girls, both body mass index and skinfold thickness were used as outcomes, the latter being a measure of fatness. During 10-years of follow-up of participants in the NGHS there was a dramatic decrease in activity and increase in the prevalence of obesity (Kimm, Barton et al., 2002; Kimm, Glynn et al., 2002). Declines in activity were associated with increased subsequent weight gain and sum of skinfold thickness among both white and back girls who were studied from ages 9–10 to ages 18–19. At the end of follow-up active girls were almost 2–3 BMI units lighter than their inactive peers (Kimm et al., 2005). Among 6,149 girls and 4,620 boys in the Growing Up Today Study, low level of activity predicted larger BMI changes among the girls, but there was no association among the boys.

At least two reasons come to mind for the lack of an association among the males First, activity may only be protective against weight gain if it is coupled with decreases in caloric intake. Second, activity may lead to loss of fat mass, but increases in muscle mass, and BMI does not distinguish between the two. The results from several studies that used both BMI and skinfold thicknesses or waist circumference, suggest that the inability of BMI to distinguish between lean and fat mass may make BMI too insensitive to use when studying the benefits of activity, at least among males.

Large prospective studies of adolescent males and females with measures of activity, inactivity, dietary intake and fatness, such as skinfolds or circumferences, as well as BMI, are needed to better understand the relationship between activity and adiposity, but these are scarce. In one such study, involving 222 boys and 214 girls in Northern France, Kettaneh et al. (Kettaneh et al., 2005) found that at baseline activity level was not related to BMI in boys or girls. However, during two years of follow-up, girls who decreased their level of moderate activity had the largest increases in BMI, percent body fat, skinfolds, and waist circumference. Among the boys, changes in moderate activity were not related to changes in BMI, but boys who increased their vigorous activity had the lowest skinfold thickness and those who decreased their vigorous activity had the highest. Among 2,834 males and 2,872 females from Finland who were assessed at age 14 and followed up when they were 31 years of age, both baseline activity and change in activity levels were independently associated with being overweight or obese (based on BMI) or having abdominal obesity at age 31 (Tammelin, Laitinen, & Nayha, 2004). Compared to their same sex peers who were active at baseline and follow-up, those who became inactive were significantly more likely to develop severe abdominal obesity. In addition, among both males and females, there was a suggestion that compared to their peers who remained active, those who became inactive were more likely to become obese adults. Among the females, but not the males, there was a suggestion that those who remained inactive were more likely than those who remained active to become obese by age 31 years.

Physical activity is notoriously difficult to measure precisely. Many self-report instruments do an adequate job at ranking subjects, but cannot precisely estimate energy expenditure. This is particularly relevant for understanding the relationship of activity and weight gain since the relevant variable is the amount of activity or energy expended through activity for a given caloric intake. Further complicating the situation is that many studies use BMI or change in BMI as the outcome measure. As previously noted, BMI does not distinguish fat mass from lean mass. It is, therefore, possible that activity decreases fat mass, but increases lean mass, so the adolescent maintains his or her BMI, but lowers his or her risk of becoming obese and developing obesity-related adverse health consequences.

Identifying Opportunities for Prevention

Parents, peers, the school environment, and the media all should play a role in the prevention of obesity. Potentially modifiable variables in each of these environments are reviewed in this section. One of the possible reasons that obesity prevention interventions have not been more successful is that they have intervened on at most two or three of these influences, but not all four.

Parental Influences

As young people become more independent they make more of their own choices about whether to participate in sports, when and what they want to eat and drink, and they may become more conscious of their weight and as a result adopt behaviors to change their weight or shape. Unlike young children who may want to adopt the behaviors that will please their parents, some adolescents may be more interested in adopting behaviors that their peers will approve of and have less interest in complying with their parents' suggestions. However, parental influences are still important at this age, particularly for preadolescents and adolescents living at home.

Eating Behavior

Parents have a major influence on home food availability and they are also both implicit and explicit role models. Parents are more likely than their children to buy and prepare food. Thus they play a key role in promoting healthy or unhealthy dietary patterns. Parental modeling of eating patterns includes what parents eat as well as which foods they purchase and keep in the home. In a study 902 adolescents and their parents and/or caregivers, Hanson et al. (Hanson, Neumark-Sztainer, Eisenberg, Story, & Wall, 2005) found that although 90% of parents/caregivers reported that fruits and vegetables were available at home, many of the parent/caregivers were not consuming the recommended number of servings of fruits and vegetables. Thus they were only partially modeling healthy dietary practices. Moreover, in over half of the homes, soft drinks were usually available. Overall, parental intake was more related to their daughter's intake than their son's intake. Among the girls, parental intake was a significant predictor of dairy, fruits, and vegetables. In contrast, parental reports of fruit and vegetable intake were unrelated to the boys' intakes.

A study of 3,957 adolescents in Minnesota underscored the importance of availability of fruits and vegetables in the home. Neumark-Sztainer et al. (Neumark-Sztainer, Wall, Perry, & Story, 2003) found that if there was low availability of fruits and vegetables in the home, intake patterns were low regardless of how much the adolescents liked or disliked the taste of fruits and vegetables. However, if availability was high, even adolescents who did not like the taste consumed more fruits and vegetables than their peers in home with low availability. Unfortunately in many economically disadvantaged communities there are few large supermarkets (Chung & Myers, 1999). In such cases, fruits and vegetables may be unavailable or too expensive for parents and caregivers to purchase in sufficient quantities.

Another possible mechanism through which parents may influence the eating patterns of their children is through encouraging the family to eat together. A variety of benefits have been associated with eating meals with family, such as having a lower likelihood of using tobacco, alcohol, and marijuana (Eisenberg, Olson, Neumark-Sztainer, Story, & Bearinger, 2004), and obesity prevention may be another. In cross-sectional studies, eating family meals is associated with following healthier dietary practices. In a cross-sectional analysis of 7,784 girls and 6,647 boy in the Growing Up Today Study (GUTS), a prospective cohort study, Gillman et al. (Gillman et al., 2000) observed that 17% of participants rarely ate dinner with their family, 40% ate with them on most days, and 43% ate with family members daily. Compared to adolescents, preadolescents ate dinner more frequently with their family. Independent of age and gender, children who frequently ate dinner with their family were significantly more likely to eat at least 5 servings per day of fruits and vegetables and were significantly less likely to drink soda or eat any fried foods away from home.

A similar positive association between frequency of eating family meals and dietary patterns was seen among 4,746 adolescents in Project EAT (Eating Among Teens). Neumark-Sztainer et al. found that frequency of family meals was positively associated with intake of fruits and vegetables and inversely associated with soft drink consumption (Neumark-Sztainer, Hannan, Story, Croll, & Perry, 2003). In addition, they found that being male, in middle-school, having a mother who was not working, and being high socioeconomic status (SES) were all related to frequency of consuming family meals. The SES findings are particularly noteworthy. Among whites and Hispanics, high SES is inversely related to obesity (Gordon-Larsen, Adair, & Popkin, 2003) thus it is possible that family meals is one mechanism through which high SES individuals decrease their risk of becoming overweight or obese. However, it is also possible that family dinner might appear to be associated with healthy eating patterns because it is a proxy for high SES. Cross-sectional studies are not sufficient for testing directionality of associations or exploring mechanisms, but in cross-sectional comparisons it appeared that family meals were associated with healthy diet patterns that should confer protection against the development of overweight.

The longitudinal data on eating family meals and subsequent weight change are limited and inconclusive. In the GUTS cohort, Taveras et al. (Taveras, Rifas-Shiman et al., 2005) observed that the more frequently a child ate dinner with their family, the less likely he/she was to be overweight at baseline. However, the frequency of eating dinner with their family was not related to whether the child became overweight during the subsequent year. The lack of prospective association has at least two possible explanations. Some children may not be eating dinner with their family because they are in sports practice, in which case their level of activity would be more protective against the development of obesity than any effects associated with family dinner. Another possible explanation is that not all family dinners are healthy or modest in portion size. Since obesity is known to cluster in families due to a combination of genetic and environmental influences, it is possible that in families with overweight parents, family dinner may be characterized by excessive calories and therefore not protective against excessive weight gain.

Physical Activity

Parents may influence their children's activity levels by modeling the behavior (i.e., being active themselves), encouraging their child to be active, and providing logistical support (i.e., driving the child to a playing field) (Hoefer, McKenzie, Sallis, Marshall, & Conway, 2001; Sallis, Prochaska, & Taylor, 2000; Trost et al., 2003). Unfortunately there are limited prospective data on this topic; most of the studies have been cross-sectional. In a multiethnic sample of 900 adolescent girls and boys, McGuire observed that parental encouragement (as reported by the parent) was positively related to physical activity among girls of all racial/ethnic groups and among white boys and black boys (McGuire, Hannan, Neumark-Sztainer, Cossrow, & Story, 2002). Moreover, there was a modest, but significant, association between the physical activity attitudes and behaviors of the adolescents and those of their parents. A stronger association between activity levels of adolescents and those of their parents was observed in a study of 3,000 12-year old students in France. Wagner et al. (Wagner et al., 2004) found that compared to children of inactive parents, girls and boys whose parents were both active were at least 50% more likely to participate in structured physical activity outside of school. It also appears that parents have a lasting influence. In a study of 947 college students and their parents who were followed for three years, prior parental influences were evident in the physical activity and other health-related behaviors of their children while at college (Lau, Quadrel, & Hartman, 1990) which suggests that parents who value activity pass along that value to their children. Taken together the results support an important role parents have in promoting activity among their children.

Given the low levels of activity among adults in the United States, it is possible that the magnitude of the possible influence of parental activity on offspring is being underestimated due to few studies having sufficient numbers of active parents. Moreover, data are lacking on whether the activity level and beliefs about activity of mothers and fathers are equally important for male and female offspring. It does appear, however, that it may be difficult for parents to motivate their preadolescent and adolescent offspring sufficiently to become more active. Fulkerson et al. (Fulkerson et al., 2004) assessed 295 preadolescent girls and their mothers and observed that although the overweight girls were more likely than non-overweight girls to report that their friends and guardians thought they should exercise more, they engaged in less activity. Overweight and non-overweight girls did not differ in terms of having the time or the logistical support to be active, but compared to their leaner peers, overweight girls more often reported liking activity less, not being good at it, and preferring to do other things. Thus, to promote activity parents may need to do more than offer support, they should try to be role models by being active themselves and they should work with their preadolescent or adolescent child to find an activity that he or she enjoys, as well as an environment in which the child feels confident to engage in activity.

Inactivity

Just as parents may help to promote activity through their beliefs, behaviors, and support, they may also inadvertently promote unhealthy lifestyle choices that increase the risk of their child becoming overweight or obese. At least 67% of preadolescents and adolescents live in a home with three or more televisions and approximately 68% have a television in their bedroom (Robert, Foehr, & Rideout, 2005). Among preadolescents, having a television in the bedroom is associated with greater time spent watching television (Wiecha, Sobol, Peterson, & Gortmaker, 2001). Some, but not all, studies have observed that having a television in the bedroom is associated with being overweight (Dennison, Erb, & Jenkins, 2002; Saelens et al., 2002).

The number and placement of televisions in the house is not the only way that parents inadvertently promote inactivity. Davison et al. (Davison, Francis, & Birch, 2005) found that among 173 white girls and their parents, girls whose parents watched a considerable amount of television watched significantly more TV than their peers and their parents were less likely to have limits placed on their access to television. Given that most Americans spend more time watching television than engaging in physical activity (*50th Anniversary of 'Wonderful World of Color' TV*, 2004; Crespo, Keteyian, Heath, & Sempos, 1996; Crespo, Smit, Andersen, Carter-Pokras, & Ainsworth, 2000) it is possible that modeling of parental behaviors is doing more to promote rather than prevent obesity among preadolescents and adolescents.

Peer Influences

During preadolescence and adolescence, acceptance by peers is highly valued. To gain this acceptance, adolescents may adopt the perceived beliefs and behaviors practiced by members of their peer group (Epstein, Botvin, & Diaz, 1999; Paxton, Schutz, Wertheim, & Muir, 1999; Sieving, Perry, & Williams, 2000; West, Sweeting, & Ecob, 1999). Although peer influences are predictors of initiation of some unhealthy behaviors (Epstein et al., 1999; Field, Camargo, Taylor, Berkey, & Colditz, 1999; McCabe, Ricciardelli, & Finemore, 2002; Paxton et al., 1999; West et al., 1999) some studies have explored the possibility of using peer-based interaction and social pressure to make a positive impact on health and risk behavior (Komro et al., 1996; Reisberg, 2000; Sciacca & Appleton, 1996). Individual values change in relation to peer-group norms and values (Pugh & Hart, 1999), thus it is likely that peers play an important role in determining diet and activity patterns of adolescents. However, only a limited number of studies have assessed peer influences on diet and activity patterns have not been studied extensively (Brown, Frankel, & Fennell, 1989; French et al., 2001; Lau et al., 1990).

Several interventions have explored using peer role models to promote consumption of fruits and vegetables in children of various ages. Lowe et al. (Lowe, Horne, Tapper, Bowdery, & Egerton, 2004) conducted a short-term intervention with 402 children who were 4 to 11 years of age. Children watched 6 videos with heroic peers (two boys and two girls who were 12–13 years of age) in them who enjoyed eating fruits and vegetables. The combination of watching the videos and receiving a small reward for consuming fruits and vegetables lead to a significant increase in consumption during the 16-day intervention on weekdays but not weekend days. The results were similar for the children who were ages 4 to 7 (2.5 portion increase) and those who were ages 7 to 11 (2.2 portion increase) years of age. The authors suggest that the lack of effect on weekend days was due to most of the intervention being delivered during the week; thus there were insufficient cues to change consumption during the weekend. Although the results are intriguing, the length of the trial was too short to address whether the changes were sustained. More promising results on the importance of peer modeling come from the Teens Eating for Energy and Nutrition at School (TEENS) intervention, which had a school environment interventions arm, a classroom plus school environment interventions arm, and a peer leaders plus a classroom and school environment interventions arm. Birnbaum et al. (Birnbaum, Lytle, Story, Perry, & Murray, 2002) found that children in the peer leaders plus classroom and school environment interventions arm made the largest positive changes in dietary intake. These results suggest that interventions to promote healthy dietary patterns would be wise to involve peers as role models and promoters of the intervention.

Social norms may be an important and understudied determinant of lifestyle related to obesity prevention. A growing body of literature suggests that social norms influence dieting and unhealthy weight control behaviors of teens. In a large study of students in 31 schools in Minnesota, Eisenberg and colleagues (Eisenberg, Neumark-Sztainer, Story, & Perry, 2005) found that among normal weight girls, friends' dieting behaviors were significantly related to a girl's use of unhealthy weight control behaviors. The relationship was not seen among underweight or overweight girls, thus suggesting that peer influences may vary by weight status, age, and other demographic factors.

Even less well studied is the role peer influences have in the decline in activity as girls progress through preadolescence and adolescence (Kimm, Glynn et al., 2002). As mentioned previously, girls progressing through preadolescence and adolescence tend to become more aware of their appearance and may become less inclined to participate in activities that could damage their hairstyles, make-up, or nails. These concerns are reported by physical education teachers, but have not been studied in qualitative or quantitative studies. Thus it is unclear how prevalent these concerns are and what impact they have on the decline in physical activity among girls. Not all peer influences are necessarily negative, however. Friends may also support health promoting behaviors. Among 354 girls who were 8–11 years of age, those whose friends and family supported exercise were more likely than their peers to engage in weight bearing physical activity (Ievers-Landis et al., 2003). This suggests that to successfully promote activity and prevent obesity among preadolescent and adolescent females, one should include a component that seeks to change peer norms to support and value being active and eating a healthy diet. However, much more research is needed to better understand the association of peer norms and influences on diet and activity patterns of preadolescent and adolescent boys.

School Environment

Preadolescents and adolescents spend a large part of their day in school, thus the school environment may play an extremely important role in promoting or preventing obesity. One of the most obviously school-based influences is food options made available to students. As one method to generate additional revenue in an era of tight funding, many schools have vending machines and/or contracts with soft drink companies and fast food vendors. The U.S. national School Health Policies and Programs Study 2000 estimated that 83% of middle schools and 94% of high schools have vending machines, a school store, or snack bar where young people can purchase foods of low nutritional value (Wechsler, Brener, Kuester, & Miller, 2001). Even more troubling is the trend in schools signing pouring rights contracts that give companies the rights to sell sugar-sweetened beverages, such as soda, as well as the right to advertise their product in the school. In the United States approximately 50% of junior high schools and 72% of high schools have such contracts (Wechsler et al., 2001). These contracts can generate considerable income since they frequently involve receiving a percentage of the sales revenue. Approximately 41% of middle schools and 57% of high schools with soft drink contracts receive incentives if certain sales goals are met (Wechsler et al., 2001). However, recently despite the lure of additional funds, some large school districts which are concerned about the widespread problem of obesity among youth have declined to sign pouring rights contracts and have moved to no longer sell soft drinks in the schools (Fried & Nestle, 2002).

Although there have been efforts to improve the federally-funded lunch programs in schools, those improvements are unlikely to have a meaningful impact on the weight status of youth if schools continue to offer fast food, sugar-sweetened beverages, and snack foods. It is estimated that approximately 20% of high schools in the United States offer Pizza Hut, Taco Bell, or other fast food brands (Wechsler et al., 2001). Not only do these fast food vendors potentially offer high calorie food options, but, as with the soft drink vendors, they may be allowed to advertise in the schools. Additional advertisements for food products of questionable nutritional value may be seen by children whose schools are connected to Channel One (Story & French, 2004). Channel One is a commercial public-affairs program designed for adolescents that includes ten minutes of news and two minutes of public service announcements or paid advertising. It is shown each in 350,000 classrooms throughout the United States (E. W. Austin, Chen, Pinkleton, & Quintero Johnson, 2006). In one study evaluating the advertisements on Channel One, it was found that 70% of the 45 food commercials shown were for fast food, soft drinks, and snack foods, all of which would be considered foods of questionable nutritional value.

There is considerable variability in the access to soda, snack foods, and fast foods in and around schools. Some schools turn off vending machines during the day, others do not. Likewise, some schools allow students to leave the school during lunchtime, others do not. Neumark-Sztainer et al. (2005) randomly sampled 1,088 high school students from 20 high schools in Minnesota and found that students in high schools with open campuses during lunch were significantly more likely than their peers at schools with closed campuses to eat fast food. Whereas, students attending schools that turned off soda machines during lunch time bought significantly fewer soft drinks than their peers in schools that did not turn off machines (Neumark-Sztainer, French, Hannan, Story, & Fulkerson, 2005). In the Chicago area, 78% of schools had at least one fast food restaurant within half a mile (Austin et al., 2005), which makes it understandable that an open campus policy would be associated with fast food intake. The fact that fast food vendors are allowed in schools and fast food restaurants are located near schools highlights the reason that there is considerable interest in fast food as a source of excess calories in the diets of young people.

At the same time that schools are offering more calories than ever, physical education classes and after-school programs are being scaled back. The School Health Policies and Programs Study in 2000 found that only 6% of middle schools and high schools provide daily physical activity for all students throughout the school year and rates of mandatory physical education class drop off steadily by grade level starting around 6th grade (Wechsler et al., 2001). Moreover, according to the Youth Risk Behavior Survey, the percentage of high school girls who attend physical education class daily decreased from 37% in 1991 to 26% in 2003. The decline was even larger for the males among whom daily physical education dropped from 46% in 1991 to 31% in 2003 (Lowry et al., 2004). Thus the current school environment may be one of the important contributors to the growing obesity epidemic among children and adolescents in the United States. In order to prevent excessive weight gain and the development of obesity, schools need to refrain from offering food and beverage choices of questionable nutritional value and high energy density, minimize the opportunities for students to buy fast food, snack foods, and soda on and off the school campus, and require more activity during or after school in order to promote energy balance among their students.

Media Use

Recent estimates are that preadolescents and adolescents watch approximately 3 hours per day of television (Robert et al., 2005). This high level of media consumption means that preadolescents and adolescents are potentially exposed to 40,000 television advertisements per year (Robert et al., 2005). Harrison and Marske observed that there was an average of 10.65 food advertisements per hour and that 36% of food advertisements on television were for candy, sweets, and soft drinks and 46.5% were for convenience foods (Harrison & Marske, 2005). Thus, the average 8–18 year old child who watches 3 hours per day of television would view 11,000 food advertisements per year and the most of these advertisements would be for foods or beverages that may promote weight gain.

Time spent watching television is a robust predictor of weight gain and obesity in both observational studies (Berkey et al., 2000; Gortmaker et al., 1996) and randomized clinical trials (Gortmaker, Peterson et al., 1999; Robinson, 1999). Moreover, clinical trials that have targeted reducing time spent watching television have observed significant reductions in obesity (Robinson, 1999; Robinson et al., 2003). Thus, limiting the number of hours preadolescents and adolescents spend watching television should help to prevent excessive weight gain and the development of obesity. Several studies have found that television-viewing patterns are related to dietary intake patterns. A national survey of approximately 2,000 children and adolescents found that 65% of preadolescents and adolescents reported that the television was on during mealtimes in their house (Robert, Foehr, Rideout, & Brodie, 1999) and a study of ten year French Canadian children observed that approximately 18% of the girls and 25% of the boys reported that they ate while watching television seven days a week. In a smaller American study, 36% of dinners and 67% of snacks during the week were consumed in front of the television (Matheson, Killen, Wang, Varady, & Robinson, 2004). The cross-sectional associations did not, however, reveal a clear pattern between eating while watching television and body mass index. In a prospective analysis of changes in television and changes in foods commonly advertised on television among 9,263 preadolescents and adolescents in the Growing Up Today Study, Gortmaker and colleagues (personal communication) observed that for each one hour increase in television viewing over the one year follow-up period, children increased their daily energy intake by approximately 50 calories and those who increased their viewing time by 2 hours increased their intake by 100 calories per day. Thus it appears that one mechanism through which television viewing promotes weight gain and obesity is through promoting increased caloric intake. Other mechanisms related to physical inactivity were discussed previously.

Table 20.2 summarizes conclusions about how elements of role modeling, policy change, and education about nutrition and physical activity and inactivity intersect with parental, peers, and school environment variables as components of obesity prevention interventions. Many of these components are discussed in detail in the Institute of Medicine Report on childhood obesity prevention (Koplan et al., 2005). Schools as settings for obesity prevention interventions are discussed in Chapter 16.

Summary and Implications

Preadolescence and adolescence are important periods to target for obesity prevention efforts. During puberty, which most often occurs during preadolescence for females and adolescence for males, females experience a growth spurt and an increase in body fat, as well as lean mass. Among males, the growth spurt occurs later, during adolescence, and is associated with increases in lean mass, but decreases in fat mass (Rico et al., 1993). Some weight change is a normal and healthy part of preadolescence and adolescence. However, for an increasing

Table 20.2 Summary of components to include in interventions to prevent obesity and recommendations to parents regarding managing their child's weight change.

	Parents	Peers	Schools
Role modeling	1. Limit having sugar-sweetened beverages and calorie dense foods at home 2. Regularly engage in activity 3. Buy less prepared foods and eat out less often	1. Encourage adolescents to become role models for their peers and younger students and siblings instead of following what others eat or do	1. Do not have nutritionally questionable foods in the school lunch room
Policy	1. Limit the amount of television viewing by household members 2. Remove or do not put a television set in the parents' or children's bedrooms 3. Do not have television on during meals		1. Mandate more physical education classes and after-school sports and include some choices that are single gender classes 2. Remove vending machines or replace sugar-sweetened beverage and calorie dense snack foods in vending machines and offered as a la carte options with more nutritious food and beverage options 3. Close school campuses so that young people cannot buy fast food or other convenience foods that are calorie dense 4. Include media literacy classes to educate preadolescents and adolescents that they are being targeted by the media to adopt or continue behaviors that may not be in their best interests
Education about dietary intake, activity, inactivity, and weight	1. Unclear whether increasing knowledge about diet and activity changes behavior , focusing on weight (parent's weight, child's weight, or weight in general) is associated with high levels of weight concerns and use of unhealthy weight control behaviors	1. Healthy and unhealthy dietary and weight control practices are learned behaviors. It is unclear whether increasing knowledge about diet and activity changes behavior, but training preadolescents and adolescents to be peer educators could potentially lead to greater behavior change	1. Unclear whether increasing knowledge about diet and activity changes behavior, but interventions that do not discuss weight per se are more successful than those that do discuss weight

number of youth, excessive amounts of body weight are being accrued during this period. Moreover, youth are highly influenced by social pressures, media images and marketing, and the beliefs and behavior of their friends and family. Thus preadolescence and adolescence are important periods to target because of a combination of social, maturational, and other developmental influences. It has been established that adolescents who are overweight are extremely likely to become overweight or obese adults. Second, it is during this period that young people start to strive for greater autonomy and want to make their own decisions. Guiding them to make healthy decisions regarding dietary intake, physical activity, and inactivity should reduce their risk for becoming overweight.

One of the limiting factors is that it is not entirely clear what type of diet should be promoted to minimize excessive weight gain. For example, efforts to promote the intake of fruits and vegetables may lead to lowering of risk for developing chronic diseases in adulthood, but it unclear whether such interventions would help to prevent adolescent obesity. Although it is not clear whether certain components of dietary intake prevent excessive weight gain, it cannot be disputed that consuming more calories than one expends will result in weight gain. To minimize unhealthy weight gain, the focus should be on energy balance rather than change in intake of specific foods or nutrients.

Since it is not realistic or even desirable to promote calorie counting among young people, it would be best to focus on changing diet and activity patterns versus specific foods or behaviors. Consumption of fast food and other quick food predicts greater weight gain. It is not clear whether the association is due to the high energy density of many fast food items, the promotion of 'value meals' that promote consumption of excess calories, or due to fast food consumption being a marker for a generally unhealthy lifestyle. Nevertheless, encouraging adolescents and their parents to reduce their visits to fast food restaurants, food courts, and other locations with high energy density prepared foods may be more effective at preventing obesity than encouraging an increase in servings of fruits and vegetables. Moreover, schools should not only limit or eliminate energy-dense snacks, sugar-sweetened soda, and fast food from inside the schools, they also should adopt a closed campus policy so that students will not purchase these poor food choices during lunchtime. Schools also need to offer more opportunities for students to be more physically active during and after school. Many preadolescents and adolescents do not participate in activities outside of school, so more should be done to promote activity during the school day and to offer free or low cost after school programs with an activity component.

It appears that parents play an important role as gatekeepers and role models, but peers may play an increasingly important role in shaping the decisions about whether young people are active and what they eat. Interventions to prevent obesity therefore must contain goals to improve the diet and activity patterns of the adults so they can be appropriate role models. Interventions should also recognize that the influence of parents will remain important, but will decrease as preadolescents become adolescents and young adults. Therefore, it is also essential that interventions attempt to sway peer norms to support and promote activity. Strategies that work well with preadolescents may not work at all with adolescents. Formative research approaches such as focus groups will be needed to understand the particular peer culture and to adapt interventions as needed, much as marketing campaigns tailor their messages for select subsets of the population. Marketers have been extremely successful at selling many foods and beverages of questionable nutritional value to children and adolescents. It is time that we learn to use some of the same tactics to promote healthy dietary and activity patterns that will help to prevent excessive weight gain.

References

50th Anniversary of 'Wonderful World of Color' TV. (2004). U.S. Census Bureau. Retrieved from http://www.census.gov/Press-Release/www/releases/archives/facts_ for_ features/001702.html

Austin, E. W., Chen, Y. C., Pinkleton, B. E., & Quintero Johnson, J. (2006). Benefits and costs of Channel One in a middle school setting and the role of media-literacy training. *Pediatrics, 117*(3), e423–e433.

Austin, S. B., Melly, S. J., Sanchez, B. N., Patel, A., Buka, S., & Gortmaker, S. L. (2005). Clustering of fast-food restaurants around schools: A novel application of spatial statistics to the study of food environments. *American Journal of Public Health, 95*(9), 1575–1581.

Austin, S. B., Ziyadeh, N., Kahn, J. A., Camargo, C. A., Jr., Colditz, G. A., & Field, A. E. (2004). Sexual orientation, weight concerns, and eating-disordered behaviors in adolescent girls and boys. *Journal of the American Academy of Child and Adolescent Psychiatry, 43*(9), 1115–1123.

Baranowski, T., Baranowski, J. C., Cullen, K. W., Thompson, D. I., Nicklas, T., Zakeri, I. E., et al. (2003). The Fun, Food, and Fitness Project (FFFP): The Baylor GEMS pilot study. *Ethnicity and Disease, 13*(1 Suppl. 1), S30–S39.

Barton, B. A., Eldridge, A. L., Thompson, D., Affenito, S. G., Striegel-Moore, R. H., Franko, D. L., et al. (2005). The relationship of breakfast and cereal consumption to nutrient intake and body mass index: The National Heart, Lung, and Blood Institute Growth and Health Study. *Journal of the American Dietetic Association, 105*(9), 1383–1389.

Beech, B. M., Klesges, R. C., Kumanyika, S. K., Murray, D. M., Klesges, L., McClanahan, B., et al. (2003). Child- and parent-targeted interventions: The Memphis GEMS pilot study. *Ethnicity and Disease, 13*(1 Suppl. 1), S40–S53.

Berkey, C. S., Rockett, H. R., Field, A. E., Gillman, M. W., & Colditz, G. A. (2004). Sugar-added beverages and adolescent weight change. *Obesity Research, 12*(5), 778–788.

Berkey, C. S., Rockett, H. R., Field, A. E., Gillman, M. W., Frazier, A. L., Camargo, C. A., Jr., et al. (2000). Activity, dietary intake, and weight changes in a longitudinal study of preadolescent and adolescent boys and girls. *Pediatrics, 105*(4), E56.

Berkey, C. S., Rockett, H. R., Willett, W. C., & Colditz, G. A. (2005). Milk, dairy fat, dietary calcium, and weight gain: A longitudinal study of adolescents. *Archives of Pediatric and Adolescent Medicine, 159*(6), 543–550.

Birnbaum, A. S., Lytle, L. A., Story, M., Perry, C. L., & Murray, D. M. (2002). Are differences in exposure to a multicomponent school-based intervention associated with varying dietary outcomes in adolescents? *Health Education and Behavior, 29*(4), 427–443.

Boutelle, K., Neumark-Sztainer, D., Story, M., & Resnick, M. (2002). Weight control behaviors among obese, overweight, and nonoverweight adolescents. *Journal of Pediatrics Psychology, 27*(6), 531–540.

Bowman, S. A., Gortmaker, S. L., Ebbeling, C. B., Pereira, M. A., & Ludwig, D. S. (2004). Effects of fast-food consumption on energy intake and diet quality among children in a national household survey. *Pediatrics, 113*(1, Pt. 1), 112–118.

Braun, D. L., Sunday, S. R., Huang, A., & Halmi, K. A. (1999). More males seek treatment for eating disorders. *International Journal of Eating Disorders, 25*(4), 415–424.

Briefel, R. R., & Johnson, C. L. (2004). Secular trends in dietary intake in the United States. *Annual Review of Nutrition, 24*, 401–431.

Brown, B., Frankel, B., & Fennell, M. (1989). Hugs or shrugs: Parental and peer influence on continuity of involvement in sport by female adolescents. *Sex Roles, 20*, 397–409.

Brug, J., & van Lenthe, F. (2005). *Environmental determinants and interventions for physical activity, nutrition, and smoking: A review.* Rotterdam: Ikenweij.

Campfield, L. A., Smith, F. J., Rosenbaum, M., & Hirsch, J. (1996). Human eating: Evidence for a physiological basis using a modified paradigm. *Neuroscience and Biobehavioral Reviews, 20*(1), 133–137.

Carruth, B. R., & Skinner, J. D. (2001). The role of dietary calcium and other nutrients in moderating body fat in preschool children. *International Journal of Obesity and Related Metabolic Disorders, 25*(4), 559–566.

Centers for Disease Control (CDC). (2002). 2000 CDC Growth Charts: United States. Retrieved December 15, 2003, from http://www.cdc.gov/growthcharts/

Chung, C., & Myers, S. L. (1999). Do the poor pay more for food? An analysis of grocery store availability and food price disparities. *Journal of Consumer Affairs, 32*(2), 276.

Crespo, C. J., Keteyian, S. J., Heath, G. W., & Sempos, C. T. (1996). Leisure-time physical activity among US adults. Results from the Third National Health and Nutrition Examination Survey. *Archives of Internal Medicine, 156*(1), 93–98.

Crespo, C. J., Smit, E., Andersen, R. E., Carter-Pokras, O., & Ainsworth, B. E. (2000). Race/ethnicity, social class and their relation to physical inactivity during leisure time: Results from the Third National Health and Nutrition Examination Survey, 1988-1994. *American Journal of Preventive Medicine, 18*(1), 46–53.

Davison, K. K., Francis, L. A., & Birch, L. L. (2005). Links between parents' and girls' television viewing behaviors: A longitudinal examination. *Journal of Pediatrics, 147*(4), 436–442.

Dennison, B. A., Erb, T. A., & Jenkins, P. L. (2002). Television viewing and television in bedroom associated with overweight risk among low-income preschool children. *Pediatrics, 109*(6), 1028–1035.

Dennison, B. A., Rockwell, H. L., & Baker, S. L. (1997). Excess fruit juice consumption by preschool-aged children is associated with short stature and obesity. *Pediatrics, 99*(1), 15–22.

Ebbeling, C. B., Feldman, H. A., Osganian, S. K., Chomitz, V. R., Ellenbogen, S. J., & Ludwig, D. S. (2006). Effects of decreasing sugar-sweetened beverage consumption on body weight in adolescents: A randomized, controlled pilot study. *Pediatrics, 117*(3), 673–680.

Ebbeling, C. B., Leidig, M. M., Sinclair, K. B., Seger-Shippee, L. G., Feldman, H. A., & Ludwig, D. S. (2005). Effects of an ad libitum low-glycemic load diet on cardiovascular disease risk factors in obese young adults. *American Journal of Clinical Nutrition, 81*(5), 976-982.

Eisenberg, M. E., Neumark-Sztainer, D., Story, M., & Perry, C. (2005). The role of social norms and friends' influences on unhealthy weight-control behaviors among adolescent girls. *Social Science and Medicine, 60*(6), 1165–1173.

Eisenberg, M. E., Olson, R. E., Neumark-Sztainer, D., Story, M., & Bearinger, L. H. (2004). Correlations between family meals and psychosocial well-being among adolescents. *Archives of Pediatric and Adolescent Medicine, 158*(8), 792–796.

Epstein, J. A., Botvin, G. J., & Diaz, T. (1999). Etiology of alcohol use among Hispanic adolescents: Sex-specific effects of social influences to drink and problem behaviors. *Archives of Pediatric and Adolescent Medicine, 153*(10), 1077–1084.

Field, A. E., Austin, S. B., Gillman, M. W., Rosner, B., Rockett, H. R., & Colditz, G. A. (2004). Snack food intake does not predict weight change among children and adolescents. *International Journal of Obesity and Related Metabolic Disorders, 28*(10), 1210–1216.

Field, A. E., Austin, S. B., Taylor, C. B., Malspeis, S., Rosner, B., Rockett, H. R., et al. (2003). Relation between dieting and weight change among preadolescents and -adolescents. *Pediatrics, 112*(4), 900–906.

Field, A. E., Camargo, C. A., Jr., Taylor, C. B., Berkey, C. S., & Colditz, G. A. (1999). Relation of peer and media influences to the development of purging behaviors among preadolescent and adolescent girls. *Archives of Pediatric and Adolescent Medicine, 153*(11), 1184–1189.

Field, A. E., Camargo, C. A., Jr., Taylor, C. B., Berkey, C. S., Frazier, A. L., Gillman, M. W., et al. (1999). Overweight, weight concerns, and bulimic behaviors among girls and boys. *Journal of the American Academy of Child and Adolescent Psychiatry*, *38*(6), 754–760.

Field, A. E., Colditz, G. A., & Peterson, K. E. (1997). Racial/ethnic and gender differences in concern with weight and in bulimic behaviors among adolescents. *Obesity Research*, *5*(5), 447–454.

Field, A. E., Cook, N. R., & Gillman, M. W. (2005). Weight status in childhood as a predictor of becoming overweight or hypertensive in early adulthood. *Obesity Research*, *13*(1), 163–169.

Field, A. E., Gillman, M. W., Rosner, B., Rockett, H. R., & Colditz, G. A. (2003). Association between fruit and vegetable intake and change in body mass index among a large sample of children and adolescents in the United States. *International Journal of Obesity and Related Metabolic Disorders*, *27*(7), 821–826.

Field, A. E., Manson, J. E., Taylor, C. B., Willett, W. C., & Colditz, G. A. (2004). Association of weight change, weight control practices, and weight cycling among women in the Nurses' Health Study II. *International Journal of Obesity and Related Metabolic Disorders*, *28*(9), 1134–1142.

Field, A. E., Peterson, K. E., Gortmaker, S. L., Cheung, L., Rockett, H., Fox, M. K., et al. (1999). Reproducibility and validity of a food frequency questionnaire among fourth to seventh grade inner-city school children: Implications of age and day-to-day variation in dietary intake. *Public Health Nutrition*, *2*(3), 293–300.

Flynn, M. A., McNeil, D. A., Maloff, B., Mutasingwa, D., Wu, M., Ford, C., et al. (2006). Reducing obesity and related chronic disease risk in children and youth: A synthesis of evidence with 'best practice' recommendations. *Obes Rev*, *7* (Suppl. 1), 7–66.

Foster-Powell, K., & Miller, J. B. (1995). International tables of glycemic index. *American Journal of Clinical Nutrition*, *62*(4), 871S–890S.

Francis, L. A., Lee, Y., & Birch, L. L. (2003). Parental weight status and girls' television viewing, snacking, and body mass indexes. *Obesity Research*, *11*(1), 143–151.

French, S. A., Story, M., Downes, B., Resnick, M. D., & Blum, R. W. (1995). Frequent dieting among adolescents: Psychosocial and health behavior correlates. *American Journal of Public Health*, *85*(5), 695–701.

French, S. A., Story, M., Neumark-Sztainer, D., Fulkerson, J. A., & Hannan, P. (2001). Fast food restaurant use among adolescents: Associations with nutrient intake, food choices and behavioral and psychosocial variables. *International Journal of Obesity and Related Metabolic Disorders*, *25*(12), 1823–1833.

Fried, E. J., & Nestle, M. (2002). The growing political movement against soft drinks in schools. *Journal of the American Medical Association*, *288*(17), 2181.

Fulkerson, J. A., French, S. A., Story, M., Hannan, P. J., Neumark-Sztainer, D., & Himes, J. H. (2004). Weight-bearing physical activity among girls and mothers: Relationships to girls' weight status. *Obesity Research*, *12*(2), 258–266.

Gillman, M. W., Rifas-Shiman, S. L., Frazier, A. L., Rockett, H. R., Camargo, C. A., Jr., Field, A. E., et al. (2000). Family dinner and diet quality among older children and adolescents. *Archives of Family Medicine*, *9*(3), 235–240.

Gordon-Larsen, P., Adair, L. S., Nelson, M. C., & Popkin, B. M. (2004). Five-year obesity incidence in the transition period between adolescence and adulthood: The National Longitudinal Study of Adolescent Health. *American Journal of Clinical Nutrition*, *80*(3), 569–575.

Gordon-Larsen, P., Adair, L. S., & Popkin, B. M. (2002). Ethnic differences in physical activity and inactivity patterns and overweight status. *Obesity Research*, *10*(3), 141–149.

Gordon-Larsen, P., Adair, L. S., & Popkin, B. M. (2003). The relationship of ethnicity, socioeconomic factors, and overweight in US adolescents. *Obesity Research*, *11*(1), 121–129.

Gortmaker, S. L., Cheung, L. W., Peterson, K. E., Chomitz, G., Cradle, J. H., Dart, H., et al. (1999). Impact of a school-based interdisciplinary intervention on diet and physical activity among urban primary school children: Eat well and keep moving. *Archives of Pediatric and Adolescent Medicine, 153*(9), 975–983.

Gortmaker, S. L., Must, A., Sobol, A. M., Peterson, K., Colditz, G. A., & Dietz, W. H. (1996). Television viewing as a cause of increasing obesity among children in the United States, 1986-1990. *Archives of Pediatric and Adolescent Medicine, 150*(4), 356–362.

Gortmaker, S. L., Peterson, K., Wiecha, J., Sobol, A. M., Dixit, S., Fox, M. K., et al. (1999). Reducing obesity via a school-based interdisciplinary intervention among youth: Planet Health. *Archives of Pediatric and Adolescent Medicine, 153*(4), 409–418.

Gunther, C. W., Legowski, P. A., Lyle, R. M., McCabe, G. P., Eagan, M. S., Peacock, M., et al. (2005). Dairy products do not lead to alterations in body weight or fat mass in young women in a 1-y intervention. *American Journal of Clinical Nutrition, 81*(4), 751–756.

Guthrie, J. F., Lin, B. H., & Frazao, E. (2002). Role of food prepared away from home in the American diet, 1977-78 versus 1994-96: Changes and consequences. *Journal of Nutrition Education and Behavior, 34*(3), 140–150.

Hanson, N. I., Neumark-Sztainer, D., Eisenberg, M. E., Story, M., & Wall, M. (2005). Associations between parental report of the home food environment and adolescent intakes of fruits, vegetables and dairy foods. *Public Health Nutrition, 8*(1), 77–85.

Harrison, K., & Marske, A. L. (2005). Nutritional content of foods advertised during the television programs children watch most. *American Journal of Public Health, 95*(9), 1568–1574.

Himes, J. H., & Faricy, A. (2001). Validity and reliability of self-reported stature and weight of US adolescents. *American Journal of Human Biology, 13*(2), 255–260.

Himes, J. H., Ring, K., Gittelsohn, J., Cunningham-Sabo, L., Weber, J., Thompson, J., et al. (2003). Impact of the Pathways intervention on dietary intakes of American Indian schoolchildren. *Preventive Medicine, 37*(6, Pt. 2), S55–S61.

Hoefer, W. R., McKenzie, T. L., Sallis, J. F., Marshall, S. J., & Conway, T. L. (2001). Parental provision of transportation for adolescent physical activity. *American Journal of Preventive Medicine, 21*(1), 48–51.

Howarth, N. C., Huang, T. T., Roberts, S. B., & McCrory, M. A. (2005). Dietary fiber and fat are associated with excess weight in young and middle-aged US adults. *Journal of the American Dietetic Association, 105*(9), 1365–1372.

Ievers-Landis, C. E., Burant, C., Drotar, D., Morgan, L., Trapl, E. S., & Kwoh, C. K. (2003). Social support, knowledge, and self-efficacy as correlates of osteoporosis preventive behaviors among preadolescent females. *Journal of Pediatrics Psychology, 28*(5), 335–345.

Jahns, L., Siega-Riz, A. M., & Popkin, B. M. (2001). The increasing prevalence of snacking among US children from 1977 to 1996. *Journal of Pediatrics, 138*(4), 493–498.

Kettaneh, A., Oppert, J. M., Heude, B., Deschamps, V., Borys, J. M., Lommez, A., et al. (2005). Changes in physical activity explain paradoxical relationship between baseline physical activity and adiposity changes in adolescent girls: The FLVS II study. *International Journal of Obesity (Lond), 29*(6), 586–593.

Kimm, S. Y., Barton, B. A., Obarzanek, E., McMahon, R. P., Kronsberg, S. S., Waclawiw, M. A., et al. (2002). Obesity development during adolescence in a biracial cohort: The NHLBI Growth and Health Study. *Pediatrics, 110*(5), e54.

Kimm, S. Y., Glynn, N. W., Kriska, A. M., Barton, B. A., Kronsberg, S. S., Daniels, S. R., et al. (2002). Decline in physical activity in black girls and white girls during adolescence. *New England Journal of Medicine, 347*(10), 709–715.

Kimm, S. Y., Glynn, N. W., Obarzanek, E., Kriska, A. M., Daniels, S. R., Barton, B. A., et al. (2005). Relation between the changes in physical activity and body-mass index during adolescence: A multicentre longitudinal study. *Lancet, 366*(9482), 301–307.

Klein-Platat, C., Oujaa, M., Wagner, A., Haan, M. C., Arveiler, D., Schlienger, J. L., & Simon, C. (2005). Physical activity is inversely related to waist circumference in 12-year old French adolescents. *International Journal of Obesity, 29*(1), 9–14.

Koh-Banerjee, P., Franz, M., Sampson, L., Liu, S., Jacobs, D. R., Jr., Spiegelman, D., et al. (2004). Changes in whole-grain, bran, and cereal fiber consumption in relation to 8-y weight gain among men. *American Journal of Clinical Nutrition*, *80*(5), 1237–1245.

Komro, K. A., Perry, C. L., Murray, D. M., Veblen-Mortenson, S., Williams, C. L., & Anstine, P. S. (1996). Peer-planned social activities for preventing alcohol use among young adolescents. *Journal of School Health*, *66*(9), 328–334.

Koplan, J. P., Liverman, C. T., Kraak, V. I., (2005). Committee on prevention of obesity in children and youth. Preventing childhood obesity: Health in balance. *Journal of the American Dietetic Association*, *105*(1), 131–138.

Labre, M. P. (2002). Adolescent boys and the muscular male body ideal. *Journal of Adolescent Health*, *30*(4), 233–242.

Lappe, J. M., Rafferty, K. A., Davies, K. M., & Lypaczewski, G. (2004). Girls on a high-calcium diet gain weight at the same rate as girls on a normal diet: A pilot study. *Journal of the American Dietetic Association*, *104*(9), 1361–1367.

Lau, R. R., Quadrel, M. J., & Hartman, K. A. (1990). Development and change of young adults' preventive health beliefs and behavior: Influence from parents and peers. *Journal of Health and Social Behavior*, *31*(3), 240–259.

Lewis, C. E., Jacobs, D. R., Jr., McCreath, H., Kiefe, C. I., Schreiner, P. J., Smith, D. E., et al. (2000). Weight gain continues in the 1990s: 10-year trends in weight and overweight from the CARDIA study. Coronary Artery Risk Development in Young Adults. *American Journal of Epidemiology*, *151*(12), 1172–1181.

Lewis, C. E., Smith, D. E., Wallace, D. D., Williams, O. D., Bild, D. E., & Jacobs, D. R., Jr. (1997). Seven-year trends in body weight and associations with lifestyle and behavioral characteristics in black and white young adults: The CARDIA study. *American Journal of Public Health*, *87*(4), 635–642.

Lin, Y. C., Lyle, R. M., McCabe, L. D., McCabe, G. P., Weaver, C. M., & Teegarden, D. (2000). Dairy calcium is related to changes in body composition during a two-year exercise intervention in young women. *Journal of American College of Nutrition*, *19*(6), 754–760.

Liu, S., Willett, W. C., Manson, J. E., Hu, F. B., Rosner, B., & Colditz, G. (2003). Relation between changes in intakes of dietary fiber and grain products and changes in weight and development of obesity among middle-aged women. *American Journal of Clinical Nutrition*, *78*(5), 920–927.

Lowe, C. F., Horne, P. J., Tapper, K., Bowdery, M., & Egerton, C. (2004). Effects of a peer modelling and rewards-based intervention to increase fruit and vegetable consumption in children. *European Journal of Clinical Nutrition*, *58*(3), 510–522.

Lowry, R., Brener, N., Lee, S., Epping, J., Fulton, J, & Eaton, D. (2004). Participation in high school physical education—United States, 1991–2003. *MMWR Morbidity Mortality Weekly Report*, *53*(36), 844–847.

Lowry, R., Galuska, D. A., Fulton, J. E., Wechsler, H., & Kann, L. (2002). Weight management goals and practices among U.S. high school students: Associations with physical activity, diet, and smoking. *Journal of Adolescent Health*, *31*(2), 133–144.

Ludwig, D. S., Majzoub, J. A., Al-Zahrani, A., Dallal, G. E., Blanco, I., & Roberts, S. B. (1999). High glycemic index foods, overeating, and obesity. *Pediatrics*, *103*(3), E26.

Ludwig, D. S., Pereira, M. A., Kroenke, C. H., Hilner, J. E., Van Horn, L., Slattery, M. L., et al. (1999). Dietary fiber, weight gain, and cardiovascular disease risk factors in young adults. *Journal of the American Medical Association*, *282*(16), 1539–1546.

Ludwig, D. S., Peterson, K. E., & Gortmaker, S. L. (2001). Relation between consumption of sugar-sweetened drinks and childhood obesity: A prospective, observational analysis. *Lancet*, *357*(9255), 505–508.

Matheson, D. M., Killen, J. D., Wang, Y., Varady, A., & Robinson, T. N. (2004). Children's food consumption during television viewing. *American Journal of Clinical Nutrition*, *79*(6), 1088–1094.

McCabe, M. P., & Ricciardelli, L. A. (2001). Parent, peer, and media influences on body image and strategies to both increase and decrease body size among adolescent boys and girls. *Adolescence*, *36*(142), 225–240.

McCabe, M. P., Ricciardelli, L. A., & Finemore, J. (2002). The role of puberty, media and popularity with peers on strategies to increase weight, decrease weight and increase muscle tone among adolescent boys and girls. *Journal of Psychosomatic Research, 52*(3), 145–153.

McGuire, M. T., Hannan, P. J., Neumark-Sztainer, D., Cossrow, N. H., & Story, M. (2002). Parental correlates of physical activity in a racially/ethnically diverse adolescent sample. *Journal of Adolescent Health, 30*(4), 253–261.

Nader, P. R., Stone, E. J., Lytle, L. A., Perry, C. L., Osganian, S. K., Kelder, S., et al. (1999). Three-year maintenance of improved diet and physical activity: The CATCH cohort. Child and Adolescent Trial for Cardiovascular Health. *Archives of Pediatric and Adolescent Medicine, 153*(7), 695–704.

Neumark-Sztainer, D., French, S. A., Hannan, P. J., Story, M., & Fulkerson, J. A. (2005). School lunch and snacking patterns among high school students: Associations with school food environment and policies. *International Journal of Behavioral Nutrition and Physical Activity, 2*(1), 14.

Neumark-Sztainer, D., Hannan, P. J., Story, M., Croll, J., & Perry, C. (2003). Family meal patterns: Associations with sociodemographic characteristics and improved dietary intake among adolescents. *Journal of the American Dietetic Association, 103*(3), 317–322.

Neumark-Sztainer, D., Hannan, P. J., Story, M., & Perry, C. L. (2004). Weight-control behaviors among adolescent girls and boys: Implications for dietary intake. *Journal of the American Dietetic Association, 104*(6), 913–920.

Neumark-Sztainer, D., Story, M., Hannan, P. J., Perry, C. L., & Irving, L. M. (2002). Weight-related concerns and behaviors among overweight and nonoverweight adolescents: Implications for preventing weight-related disorders. *Archives of Pediatric and Adolescent Medicine, 156*(2), 171–178.

Neumark-Sztainer, D., Story, M., Hannan, P. J., & Rex, J. (2003). New Moves: A school-based obesity prevention program for adolescent girls. *Preventive Medicine, 37*(1), 41–51.

Neumark-Sztainer, D., Wall, M., Perry, C., & Story, M. (2003). Correlates of fruit and vegetable intake among adolescents. Findings from Project EAT. *Preventive Medicine, 37*(3), 198–208.

Ogden, C. L., Carroll, M. D., Curtin, L. R., McDowell, M. A., Tabak, C. J., & Flegal, K. M. (2006). Prevalence of overweight and obesity in the United States, 1999–2004. *Journal of the American Medical Association, 295*(13), 1549–1555.

Ogden, C. L., Flegal, K. M., Carroll, M. D., & Johnson, C. L. (2002). Prevalence and trends in overweight among US children and adolescents, 1999–2000. *Journal of the American Medical Association, 288*(14), 1728–1732.

Paxton, S. J., Schutz, H. K., Wertheim, E. H., & Muir, S. L. (1999). Friendship clique and peer influences on body image concerns, dietary restraint, extreme weight-loss behaviors, and binge eating in adolescent girls. *Journal of Abnormal Psychology, 108*(2), 255–266.

Pereira, M., Kartashov, A., Slattery, M., Van Horn, L., Jacobs, D. J., & Ludwig, D. S. (2003). Reported breakfast habits and incidence of obesity and the insulin resistance syndrome in young black and white adults: The CARDIA Study. *Circulation. 107*(e7001). (http://circ.ahajournals.org/cgi/reprint/107/7/e7001; Feb. 25, 2003 issue)

Phillips, S. M., Bandini, L. G., Cyr, H., Colclough-Douglas, S., Naumova, E., & Must, A. (2003). Dairy food consumption and body weight and fatness studied longitudinally over the adolescent period. *International Journal of Obesity and Related Metabolic Disorders, 27*(9), 1106–1113.

Phillips, S. M., Bandini, L. G., Naumova, E. N., Cyr, H., Colclough, S., Dietz, W. H., et al. (2004). Energy-dense snack food intake in adolescence: Longitudinal relationship to weight and fatness. *Obesity Research, 12*(3), 461–472.

Pirozzo, S., Summerbell, C., Cameron, C., & Glasziou, P. (2003). Should we recommend low-fat diets for obesity? *Obesity Reviews, 4*(2), 83–90.

Pugh, M. J., & Hart, D. (1999). Identity development and peer group participation. *New Directions for Child and Adolescent Development*, (84), 55–70.

Rampersaud, G. C., Pereira, M. A., Girard, B. L., Adams, J., & Metzl, J. D. (2005). Breakfast habits, nutritional status, body weight, and academic performance in children and adolescents. *Journal of the American Dietetic Association*, *105*(5), 743–760; quiz 761–742.

Reisberg, L. (2000, July 28). Colleges use peer presure to encourage healthy behavior. *Chronicle of Higher Education*, *46*, A60–A61.

Rico, H., Revilla, M., Villa, L. F., Hernandez, E. R., Alvarez de Buergo, M., & Villa, M. (1993). Body composition in children and Tanner's stages. A study with dual-energy x-ray absorptiometry. *Metabolism*, *42*, 967–970.

Rimm, E. B., Ascherio, A., Giovannucci, E., Spiegelman, D., Stampfer, M. J., & Willett, W. C. (1996). Vegetable, fruit, and cereal fiber intake and risk of coronary heart disease among men. *Journal of the American Medical Association*, *275*(6), 447–451.

Robert, D., Foehr, U., & Rideout, V. (2005). *Generation M: Media in the lives of* 8–18 *year olds*. Menlo Park, CA: Kaiser Family Foundation.

Robert, D., Foehr, U., Rideout, V., & Brodie, M. (1999). *Kids & media @ the new millenium*. Menlo Park, CA: Kaiser Family Foundation.

Robinson, T. N. (1999). Reducing children's television viewing to prevent obesity: A randomized controlled trial. *Journal of the American Medical Association*, *282*(16), 1561–1567.

Robinson, T. N., Killen, J. D., Kraemer, H. C., Wilson, D. M., Matheson, D. M., Haskell, W. L., et al. (2003). Dance and reducing television viewing to prevent weight gain in African-American girls: The Stanford GEMS pilot study. *Ethnicity and Disease*, *13*(1 Suppl. 1), S65–S77.

Rochon, J., Klesges, R. C., Story, M., Robinson, T. N., Baranowski, T., Obarzanek, E., et al. (2003). Common design elements of the Girls health Enrichment Multi-site Studies (GEMS). *Ethnicity and Disease*, *13*(1 Suppl. 1), S6–S14.

Saelens, B. E., Sallis, J. F., Nader, P. R., Broyles, S. L., Berry, C. C., & Taras, H. L. (2002). Home environmental influences on children's television watching from early to middle childhood. *Journal of Developmental and Behavioral Pediatrics*, *23*(3), 127–132.

Sallis, J. F., Prochaska, J. J., & Taylor, W. C. (2000). A review of correlates of physical activity of children and adolescents. *Medicine and Science in Sports and Exercise*, *32*(5), 963–975.

Schmitz, K. H., Jacobs, D. R., Jr., Leon, A. S., Schreiner, P. J., & Sternfeld, B. (2000). Physical activity and body weight: Associations over ten years in the CARDIA study. Coronary Artery Risk Development in Young Adults. *International Journal of Obesity and Related Metabolic Disorders*, *24*(11), 1475–1487.

Schulze, M. B., Manson, J. E., Ludwig, D. S., Colditz, G. A., Stampfer, M. J., Willett, W. C., et al. (2004). Sugar-sweetened beverages, weight gain, and incidence of type 2 diabetes in young and middle-aged women. *Journal of the American Medical Association*, *292*(8), 927–934.

Sciacca, J., & Appleton, T. (1996). Peer helping: A promising strategy for effective health education. *Peer Facilitator Quarterly*, *13*, 322–328.

Sieving, R. E., Perry, C. L., & Williams, C. L. (2000). Do friendships change behaviors, or do behaviors change friendships? Examining paths of influence in young adolescents' alcohol use. *Journal of Adolescent Health*, *26*(1), 27–35.

Skinner, J. D., Bounds, W., Carruth, B. R., & Ziegler, P. (2003). Longitudinal calcium intake is negatively related to children's body fat indexes. *Journal of the American Dietetic Association*, *103*(12), 1626–1631.

Skinner, J. D., Carruth, B. R., Moran, J., 3rd, Houck, K., & Coletta, F. (1999). Fruit juice intake is not related to children's growth. *Pediatrics*, *103*(1), 58–64.

Stice, E., Cameron, R. P., Killen, J. D., Hayward, C., & Taylor, C. B. (1999). Naturalistic weight-reduction efforts prospectively predict growth in relative weight and onset of obesity among female adolescents. *Journal of Consulting and Clinical Psychology*, *67*(6), 967–974.

Story, M., & French, S. (2004). Food Advertising and Marketing Directed at Children and Adolescents in the US. *International Journal of Behavioral Nutrition and Physical Activity, 1*(1), 3.

Story, M., Sherwood, N. E., Himes, J. H., Davis, M., Jacobs, D. R., Jr., Cartwright, Y., et al. (2003). An after-school obesity prevention program for African-American girls: The Minnesota GEMS pilot study. *Ethnicity and Disease, 13*(1 Suppl. 1), S54–S64.

Strong, W. B., Malina, R. M., Blimkie, C. J., Daniels, S. R., Dishman, R. K., Gutin, B., et al. (2005). Evidence based physical activity for school-age youth. *Journal of Pediatrics, 146*(6), 732–737.

Sun, S. S., Schubert, C. M., Chumlea, W. C., Roche, A. F., Kulin, H. E., Lee, P. A., et al. (2002). National estimates of the timing of sexual maturation and racial differences among US children. *Pediatrics, 110*(5), 911–919.

Swinburn, B., Gill, T., & Kumanyika, S. (2005). Obesity prevention: A proposed framework for translating evidence into action. *Obesity Reviews, 6*(1), 23–33.

Tammelin, T., Laitinen, J., & Nayha, S. (2004). Change in the level of physical activity from adolescence into adulthood and obesity at the age of 31 years. *International Journal of Obesity and Related Metabolic Disorders, 28*(6), 775–782.

Taveras, E. M., Berkey, C. S., Rifas-Shiman, S. L., Ludwig, D. S., Rockett, H. R., Field, A. E., et al. (2005). Association of consumption of fried food away from home with body mass index and diet quality in older children and adolescents. *Pediatrics, 116*(4), e518–e524.

Taveras, E. M., Rifas-Shiman, S. L., Berkey, C. S., Rockett, H. R., Field, A. E., Frazier, A. L., et al. (2005). Family dinner and adolescent overweight. *Obesity Research, 13*(5), 900–906.

Thompson, O. M., Ballew, C., Resnicow, K., Must, A., Bandini, L. G., Cyr, H., et al. (2004). Food purchased away from home as a predictor of change in BMI z-score among girls. *International Journal of Obesity and Related Metabolic Disorders, 28*(2), 282–289.

Trost, S. G., Sallis, J. F., Pate, R. R., Freedson, P. S., Taylor, W. C., & Dowda, M. (2003). Evaluating a model of parental influence on youth physical activity. *American Journal of Preventive Medicine, 25*(4), 277–282.

Wagner, A., Klein-Platat, C., Arveiler, D., Haan, M. C., Schlienger, J. L., & Simon, C. (2004). Parent-child physical activity relationships in 12-year old French students do not depend on family socioeconomic status. *Diabetes and Metabolism, 30*(4), 359–366.

Wechsler, H., Brener, N. D., Kuester, S., & Miller, C. (2001). Food service and foods and beverages available at school: Results from the School Health Policies and Programs Study 2000. *Journal of School Health, 71*(7), 313–324.

West, P., Sweeting, H., & Ecob, R. (1999). Family and friends' influences on the uptake of regular smoking from mid-adolescence to early adulthood. *Addiction, 94*(9), 1397–1411.

Whitaker, R. C., Wright, J. A., Pepe, M. S., Seidel, K. D., & Dietz, W. H. (1997). Predicting obesity in young adulthood from childhood and parental obesity. *New England Journal of Medicine, 337*(13), 869–873.

Wiecha, J. L., Sobol, A. M., Peterson, K. E., & Gortmaker, S. L. (2001). Household television access: Associations with screen time, reading, and homework among youth. *Ambulatory Pediatrics, 1*(5), 244–251.

Willett, W. C. (1994). Diet and health: What should we eat? *Science, 264*(5158), 532–537.

Willett, W. C., & Leibel, R. L. (2002). Dietary fat is not a major determinant of body fat. *American Journal of Medicine, 113* (Suppl. 9B), 47S–59S.

Wolever, T. M., Jenkins, D. J., Jenkins, A. L., & Josse, R. G. (1991). The glycemic index: Methodology and clinical implications. *American Journal of Clinical Nutrition, 54*(5), 846–854.

Young, L. R., & Nestle, M. (2003). Expanding portion sizes in the US marketplace: Implications for nutrition counseling. *Journal of the American Dietetic Association, 103*(2), 231–234.

Chapter 21

Obesity Prevention During Adulthood

Suzanne Phelan, Meghan Butryn, and Rena R. Wing

The weight distribution of the U.S. population has been shifting upwards, and overweight and obesity have increased steadily across all ages. As discussed in Chapters 18 through 20, it is important that obesity prevention efforts begin during childhood. However, the importance of obesity prevention in children should not overshadow the need and potential for prevention of excess weight gain in adults (Seidell, Nooyens & Visscher, 2005). The need for obesity prevention in U.S. adults is clear in recent trend data from national surveys conducted over the past 20 years. Based on data from the 1999–2002 National Health and Nutrition Examination Survey (NHANES), 65% of the U.S. population aged 20 years and older is overweight or obese (defined as having a body mass index [BMI] of 25 kg/m² or more) compared with 46% seen in NHANES I, conducted between 1971 and 1974 (A.A. Hedley et al., 2004; National Center for Health Statistics/Division of Data Services, 2005). During the same time span, the percent obese (BMI $\geq$30 kg/m²) more than doubled—from about 15% in 1971–1974 (Flegal, Carroll, Ogden, & Johnson, 2002) to more than 30% in 1999–2002 (Hedley, 2004 #5741).

Although some obese adults were obese as children, currently the high prevalence of obesity in U.S. adults is largely due to major weight gains that occur during adulthood. This is of concern as weight gain during adulthood contributes substantially to increased mortality and morbidity from obesity and has been related prospectively to the development of major health problems. For example, in the Nurses Health Study, regardless of BMI at baseline, women gaining $\geq$10 kg after the age of 18 were found to have a 70–150% increased risk of developing coronary heart disease and 20–60% greater risk of death from all causes compared with those who gained < 3 kg (Manson et al., 1990; Manson et al., 1995). Prevention of weight gain in adults might significantly reduce the overall rates of mortality and morbidity associated with obesity. Table 21.1 identifies several other elements of the rationale for targeting adults with obesity prevention programs, based on a review of this issue by Seidell, Nooyens, and Visscher (2005).

This chapter provides a perspective on how obesity prevention can be approached from young adulthood and, in women, through the perimenopause

Table 21.1. Rationale for obesity prevention during adulthood (Adapted from Seidell, Nooyens, & Visscher, 2005).

Issue	Explanation
High incidence of obesity	Continued weight gain leads to sharp increases in obesity incidence during adulthood
Health risks associated with weight gain	Independent of the extent of overweight, weight gain during adulthood is a risk factor for many chronic diseases, including heart disease and diabetes
High absolute risks of obesity-related disease	Health outcomes that are associated with obesity are common during adulthood. On a population basis, the *relative* contribution of obesity to these diseases may decrease with age, but the absolute numbers of people affected by these diseases is large
Benefits of preventing weight gain	Several interventions have demonstrated the reduction in disease incidence associated with preventing weight gain and weight loss in adults, e.g., diabetes prevention
Immediate payoff	Effective weight gain prevention in adults may yield benefits immediately (e.g., compared to the longer time horizon for prevention in childhood) with respect to reducing disease burden
Ancillary effects on others	Obesity prevention in adults might, therefore, have benefits on other household members, including children

period. We begin by identifying the populations groups for which obesity prevention efforts are most needed. We then review evidence on behavioral determinants of excess weight gain and on the effectiveness of individually-focused interventions, followed by discussion of the research directions implied by the literature to date. Environmental variables that influence individuals' ability to control their weight, and ways to intervene on these factors that are complementary to more intensive individually focused interventions, are discussed in Chapters 13 through 16.

Risk for Weight Gain in Adulthood

There are several risk factors associated with weight gain in adulthood, including ethnicity, age, and BMI. As discussed in Chapter 3, African American women and Mexican American men and women are more likely to become obese or extremely obese compared to their sex-age peers in the non-Hispanic white population (A. A. Hedley et al., 2004), and American Indians and Pacific Islander adults are also at higher risk of obesity compared to U.S. adults in general. Across ethnicity, immigrants to the United States—who are often less obese than the U.S. average when they arrive—may also experience major weight gains with increasing duration of U.S. residence (Dey & Lucas, 2006; Goel, McCarthy, Phillips, & Wee, 2004; Lauderdale & Rathouz, 2000). Low socioeconomic status is also associated with higher levels of obesity in adult women in affluent countries (Lahmann, Lissner, Gullberg, & Berglund, 2000; Sobal & Stunkard, 1989). For example, in an epidemiologic study of

Swedish women aged 45–73 years, Lahmann et al (2000) found that socioeconomic status was one of the strongest predictors of large weight gain during adult life.

Both low initial body weight (BMI <20) (Bild et al., 1996; French et al., 1994) and being overweight/obese (BMI >25) (Williamson, Kahn, Remington, & Anda, 1990) are also significant predictors of weight gain. In the Swedish study by Lahmann et al. (2000), individuals with a BMI <20 at age 20 gained significantly more during adult life than those who had a BMI ≥20 (14 vs. 11 kg weight gain, respectively). Despite the higher weight gain in individuals with a lower initial BMI, they remained significantly leaner later in life (ages 45–73) compared with those who had a higher initial BMI (24 vs. 27 kg/m², respectively). However, individuals who are initially overweight or obese (BMI ≥25) also are at greater risk of substantial weight gain. For example, in a representative sample of the U.S. population (NHANES I), initially overweight women aged 25 to 44 years had the highest incidence (14.2%) of major weight gain (>10 kg) over 10 years compared with any other subgroup (Williamson et al., 1990).

Within the adult population, the greatest risk for major weight gain over time occurs during young adulthood. In the NHANES Follow Up Study of U.S. adults initially surveyed in 1971–1975, major weight gain over 10 years (defined as increased BMI ≥5 kg/m² or approximately 30 pounds) was highest at ages 25–34 (Williamson et al., 1990). Similarly, in a large bi-racial cohort of young adults (the Coronary Artery Risk Development in Young Adults [CARDIA] study), aging-related weight gain was larger in the early to mid-20s than for older ages (Lewis, Jacobs, & McCreath, 2000). On average, participants in the study gained approximately 1 kg/year. However, those aged 18–30 gained about half a kilogram more per year than other individuals (i.e., those aged ≥30.). The average 15-year weight gain was 16 kg in African American women, 14 kg in African-American men, 10 kg in white women, and 11 kg in white men, with a ≥15 kg gain in 48%, 41%, 26%, and 29%, respectively (Lewis et al., 2000). The NHANES Follow Up Study also found that African-Americans were more likely than Caucasians to have experienced major weight gain and to have become obese over 10 years of follow-up (Williamson, Kahn, & Byers, 1991). Weight gain continues at a slower rate (i.e., less than the ~1–2 kg/year observed at ages 25 to 34) during later adulthood (ages 35–65), and starts to decline after age 65 (Bild et al., 1996; Colditz, Willett, Stampfer, Manson et al., 1990; French et al., 1994; Lahmann et al., 2000).

Genetic markers (Bouchard & Perusse, 1996), low metabolic rate, a high respiratory quotient (indicating carbohydrate oxidation), and increased insulin sensitivity (Ravussin & Swinburn, 1992) have also been associated with excess risk of weight gain. Identifying individuals at higher risk because of their genetic or physiologic makeup may ultimately provide the basis for a preventive strategy by targeting overweight families and screening their children.

As will become evident in the review of intervention data, there are also several periods in adulthood (e.g., pregnancy, menopause) that are associated with life transitions that pose a potential for excess weight gain and, consequently, opportunities for prevention. Before reviewing this literature, however, we will address potential behavioral targets for intervention.

Behaviors Associated with Weight Gain

In this section we examine behavioral predictors of weight gain and obesity in observational, prospective studies of the general population in an effort to guide future prevention and treatment efforts. Variables considered are high total caloric intake, consumption of sweets and high fat foods, consumption of sugar-sweetened beverages, physical inactivity, television (TV) viewing, and psychological factors. Strategies for controlling obesity via food industry interventions are covered in Chapter 9.

High Calorie, High Fat Food Intake

Findings on the effects of calorie and fat intake on weight gain in population-based studies have been largely inconsistent, and often counter to those expected on the basis of the experimental literature. Time trend analyses of the relationships between the proportion of individuals in the population who are obese and the preceding diet have found marked parallels between the increase in percentage of energy from fat and the subsequent increases in obesity (Lissner & Heitmann, 1995; Price, Charles, Pettitt, & Knowler, 1993; Sonne-Holm & Sorensen, 1977). However, several prospective studies of the general population have found that neither total calorie intake nor total fat intake was statistically associated with subsequent weight gain in either men or women (Colditz, Willett, Stampfer, London et al., 1990; Kant, Graubard, Schatzkin, & Ballard-Barbash, 1995). Other studies have found effects for macronutrient composition in women but not men (Klesges, Klesges, Haddock, & Eck, 1992b; Rissanen, Heliovaara, Knekt, Reunanen, & Aromaa, 1991).

These contradictory and often negative findings likely result from the limited techniques available for assessing diet in the general population. Weight gain of one kilogram a year would occur with increased calorie intake of just 20 calories per day, a level of precision that far exceeds current diet methods. Given this difficulty, the question arises as to whether the focus should be on energy density or on more practical characteristics of diet, such as the choice of specific foods or food groups.

Consumption of Sweets and High Fat Foods

Rather than examine associations between weight change and intake of macronutrients, several authors have estimated the associations between weight gain and intake of specific foods. For example, in the epidemiologic study of the European Prospective Investigation into Cancer and Nutrition (EPIC)-Potsdam cohort (Schulz et al., 2002), reported intake of food groups that were characterized by a high content of energy and fat, namely, cooking and spreading fats, sauces, meat and sweets, was found to be predictive of weight gain. Moreover, a clear gender difference in associations of food group intake with weight change was observed; in women, several high fat food groups were strongly related to weight gain, whereas among men, reported intake of sweets was the strongest predictor of weight gain.

Similar observations have been found in other studies. French et al. (1994) used data originally collected in worksites as part of randomized controlled intervention study of smoking cessation and weight control (i.e., the Healthy Worker Project). In both genders, consumption of sweets was associated with a modest increase in weight. In women, there was a direct association between weight gain and consumption of dairy products, meat, and especially French fries. In a Mediterranean cohort (Bes-Rastrollo et al., 2006), increased consumption of hamburgers, pizza, and sausages was associated with a higher risk of weight gain. Quatromoni et al. (2002) examined the non-overweight offspring/spouse cohort of women in the Framingham study. They found that women who ate a diet that was rich in sweets and fats with fewer servings of nutrient-dense fruits, vegetables, and lean food choices were at the highest risk for developing overweight, after adjusting for other known risk factors. Finally, in the Nurses Health Study, inverse associations were observed between intake of fruits and vegetables (He et al., 2004) and whole grain foods and fiber (Liu et al., 2003) and risk of subsequent obesity or weight gain.

These findings suggest that focusing on the food groups in the diet rather than total calories or overall fat intake may help in identifying predictors of weight gain and provide potential targets for prevention efforts.

Sugar-Sweetened Beverages

Coinciding with the increasing prevalence of obesity, soft drink consumption in the United States increased by 131% since 1977 (Putnam & Gerrior, 1999). This huge increase has contributed to the added sugars that now comprise 16% of total energy intake in the American diet. Soft drinks are the leading source of added sugars in the U.S. diet (Bray, Nielsen, & Popkin, 2004) and have been found to predict weight gain in several population studies. For example, in the 8-year follow-up of women in the Nurses Health Study (Schulz et al., 2004), positive associations between sugar-sweetened beverage consumption at baseline and greater weight gain and risk of type 2 diabetes was observed, independent of known risk factors. Similar findings have been reported elsewhere (Bes-Rastrollo et al., 2006).

Interestingly, low calorie soft drinks sweetened with artificial sweeteners do not appear to prevent weight gain. Several long-term epidemiological prospective studies have reported positive relationships between saccharin intake (Bolton-Smith & Woodward, 1994), or artificial sweeteners (Parker et al., 1997) and subsequent weight change. These finding suggests that artificial sweeteners may not prevent weight gain, but the apparent relationship is confounded by the fact that those choosing artificial sweeteners may have more of a susceptibility to weight gain.

Fast Food Consumption

Fast food is a growing component of the American diet, with a current estimate of about 247,115 restaurants in the U.S. (Tecnomic Information Services, 2002). Since 1970, fast food sales have increased by 300% (Sheridan & McPherrin, 1983). Recent studies have found that fast food consumption is related to weight gain in the general population. For example, among the 891 women in the Pound of Prevention study (French, Harnack, & Jeffery, 2000), frequency of fast food restaurant use was associated with a variety of other eating behaviors including, more frequent intake of hamburgers, French fries and soft drinks, less frequent intake of vegetables, less restrained eating, and fewer low-fat eating behaviors. Moreover, frequency of fast food restaurant use was prospectively associated with higher fat and energy intake and greater body weight. Increases in the frequency of fast food restaurant use were also associated with increases in body weight over a 3 y period, during which the average weight gain was 1.7 kg. Women in the highest tertile of fast food restaurant use gained an additional 0.72 kg more than women in the lowest tertile of fast food restaurant use.

Similarly, data from the CARDIA study also suggest an association between fast food consumption and later weight gain (Pereira et al., 2005). Over 15 years, change in fast food consumption was directly associated with changes in body weight. Those with frequent (more than twice a week) visits to fast-food restaurants at baseline and follow-up gained 4.5 kg more over 12 years than participants with infrequent (less than once a week) fast-food restaurant use at baseline and follow-up.

These findings suggest that frequent fast food restaurant use could be a risk factor for excess weight gain over time.

Physical Inactivity

In population-based studies, an inverse association between reported physical activity and body weight has been fairly consistently reported from both cross-sectional and longitudinal studies of older (Dannenberg, Keller, Wilson, & Castelli, 1989; DiPietro, Williamson, Caspersen, & Eaker, 1993; Folsom et al., 1985; French et al., 1994) and younger adult populations (Schmitz, Jacobs, Leon, Schreiner, & Sternfeld, 2000). Most studies reported an association between increases in physical activity and corresponding decreases in magnitude of weight gain. For example, in the young adults of the CARDIA cohort, the mean weight gain attenuation was about 1 kg per year for a modest increase in self-reported physical activity (Schmitz et al., 2000).

Studies examining baseline physical activity as predictors of subsequent weight gain have yielded less conclusive findings, perhaps partly because of differences in the type of physical activity assessment or study population. Klesges et al. (1992) found that, in women, participation in work and leisure time physical activities reported at baseline were inversely related to subsequent weight gain, as was increased work-related physical activity that occurred during the follow-up period. Williamson et al. (1993) found no association between baseline recreational physical activity and subsequent weight gain in the NHANES Follow Up Study. Thus, the predictive value of physical activity, as measured before the follow-up (at baseline), remains uncertain; however, change in physical activity is consistently associated with weight change.

TV Viewing

Television (TV) watching is a major sedentary behavior in the United States. In a survey conducted in 1997, adult males spent approximately 28 hours per week watching TV, and adult females spent 34 hours per week (Nielsen Media Research, 2000). In recent decades, in parallel with increasing obesity, there has been a steady increase in the number of homes with multiple TV sets, videocassette recorders (VCRs), cable TV, and remote controls, as well as the number of hours spent watching TV (Nielsen Media Research, 2000).

Several prospective, population-based studies have shown associations between TV viewing and subsequent weight gain. In the large prospective cohort of females in the Nurses Health Study (Hu, Li, Colditz, Willett, & Manson, 2003), sedentary behaviors, especially TV watching, were significantly associated with risk of obesity and type 2 diabetes. Employment in sedentary occupations, reflected by long hours of sitting or standing at work, was also significantly associated with risk of obesity. In contrast, even light activities such as standing or walking around at home and brisk walking were associated with a significantly lower risk of obesity and diabetes. The authors concluded that 30% of obesity cases could be potentially prevented by following a relatively active lifestyle (<10 h/wk TV watching). These findings are consistent with previous studies of TV watching in relation to obesity and weight gain in adults (Ching et al., 1996; Sidney et al., 1996; Tucker & Bagwell, 1991; Tucker & Friedman, 1989), suggesting that TV viewing may be another important target for prevention efforts.

Psychological Factors

Several psychological factors have also been identified as predictors of weight gain, including depression, anxiety, dietary restraint, dietary disinhibition, and weight cycling. In a study of 336 African American and Caucasian American women, randomly selected from among urban residents aged 35–47 years at baseline, depressed mood scores, anxiety, and reduced quality of life were the major predictors of gaining ≥10 lb over a 4 year period. These factors remained independent predictors of weight gain after adjusting for a variety of other demographic and lifestyle measures (e.g., age, diet, physical activity). Of note, depressive symptoms were the strongest predictor, with the odds of gaining ≥10 lb over the 4-year period being twice as high for subjects presenting with depressive symptoms compared to those without symptoms.

Several studies have also found that high levels of dietary disinhibition and low levels of dietary restraint may be important contributors to the current high levels of adult weight gain (Hays et al., 2002; Westenhoefer, Pudel, & Maus, 1990; Williamson, Lawson, & Brooks, 1995). However, whether these variables may be used to prospectively predict weight gain remains unclear. In a recent study of 466 adults living in France, Lauzon-Guillain et al. (Lauzon-Guillain et al., 2006) found that dietary restraint did not significantly predict subsequent 2-year weight change. By contrast, in a sample of 638 American women, Hays et al. (Hays et al., 2002) reported that high dietary restraint did appear to prevent subsequent weight gain over 10 years of follow-up, but only in those individuals with high levels of dietary disinhibition. Higher disinhibition was strongly associated with greater adult weight gain, and dietary restraint appeared to attenuate this association when disinhibition was high.

Dieting history has also been identified as a significant predictor of weight gain. For example, in a 6-year follow-up of risk factors for weight gain in twins, Korkeila et al. (1998) found that dieting at baseline in both men and women was associated with greater risk of subsequent weight gain. Other studies have reported similar findings (Bild et al., 1996; Colditz, Willett, Stampfer, Manson et al., 1990). These findings suggest that these individuals may be more prone to obesity and, despite dieting efforts, will experience the greatest weight gains over time.

Opportunities for Preventive Intervention

Since weight gain occurs commonly during adulthood and is associated with increased morbidity and mortality, it is important to develop interventions to prevent or reduce this weight gain. In the following section, we consider individual-level interventions that have been designed to reduce the incidence and magnitude of weight gain. One approach to such weight gain prevention efforts is to identify times that create a high risk for weight gain and then develop interventions for these times. College years, the period surrounding pregnancy, young adulthood (age 25–45), and menopause are examples of such times.

(a) *Intervention in college students.* Obesity in young adults has been increasing more quickly than in any other age group. Based on self-reported height and weight data collected in the National College Health Risk Behavior Survey, 35% of college students are overweight or obese (Lowry et al., 2000). In addition, weight gain occurs frequently in this age group. One large study of women 18 to 23 years of age at baseline found that after 4 years, only 44% maintained a BMI within 5% of their baseline BMI, whereas 41% gained weight; 15% lost weight (Ball, Brown, & Crawford, 2002).

College students may be an important group to target for weight gain prevention: two-thirds of students who graduated from high school in 2004 subsequently enrolled in colleges or universities (Bureau of Labor Statistics, 2005). Weight gain appears especially likely to occur in the first year of college. Average weight gain during the first semester of study for females has been reported to range from 1.3 kg to 3.1 kg (Anderson, Shapiro, & Lundgren, 2003; Levitsky, Halbmaier, & Mrdjenovic, 2004; Levitsky, Garay, Nausbaum, Neighbors, & Dellavalle, 2006; Lowe et al., 2006). When students are assessed at the end of the freshman year, similar amounts of weight gain have been reported, suggesting that the changes that occur during the first semester are not subsequently reversed (Cooley & Toray, 2001; Hovell, Mewborn, Randle, & Fowler-Johnson, 1985; Megal, Wade, Hawkins, & Norton, 1994). In one study of freshman women, 20% of weight gain could be attributed to eating in all-you-can-eat dining halls, 10% to evening snacks, and 12% to consumption of high fat foods (Levitsky et al., 2004). In the college environment, students prepare few of their meals themselves and many of the venues at which they eat offer individually-determined portions and high-energy density foods. The features of this environment or other aspects of the developmental transition to college or adulthood may increase the risk of weight gain dramatically.

Several characteristics of this time period may make it an opportune time for weight gain prevention efforts. Students entering college are excellent targets for weight gain prevention programs, as their adjustment to a new environment and increased independence offer a critical period for adoption of healthy eating and activity behaviors. At the same time, social and personal concerns about body weight that are common during this period could help motivate students to adopt and maintain eating and physical activity changes to prevent weight gain.

The effectiveness of several weight gain prevention programs for college students has been tested. These preliminary studies suggest that some minimal-intensity interventions can have a surprisingly powerful effect on weight gain during this time.

Weight monitoring is one such approach. Providing individuals with the tools necessary to monitor their weight requires relatively few resources, which is appealing because weight gain prevention programs that have demonstrated efficacy will likely need to be of low cost if they are to be widely disseminated. Most self-regulation theories consider self-monitoring, the systematic observation of target behaviors, an essential element of self-regulation (Kanfer & Karoly, 1972; Kirschenbaum, 1987). Research on self-monitoring has focused primarily on recording eating behaviors and food intake and, to a lesser extent, physical activity. Self-monitoring these behaviors is strongly associated with improved weight control (Baker & Kirschenbaum, 1998; Boutelle, Baker, Kirschenbaum, & Mitchell, 1999; Sperduto, Thompson, & O'Brien, 1986). Monitoring of body weight has also been associated with successful weight loss and weight maintenance (Wing & Hill, 2001; Linde, Jeffery, French, Pronk, & Boyle, 2005; Wadden et al., 2005).

Two experiments conducted by Levitsky, Garay, Nausbaum, Neighbors, and DellaValle (2006) demonstrated that weight-monitoring successfully reduced weight gain in female participants during the first semester of college. In these experiments, participants who were randomly assigned to the weight monitoring intervention were provided with bathroom scales and instructed to weigh themselves each morning immediately upon waking. Participants emailed their daily weights to research staff, who in turn emailed automated feedback about weight changes to the participants. A linear regression was performed on the most recent 7 days and information about weight change was provided to participants. In the first study, participants were simply provided with the slope of this linear regression line and instructions about how to interpret the slope (e.g., that a positive slope indicated weight gain). In the second study, the difference between initial weight and current weight was calculated and used to determine the values included in the following message, which was sent to participants: "In order for you to maintain the average weight of your first 7 days, you should [increase/decrease] your intake by __ calories."

In the first experiment, 32 participants were randomly assigned to the control or intervention condition. After 12 weeks, 15 of 16 participants in the control group and 11 of 16 in the intervention condition provided post-treatment data. At post-treatment, participants in the control group gained an average of 3.1 kg, whereas participants in the intervention group lost an average of 0.7 kg. In the second experiment, 41 participants were randomly assigned to the control or intervention condition. After 10 weeks, 16 of 24 participants in the control group provided post-treatment data and 16 of 17 participants in the experimental group did. Participants in the control group gained an average of 2.0 kg, while those in the weight monitoring intervention lost 0.8 kg. In both experiments, weight change between groups was significantly different.

Although the results obtained by Levitsky et al. (2006) are promising, the small sample size, attrition rates, and large weight gains in the control groups make these studies difficult to interpret. Moreover, these results were not replicated in another investigation of weight monitoring for college students. In that pilot study (Butryn, Lowe, & Marcowitz, 2005), normal weight, female freshmen were randomly assigned to one of the following intervention conditions: (1) an assessment-only control group (n = 21); (2) a weight monitoring intervention (n = 26); or (3) a weight monitoring plus healthy eating intervention (n = 23). Participants assigned to do weight monitoring were asked to weigh themselves daily using a digital scale that was provided to them and e-mail their weights to the researchers each day. Every seven days, each participant was given information via e-mail about her weight trajectory for the past week and for the period of time since enrolling in the study. Information consisted of the following: "Your weight increased/ decreased—pounds since last week, as depicted in graph A below. Your weight has increased/decreased _ pounds since the beginning of the Fall term, as depicted in graph B below." Participants in the weight monitoring plus healthy eating intervention were asked to follow all of the procedures for the weight monitoring, plus attend four, 1-hour group sessions that focused on increasing skills for healthy eating. The group sessions consisted of discussion of barriers to behavior change, goal setting, problem solving, and weekly homework assignments (e.g., keeping food records). At the end of the 8-week intervention period, 91% of participants completed post-intervention assessments. There was no evidence of differential weight gain between the control, weight monitoring, and weight monitoring plus healthy eating groups (1.0 kg, 1.2 kg, and 1.1 kg, respectively). However, positive changes in some weight control behaviors were observed in the weight monitoring plus healthy eating participants who were most compliant with intervention activities. Because of common concerns that promoting weight control behaviors could increase risk for eating disorders, this study also examined changes in disordered eating during the intervention period through both semi-structured clinical interview and self-report measures of body dissatisfaction and dieting behaviors, and also assessed mood. All measures indicated that the interventions did not have any iatrogenic effects on the young women enrolled in this study.

Psycho-education interventions have also been demonstrated to be surprisingly effective in college students. One study found that simply participating in a conventional one-semester college nutrition course that taught principles of human physiology, energy metabolism, and genetics could prevent weight gain in students who are most predisposed to overweight or obesity. Those with a BMI greater than 24 kg/m^2 lost an average of 0.6 kg at 1-year follow-up, whereas comparable participants in a control group gained 4.2 kg during the same period (Matvienko, Lewis, & Schafer, 2001).

Education focused on disordered eating also has been demonstrated to be effective for weight gain prevention in college students (Stice, Orjada, & Tristan, 2006). Participants were female undergraduates enrolled in a 15-week eating disorders seminar and matched comparison students. The seminar leader provided didactic material on eating disorders and led therapeutic discussions about topics such as internalization of the thin-ideal of beauty; critical viewing of mass media; and perceptions of weight, shape, and attractiveness norms. At both post-test and 6-month follow-up, intervention participants showed greater reductions in thin-ideal internalization, body dissatisfaction, and eating disorder symptoms than matched controls. There was a significant difference between groups for changes in BMI, based on self-reported weight and height. BMI increased significantly in the matched controls (by an average of 1.6 BMI units over the 10-month study period), whereas BMI did not change in the intervention subjects. These results are consistent with other studies with young women that have found that a brief intervention that promotes weight maintenance by building skills for healthy weight management can reduce the risk of obesity and level of disordered eating (Stice, Presnell, Groesz, & Shaw, 2005).

(b) *Intervention in young adults.* Since young adults, aged 20–44, are at high risk for weight gain, several interventions have targeted this group. The largest weight gain prevention study conducted to date was the Pound of Prevention Study reported by Jeffery and French (Jeffery & French, 1999). Extending an earlier study by Forster and colleagues (Forster, Jeffery, Schmid, & Kramer, 1988), these investigators recruited 228 men and 594 women employed at the University of Minnesota and 404 women of lower socioeconomic status (household income ≤$25,000/year). Participants were required to be age 20–45 and healthy. As noted above, young adults who are already overweight have high rates of weight gain with age. Therefore, no weight criterion was used since prevention of further weight gain was considered important even in already overweight individuals.

The Pound of Prevention Program utilized a public health model of a low intensity intervention that could be delivered inexpensively to large numbers of participants. Participants in Pound of Prevention were randomly assigned to a control group or to an intervention involving education only or education plus incentives. The education program emphasized regular weighing (at least once a week), eating more fruit (2 servings/day), eating more vegetables (3 servings/day), reducing consumption of high fat foods, and increasing exercise, particularly walking. These messages were delivered through monthly newsletters; a postcard was included with each newsletter asking participants to report their weight and to indicate whether in the last 24 hours, they had achieved each of the above goals. Other low-cost weight or exercise related activities were also offered over the 3-year program, but were used by few individuals. Both groups received the same education intervention; the participants in the intervention condition were also entered into a monthly $100 raffle if they returned their post cards. Thus, the intervention required no face-to-face or telephone contact.

At baseline, participants were an average of 38 years old, with a mean BMI of 26.6. Eighty percent were female, and over 90% were Caucasian. Participants were assessed annually and 72% completed data collection visits at baseline and 1, 2, and 3-year follow-up. On average, 68% of the newsletter postcards were returned; 25% of the intervention group members participated in at least 1 additional activity offered during the program.

Unfortunately, the intervention had no effect on weight gain. Participants gained 0.6 lb per year in each of the 3 conditions (total = 1.7 kg over the 3 years). Sixty-three percent of participants were above baseline at the end of the 3-year trial, with no differences among conditions. There was also no effect of treatment on reported caloric intake or physical activity. The primary effect was an increase in frequency of self-weighing in the intervention group compared to a decreased frequency in controls. However, correlational data supported the expected relationship between behavior change and weight change. Changes in reported intake, activity, frequency of weighing, and reported use of healthy weight control practices were all associated with weight change in the expected directions.

Other interventions for young adults have utilized more intensive approaches. However, a large randomized trial for women aged 25–44 that focused on weight gain prevention revealed many difficulties/obstacles to conducting such interventions (Levine et al., 2006).

First, recruitment for a trial focused on preventing weight gain proved quite difficult. Initially the study was designed for normal weight women with a BMI of 21–25; however the upper BMI criterion had to be increased to 30 in order to attract more participants. Even with this modification, it was necessary to screen 1,816 women to recruit 284 eligible participants. The major reasons for ineligibility (n = 837) were that the woman's BMI was too high or the woman was interested in weight loss (not weight gain prevention). In addition, after hearing about the study, 695 women were not interested in participation. Thus, it appears that these young women have little interest in weight gain prevention and are far more focused on weight loss.

The 284 women who were randomized were age 36 on average, with a mean BMI of 25; 42 % reported gaining weight during the past year and 32% were currently dieting. Again, these findings suggest that the program attracted mainly women who were interested in achieving weight loss, rather than preventing weight gain.

The women were randomly assigned to receive a clinic-based intervention, a correspondence program, or a newsletter control group. The two interventions were conducted over 2 years and were identical in content and frequency of contact. Both involved biweekly contacts for the first 2 months followed by bimonthly contacts. The interventions taught women to make modest changes in their diet and physical activity and encouraged self-monitoring of these behaviors. The program stressed regular self-weighing with increased therapist attention if weight gain was observed. Seventy two percent of the women completed the 3-year trial.

This study found no effect of the intervention on weight change at 1, 2 or 3 years. Weight gain over the 3 years averaged approximately .5 kg (which is somewhat lower than .5–1 kg/year gain typically seen in the general population). Women with a BMI of 25 or greater gained .2 + 5.2 kg over 3 years and those with a BMI <25 gained .9 + 4.8 kg. There was a trend (p = .10) for BMI to decrease more in the clinic based intervention than in the correspondence or control group at 2 years, but none of the other comparisons approached significance. Thus a second concern is the limited effect of intervention on prevention of weight gain.

Overall, 28% of the women lost 2 lbs or more over the 3-year trial; 12% stayed within 2 lbs, and 60% gained >2 lbs. Thus, another difficulty of such an intervention is that many women do not gain excessive amounts of weight and, thus, do not need this intervention. Moreover, it is hard to know ahead who is likely to gain weight and would benefit from such an intervention. The only baseline factors associated with subsequent weight change were age, hunger at baseline, and being on a diet at baseline. Women who were younger, felt more hunger, and were on a diet at baseline were more likely to gain weight over the 3-year trial. Again these findings suggest that weight gain prevention may be best focused on those who are already having difficulty with weight management as evidenced by their hunger and current use of a diet.

The age period of 25–44 poses the greatest risk for weight gain not only among women, but also among men. Weight gain occurs most commonly among men who are already somewhat overweight, making it important to try to prevent weight gain in both normal weight and slightly overweight individuals. Leermakers et al. (1998) studied 67 sedentary men with a BMI of 22–30. These participants were randomly assigned to a control condition or to receive a clinic based or correspondence based program. To try to be most responsive to the male participants, the intervention focused primarily on increasing physical activity; consuming a healthy diet, rather than calorie restriction, per se, was the other target of the intervention. The exercise goal was gradually increased over the course of the intervention, to a final goal of 3 miles/day on 4 days/week with exercise at 60–70% of maximum heart rate reserve. The diet intervention focused on lowering fat to less than 20% of calories. The intervention included 12 sessions over 4 months; the clinic based group attended 30-minute lessons followed by supervised walks or runs weekly for 8 weeks and then every other week for 8 weeks. The correspondence group attended an initial face-to-face meeting but subsequently were sent news- letters, asked to return homework by mail, and called weekly or bimonthly by therapy staff. Members of both intervention groups were eligible to receive small exercise incentives by meeting the physical activity goals.

The 4-month program was completed by 92.5% of subjects. Sixty-eight percent of the participants in the intervention condition lost weight or maintained their weight over the 4 months, compared to 38.9% of controls (p < .05). Actual weight changes were also greater in the clinic (−1.9 kg) and correspondence (−1.3 kg) interventions than in the control (+.22 kg). Although the two interventions produced comparable outcomes, the clinic-based group had better adherence to self-monitoring and to physical activity than the correspondence group. Of particular interest was the fact that the intervention was more effective in men with a BMI of 27–30 than in men with lower BMI. This study suggests that a weight gain prevention intervention targeting physical activity can be attractive and effective in young men; however, the program appeared to serve largely as a weight loss program for those who were moderately overweight.

(c) *Pregnant women.* Pregnancy represents another high-risk period for the development of obesity. Although on average women gain only about 2 kg as a result of a pregnancy, 25% will retain >5 kg one year after delivery (Greene, Smiciklas-Wright, Scholl, & Karp, 1988; Kac, Benicio, Velasquez-Melendez, Valente, & Struchiner, 2004; Keppel & Taffel, 1993; Ohlin & Rossner, 1990). Moreover, a recent study has found that nearly 44% of normal weight women who had retained significant amounts of weight (*M* = 4.8 kg) at 12 months postpartum became overweight later in life (Linne, Dye, & Rossner, 2004). Thus, intervening during the period surrounding pregnancy may be an effective approach to prevention of future obesity.

The strongest predictor of weight retention after pregnancy is the amount of weight gained during pregnancy (Gore, Brown, & Smith-West, 2003). The Institute of Medicine recommends that normal weight women (BMI of 19.8–26.0 kg/m^2) gain 25–35 lb (11.4–15.9 kg) during pregnancy, and that overweight women (BMI 26.1–29.0) gain 15–25 lb (6.8–11.4 kg) (Institute of Medicine, 1990). These recommendations are based on ensuring healthy fetal and maternal outcomes. However, large proportions of women exceed these weight gain recommendations (Keppel & Taffel, 1993; Olson, Strawderman, Hinton, & Pearson, 2003). Based on data from the National Maternal and Infant Health Survey (Keppel & Taffel, 1993), a representative sample of U.S. women with live births in 1988, 37% of normal weight women and 64% of overweight women exceed these goals. Women who exceed the weight gain recommendations retain twice as much weight as those who gain within the recommended level. In the National Maternal and Infant Health Survey (Keppel & Taffel, 1993) white women who exceeded the weight gain goal retained 2.2 kg at 10–18 months postpartum, whereas those who gained the recommended level retained only 0.7 kg. Weight retention was even greater among African Americans; those who exceeded the IOM levels retained 5.8 kg, and those who gained within the levels, retained 3.3 kg.

There are advantages and disadvantages to conducting a weight gain prevention intervention during pregnancy. The greatest disadvantage is that weight control efforts during this period must be carefully regulated to ensure optimal growth and safety for the fetus. Concern is raised about possible adverse effects of caloric restriction and vigorous exercise. Although few would argue with the benefits of promoting healthy eating choices and moderate lifestyle activity, the more intense approaches to weight control are often contraindicated. However, there are also some advantages to intervening during pregnancy when this can be done safely; this time period may well be a "teachable moment" when mothers are concerned about doing what is best for their baby. Healthy habits that mothers develop during pregnancy may also persist post-pregnancy.

To date, there have been few interventions designed to help women gain the appropriate amount of weight within pregnancy. Polley et al. (Polley, Wing, & Sims, 2002) recruited 120 women (on average, 25.5 years of age), who were <20 weeks gestation, and randomly assigned them to either a control condition that received usual care or to an intervention designed to help women stay within the IOM weight gain recommendations. The intervention included biweekly newsletters, which provided helpful information about healthy eating and exercise during pregnancy. In addition, after each clinic visit, women were sent a letter, which included a personalized weight gain graph, showing how the participant was doing compared to the recommendation. Those women who were gaining the appropriate amount received reinforcing messages. Those who were exceeding the weight gain goals were given additional counseling at regularly scheduled clinic visits or via phone using a stepped-care approach.

The intervention was effective in reducing the prevalence of excessive weight gain among the normal weight women. Among normal weight women, 58% of the control group exceeded the IOM recommendations compared to 33% of the intervention women (p < .05). Among overweight women, the effect was non-significant, but in the opposite direction. Thirty-two percent of the control women exceeded the IOM recommendation compared to 59% of intervention. Moreover, weight gain in pregnancy was highly related (r = 0.89) to postpartum weight retention. The intervention tested by Polley et al. (Polley et al., 2002) appeared to work by preventing excessive weight gain in the normal weight women. Once women exceeded the weight goals, the intervention was less effective in helping them "recover". This finding suggests that the less costly parts of the intervention, such as the newsletter and weight graphs, may have been more potent than the more costly stepped-care treatment components.

The findings related to obese participants are of concern and require further investigation. In this pilot study, the prevalence of excessive weight gain was very low in overweight women in the control group; only 32% of these women exceeded the goal compared to previous reports suggesting that two-thirds of overweight women exceed the goal. Thus the finding may have been due just to the small sample size in this study. Alternatively, intervening to promote appropriate weight gain during pregnancy may not be positively received by overweight women and may cause them to gain more. Replication of this study with a larger sample size is clearly warranted to re-examine the effects of the intervention in both normal and overweight women.

(d) *Postpartum women*. Gestational weight gain and weight gain during the year postpartum are both independently related to the risk of subsequent weight gain and development of obesity at 10–15 year follow-up (Linne et al., 2004; Rooney & Schauberger, 2002). As described above, interventions during pregnancy can be effective in helping women gain an appropriate amount of weight and thus reduce postpartum weight retention. However, given the safety concerns about interventions during pregnancy, intervening after childbirth and helping women lose the weight they have gained is an important alternative approach. In addition, this approach can address factors related to weight gain during the year postpartum.

Greater weight retention among African American compared to white women has been documented, for example, in the CARDIA study data (Smith et al., 1994). Findings are mixed on the mechanism for this effect of ethnicity on postpartum weight retention (Boardley, Sargent, Coker, Hussey, & Sharpe, 1995; Gore et al., 2003; Gunderson, Abrams, & Selvin, 2000; Wolfe, Sobal, Olsen, Frongillo, & Williamson, 1997), that is, whether it is due to confounding factors, such as socioeconomic status or stress or to culturally-mediated behavioral influences (Gore et al., 2003). Changes in the amount of food eaten and low levels of physical activity have also been associated with postpartum weight gain (Olson et al., 2003). Although breastfeeding is considered an important factor in helping women return to pre-pregnancy weights, the research on the effects of breastfeeding is quite inconsistent (Boardley et al., 1995; Brewer, Bates, & Vannoy, 1989; Gore et al., 2003; Harris, Ellison, Hollliday, & Lucassen, 1997; Muscati, Gray-Donald, & Koski, 1996; Parker & Abrams, 1993; Thorsdottir & Birgisdottir, 1998). In addition, the sooner mothers return to work the less weight they retain at 6 months postpartum (Schauberger, Rooney, & Brimer, 1990), perhaps because employment reduces their exposure to food cues in the home.

Intervening in the postpartum period is problematic because women are typically very busy and attending group meetings is therefore difficult. Consequently, correspondence approaches may be most appropriate. Leermakers et al. (Leermakers, Anglin, & Wing, 1998) recruited 90 women who had delivered within the past 3–12 months and currently exceeded their prepregnancy weight by at least 6.8 kg. These women were randomly assigned to a no-treatment control group or to a 6-month correspondence behavioral weight loss program. The intervention included 2 face-to-face group sessions, 16 written lessons which were mailed weekly or biweekly, and brief phone contacts. The lessons helped women learn to adopt a low calorie, low fat eating plan and to increase their physical activity; all lessons were tailored to the special needs of new mothers.

The 6-month assessments were completed by 62 of the 90 women (69%). Women in the correspondence group lost 7.8 kg over the 6 months compared to 4.9 kg in the control group. Moreover, correspondence subjects lost 79% of their excess postpartum weight and 33% returned to (or below) their prepregnancy weight. In contrast the control group lost only 44% of their excess weight and 11.5% returned to their prepregnancy weight.

The substantial weight losses achieved in this study suggest that the postpartum period may be a good time for intervention. However, the attrition rate (27%) was relatively high, and women in the intervention group returned only 10 of the 25 self-monitoring records. These findings suggest that adherence to even a correspondence-based weight loss program may be difficult in the postpartum period. In addition, 5 women became pregnant again during this trial, another limitation of intervening at this time in a women's life.

(e) *Perimenopausal women* The most successful intervention for weight gain prevention was reported by Kuller and colleagues (Kuller, Simkin-Silverman, Wing, Meilahn, & Ives, 2000; Simkin-Silverman, Wing, Boraz, & Kuller, 2003). This intervention focused on the menopausal transition period and targeted both weight and LDL cholesterol levels. Epidemiological studies have shown that women aged 44–50 gain approximately .7 kg per year. This weight gain appears to be due primarily to age-related, rather than to the menopause per se, with decreases in physical activity being the strongest predictor of weight gain (Owens, Matthews, Wing, & Kuller, 1992; Wing, Matthews, Kuller, Meilahn, and Plantinga, 1991). The increase in body weight in menopausal women is associated with increased central adiposity and worsening in cardiovascular disease risk factors (Matthews et al., 1989); thus efforts to prevent this weight gain would have an important health impact.

The Women's Healthy Lifestyle Project (Kuller, et al., 2000; Simkin-Silverman et al., 2003) was designed to prevent weight gain and increases in LDL-cholesterol during the menopausal transition. A total of 535 women, who were aged 44–50, premenopausal, with a BMI of 20–34 and with normal cholesterol, blood pressure, and glucose were recruited. The women were randomly assigned to an assessment-only control group or lifestyle intervention condition. The intervention was far more intensive than the other weight-gain prevention approaches described above. The intervention involved 15 group meetings over the first 20 weeks. In addition, women were given a weight loss goal in order to prevent any weight gain above baseline. Women who were normal weight (BMI 20–24) were encouraged to lose 5 lbs (2.2 kg); those with a BMI of 25–26 were encouraged to lose 10 lbs (4.5 kg) and those with a BMI $\geq$27 were encouraged to lose 15 lbs (6.8 kg). To accomplish these weight losses, the women were prescribed a specific meal plan (1,300 kcal/day, 25% of calories from fat with 7% from saturated fat and 100 mg cholesterol) for the first month of this trial. Subsequently the women modified the plan to accommodate their personal preferences. Women were also encouraged to gradually increase their physical activity to 1,000–1,500 kcal/week. Standard behavioral strategies were utilized throughout the program.

From month 6 to 54 of the program, women attended periodic group meetings, with 6-week refresher programs and mail and phone contact. Women who were experiencing increased weight or LDL cholesterol, or decreased physical activity were offered 3–6 individual sessions to help them reinstate their behavior changes.

The mean weight loss in the intervention group was .01 $\pm$ 5.2 kg at 54 months, compared with an average gain of 2.4 $\pm$ 4.9 kg in the control group. Moreover, 55% of the intervention group were at or below baseline after 4.5 years compared with 26% of controls.

The intervention was effective in increasing the level of physical activity and changing dietary intake. At 54 months, the intervention group reported higher physical activity (due primarily to increased walking), and lower calorie and dietary fat intake. Moreover, weight changes within the intervention group were associated with changes in physical activity and fat intake. Specifically, the quartile of women who reported the largest weight losses (-3.2 to -17 kg) had increases of physical activity of 565 kcal/week and an 8.9% decrease in percent of calories from fat. In contrast, the quartile of women with greatest weight gains (2.5–25.1 kg) reported decreased physical activity (-90 kcal/week) and decreases in percent of calories from fat of only 4.4%.

Women in the Women's Healthy Lifestyle Project (WHLP) were asked to complete measures of dietary restraint, perceived stress, depressive symptoms, and binge eating at baseline and 6 months. Women in the intervention group reported more favorable changes than control women on measures of depressive symptoms and perceived stress. Normal weight women and overweight women experienced comparable positive changes on these measures. This is of interest since normal weight women in the intervention group achieved a mean weight loss of 8 lb at 6 months (Klem, Wing, Simkin-Silverman, & Kuller, 1997) and thus provide a good test of the hypothesis that a focus on weight loss among normal weight women might have iatrogenic effects. Scores on the Binge Eating Scale also declined in both normal weight and overweight women and in both the intervention and control groups; overweight women in the intervention group experienced the greatest improvements, but normal weight women also experienced improvements (not worsening) in these symptoms. At baseline .05% of control subjects and 1.8% of intervention subjects were classified as binge eaters; at 6 months, .05% of both conditions were classified as binge eaters. Thus this more intensive intervention to prevent weight gain during the menopausal transition produced positive changes in weight, eating and activity, and psychological parameters, with no evidence of any adverse effects.

Research Directions

Adult weight gain is clearly of concern. It has been well documented that, on average, there is about a .5–1 kg gain per year (Lewis et al., 2000; Williamson et al., 1990) that is associated with worsening of CVD risk factors (Manson et al., 1990; Manson et al., 1995). However, our review suggests that most interventions designed to prevent or reduce this weight gain have been unsuccessful. In this section, we will consider several possible explanations for the failure to demonstrate greater effectiveness of these interventions.

Increasing Program Effect Size

One explanation is that the sample sizes used in these studies are not sufficient to detect differences between conditions. In the largest weight gain prevention study to date, Jeffery et al. (Jeffery & French, 1999) found that the control group had a 1.8 kg weight gain over 3 years with a standard deviation of 6.5 kg. To detect a 50% reduction in magnitude of gain (i.e. 0.9 kg weight gain in the intervention group) would require a sample size of over 700/group. In order to reduce the required sample size, it is necessary to either increase the difference between the weight gain of the treatment and control group and/or reduce the standard deviation of weight change. Thus, using the above example, if treatment was successful in preventing weight gain (i.e., achieved 0 lb average weight gain), only 200 subjects per group would be required.

Since the goal of weight gain prevention studies is to reduce the magnitude of weight gain (and not to produce weight loss), it is difficult to detect the difference between the treatment and control group if the control group gains only 1.8 kg on average. One solution to this problem is to make prevention studies longer. With longer studies, the control group would be expected to experience larger average weight gains and there would be more opportunity to see mean differences between groups. In a 10-year trial, for example, the average weight gains might be 5–10 kg, and (assuming the standard deviations of weight gain remained the same), a 50% reduction in magnitude of weight gain could be detected with sample sizes of 50 to 100 subjects.

Another approach to the sample size problem is to somehow reduce the variability in weight gain, perhaps by better selecting those individuals who are expected to gain large amounts. In the Jeffery study (Jeffery & French, 1999), weight changes over 3 years ranged from − 45 kg to + 30 kg. Forty percent of the control group remained at or below baseline at study end and, thus, did not need a weight gain prevention effort. Identifying individuals who will gain large amounts of weight and focusing our weight gain prevention efforts on these individuals would reduce the number of individuals we need to study.

Alternatively, weight gain prevention efforts could target time periods where the weight gain averages more than 5 kg a year and affects a greater proportion of the population. Freshman year in college and the period surrounding pregnancy are such time periods. Other time periods where larger weight gain would be expected include the year following smoking cessation and the years following successful weight loss. On average, individuals gain 3.3 kg after stopping smoking (D. F. Williamson et al., 1991). There have been several interventions designed to reduce weight gain after smoking cessation (Hall, Tunstall, Vila, & Duffy, 1992; Perkins et al., 2001; Pirie et al., 1992; Spring, Doran, Pagoto, Schneider, & Pigitore, 2004). However, evidence has been mixed regarding whether weight control intervention combines efficaciously with smoking cessation treatment. In some of the interventions, emphasizing weight gain prevention led to poorer rates of smoking cessation (Hall et al., 1992). Likewise, in weight control interventions, participants lose weight for approximately 6 months and then typically begin to regain; on average, individuals regain one third of their weight loss within the next year (Wadden & Foster, 2000). A number of intervention strategies have been tested as ways to minimize this weight regain after intentional weight loss (Perri & Corsica, 2002; Wing, 2004), but further research in this area is clearly needed.

Behavioral Targets

Another explanation for the limited results could be that the interventions used thus far may have focused on the wrong behavioral targets. The observational studies on weight gain have shown consistent associations between specific eating behaviors and weight gain (e.g. fast food consumption) but have not found significant associations with overall caloric intake. In contrast, intervention studies have typically targeted overall caloric intake. Is this a mistake? Unfortunately, there are limited data to address this question. The Pound of Prevention Study (Jeffery & French, 1999) is the only study that used more specific behavioral intervention targets; this study found no effects of the intervention on weight gain. However, Pound of Prevention presented these strategies through newsletters, rather than face-to-face meetings, and this low-intensity approach may have weakened the effects. It remains unclear whether specific behavior changes, such as decreasing fast food consumption, will be sufficient to prevent weight gain. Theoretically, they should be; since the average weight gain is only .5 – 1 kg per year, a decrease of 10–20 calories/day should be sufficient. However, it would be very easy for people to slightly increase other sources of caloric intake and thereby reduce the efficacy of this change. Thus far, weight gain prevention studies that have given participants specific calorie goals for intake and activity and recommended much larger calorie reductions (approximately 500–1,000 calories/day reductions in intake and 1,500 kcal/week increases in activity) have been the most successful in preventing weight gain.

Program Intensity

Along with the issue of the magnitude and type of behavior change that is recommended is the question of the intensity of the approach. The weight gain prevention trials cited above, and those that have used population-level approaches directed at whole communities, schools, or worksites (Schmitz & Jeffery, 2002), have had very limited effects. Far better results occur with more intensive approaches. Of note is the fact that Kuller's study (Kuller, et al., 2000) is the only large weight gain prevention study to show significant differences between treatments at 3–5 years. We strongly recommend that further research on weight gain prevention adopt this model. Key elements of the intervention were as follows: Participants attended 15 group meetings over 15 weeks; all participants (even normal weight individuals) were encouraged to lose weight (5–15 pounds) to prevent anticipated weight gain; the intervention included a caloric intake goal of 1,000 kcal below baseline, an exercise goal of 150 minutes per week, and training in behavioral strategies; participants who experienced weight gains over the follow-up received more intensive individualized treatment. This intensive level of intervention produced maintenance of body weight; on average the intervention condition had a mean weight loss of −.01 kg.

Summary and Implications

Given the prevalence of weight gain during adulthood and its negative health consequences, successful approaches for preventing weight gain are urgently needed. As reviewed in this chapter, key factors to consider in designing obesity prevention interventions include:

• Targeting specific subgroups of individuals at risk of major weight gain, including young adults, minority populations, and/or individuals of low socioeconomic status;

- Targeting specific behavioral factors shown to predict major weight gain, including food groups in the diet, sugar-sweetened beverages, fast food consumption, and TV viewing;
- Intervening during critical times that create high risk for weight gain, including college, pregnancy/postpartum, and perimenopause.

Although minimal-intensity interventions have been found to work in some subgroups of the population (e.g., weight monitoring in college students), at present, it appears that the goal of weight gain prevention in the general population will not be as simple as some might have anticipated; rather intensive approaches may be needed to help adults remain weight stable and healthy as they age. Further studies are needed to develop and test such approaches.

References

Anderson, D. A., Shapiro, J. R., & Lundgren, J. D. (2003). The freshman year of college as a critical period for weight gain: An initial evaluation. *Eating Behaviors*, *4*(4), 363–367.

Baker, R. C., & Kirschenbaum, D. S. (1998). Weight control during the holidays: Highly consistent self-monitoring as a potentially useful coping mechanism. *Health Psychology*, *17*(4), 367–370.

Ball, K., Brown, W., & Crawford, D. (2002). Who does not gain weight? Prevalence and predictors of weight maintenance in young women. *International Journal of Obesity and Related Metabolic Disorders*, *26*(12), 1570–1578.

Bes-Rastrollo, M., Sanchez-Villegas, A., Gomez-Garcia, E., Martinez, J. A., Parjares, R. M., & Martinez-Gonzalez, M. A. (2006). Predictors of weight gain in a Mediterranean cohort: The Seguimiento Universidad de Navarra Study. *American Journal of Clinical Nutrition*, *83*, 362–370.

Bild, D. E., Sholinksy, P., Smith, D. E., Lewis, C. E., Hardin, J. M., & Burke, G. L. (1996). Correlates and predictors of weight loss in young adults: The CARDIA study. *International Journal of Obesity*, *20*, 47–55.

Boardley, D. J., Sargent, R. G., Coker, A. L., Hussey, J. R., & Sharpe, P. A. (1995). The relationship between diet, activity, and other factors, and postpartum weight change. *Obstetrics and Gynecolology*, *86*, 834–838.

Bolton-Smith, C., & Woodward, M. (1994). Dietary composition and fat to sugar ratios in relation to obesity. *International Journal of Obesity*, *18*(12), 820–828.

Bouchard, C., & Perusse, L. (1996). Current status of the human obesity gene map. *Obesity Research*, *4*, 80–89.

Boutelle, K., Baker, R., Kirschenbaum, D., & Mitchell, M. (1999). How can obese weight controllers minimize weight gain during the high risk holiday season? By self-monitoring very consistently. *Health Psychology*, *18*(4), 364–368.

Bray, G. A., Nielsen, S. J., & Popkin, B. M. (2004). Consumption of high-fructose corn syrup in beverages may play a role in the epidemic of obesity. *American Journal of Clinical Nutrition*, *79*, 537–543.

Brewer, M. M., Bates, M. R., & Vannoy, L. P. (1989). Postpartum changes in maternal weight and body fat deposits in lactating versus nonlactating women. *American Journal of Clinical Nutrition*, *49*, 259–265.

Bureau of Labor Statistics. (2005). College enrollment and work activity of 2004 high school graduates.

Butryn, M. L., Lowe, M. R., & Marcowitz, J. T. (2005). *A randomized trial of weight gain prevention interventions in young women*. Vancouver, BC: North American Association for the Study of Obesity.

Ching, P. I. Y. H., Willett, W. C., Rimm, E. B., Colditz, G. A., Gortmaker, S. L., & Stampfer, M. J. (1996). Activity level and risk of overweight in male health professionals. *American Journal of Public Health, 86*(1), 25–30.

Colditz, G. A., Willett, W. C., Stampfer, M. J., London, S. J., Segal, M. R., & Speizer, F. E. (1990). Patterns of weight change and their relation to diet in a cohort of healthy women. *American Journal of Clinical Nutrition, 51*, 1100–1105.

Colditz, G. A., Willett, W. C., Stampfer, M. J., Manson, J. E., Hennekens, C. H., Arky, R. A., & Speizer, F. E. (1990). Weight as a risk factor for clinical diabetes in women. *American Journal of Epidemiology, 132*, 501–513.

Cooley, E., & Toray, T. (2001). Body image and personality predictors of eating disorder symptoms during the college years. *International Journal of Eating Disorders, 30*(1), 28–36.

Dannenberg, A. L., Keller, J. B., Wilson, P. W. F., & Castelli, W. P. (1989). Leisure time physical activity in the Framingham Offspring Study. Description, seasonal variation, and risk factor correlates. *American Journal of Epidemiology, 129*, 76–88.

Dey, A. N., & Lucas, J. W. (2006). Physical and mental health characteristics of U.S. –and foreign-born adults: United States, 1998-2003. *Adv Data* (369), 1–19.

DiPietro, L., Williamson, D. F., Caspersen, C. J., & Eaker, E. (1993). The descriptive epidemiology of selected physical activities and body weight among adults trying to lose weight: The Behavioral Risk Factor Surveillance System survey, 1989. *International Journal of Obesity and Related Metabolic Disorders, 17*(2), 69–76.

Flegal, K. M., Carroll, M. D., Ogden, C. L., & Johnson, C. L. (2002). Prevalence and trends in obesity among US adults, 1999-2000. *JAMA, 288*(14), 1723–1727.

Folsom, A. R., Caspersen, C. J, Taylor, H. L., Jacobs, D. R., Luepker, R. V., Gomez-Marin, O., Gillum, R. F., & Blackburn, H. (1985). Leisure time physical activity and its relationship to coronary risk factors in a population-based sample. The Minnesota Heart Survey. *American Journal of Epidemiology, 121*, 570–579.

Forster, J. L., Jeffery, R. W., Schmid, T. L., & Kramer, M. (1988). Preventing weight gain in adults: A pound of prevention. *Health Psychology, 7*, 515–525.

French, S. A., Harnack, L., & Jeffery, R. W. (2000). Fast food restaurant use among women in the Pound of Prevention study: Dietary, behavioral and demographic correlates. *International Journal of Obesity, 24*(10), 1353–1359.

French, S. A., Jeffery, R. W., Forster, J. L., McGovern, P. G., Kelder, S. H., & Baxter, J. (1994). Predictors of weight change over two years among a population of working adults: The Healthy Worker Project. *International Journal of Obesity and Related Metabolic Disorders, 18*, 145–154.

Goel, M. S., McCarthy, E. P., Phillips, R. S., & Wee, C. C. (2004). Obesity among US immigrant subgroups by duration of residence. *JAMA, 292*(23), 2860–2867.

Gore, S., Brown, D. M., & Smith-West, D. (2003). The role of postpartum weight retention in obesity among women: A review of evidence. *Annals of Behavioral Medicine, 26*(2), 149–159.

Greene, G. W., Smiciklas-Wright, H., Scholl, T. O., & Karp, R. J. (1988). Postpartum weight change: How much of the weight gained in pregnancy will be lost after delivery? *Obstetrics and Gynecolology, 71*, 701–707.

Gunderson, E. P., Abrams, B., & Selvin, S. (2000). The relative importance of gestational gain and maternal characteristics associated with the risk of becoming overweight after pregnancy. *International Journal of Obesity and Related Metabolic Disorders, 24*(12), 1660–1668.

Hall, S. M., Tunstall, C. D., Vila, K. L., & Duffy, J. (1992). Weight gain prevention and smoking cessation: Cautionary findings. *American Journal of Public Health, 82*(6), 799–803.

Harris, H. E., Ellison, G. T. H., Hollliday, M., & Lucassen, E. (1997). The impact of pregnancy on the long term weight gain of primiparous women in England. *International Journal of Obesity and Related Metabolic Disorders, 21*, 747–755.

Hays, N. P., Bathalon, G. P., McCrory, M. A., Roubenoff, R., Lipman, R., & Roberts, S. B. (2002). Eating behavior correlates of adult weight gain and obesity in healthy women aged 55–65 y. *American Journal of Clinical Nutrition, 75*, 476–486.

He, K., Hu, F. B., Colditz, G. A., Manson, J. E., Willett, W. C., & Liu, S. (2004). Changes in intake of fruits and vegetables in relation to risk of obesity and weight gain among middle-aged women. *International Journal of Obesity, 28*, 1569–1574.

Hedley, A. A., Ogden, C. L., Johnson, C. L., Carroll, M. D., Curtin, L. R., & Flegal, K. M. (2004). Prevalence of overweight and obesity among US children, adolescents, and adults, 1999–2002. *Journal of the American Medical Association, 291*(23), 2847–2850.

Hovell, M. F., Mewborn, C. R., Randle, Y., & Fowler-Johnson, S. (1985). Risk of excess weight gain in university women: A three-year community controlled analysis. *Addictive Behaviors, 10*(1), 15–28.

Hu, F. B., Li, T. Y., Colditz, G. A., Willett, W. C., & Manson, J. E. (2003). Television watching and other sedentary behaviors in relation to risk of obesity and type 2 diabetes mellitus in women. *Journal of the American Medical Association, 289*(14), 1785–1791.

Institute of Medicine. (1990). *Subcommittee on nutritional status and weight gain during pregnancy. Nutrition during pregnancy.* Washington, DC: National Academy of Sciences.

Jeffery, R., & French, S. (1999). Preventing weight gain in adults: The pound of prevention study. *American Journal of Public Health, 89*(5), 747–751.

Kac, G., Benicio, M. H., Velasquez-Melendez, G., Valente, J. G., & Struchiner, C. J. (2004). Gestational weight gain and prepregnancy weight influence postpartum weight retention in a cohort of Brazilian women. *Journal of Nutrition, 134*(3), 661–666.

Kanfer, F. H., & Karoly, P. (1972). Self-control: A behavioristic excursion into the lion's den. *Behavior Therapy, 3*, 398–416.

Kant, A. K., Graubard, B. I., Schatzkin, A., & Ballard-Barbash, R. (1995). Proportion of energy intake from fat and subsequent weight change in the NHANES I Epidemiologic follow-up study. *Journal of Clinical Nutrition, 61*, 11–17.

Keppel, K., & Taffel, S. (1993). Pregnancy -related weight gain and retention: Implications of the 1990 Institute of Medicine guidelines. *American Journal of Public Health, 83*, 1100–1103.

Kirschenbaum, D. S. (1987). Self-regulatory failure: A review with clinical implications. *Clinical Psychology Review, 7*, 77–104.

Klem, M. L., Wing, R. R., Simkin-Silverman, L., & Kuller, L. H. (1997). The psychological consequences of weight gain prevention in healthy, premenopausal women. *International Journal of Eating Disorders, 21*(2), 167–174.

Klesges, R. C., Klesges, L. M., Haddock, C. K., & Eck, L. H. (1992). A longitudinal analysis of the impact of dietary intake and physical activity on weight change in adults. *American Journal of Clinical Nutrition, 55*, 818–822.

Korkeila, M., Kaprio, J., Rissanen, A., Koskenvuo, M., & Sorensen, T. I. A. (1998). Predictors of major weight gain in adult Finns: Stress, life satisfaction and personality traits. *International Journal of Obesity Related Metabolic Disorders, 22*(10), 949–957.

Kuller, L. H., Simkin-Silverman, L. R., Wing, R. R., Meilahn, E. N., Ives, D. G. (2000). Women's healthy lifestyle project; A randomized clinical trial. *Circulation, 1*(103), 32–37.

Lahmann, P. H., Lissner, L., Gullberg, B., & Berglund, G. (2000). Sociodemographic factors associated with long-term weight gain, current body fatness and central adiposity in Swedish women. *International Journal of Obesity, 24*(6), 685–694.

Lauderdale, D. S., & Rathouz, P. J. (2000). Body mass index in a US national sample of Asian Americans: Effects of nativity, years since immigration and socioeconomic status. *International Journal of Obesity and Related Metabolic Disorders, 24*(9), 1188–1194.

Lauzon-Guillain, B., Basdevant, A., Romon, M., Karlsson, J., Borys, J. M., & Charles, M. A. (2006). Is restrained eating a risk factor for weight gain in a general population? *American Journal of Clinical Nutrition, 83*, 132–138.

Leermakers, E. A., Anglin, K., & Wing, R. R. (1998). Reducing postpartum weight retention through a correspondence intervention. *International Journal of Obesity, 22*, 1103–1109.

Leermakers, E. A., Jakicic, J. M., Viteri, J., & Wing, R. R. (1998). Clinic-based vs. home-based interventions for preventing weight gain in men. *Obesity Research, 6*(5), 346–352.

Levine, M. D., Klem, M. L., Kalarchian, M. A., Wing, R. R., Weissfeld, L., Qin, L., et al. (2007). Weight gain prevention among women. *Obesity, 15*(5): 1267–1277.

Levitsky, D. A., Garay, J., Nausbaum, M., Neighbors, L., & Dellavalle, D. M. (2006). Monitoring weight daily blocks the freshman weight gain: A model for combating the epidemic of obesity. *International Journal of Obesity, 30*(6), 1003–1010.

Levitsky, D. A., Halbmaier, C. A., & Mrdjenovic, G. (2004). The freshman weight gain: A model for the study of the epidemic of obesity. *International Journal of Obesity and Related Metabolic Disorders, 28*(11), 1435–1442.

Lewis, C. E., Jacobs, D. R., & McCreath, H. (2000). Weight gain continues in the 1990s: 10-year trends in weight and overweight from the CARDIA study. Coronary Artery Risk Development in Young Adults. *American Journal of Epidemiology, 151*, 1172–1181.

Linde, J. A., Jeffery, R. W., French, S. A., Pronk, N. P., & Boyle, R. G. (2005). Self-weighing in weight gain prevention and weight loss trials. *Annals of Behavioral Medicine, 30*(3), 210–216.

Linne, Y., Dye, L., & Rossner, S. (2004). Long-term weight development in women: A 15-year follow-up of the effects of pregnancy. *Obesity Research, 12*(7), 1116–1178.

Lissner, L., & Heitmann, B. L. (1995). Dietary fat and obesity: Evidence from epidemiology. *European Journal of Clinical Nutrition, 49*, 79–90.

Liu, S., Willett, W. C., Manson, J. E., Hu, F. B., Rosner, B., & Colditz, G. A. (2003). Relation between changes in intakes of dietary fiber and grain products and changes in weight and development of obesity among middle-aged women. *American Journal of Clinical Nutrition, 78*, 920–927.

Lowe, M. R., Annunziato, R. A., Markowitz, J. T., Didie, E., Bellace, D. L., Riddell, L., et al. (2006). Multiple types of dieting prospectively predict weight gain during the freshman year of college. *Appetite, 47*(1): 83–90.

Lowry, R., Galuska, D. A., Fulton, J. E., Wechsler, H., Kann, L., & Collins, J. L. (2000). Physical activity, food choice, and weight management goals and practices among US college students. *American Journal of Preventive Medicine, 18*(1), 18–27.

Manson, J. E., Colditz, G. A., Stampfer, M. J., Willett, W. C., Rosner, B., Monson, R. R., et al. (1990). A prospective study of obesity and risk of coronary heart disease in women. *New England Journal of Medicine, 322*, 882–889.

Manson, J. E., Willett, W. C., Stampfer, M. J., Colditz, G. A., Hunter, D. J., Hankinson, S. E. et al. (1995). Body weight and mortality among women. *New England Journal of Medicine, 333*(11), 677–685.

Matthews, K. A., Meilahn, E., Kuller, L. H., Kelsey, S. F., Caggiula, A. W., & Wing, R. R. (1989). Menopause and risk factors for coronary heart disease. *New England Journal of Medicine, 321*, 641–646.

Matvienko, O., Lewis, D. S., & Schafer, E. (2001). A college nutrition science course as an intervention to prevent weight gain in female college freshmen. *Journal of Nutrition and Education, 33*(2), 95–101.

Megal, M. E., Wade, F., Hawkins, P., & Norton, J. (1994). Health promotion, self-esteem, and weight among female college freshman. *Health Values, 18*, 10–19.

Muscati, S. K., Gray-Donald, K., & Koski, K. G. (1996). Timing of weight gain during pregnancy: Promoting fetal growth and minimizing maternal weight retention. *Obstetrics and Gynecolology*, *86*, 834–838.

National Center for Health Statistics/Division of Data Services. (2005). "Health, United States, 2005 with chartbook on trends in the health of Americans www.cdc.gov/nchs/data/hus/hus05.pdf#chartbookontrends.

Nielsen Media Research. (2000). 2000 *Report on Television: The First 50 Years*. New York: AC Nielsen Co.

Ohlin, A., & Rossner, J. (1990). Maternal body weight development after pregnancy. *International Journal of Obesity and Related Metabolic Disorders*, *14*, 159–173.

Olson, C. M., Strawderman, M. S., Hinton, P. S., & Pearson, T. A. (2003). Gestational weight gain and postpartum behaviors associated with weight change from early pregnancy to 1 y postpartum. *International Journal of Obesity*, *27*, 117–127.

Owens, J. F., Matthews, K. A., Wing, R. R., & Kuller, L. H. (1992). Can physical activity mitigate the effects of aging in middle-aged women? *Circulation*, *85*, 1265-1270.

Parker, D. R., Gonzalez, S., Derby, C. A., Gans, K. M., Lasater, T. M., & Carleton, R. A. (1997). Dietary factors in relation to weight change among men and women from two southeastern New England communities. *International Journal of Obesity*, *21*, 103–109.

Parker, J. D., & Abrams, B. (1993). Differences in postpartum weight retention between black and white mothers. *Obstetrics and Gynecolology*, *81*, 768–774.

Pereira, M. A., Kartashov, A. B., Ebbeling, C. B., Van Horn, L., Slattery, M. L., Jacobs, D. R.et al. (2005). Fast-food habits, weight gain, and insulin resistance (the CARDIA study): 15-year prospective analysis. *Lancet*, *365*, 36–42.

Perkins, K. A., Marcus, M. D., Levine, M. D., D'Amico, D., Miller, A., & Broge, M. (2001). Cognitive-behavioral therapy to reduce weight concerns improves smoking cessation outcome in weight-concerned women. *Journal of Consulting and Clinical Psychology*, *69*, 604–613.

Perri, M. G., & Corsica, J. A. (2002). Improving maintenance of weight loss in behavioral treatment of obesity. In T. A. Wadden & A. J. Stunkard (Eds.), *Handbook of obesity treatment*. New York: The Guilford Press.

Pirie, P. L., McBride, C. M., Hellerstedt, W., Jeffery, R. W., Hatsukami, D., Allen, S., et al. (1992). Smoking cessation in women concerned about weight. *American Journal of Public Health*, *82*, 1238–1243.

Polley, B. A., Wing, R. R., & Sims, C. J. (2002). Randomized controlled trial to prevent excessive weight gain in pregnant women. *International Journal of Obesity and Related Metabolic Disorders*, *26*, 1494–1502.

Price, R. A., Charles, M. A., Pettitt, D. J., & Knowler, W. C. (1993). Obesity in Pima Indians: Large increases among post-World War II birth cohorts. *American Journal of Physical Anthropology*, *92*, 473–479.

Putnam, J. J., & Gerrior, S. (1999). Trends in the US Food Supply, 1970-1997. *America's eating habits: Changes and consequences*. Washington DC: USDA Economic Research Service.

Quatromoni, P. A., Copenhafer, D. L., D'Agostino, R. B., & Millen, B. E. (2002). Dietary patterns predict the development of overweight in women: The Framingham Nutrition Studies. *Journal of the American Dietetic Association*, *102*(9), 1240–1246.

Ravussin, E., & Swinburn, B. A. (1992). Pathophysiology of obesity. *Lancet*, 340, 404–408.

Rissanen, A., Heliovaara, M., Knekt, P., Reunanen, A., & Aromaa, A. (1991). Determinants of weight gain and over-weight in adult Finns. *European Journal of Clinical Nutrition*, *45*, 419–430.

Rooney, B. L., & Schauberger, C. W. (2002). Excess pregnancy weight gain and long-term obesity: One decade later. *Obstetrics and Gynecology*, *100*(2), 245–252.

Schauberger, C. W., Rooney, B. L., & Brimer, L. M. (1990). Factors that influence weight loss in the puerperium. *International Journal of Obesity*, *14*, 159–173.

Schmitz, K. H., Jacobs, D. R., Leon, A. S., Schreiner, P. J., & Sternfeld, B. (2000). Physical activity and body weight: Associations over ten years in the CARDIA study. Coronary Artery Risk Development in Young Adults. *International Journal of Obesity, 24*(11), 1475–1487.

Schmitz, K. H., & Jeffery, R. W. (2002). Prevention of obesity. In T. Wadden & A. Stunkard (Eds.), *Handbook of obesity treatment* (pp. 556–593). New York: Guilford Press.

Schulz, M., Kroke, A., Liese, A. D., Hoffmann, K., Bergmann, M. M., & Boeing, H. (2002). Food groups as predictors for short-term weight changes in men and women of the EPIC-Potsdam Cohort. *Journal of Nutrition, 132*, 1335–1340.

Schulz, M. B., Manson, J. E., Ludwig, D. S., Colditz, G. A., Stampfer, M. J., Willett, W. C., & Hu, F. B. (2004). Sugar-sweetened beverages, weight gain, and incidence of type 2 diabetes in young and middle-aged women. *Journal of the American Medical Association, 292*(8), 927–934.

Seidell, J. C., Nooyens, A. J., & Visscher, T. L. (2005). Cost-effective measures to prevent obesity: Epidemiological basis and appropriate target groups. *Proc Nutr Soc, 64*(1), 1–5.

Sheridan, M., & McPherrin, E. (1983). *Fast food and the American diet.* New York: American Council of Science and Health.

Sidney, S., Sternfeld, B., Haskell, W. L., Jacobs, D. R., Chesney, M. A., & Hulley, S. B. (1996). Television viewing and cardiovascular risk factors in young adults: The CARDIA study. *Annals of Epidemiology, 6*(2), 154–159.

Simkin-Silverman, L. R., Wing, R. R., Boraz, M. A., & Kuller, L. H. (2003). Lifestyle intervention can prevent weight gain during menopause: Results from a 5-year randomized clinical trial. *Annals of Behavioral Medicine, 26*(3), 212–220.

Sobal, J., & Stunkard, A. J. (1989). Socioeconomic status and obesity: A review of the literature. *Psychological Bulletin, 105*(2), 260–275.

Sonne-Holm, S., & Sorensen, T. I. (1977). Post-war course of the prevalence of extreme overweight among Danish young men. *Journal of Chronic Diseases, 30*, 351–358.

Sperduto, W. A., Thompson, H. S., & O'Brien, R. M. (1986). The effect of target behavior monitoring on weight loss and completion rate in a behavior modification program for weight reduction. *Addictive Behaviors, 11*(3), 337–340.

Spring, B., Doran, N., Pagoto, S., Schneider, K., & Pigitore, R. (2004). Randomized controlled trial for behavioral smoking and weight control treatment: Concurrent versus sequential intervention. *Journal of Consulting and Clinical Psychology, 72*(5), 785–796.

Stice, E., Orjada, K., & Tristan, J. (2006). Trial of a psychoeducational eating disturbance intervention for college women: A replication and extension. *International Journal of Eating Disorders, 39*(3), 233–239.

Stice, E., Presnell, K., Groesz, L., & Shaw, H. (2005). Effects of a weight maintenance diet on bulimic symptoms in adolescent girls: An experimental test of the dietary restraint theory. *Health Psychology, 24*(4), 402–412.

Tecnomic Information Services. (2002). *US Food Service Industry Forecast.* Chicago, IL: Tecnomic.

Thorsdottir, I., & Birgisdottir, B. E. (1998). Different weight gain in women of normal weight before pregnancy: Postpartum weight and birth weight. *Obstetrics and Gynecolology, 92*, 377–383.

Tucker, L. A., & Bagwell, M. (1991). Television viewing and obesity in adult females. *American Journal of Public Health, 81*, 908–911.

Tucker, L. A., & Friedman, G. M. (1989). Television viewing and obesity in adult males. *American Journal of Public Health, 79*(4), 516–518.

Wadden, T. A., Berkowitz, R. I., Womble, L. G., Sarwer, D. B., Phelan, S., Cato, R. K., et al. (2005). Randomized trial of lifestyle modification and pharmacotherapy for obesity. *New England Journal of Medicine, 353*(20), 2111–2120.

Wadden, T. A., & Foster, G. D. (2000). Behavioral treatment of obesity. *Medical Clinics of North America, 84*(2), 441–462.

Westenhoefer, J., Pudel, V., & Maus, N. (1990). Some restrictions on dietary restraint. *Appetite, 14*, 137–141.

Williamson, D. A., Lawson, O. J., & Brooks, E. R. (1995). Association of body mass with dietary restraint and disinhibition. *Appetite, 25*, 31–41.

Williamson, D. F., Kahn, H. S., & Byers, T. (1991). The 10-y incidence of obesity and major weight gain in black and white US women aged 30-55 y. *American Journal of Clinical Nutrition, 53*, 151S–158S.

Williamson, D. F., Kahn, H. S., Remington, P. L., & Anda, R. F. (1990). The 10-year incidence of overweight and major weight gain in US adults. *Archives of Internal Medicine, 150*, 665–672.

Williamson, D. F., Madans, J., Anda, R. F., Kleinman, J. C., Giovino, G. A., & Byers, T. (1991). Smoking cessation and severity of weight gain in a national cohort. *New England Journal of Medicine, 324*(11), 739–745.

Williamson, D. F., Madans, J., Anda, R. F., Kleinman, J. C., Kahn, H. S., & Byers, T. (1993). Recreational physical activity and ten-year weight change in a US national cohort. *International Journal of Obesity, 17*, 279–286.

Wing, R., & Hill, J. O. (2001). Successful weight loss maintenance. *Annual Review of Nutrition, 21*, 323–341.

Wing, R. R. (2004). Behavioral approaches to the treatment of obesity. In G. Bray & C. Bouchard (Eds.), *Handbook of Obesity: Clinical Applications* (2nd ed.). New York: Marcel Dekker, Inc.

Wing, R. R., Matthews, K. A., Kuller, L. H., Meilahn, E. N., & Plantinga, P. L. (1991). Weight gain at the time of menopause. *Archives of Internal Medicine, 151*, 97–102.

Wolfe, W. S., Sobal, J., Olsen, C. M., Frongillo, E. A., & Williamson, D. F. (1997). Parity-associated weight gain and its modification by sociodemographic and behavioral factors: A prospective analysis in US women. *International Journal of Obesity and Related Metabolic Disorders, 21*(9), 802–810.

Chapter 22

Obesity Prevention: Charting a Course to a Healthier Future

Ross C. Brownson and Shiriki Kumanyika

Introduction

Described in this book are the importance and complexity of the obesity problem and the need for an increased focus on obesity prevention rather than only on treatment in order to curb the epidemic prevalence levels. Treatment issues are covered extensively in other texts (Cooper, Fairburn, & Hawker, 2003; Fairburn & Brownell, 2002; Wadden & Stunkard, 2002) and dominate the current obesity literature. As illustrated throughout the chapters in this book, the obesity epidemic is among the most pressing public health concerns in the United States and globally. While our understanding of the epidemic itself and underlying determinants has grown considerably in the past few decades, knowledge about effective and externally valid interventions is lacking for many settings and populations. It is essential to keep in mind both the rapid change in our knowledge about causes and effective methods of obesity prevention and the continuing change in the physical, economic, policy, and socio-cultural environments in which obesity develops. Therefore, solutions to this problem need to be adapted to fit our evolving knowledge about this changing landscape.

When the chapters in this book are considered as a group, several important themes emerge.

1. We now have many studies documenting the nature and scope of the obesity epidemic, yet a number of areas need more emphasis including economic evaluation, building surveillance systems to monitor population weight trends, and developing intermediate outcomes to complement established measures such as BMI.
2. Although population-wide risk is important, various subgroups (e.g., racial/ethnic minorities, individuals of lower socioeconomic status) bear disproportionate burden. Special emphasis is needed to eliminate these disparities.
3. While some interventions are now known to be effective, more research is needed in "real world" settings to determine approaches with long-lasting impact.

4. To effectively address the obesity epidemic, we will likely need multilevel and societal changes that includes alterations of:

- the physical ("built") environment (e.g., design or re-design of neighborhoods in ways that encourage more physical activity);
- social environments (e.g., how healthy eating and physical activity can be supported within families and social networks);
- policy settings (e.g., more regulations that guarantee certain minimal, health-promotion qualities of worksites, schools, and communities)
- health care delivery (e.g., more effective counseling for obesity prevention as part of reimbursable services), and
- private industry practices (e.g., making healthy foods more attractive).

In this chapter, we highlight several essential topics that touch on the themes above. The issues covered are not meant to be exhaustive; rather, we seek to identify the most pressing and promising areas that will move obesity prevention and control forward.

Understanding Risk Pathways

Incorporate a Developmental Perspective

Obesity prevention is relevant at life stages from gestation through adulthood. Obesity prevalence is higher in school age children and adolescents compared to younger children and increases with age during adulthood. Therefore, prevention measures at any age may reduce the proportion of the population who enter the next life stage with excess weight. Prevention instituted in the earliest life stages has the highest potential to facilitate healthy weight over a lifetime. Prevention during young and mid adulthood can yield immediate benefits in reducing the health and societal cost burdens associated with obesity-related diseases.

The challenges associated with obesity prevention vary markedly by developmental or life stage, with major gaps in knowledge about potential efficacy and safety. For example, the potential for obesity development is influenced by the gestational and postnatal environments, yet the possibility for interventions to have adverse effects is also high during these sensitive developmental periods. The contexts for interventions in children and adolescents vary with changes in cognitive ability, personal autonomy, parenting practices, school environments, and many aspects of community and media environments, which are different for children of different ages, ethnicity, and gender. Contexts for interventions in adults vary by social and occupational circumstances, reproductive status, health status, and broader environmental influences. Population-wide interventions will reach these different life stage groups concurrently but differentially. Potential effects across the age spectrum should be anticipated.

Improve Measurement of Intermediate Indicators of Obesity

As described in Chapter 2, BMI-based classification is the current "gold standard" for measuring obesity on a population level. While this classification scheme has its limitations and measurement error, it is adequate as an outcome measure for population-based surveillance and evaluation. Perhaps most pressing in the area of measurement is the need for intermediate indicators of success in preventing obesity and its associated risk factors. We need more intermediate markers because evaluators tend to assess program or policy-related changes in periods of months or a few years, rather than the many years or decades that some outcomes will require. These measures may include both behavioral end-points (e.g., changes in eating and physical activity) or environmental/policy indicators (measures of the extent to which recommended behaviors such as walking or eating fruits and vegetables are facilitated or constrained). Environmental indicators might include the miles of walking trails or the density or sales volumes of fast food restaurants in a particular community. New tools can be used to measure these attributes. For example, Geographic Information Systems (GIS) have been used to objectively measure factors in the built environment that are likely to influence obesity risk (Zhang, Christoffel, Mason, & Liu, 2006). GIS data can also be used to guide direct assessments of physical activity or food environments in conjunction with intervention planning and implementation (Lewis et al., 2005; Sloane et al., 2006).

Understand Neighborhood and Community-Level Correlates of Obesity

The identification of specific 'obesogenic' features of neighborhood and community environments is an emerging field of research and involves an understanding of correlates (i.e., statistical association between measured explanatory factors and obesity (Bauman, Sallis, Dzewaltowski, & Owen, 2002)). Less favorable neighborhood characteristics are associated with unhealthy dietary behaviors and physical inactivity (Brownson, Baker, Housemann, Brennan, & Bacak, 2001; Morland, Wing, & Diez Roux, 2002). In addition, neighborhood availability of food and physical activity options is less favorable in populations that are at higher than average risk of obesity (e.g., ethnic minority or low income communities) (Baker, Schootman, Barnidge, & Kelly, 2006; Powell, Slater, Chaloupka, & Harper, 2006; Powell, Slater, Mirtcheva, Bao, & Chaloupka, 2006).

As noted in Chapter 8, there is growing evidence that features of the built environment (e.g., land use mix) are associated with the prevalence of obesity in urban and suburban settings and similar findings are emerging to link obesity and neighborhood determinants of healthy eating (e.g., density of fast food restaurants, access to fresh fruits and vegetables) (Morland, Diez Roux, & Wing, 2006).

A range of policy influences at the community level may also be important for obesity. For example, in a recent study of correlates of obesity across 24 European countries, statistically significant inverse associations were observed between overall and female obesity prevalence and variables from the following domains: economic (real domestic product), food supply (available fat), urbanization (urban population), transport (passenger cars, price of gasoline, motorways), and policy (governance indicators) (Rabin, Boehmer, & Brownson, 2006). Methods for studying these relationships are also evolving. For example, multilevel models are increasingly being used to identify physical and social characteristics of neighborhoods (contextual effects) that influence health outcomes independently of (or in addition to) characteristics of the people who live there (compositional effects) (Diez Roux, 2001) and also to design interventions (Peterson et al., 2002).

Improve Surveillance Policy-Related Variables

Public health surveillance, i.e., the ongoing systematic collection, analysis, and interpretation of outcome-specific health data, is a cornerstone of public health (Thacker & Berkelman, 1988). In the United States we now have excellent epidemiologic data for estimating which population groups and which regions of the country are affected and how patterns are changing over time with respect to the obesity epidemic. To supplement these data, we need better information on a broad array of environmental and policy factors that determine these patterns. These factors may include both objective and perceived access to healthy foods or places for physical activity. When implemented properly, policy surveillance systems can be an enormous asset for policy development process and evaluation. For example, we know that there were nearly 1,000 obesity-related bills and resolutions introduced and adopted from 2003–2005 across the 50 states and the District of Columbia (Boehmer, Brownson, Haire-Joshu, & Dreisinger, 2007). These data allow us to compare progress among states, determine the types of bills that are being introduced and passed (e.g., school nutrition standards, safe routes to school programs), and begin to track progress over time.

Sporadic efforts to track policy progress have begun via obesity report cards (e.g., http://www.ubalt.edu/experts/obesity/index.html). In addition, the Robert Wood Johnson Foundation has sponsored the tracking of state-level policy initiatives to prevent childhood obesity (Health Policy Tracking Service, 2006). We need expanded policy surveillance that will enhance our ability to examine time trends in policies and to conduct more sophisticated research on the determinants, implementation, and effectiveness of obesity prevention policy. In addition, by triangulating various surveillance data, hypotheses can be developed (e.g., examining whether state-level physical education policy influences rates of activity in children), which can in turn be tested in intervention studies.

Understanding Intervention Effectiveness

Build more Evidence on Intervention Effectiveness

Various forms of evidence inform our knowledge about the etiology and prevention of obesity. The first type of evidence involves data from analytic epidemiology showing the importance of a particular health condition and its link with some preventable risk factor. For example, a large body of research shows that a lack of physical activity is linked with higher risk of cardiovascular disease, diabetes, and certain cancers (U.S. Department of Health and Human Services, 1996). This type of evidence may lead one to conclude that "*something* should be done" about a condition or preventable risk factors (type 1 evidence).

A second type of evidence focuses on the relative effectiveness of specific interventions to address a particular health condition. For example, worksite interventions to reduce obesity rates that involve multiple components (e.g., nutrition education; prescriptions for aerobic/strength training exercise; training in behavioral techniques) have been shown to be effective (Katz et al., 2005). This type of evidence points the researcher or practitioner toward "*specifically*, this should be done" (type 2 evidence). For obesity, we have an abundance of type 1 evidence on the health consequences of obesity and its related risk factors (lack of activity, unhealthy eating). Yet we have relatively little type 2 evidence on effective methods of obesity prevention. We have even less rigorous research on how best to disseminate type 2 evidence to benefit large populations. Many existing interventions have short-term follow-up periods (a few weeks to 12 months); therefore, studies with long-term follow up are needed. These evaluations need to include multiple outcomes in addition to behavioral endpoints including descriptions of specific programs and policies that might prevent obesity (Swinburn, Gill, & Kumanyika, 2005).

Several other concepts are important to consider when developing and implementing interventions. We use the term "intervention" broadly to include a range of activities from individual-level behavioral change (e.g., physician counseling on dietary change) to macro-level environmental change (e.g., a new mass transit system in an urban setting). Some of these interventions reach individuals directly, whereas others work indirectly by changing environmental and policy variables that influence the options and ease of access to healthy options. Assessment of a body of literature on intervention effectiveness needs to take into account the full context of factors that shape behavior including theory and evidence from other disciplines such as policy analysis and systems theory (Pawson, Greenhalgh, Harvey, & Walshe, 2005). Finally, Robinson has suggested that our reductionist approach to understanding the obesity issue (e.g., over-reliance on etiologic research) needs to give way to more solution-oriented research that seeks to quickly answer questions to inform obesity prevention (Robinson & Sirard, 2005).

Describe Cost and Cost-Effectiveness

As described in Chapter 4, the economic burden of obesity is enormous (up to 7% of total healthcare expenditure in some developed countries (Colditz, 1999)). These costs fail to account for all endpoints from obesity (e.g., decreased physical functioning) and are therefore under-estimates. As effective interventions to prevent obesity are identified, cost-effectiveness analysis (CEA) will become an increasingly important tool for researchers, practitioners, and policy makers. CEA attempts to describe how much health improvement can be gained when an intervention is compared, dollar for dollar, with an alternative. This allows policy makers to determine how money can be spent with maximum public health benefit. A recent CEA examined 13 interventions for the prevention of obesity in youth (Haby et al., 2006). Haby and colleagues use of consistent methods and outcomes, as well as evidence from non-traditional study designs is an advancement for the field. Economic influences also need more attention as routes of intervention. For example, economic policies may make active-living choices easier or more desirable by increasing the tax on gasoline, providing parking cash-outs, or adding extra charges for automobiles entering congested city areas (Pratt, Macera, Sallis, O'Donnell, & Frank, 2004).

Develop Additional Environmental and Policy Interventions

Building on the notion of understanding obesity correlates, we have a great deal to learn about environmental and policy approaches. These interventions affect energy balance and are aimed at changing the physical and socio-political environments (Brownson, Haire-Joshu, & Luke, 2006; Schmid, Pratt, & Howze, 1995). Environmental and policy approaches are designed to provide opportunities, support, and cues to help people develop healthier behaviors. They can serve as an important complement to individual-level programs. For example, policy changes can benefit all people exposed to the environment rather than focusing on changing the behavior of one person at a time. Alterations in the policy environment may directly affect behaviors (e.g., the price of high fat foods influencing consumption) or they may alter social norms (e.g., social support for a worksite intervention to promote activity) (Matson-Koffman, Brownstein, Neiner, & Greaney, 2005). Yet there is a paradox regarding policy interventions to prevent obesity. They hold high face validity, and analogy from other areas of public health support their use, yet the empirical data supporting their effectiveness is limited (Chapter 13).

Conduct More Research on "Natural Experiments"

In mainstream epidemiology, the most rigorous design for hypothesis testing is the randomized controlled trial (Last, 2001). However, in many examples of obesity interventions, a randomized design is not feasible because the evaluator cannot randomly assign exposure (e.g., a policy). Therefore, we need to conduct more frequent and rigorous evaluations of "natural experiments." A "natural experiment" involves naturally occurring circumstances where different populations are exposed or not exposed to a potentially causal factor (e.g., a stringent new school food policy) such that it resembles a true experiment in which study participants are assigned to exposed and unexposed groups (Committee on Progress in Preventing Childhood Obesity, 2006). Even in the absence of randomization, quasi-experimental designs (e.g., time-series designs, multilevel studies) can be sophisticated and rigorous when the evaluation is well-executed. Most of the traditional federal funding mechanisms are too slow to be useful in evaluating many natural experiments. Therefore, alternative funding mechanisms (e.g., foundation support such as Active Living Research (Sallis, Kraft, & Linton, 2002)) and Healthy Eating Research (Story & Orleans, 2006) are more useful in studying the effects of relatively rapid changes in the environment that may affect obesity risk.

Translate Effective Programs into Practice

As the body of literature on effective approaches for obesity prevention accumulates, a continuing challenge involves the translation of this evidence-based information into meaningful public health programs and policies. For example, recommendations in systematic reviews like the Community Guide provide science-based guidance on what works to promote energy balance at the population level (Zaza, Briss, & Harris, 2005). Awareness and use of these recommendations at the state and local levels are limited. Data on use of evidence-based physical activity recommendations were collected from 154 state and local health departments in 2003 (two years after publication of the Community Guide). In these data, only 30% of local health respondents were aware of the Community Guide and even fewer (11%) believed the leadership of their agency was aware of the Community Guide (Brownson, Ballew, Brown, Elliott, Haire-Joshu, Heath, & Kreuter, 2007). Evidence-based information on intervention effectiveness tells what is effective but provides sparse information on *how* to implement and evaluate potentially effective interventions (Rychetnik, Hawe, Waters, Barratt, & Frommer, 2004).

The "how" in translational research often relates to context for the intervention—i.e., What factors need to be taken into account when an internally-valid program or policy is implemented in a different setting or with a different population subgroup? If the adaptation process changes the original intervention to such an extent that the original efficacy data may no longer apply, then the program may be viewed as a new intervention under very different contextual conditions. Green has recommended that the implementation of evidence-based approaches requires careful consideration of the "best processes" needed when generalizing research to alternate populations, places, and times (Green, 2001). Effectiveness of the same obesity prevention program or policy may change over time due to context. For example, as rates of physical activity improve, the group remaining inactive may be quite different from the active population, thus requiring new approaches. As new electronic media define new patterns of communication (e.g., use of the Internet among youth), novel channels for intervention become available for advertising food and other products or delivering tailored interventions.

A number of ready-made tools are now available that are beneficial in program planning, implementation, and evaluation (http://www.cdc.gov/nccdphp/dnpa). The purpose of these tools is to provide resources on how to best implement an intervention after a potentially effective program has been chosen from the "menu" in the Community Guide or another source of scientific information. Another useful tool is the Environmental Nutrition and Activity Tool (ENACT), which provides a menu of strategies for use at a local level (http://www.preventioninstitute.org/sa/enact/enact/index.htm). When planning and implementing programs, conceptual frameworks such as RE-AIM help program planners and evaluators to pay explicit attention to *R*each, *E*fficacy/Effectiveness, *A*doption, *I*mplementation, and *M*aintenance (Glasgow, Vogt, & Boles, 1999) (http://www.re-aim.org/).

Understanding Levels and Systems of Effect

Understand the Relationships Between Process, Impact, and Outcome

As described in Chapters 5 and 12, solving the obesity problem will require changes at many levels and within many systems. For example, if a large employer seeks to address obesity prevention among its employees, initiatives may involve some combination of the following: new facilities for physical activity or healthy eating, incentives to walk or bicycle to work, discounts on health club memberships, reduced prices for healthy foods, health care coverage that supports provider counseling for energy balance, and informational campaigns to encourage activity and healthy eating among an employee's family. The main outcome for such a comprehensive worksite intervention might be the mean BMI in the workforce. However, such an outcome is downstream to many important process and impact measures such as: use of exercise equipment, intentions to change behavior, or rates of provider counseling. Future work in obesity prevention must do a better job of tying process measures to various long-term outcomes. The literature shows useful process measures for dietary interventions (Baranowski & Stables, 2000). In developing evaluation plans and tracking progress, the use of logic frameworks (aka, logic models or analytic frameworks) can be highly useful. These are diagrams depicting the inter-relationships between sectors, inputs, activities, and outcomes. Examples of these frameworks can be found in the recent Institute of Medicine report on progress in preventing childhood obesity (Committee on Progress in Preventing Childhood Obesity, 2006) and in the ongoing work of the Task Force on Community Preventive Services, which has produced the Community Guide (Zaza et al., 2005).

Apply Multi-Level and Systems Models

When implementing interventions, multilevel frameworks are often useful. These are described in Chapters 1, 5, and 12 in detail. These frameworks have been applied across a variety of settings and public health issues. An ecological framework is a useful way to organize objectives and intervention approaches. A five-level ecological model might include the following: (McLeroy, Bibeau, Steckler, & Glanz, 1988; Stokols, Allen, & Bellingham, 1996):

1. Individual factors include characteristics of the individual such as knowledge, attitudes, skills, and a person's developmental history.
2. Interpersonal factors are formal and informal social networks and social support systems, including family and friends.
3 Organizational factors involve social institutions, organizational characteristics, and rules or regulations for operation.
4. Community factors include relationships between organizations, economic forces, the physical environment, and cultural variables that shape behavior.
5. Health policy factors include local, state, and national laws, rules, and regulations.

The most effective interventions are likely to act at multiple levels since communities are made up of individuals who interact in a variety of social networks and within a particular context. We suggest that obesity prevention programs should focus on at least two ecological levels and should seek to make community- and policy-level changes that will be long-lasting. In general, the use of ecological models has outpaced evaluation studies attempting to document the effectiveness of these frameworks and the mechanisms by which changes in health behaviors occur.

Work Across Sectors and Systems

As illustrated at numerous points in this book, effective approaches to obesity prevention will require attention from many sectors including government, private industry, and academe. This concept was aptly summarized in a recent report from the Institute of Medicine suggesting, "There is no one segment of society that's going to solve this alone. It has to be a concerted, coordinated effort. That's one of the things that's missing now" (Committee on Prevention of Obesity in Children and Youth, 2004). An excellent illustration of this intersectoral potential involves the role of the built environment and obesity (Chapter 13). The public health field is concerned about the high prevalence of inactivity, obesity, and associated chronic diseases. Urban planners are largely concerned about congestion, the environmental impacts of automobile use, and quality of life. Together, these and other sectors can collaborate to address a number of environmental and policy factors that influence inactivity. Change will not always come quickly—it has taken decades to build the current (largely activity "unfriendly") urban environment and therefore a sustained commitment is needed from researchers, practitioners, and policy makers to effect changes.

Understanding High-Risk Populations

Understand How Context is Shaped by Racial/Ethnic and Socioeconomic Differences

The need for special attention to ethnic minority and low income populations to address the above-average risks of obesity development was explained in Chapter 1. The task of obesity prevention is more challenging in these high risk populations. Environments are more obesogenic, and adverse social and health conditions other than obesity compete for attention and resources (e.g., substandard housing), and resources are often insufficient. The environment favoring obesity includes both food and physical activity related variables such as: reliance on low-cost foods, of which many are high in calories and fat and heavily marketed; greater ease of access to fast food restaurants; lesser ease of access to recreational facilities; greater dependence on television and other indoor sedentary recreation to entertain children, associated with single-parenting and fears about neighborhood safety; and cultural attitudes that are relatively tolerant of large body size (Block, Scribner, & DeSalvo, 2004; Drewnoski & Darmon, 2005; Henderson & Kelly, 2005; Kumanyika, 2002; Kumanyika & Grier, 2006; Taylor, Poston, Jones, & Kraft, 2006).

Health professionals may be less motivated to advocate for environmental and policy changes in minority communities based on erroneous beliefs that the excess of obesity is genetically determined or due primarily to adverse personal choices. The methodological issues discussed in Chapter 2 related to the applicability of obesity definitions across race and ethnicity may also weaken certainty about the need for action. Policy attention may be more difficult to obtain overall for communities with low social capital. In addition, significant challenges to changing the environment are often present in low resource, socially disadvantaged communities—requiring a greater commitment of time and other resources. The greater difficulty and cost may be a deterrent to taking action. On the other hand, any broad environmental and policy change undertaken to enable obesity prevention in the society at large will probably yield a greater than average return in high risk communities.

Identify Opportunities for Maximum Impact on High Risk Groups

To accelerate obesity prevention in high risk groups requires creativity and strategic thinking to identify the most productive areas for focus. For example, low income populations are reached by federal nutrition safety net programs. This includes the Supplemental Nutrition Program for Women, Infants, and Children (WIC), federally funded subsidized meal programs, the Head Start Program, and the Food Stamp program. These programs provide potential opportunities for policy changes that would selectively reach high risk populations (Kumanyika & Grier, 2006). Developing equitable policies in these settings will not be easy given the risks of compromising personal freedoms of those who depend on these programs and given the commercial vested interests of the suppliers associated with some of these programs. Yet, the potential for selective benefit does exist. We also recommend looking beyond programs that are currently focused on eating and physical activity to other services provided selectively to populations that are at high risk for obesity (e.g., housing services, job training, academic support). Intersectoral cooperation could allow programs designed to improve access to healthy eating and physical activity to be integrated with programs in these other domains.

Learn from Global Efforts

As noted in Chapter 11, obesity has become an issue of global importance (Chopra, Galbraith, & Darnton-Hill, 2002). There are at least two key aspects relevant to prevention. First, globalization is leading the relatively rapid spread of the obesity epidemic. This is illustrated by the recent finding that obesity in China has increased fourfold in children aged 7–18 years from 1985 to 2000 and there are now 31 million obese Chinese people (Wu, 2006). Importantly, obesity-related challenges in less developed countries are compounded by poverty and hunger, diminished public infrastructure, and the epidemiologic transition to behaviors that pose risks more typically found in higher income countries (Institute for Alternative Futures, 2003). This means that the need for and means to obesity prevention in different countries must be linked through actions of international agencies and organizations (Epping-Jordan, Galea, Tukuitonga, & Beaglehole, 2005; World Health Organization, 2005).

Second, more effort is needed to transfer lessons learned from effective intervention approaches across countries more rapidly. Efforts of the WHO Collaborating Center for Obesity at Deakin University in Australia to link researchers involved in community-based obesity prevention studies globally may both contribute to this effort and also provide a model for similar efforts in respect to other types of strategies (http://www.deakin.edu.au/hmnbs/who-obesity/ico-satellite/ico-satellite-index.php). The International Association for the Study of Obesity, through its International Obesity Task Force, is coordinating a Global Prevention Alliance to develop the first global action program to tackle prevention, with a special focus on childhood obesity (Rigby & Baillie, 2006). This Global Alliance incorporates five major non-governmental organizations (NGOs) who are working with the World Health Organization (WHO), leveraging their networks around the world: the World Heart Federation, the International Diabetes Federation, the International Pediatric Association, the International Union of Nutritional Sciences, and the International Association for the Study of Obesity (http://www.preventionalliance.net/).

A Crossroads to the Future

In light of the issues discussed in this chapter and book, the central overarching need in obesity prevention and control is the need for strong and sustained leadership that spans research, policy and public health practice. Numerous public health movements (e.g., tobacco control, seat belt use) consistently show that one or more "spark plug" leaders are needed to stimulate action. These may be individuals working in health fields, policy makers, or the general public. The characteristics of "sparkplugs" include knowledge, competence, cunning, and charisma (Economos et al., 2001).

Public health history teaches us that a long "latency period" often exists between the scientific understanding of a viable chronic disease control method and its widespread application on a population basis (Brownson & Bright, 2004). For example, the Papanicolaou (Pap) test was perfected in 1943, but was not widely used until the early 1970s. Not until 1993 were programs available in all states to provide Pap testing to low income women. As stated in the reports of the Institute of Medicine (Committee on Prevention of Obesity in Children and Youth, 2004; Committee on Progress in Preventing Childhood Obesity, 2006), the trajectory of the obesity epidemic is rapid, thus calling for quick action. Yet, the public health resources devoted to obesity prevention are vastly low in proportion to the scope of the problem.

Without developing effective strategies to modify the current obesogenic environment in the United States, it is likely that the obesity epidemic will continue and accelerate. Government agencies, industry, public health workers, and individuals all need to play an active role in the growing efforts to combat the obesity epidemic. As discussed throughout this book, population-based approaches that emphasize environmental and policy changes are critical for addressing the obesity epidemic by changing the landscape and complementing individual-level interventions.

References

Baker, E. A., Schootman, M., Barnidge, E., & Kelly, C. (2006). The role of race and poverty in access to foods that enable individuals to adhere to dietary guidelines. *Prev Chronic Dis*, *3*(3), A76.

Baranowski, T., & Stables, G. (2000). Process evaluations of the 5-a-day projects. *Health Educ Behav*, *27*(2), 157–166.

Bauman, A. E., Sallis, J. F., Dzewaltowski, D. A., & Owen, N. (2002). Toward a better understanding of the influences on physical activity: The role of determinants, correlates, causal variables, mediators, moderators, and confounders. *Am J Prev Med*, *23*(Suppl. 2), 5–14.

Block, J. P., Scribner, R. A., & DeSalvo, K. B. (2004). Fast food, race/ethnicity, and income: A geographic analysis. *Am J Prev Med*, *27*(3), 211–217.

Boehmer, T. K., Brownson, R. C., Haire-Joshu, D., Dreisinger, M. L. (2007). Patterns of childhood obesity prevention legislation in the United States. *Preventing Chronic Disease*, *4*(3), A56.

Brownson, R. C., Baker, E. A., Housemann, R. A., Brennan, L. K., & Bacak, S. J. (2001). Environmental and policy determinants of physical activity in the United States. *Am J Public Health*, *91*(12), 1995–2003.

Brownson, R. C., Ballew, P., Brown, K., Elliott, M., Haire-Joshu, D., Heath, G. W.,et al. (2007). Disseminating evidence-based interventions to promote physical activity in state and local health departments. *Am J Public Health*, (in press).

Brownson, R. C., & Bright, F. S. (2004). Chronic disease control in public health practice: Looking back and moving forward. *Public Health Rep*, *119*(3), 230–238.

Brownson, R. C., Haire-Joshu, D., & Luke, D. A. (2006). Shaping the context of health: A review of environmental and policy approaches in the prevention of chronic diseases. *Annu Rev Public Health*, *27*, 341–370.

Chopra, M., Galbraith, S., & Darnton-Hill, I. (2002). A global response to a global problem: The epidemic of overnutrition. *Bull World Health Organ*, *80*(12), 952–958.

Colditz, G. A. (1999). Economic costs of obesity and inactivity. *Med Sci Sports Exerc*, *31*(Suppl. 11), S663–S667.

Committee on Prevention of Obesity in Children and Youth. (2004). *Preventing childhood obesity. Health in the balance.* Washington, DC: The National Academies Press.

Committee on Progress in Preventing Childhood Obesity. (2006). *Progress in Preventing childhood obesity. How do we measure up?* Washington, DC: Institute of Medicine of The National Academies.

Cooper, Z., Fairburn, C., & Hawker, D. (2003). *Cognitive-behavioral treatment of obesity: A* clinician's *guide*. New York: The Guilford Press.

Diez Roux, A. V. (2001). Investigating neighborhood and area effects on health. *Am J Public Health, 91*(11), 1783–1789.

Drewnoski, A., & Darmon, N. (2005). Food choices and diet costs: An economic analysis. *American Society for Nutritional Sciences, 135*(4), 900–904.

Economos, C. D., Brownson, R. C., DeAngelis, M. A., Novelli, P., Foerster, S. B., Foreman, C. T.,et al. (2001). What lessons have been learned from other attempts to guide social change? *Nutr Rev, 59*(3, Pt. 2), S40–S56; discussion S57–S65.

Epping-Jordan, J. E., Galea, G., Tukuitonga, C., & Beaglehole, R. (2005). Preventing chronic diseases: Taking stepwise action. *Lancet, 366*(9497), 1667–1671.

Fairburn, C., & Brownell, K. (2002). *Eating disorders and obesity: A comprehensive handbook* (2nd ed.). New York: The Guilford Press.

Glasgow, R. E., Vogt, T. M., & Boles, S. M. (1999). Evaluating the public health impact of health promotion interventions: The RE-AIM framework. *Am J Public Health, 89*(9), 1322–1327.

Green, L. W. (2001). From research to "best practices" in other settings and populations. *Am J Health Behav, 25*(3), 165–178.

Haby, M. M., Vos, T., Carter, R., Moodie, M., Markwick, A., Magnus, A., et al. (2006). A new approach to assessing the health benefit from obesity interventions in children and adolescents: The assessing cost-effectiveness in obesity project. *Int J Obes (Lond), 30*(10), 1463–1475.

Health Policy Tracking Service. (2006). *State actions to promote nutrition, increase physical activity and prevent obesity: A 2006 first quarter legislative overview.* Falls Church, VA: NetScan.

Henderson, V. R., & Kelly, B. (2005). Food advertising in the age of obesity: Content analysis of food advertising on general market and African American television. *J Nutr Educ Behav, 37*(4), 191–196.

Institute for Alternative Futures. (2003). *Survey on key levers of change to prevent and control chronic disease: Preliminary summary.* Copenhagen, Denmark: WHO NCD Strategy Development and Oxford Vision 2020.

Katz, D. L., O'Connell, M., Yeh, M. C., Nawaz, H., Njike, V., Anderson, L. M.,et al. (2005). Public health strategies for preventing and controlling overweight and obesity in school and worksite settings: A report on recommendations of the Task Force on Community Preventive Services. *MMWR Recomm Rep, 54*(RR-10), 1–12.

Kumanyika, S. (2002). Obesity treatment in minorities. In T. Wadden & A. Stunkard (Eds.), *Handbook of obesity treatment* (3rd ed., pp. 416–446). New York: The Guilford Press.

Kumanyika, S., & Grier, S. (2006). Targeting interventions for ethnic minority and low-income populations. *Future Child, 16*(1), 187–207.

Last, J. M. (Ed.). (2001). *A dictionary of epidemiology* (4th ed.). New York: Oxford University Press.

Lewis, L. B., Sloane, D. C., Nascimento, L. M., Diamant, A. L., Guinyard, J. J., Yancey, A. K.,et al. (2005). African Americans' access to healthy food options in South Los Angeles restaurants. *Am J Public Health, 95*(4), 668–673.

Matson-Koffman, D. M., Brownstein, J. N., Neiner, J. A., & Greaney, M. L. (2005). A site-specific literature review of policy and environmental interventions that promote physical activity and nutrition for cardiovascular health: What works? *Am J Health Promot, 19*(3), 167–193.

McLeroy, K. R., Bibeau, D., Steckler, A., & Glanz, K. (1988). An ecological perspective on health promotion programs. *Health Educ Q, 15*, 351–377.

Morland, K., Diez Roux, A. V., & Wing, S. (2006). Supermarkets, other food stores, and obesity: The atherosclerosis risk in communities study. *Am J Prev Med, 30*(4), 333–339.

Morland, K., Wing, S., & Diez Roux, A. (2002). The contextual effect of the local food environment on residents' diets: The atherosclerosis risk in communities study. *Am J Public Health, 92*(11), 1761–1767.

Pawson, R., Greenhalgh, T., Harvey, G., & Walshe, K. (2005). Realist review—a new method of systematic review designed for complex policy interventions. *J Health Serv Res Policy, 10* (Suppl. 1), 21–34.

Peterson, K. E., Sorensen, G., Pearson, M., Hebert, J. R., Gottlieb, B. R., & McCormick, M. C. (2002). Design of an intervention addressing multiple levels of influence on dietary and activity patterns of low-income, postpartum women. *Health Educ Res, 17*(5), 531–540.

Powell, L. M., Slater, S., Chaloupka, F. J., & Harper, D. (2006). Availability of physical activity-related facilities and neighborhood demographic and socioeconomic characteristics: A national study. *Am J Public Health, 96*(9), 1676–1680.

Powell, L. M., Slater, S., Mirtcheva, D., Bao, Y., Chaloupka, F. J. (2007). Food store availability and neighborhood characteristics in the United States. *Preventive Medicine, 44*(3), 189–195.

Pratt, M., Macera, C. A., Sallis, J. F., O'Donnell, M., & Frank, L. D. (2004). Economic interventions to promote physical activity: Application of the SLOTH model. *Am J Prev Med, 27*(Suppl. 3), 136–145.

Rabin, B. A., Boehmer, T. K., Brownson, R. C. (2007). Cross-national comparison of environmental and policy correlates of obesity in Europe. *European Journal of Public Health, 17*(1), 53–61.

Rigby, N., & Baillie, K. (2006). Challenging the future: The Global Prevention Alliance. *Lancet,* 368(9548), 1629–1631.

Robinson, T. N., & Sirard, J. R. (2005). Preventing childhood obesity: a solution-oriented research paradigm. *Am J Prev Med, 28*(2 Suppl. 2), 194–201.

Rychetnik, L., Hawe, P., Waters, E., Barratt, A., & Frommer, M. (2004). A glossary for evidence based public health. *J Epidemiol Community Health, 58*(7), 538–545.

Sallis, J. F., Kraft, K., & Linton, L. S. (2002). How the environment shapes physical activity. A transdisciplinary research agenda (1). *Am J Prev Med, 22*(3), 208.

Schmid, T. L., Pratt, M., & Howze, E. (1995). Policy as intervention: Environmental and policy approaches to the prevention of cardiovascular disease. *Am J Public Health, 85*(9), 1207–1211.

Sloane, D., Nascimento, L., Flynn, G., Lewis, L., Guinyard, J. J., Galloway-Gilliam, L., et al. (2006). Assessing resource environments to target prevention interventions in community chronic disease control. *J Health Care Poor Underserved, 17*(Suppl. 2), 146–158.

Stokols, D., Allen, J., & Bellingham, R. L. (1996). The social ecology of health promotion: Implications for research and practice. *Am J Health Promot, 10*(4), 247–251.

Story, M., & Orleans, C. T. (2006). Building evidence for environmental and policy solutions to prevent childhood obesity: The Healthy Eating Research Program. *Am J Prev Med, 30*(1), 96–97.

Swinburn, B., Gill, T., & Kumanyika, S. (2005). Obesity prevention: A proposed framework for translating evidence into action. *Obes Rev, 6*(1), 23–33.

Taylor, W., Poston, W., Jones, L., & Kraft, M. (2006). Environmental justice. Obesity, physical activity, and healthy eating. *Journal of Physical Activity and Health,* 3(Suppl. 1), S30–S54.

Thacker, S. B., & Berkelman, R. L. (1988). Public health surveillance in the United States. *Epidemiol Rev, 10*, 164–190.

US Department of Health and Human Services. (1996). *Physical activity and health. A report of the Surgeon General.* Atlanta, GA: US Department of Health and Human Services; Centers for Disease Control and Prevention.

Wadden, T., & Stunkard, A. (2002). *Handbook of obesity treatment* (2nd ed.). New York: The Guilford Press.

World Health Organization. (2005). *Global strategy on diet, physical activity and health.* WHO. Retrieved April 30, 2005, from the World Wide Web: http://www.who.int/dietphysicalactivity/goals/en/

Wu, Y. (2006). Overweight and obesity in China. *BMJ, 333*(7564), 362–363.

Zaza, S., Briss, P. A., & Harris, K. W. (Eds.). (2005). *The guide to community preventive services: What works to promote health?* New York: Oxford University Press.

Zhang, X., Christoffel, K. K., Mason, M., & Liu, L. (2006). Identification of contrastive and comparable school neighborhoods for childhood obesity and physical activity research. *Int J Health Geogr, 5*, 14.

Index

9 780387 478593